Schizophrenia

In memory of
Nicholas and Dimitra Pantelis
and Dick Barnes

Schizophrenia

A Neuropsychological Perspective

Edited by

CHRISTOS PANTELIS

Mental Health Research Institute and
Department of Psychiatry, The University of
Melbourne, Australia

HAZEL E. NELSON

Horton Hospital, Epsom, Surrey and
Charing Cross & Westminster Medical School,
Department of Psychiatry, London, UK

THOMAS R.E. BARNES

Charing Cross & Westminster Medical School,
Department of Psychiatry, London, UK

JOHN WILEY & SONS

Chichester · New York · Brisbane · Toronto · Singapore

Copyright © 1996 by   John Wiley & Sons Ltd,
                       Baffins Lane, Chichester,
                       West Sussex PO19 1UD, England

                       National   01243 779777
                       International   (+44) 1243 779777
                       e-mail (for orders and customer service enquiries): cs-books@wiley.co.uk
                       Visit our Home Page on http://www.wiley.co.uk
                              or http://www.wiley.com

Other Wiley Editorial Offices

John Wiley & Sons, Inc., 605 Third Avenue,
New York, NY 10158-0012, USA

Jacaranda Wiley Ltd, 33 Park Road, Milton,
Queensland 4064, Australia

John Wiley & Sons (Canada) Ltd, 22 Worcester Road,
Rexdale, Ontario M9W 1L1, Canada

John Wiley & Sons (Asia) Pte Ltd, 2 Clementi Loop #02-01,
Jin Xing Distripark, Singapore 0512

Library of Congress Cataloging-in-Publication Data

Schizophrenia : a neuropsychological perspective / edited by Christos
   Pantelis, Hazel E. Nelson, and Thomas R.E. Barnes.
      p. cm.
   Includes bibliographical references and index.
   ISBN 0-471-96644-4
   1. Schizophrenia. 2. Cognition disorders. 3. Neuropsychological
tests. I. Pantelis, Christos. II. Nelson, Hazel E. III. Barnes,
Thomas R.E.
   [DNLM: 1. Schizophrenic Psychology. 2. Cognition Disorders. WM
203 S337237 1996]
RC514.S334227   1996
616.89′82—dc20
DNLM/DLC
for Library of Congress   96–25494
                                                              CIP

British Library Cataloguing in Publication Data

A catalogue record for this book is available from the British Library

ISBN 0-471-96644-4

Typeset in 10/11½pt Times by Acorn Bookwork, Salisbury, Wiltshire
Printed and bound in Great Britain by Bookcraft (Bath) Ltd, Midsomer Norton, Somerset
This book is printed on acid-free paper responsibly manufactured from sustainable forestation,
for which at least two trees are planted for each one used for paper production.

Contents

Contributors

Barber, Fiona — Cognitive Neuropsychiatry Unit, Mental Health Research Institute of Victoria, Locked Bag 11, Parkville, Victoria 3052, Australia

Barnes, Thomas R.E. — Department of Psychiatry, Charing Cross and Westminster Medical School, St Dunstan's Rd, London W6 8RP, UK

Bilder, Robert M. — Albert Einstein College of Medicine, Long Island Jewish Medical Center, Hillside Hospital, Glen Oaks, NY 11004, and The Nathan S. Kline Institute for Psychiatric Research, Orangeburg, NY 10962, USA

Bodger, Susan — Department of Psychology, Horton Hospital, Long Grove Rd, Epsom, Surrey KT19 8PZ, UK

Brewer, Warrick — Cognitive Neuropsychiatry Unit and Schizophrenia Research Unit, Mental Health Research Institute of Victoria, and the University of Melbourne, Locked Bag 11, Parkville, Victoria 3052, Australia

Cahill, Connie — Medical Research Council, Clinical Research Centre, Division of Psychiatry, Watford Road, Harrow, Middlesex HA1 3UJ, UK

Chen, Eric Y.H. — University of Hong Kong, Department of Psychiatry, Queen Mary Hospital, Pokfulam, Hong Kong

Collinson, Simon L. — Macquarie University, Balaclava Rd, North Ryde, Sydney, NSW, Australia

Cornblatt, Barbara A. — Psychiatry Research, Hillside Hospital, 75-59 263rd Street, Glen Oaks, NY 11004, USA

Crawford, Trevor J. — Department of Psychology, Lancaster University, Lancaster, LA1 4YF, UK

Currie, Jon — Brain Research Unit, Drug and Alcohol Services, Westmead Hospital, Westmead, Sydney, Australia, and

Neurophysiology and Neurovisual Research Unit, Mental Health Research Institute of Victoria, Locked Bag 11, Melbourne, Parkville, Victoria 3052, Australia

David, Anthony   Department of Psychological Medicine, King's College School of Medicine & Dentistry and the Institute of Psychiatry, Denmark Hill, London SE5 8AZ, UK

Delahunty, Ann   Greater Murray Health Service, Mental Health Unit, Albury Base Hospital, 201 Borella Rd, Albury, NSW 2640, Australia

Ellis, Hadyn D.   University of Wales College of Cardiff, PO Box 901, Cardiff CF1 3YG, UK

Frith, Chris   Wellcome Department of Cognitive Neurology, Leopold Müller Functional Imaging Laboratory, National Hospital for Neurology & Neurosurgery, Queen Square, London WC1N 3BG, UK

Goldberg, Terry E.   Clinical Brain Disorders Branch, National Institute of Mental Health, Division of Intramural Research Programs, NIMH Neuroscience Centre at St Elizabeth's, Washington, DC 20032, USA

Goldstein, Gerald   Department of Veterans Affairs, Medical Center, Highland Drive, Pittsburgh, PA 15206, USA

Gourovitch, Monica L.   Clinical Brain Disorders Branch, National Institute of Mental Health, Division of Intramural Research Programs, NIMH Neuroscience Centre at St Elizabeth's, Washington, DC 20032, USA

Green, Jonathan F.   Department of Therapeutics and Pharmacology, the Queen's University of Belfast, Whitla Medical Building, 97 Lisburn Road, Belfast BT9 7BL, UK

Gruzelier, John   Department of Psychiatry, Charing Cross and Westminster Medical School, St Dunstan's Rd, London W6 8RP, UK

Henderson, Leslie   University of Hertfordshire, Hatfield, AL10 9AB, Hertfordshire, and Charing Cross Hospital and Medical School, St Dunstan's Rd, London W6 8RP, UK

Kennard, Christopher   Academic Unit of Neuroscience, Charing Cross and Westminster Medical School, St Dunstan's Rd, London W6 8RP, UK

King, David J.   Department of Therapeutics and Pharmacology, the Queen's University of Belfast, Whitla Medical Building, 97 Lisburn Road, Belfast BT9 7BL, UK

Liddle, Peter F.   Department of Psychiatry, University of British Columbia, 2255 Westbrook Mall, Vancouver, BC, Canada V6T 2A1

Maruff, Paul   Neurophysiology and Neurovisual Research Unit, Mental Health Research Institute of Victoria, Locked Bag 11, Parkville, Victoria 3052, Australia

McGrath, John   Clinical Studies Unit, Wolston Park Hospital, Wolston Park Rd, Wacol, Queensland 4076, Australia

McKenna, Peter J.   Fulbourn Hospital, Cambridge Health Authority, Fulbourn, Cambridge CB1 5EF, UK

Morice, Rodney   Greater Murray Health Service, Mental Health Unit, Albury Base Hospital, 201 Borella Rd, Albury, NSW 2640, Australia

Nayani, Tony   Gordon Hospital, Bloomburg St, London SW1V 2RH, UK

Nelson, Hazel E.   Department of Psychology, Horton Hospital, Epsom KT19 8PZ, and Charing Cross and Westminster Medical School, St Dunstan's Rd, London W6 8RP, UK

Neufeld, Richard W.J.   Faculty of Social Science, Department of Psychology, University of Western Ontario, London, ON N6A 5C2, Canada

Pantelis, Christos   Cognitive Neuropsychiatry Unit and Schizophrenia Research Unit, Mental Health Research Institute of Victoria, and The University of Melbourne, Locked Bag 11, Parkville, Victoria 3052, Australia

Rogers, Daniel G.C.   Directorate of Neurosciences, Burden Neurological Hospital, Stoke Lane, Stapleton, Bristol BS16 1QT, UK

Szeszko, Philip R.   Albert Einstein College of Medicine, Long Island Jewish Medical Center, Hillside Hospital, Glen Oaks, NY 11004, USA

Williamson, Peter C.   London Psychiatric Hospital, London, Ontario, Canada

Wolf, Lorraine E.   Columbia University College of Physicians and Surgeons, New York, and Neuropsychology Service, Division of Child and Adolescent Psychiatry, Department of Psychiatry, St Luke's–Roosevelt Hospital Center, New York, NY 10025, USA

Young, Andrew W.   University of Durham, Science Laboratories, South Rd, Durham DH1 3LE, UK

Preface

The impetus to write this book was the burgeoning interest in the neuropsychological deficits that characterise schizophrenia. In recent years, this has been reflected in numerous international conferences and satellite meetings specifically addressing this subject. The growing importance of the area is also reflected in the number of recent research papers that have examined the nature and extent of neuropsychological impairments in schizophrenia and other disorders and their relationship to clinical and neurobiological measures.

The aim of this volume was to provide an overview of schizophrenia from a neuropsychological perspective. The contributors were drawn from various relevant disciplines, and include clinical and experimental psychologists, and psychiatrists. All are established investigators in this area of schizophrenia research and we are grateful to them for their hard work and patience.

We believe this volume will not only be of particular interest and relevance to those beginning their exploration of the neuropsychology of schizophrenia but also provide a comprehensive overview of the subject for those already engaged in such research. In addition, many of the chapters will be of direct relevance to students of neuropsychology and psychiatry and to those clinicians who wish to understand in more detail the neuropsychological deficits associated with the schizophrenic illness, particularly as such impairments may be important determinants of treatment outcome.

We are grateful to the publishers for recognising the need for a book on this subject. We are most indebted to those people who have helped with the preparation of this book, particularly Fiona Barber and Susan Hancox for their assistance with proof-reading and editing, and the many hours spent searching for references, and Barbara Stachlewski for typing some of the manuscript. We thank Matt O'Brien, Joanne Jones and Penny Smith. We would also like to thank Dr Paul Maruff, Dr Dennis Velakoulis, Rosie Purcell, Warrick Brewer and Deidre Smith for their helpful comments on several of the chapters. Chris Pantelis is very appreciative of the patience and encouragement of his wife, Kimberley. Special thanks are also due to Associate Professor Norman James for his support. Lastly, we are grateful to the staff of the libraries at Horton Hospital (Epsom) and Royal Park Hospital (Melbourne) for all their efforts on our behalf.

C.P.
H.E.N.
T.R.E.B.

Part A
INTRODUCTION

1

Overview: Towards a Neuropsychology of Schizophrenia

CHRISTOS PANTELIS

I can still only too well remember the perplexity with which I faced, throughout very many years, the vast number of states of mental weakness harboured by every large asylum. Their manifold manifestations were to a certain extent grouped together, but, in spite of all variety in outward form, definite characteristic features recurred with surprising uniformity.

(Kraepelin, 1899/1904, p. 200)

INTRODUCTION

The influential early investigators, such as Kraepelin and Bleuler, drew their conclusions about schizophrenia from very detailed and extensive clinical observations of their patients. These clinicians sought to identify features which distinguished the various psychiatric illnesses. Kraepelin distinguished the psychoses with good prognosis, which he called "maniacal-depressive insanity", from those with a deteriorating course, which he named "dementia praecox" (5th edition of his textbook in 1896). While Kraepelin attributed this term to Pick in 1891, it was Morel who first introduced the term "demence precoce" in 1852–3, a condition equivalent to hebephrenia (Morel, 1857). Kraepelin, whose ideas evolved over time, distinguished acquired and constitutional psychiatric illness and he originally viewed dementia praecox as an acquired organic psychosis due to auto-intoxication.

Like his contemporary, Bleuler, Kraepelin considered that the core symptoms of this disorder were those which we now term the negative symptoms of schizophrenia. Thus, Kraepelin described dementia praecox as characterised by "fundamental symptoms of emotional dullness, absence of independent impulses of the will, and increased susceptibility of the will to influence . . ." (Kraepelin, 1899/1904, p. 28). However, Kraepelin continued to struggle with the evident hetero-

Schizophrenia: A Neuropsychological Perspective. Edited by C. Pantelis, H.E. Nelson and T.R.E. Barnes
© 1996 John Wiley & Sons Ltd

geneity of the disorder and was unable to draw conclusions about the underlying pathological processes that might be involved. Although he used the term dementia, he was unclear about the presence of cognitive impairments. In the 6th edition of his textbook he stated that ". . . the faculty of comprehension and the recollection of knowledge previously acquired are much less affected than the judgement, and especially than the emotional impulses and the acts of volition . . ." (Kraepelin, 1899/1904, p. 26). He later considered that there was a characteristic and progressive memory impairment (7th edn, 1903–4/1918), while he again changed his views and, in the penultimate edition (8th, 1909–1915) of his book, he concluded that there was no evidence of memory impairment, instead attributing poor performance to impairments of attention.

Bleuler (1911/1950), who introduced the term "the schizophrenias", was reconciled to the notion that there were certain fundamental "primary" features of schizophrenia, characterised by autism, ambivalence, and disturbances of association and affect. He considered that other features, including positive symptoms and cognitive changes, were secondary phenomena. Indeed, Bleuler argued that the cognitive changes in schizophrenia were not enduring features of the disorder but were psychological consequences of the negative symptoms manifest in patients with schizophrenia (see Rogers, chapter 2). These early and influential thinkers worked within a predominantly psychological framework, which necessarily limited their understanding of the underlying basis for the disorder and its many features.

In trying to understand schizophrenia today we are confronted with similar dilemmas and questions, particularly in our consideration of the neuropsychological consequences of the disorder. The condition is multifaceted and characterised by a range of phenomena, including neurocognitive deficits. Such heterogeneity continues to present a major challenge. It is only recently that attempts to address the issue of heterogeneity from a different perspective have provided some useful insights. We now consider that the neuropsychological deficits of schizophrenia are not merely secondary phenomena arising from other symptoms but, rather, that such deficits in neurocognitive function may be related in some important way to the symptoms of schizophrenia. Further, such deficits may be important in providing clues to underlying brain dysfunction, providing another avenue to help unravel the heterogeneity of the illness.

As with these early pioneers, whose detailed observations informed their understanding of the illness, the exploration of the neuropsychological deficits in schizophrenia must first be descriptive, based on careful observation and assessment. This approach is apparent in the first three sections of this book in which the neuropsychological deficits in schizophrenia are described. In the next section the identification of patterns of neuropsychological deficits and their clinicopathological correlates is examined. It is at this stage that models begin to emerge as to the underlying nature of these impairments and their possible neurobiological significance. In the fourth section of the book some possible models are presented which attempt to link behaviour, cognition and neuroanatomy. Such models generate testable hypotheses and a framework to help elucidate the underlying pathophysiological mechanisms involved. In the final section of the book the effects of drug treatments on neuropsychological function and possible strategies for their rehabilitation are examined.

OVERVIEW

An examination of neuropsychological function in schizophrenia from a historical perspective (Rogers, chapter 2) provides a starting point for the chapters that follow and places this latter work in context. This is particularly useful when the vantage point is separated by a considerable period of time and our assumptions about mental illness have changed. In his chapter, Rogers suggests that there has been a "paradigm shift", from a predominantly "psychological" understanding of functional disorders, to a more "brain-based" approach. He suggests that the views of earlier writers were a consequence of their predominantly "psychological" rather than "brain-based" view of mental illness. This is exemplified in the writings of Kraepelin and of Bleuler, as indicated above, who understood the intellectual decline in schizophrenia as a consequence of functional decline rather than a true cognitive deterioration. Rogers suggests that the attempts by earlier investigators to provide a distinction between psychiatric illness and cerebral disorders were non-productive. From his re-evaluation of the earlier work the evidence for decline of intellectual functions seems clear. Rogers concludes that this conceptual shift has paved the way for exploring the neurological basis of psychiatric illness and provided us with the necessary direction in this endeavour.

Although this historical chapter allows us to rethink the early work in this area, a number of methodological issues have been raised as complicating the interpretation of neuropsychological findings in functional disorders. In the third chapter, Goldstein discusses methodological issues in the assessment of neuropsychological function in schizophrenia. He first discusses these issues as they apply to neuropsychology in general and he then considers each with respect to schizophrenia. In particular, issues of validity and reliability, as well as sensitivity and specificity are addressed. The difficulty associated with identifying a specific pattern of deficits which are more than simply a manifestation of a general deficit are highlighted and methodologies to address this important issue are considered. Goldstein also discusses the importance of appropriate matching of patients with comparison groups and the controversies and methodological implications surrounding the use of standardised versus flexible batteries of tests. Methodological issues are also taken up by a number of other authors.

Barber and colleagues review the various studies investigating intellectual decline in schizophrenia by examining the different types of methodologies employed, such as cross-sectional or longitudinal designs. The studies in this area provide consistent support for the presence of IQ deficits in schizophrenia. Further, they suggest that such deficits exist prior to illness onset, that higher IQ premorbidly may be protective and that there is further decline in IQ from premorbid levels after illness onset. Indeed, the evidence suggests that low premorbid intellectual functioning may be one risk factor which increases the likelihood of developing the disease early in life and is predictive of a poor outcome. The available research does not support the notion of a progressive decline of intellectual function in the majority of patients, although there are few adequate prospective follow-up studies in this area. Nonetheless, in some patients with schizophrenia there are changes in performance as the illness fluctuates. Further, the available research has identified a subgroup of patients in whom there may be an interaction between the illness and age-related changes in cognitive decline. One implication is that the schizophrenic illness may bring forward in time any effects due to ageing. This notion is discussed in the chapter by Collinson and his colleagues, who consider the neuropsychology of tardive dyskinesia (chapter 12). Barber and colleagues also consider the important question of specific versus global deficits, particularly as this question has an important bearing on the evaluation of the neuropsychological profile of impairments in schizophrenia. Thus, the extent of general intellectual decline observed in schizophrenia needs to be taken into account when evaluating the extent of any specific deficits discussed in later chapters.

This chapter by Barber et al should be considered together with the chapters on high-risk samples by Wolf and Cornblatt (chapter 9), and the findings relating to cerebral asymmetry as summarised by Bilder and Szeszko (chapter 14). In these latter chapters evidence is presented for the presence of verbal rather than performance IQ deficits prior to illness onset, while studies in patients with existing illness have generally found the reverse pattern. Such apparent discrepancies may provide important clues to understanding the nature of the underlying deficits in schizophrenia.

Gourovitch and Goldberg (chapter 5) provide an overview of the specific deficits of attention, executive function, memory and language and put forward important questions requiring further study in each of these areas. The comments of Gourovitch and Goldberg should be considered together with the chapters covering each of these areas separately (Maruff and Currie, chapter 6; Chen and McKenna, chapter 7; Gruzelier, chapter 8; Wolf and Cornblatt, chapter 9; McGrath, chapter 10). Gourovitch and Goldberg conclude that these neurocognitive impairments may represent a central feature of the disease process and that, taken together with the evidence from neuropathology and neuroimaging, the temporal and prefrontal cortical systems are implicated, as has been argued by Weinberger (1991). Gourovitch and Goldberg also suggest that the neurocognitive deficits observed in schizophrenia should be the target for future drug and rehabilitative interventions, issues which are taken up later in this volume (King and Green, chapter 20; Morice and Delahunty, chapter 21).

Maruff and Currie (chapter 6) review the work examining attentional deficits in schizophrenia, an area which has been the focus of research for decades. They discuss the strengths and limitations of the various theories and models of attention which have been influential in research to date, such as the "filter theory" of Broadbent and the more recent "attentional resource model". Because of the limitations of such models, which view attention as a limited capacity selection process, the authors propose that models which specify brain–behaviour relationships are more informative in understanding the nature of the attentional disturbance in schizophrenia. In this regard they argue that defining attention as the goal-directed selection of information is more instructive in understanding underlying brain changes. These authors examine the evidence from experiments which contend that impairments in visual spatial attention result from a disturbance of a distributed cortical–subcortical neural network. Further, it is suggested that individual nodes within such a network are responsible for elementary cognitive operations of an attentional task. Thus, it is possible to examine the integrity of components by varying the task according to these more elementary cognitive operations. The strength of this approach is that it provides the possibility of identifying the brain areas which underlie the disruption in attention. A related approach is described in the chapter by Pantelis and Brewer (chapter 16), who discuss "component-specific" and "network-specific" functions (see below). Future studies examining other neuropsychological deficits in schizophrenia would benefit from the development of such brain-behaviour models.

In chapter 7, Chen and McKenna discuss memory function in schizophrenia. They first discuss the various types of memory and then examine the evidence for dysfunction of each memory system in schizophrenia. Importantly, Chen and McKenna discuss the notion of working memory, which has been considered particularly relevant to the types of deficit demonstrated in these patients (Weinberger, 1991; Goldman-Rakic, 1987). Extrapolating from the animal work, Goldman-Rakic (1987) and Weinberger (1991) have proposed that the deficits of visual spatial working memory implicate medial temporal structures and their connections with prefrontal areas. Weinberger (Weinberger, 1991; Weinberger et al, 1992), who has been a keen proponent of dysfunction of the dorsolateral prefrontal cortex (DLPFC), proposes that the functional deficit observed in the DLPFC is explained within this model. He suggests that the primary pathology lies in the hippocampus and that the apparent frontal deficits are a consequence of disruption to the pathways connecting these areas to prefrontal cortex, particularly the DLPFC. Others have similarly proposed that the observed deficits of prefrontal function are due to deafferentation from subcortical structures, such as the basal ganglia and thalami (Pantelis et al, 1992). It is also relevant here that memory function implicates frontal systems, a theme that emerges from a number of different areas of investigation and which is discussed in a number of other chapters (e.g. Gourovitch and Goldberg, chapter 5; Maruff and Currie, chapter 6; McGrath, chapter 10; Henderson et al, chapter 13; Liddle, chapter 15; Pantelis and Brewer, chapter 16; Cahill and Frith, chapter 18). For example, Maruff and Currie (chapter 6) consider that attentional deficits result from disruption to prefrontal cortical areas and their connections subcortically.

Although Baddeley's (1986) original formulation of working memory was cast very much within the context of a memory system, his description of the components of working memory closely resemble "frontal" executive functions. It is not surprising therefore that working memory implicates these areas, and that deficits of working memory are consistently shown in schizophrenia.

Chen and McKenna also highlight the importance of making comparisons between patients with schizophrenia and those with neurological disorders in which the pathology is known. Such an approach was popular in early studies of schizophrenia (see Rogers, chapter 2; Henderson et al, chapter 13) and has become important again recently (Gold et al, 1994; Hanes et al, 1995). The strength of this approach is that it allows theories regarding postulated pathophysiological changes to be examined. Further work in this area should be extended to neuroimaging studies, an example of which was the PET activation study by Goldberg and colleagues (1990) comparing schizophrenia and Huntington's disease. A continuing problem in schizophrenia research has been the absence of adequate models, such as animal models of the disorder. In this context, modelling of specific components of the illness, such as neuropsychological function, may help to generate testable hypotheses.

Gruzelier (chapter 8) reviews the literature regarding laterality and schizophrenia, work which has spanned a number of decades. That the schizophrenic illness may be lateralised is considered by a number of other authors in this volume (e.g. Gourovitch and Goldberg, chapter 5; Maruff and Currie, chapter 6; Wolf and Cornblatt, chapter 9; Neufeld and Williamson, chapter 11; Henderson et al, chapter 13; Bilder and Szeszko, chapter 14; Nayani and David, chapter 17; Ellis and Young, chapter 19). Gruzelier presents an argument that certain features of schizophrenia may be related to either right or left hemisphere and that lateralised differences are related to these different symptom profiles. He proposes that the positive symptoms of schizophrenia are associated with an imbalance in the direction of higher (over) activation of the left hemisphere and underactivation of the right hemisphere, while the negative symptoms are associated with the opposite state of imbalance. Gruzelier suggests that the links between the hemispheres are relevant and he examines the evidence for lateralised deficits of interhemispheric transmission. He concludes that, from the available evidence, in those patients with predominantly positive symptoms there is a deficit in the transmission of information across the corpus callosum from right to left. In contrast, the opposite pattern is observed in those patients with predominantly negative symptoms. Further, Gruzelier also considers relevant evidence from structural neuroimaging, evoked potential studies, the evidence for asymmetry of attention and the literature on hemineglect, and summarises the extensive literature covering overt and covert visual and auditory attentional asymmetries. He concludes that the asymmetries of attention operate at both subcortical and cortical levels and that hemispheric imbalance contributes to the symptoms in schizophrenia.

Wolf and Cornblatt (chapter 9) examine potential early markers which precede the onset of illness. As they point out, such markers may provide clues to aetiology as they are not a consequence of the illness. The high-risk study methodology is examined and some of the problems with this approach mentioned. It is relevant to the present volume that because such studies commenced almost three decades ago few neuropsychological tasks were included in the assessment of this population, apart from measures of attention. Wolf and Cornblatt review the limited evidence available from these high-risk studies to date to assess the evidence for executive (frontal) dysfunction in high-risk populations. The evidence of frontal dysfunction comes from studies using tasks similar to standard tasks of executive function (e.g. WCST, Stroop and Trails tasks). One possibility for the lack of correlation between these measures is that there exists some independence of function and possibly neuroanatomical specificity.

The findings from memory tasks in the high-risk samples again reflect the paucity of such studies in this area. However, children at risk for schizophrenia appear to have a specific deficit of encoding of information presented. Wolf and Cornblatt propose that "the memory deficit indicating a vulnerability to schizophrenia is better conceptualised by stage of information processing (early versus late) rather than type (recognition versus recall) of process". How these observations translate into the type of memory deficit observed in adult patients with schizophrenia will require further systematic study, not only of high-risk groups, but should also inform our investigations of adult patients with the condition. These authors also review language function in high-risk populations and examine issues of laterality (see also Gruzelier, chapter 8; McGrath, chapter 10). They suggest that the findings to date support the hypothesis that children at high risk for developing schizophrenia are characterised by left hemisphere dysfunction. Such a suggestion is in keeping with other evidence of dysfunction in the left brain in this disorder, although, as already mentioned, others consider that both hemispheres may be implicated in different ways (e.g. Gruzelier, chapter 8). Wolf and Cornblatt conclude that the neuropsychological markers identified as candidate markers for the later development of schizophrenia suggest that dysfunction in frontal and dominant temporal lobe and subcortical systems may play a role in the pathophysiology of schizophrenia. Indeed, these areas are identified as candidate sites by a number of authors in this volume.

Further, the findings of "neuromotor soft-signs" in high-risk samples supports the neurodevelopmental hypothesis for schizophrenia. The latter hypothesis (see Weinberger, 1987; Walker, 1991), which views schizophrenia as a manifestation of some insult early in life, has provided an important paradigm for recent research endeavour. If, as this hypothesis suggests, schizophrenia results from an early insult even prior to birth or around the time of birth, then abnormal functioning prior to illness onset may provide the window to examine these aetiological factors.

As well as the prospective high-risk studies, twin studies (Torrey et al, 1994) and studies of other groups at risk may provide further methodologies to investigate the neuropsychology of schizophrenia. The first-episode patients provide a window into the very early stage of the illness but it is also necessary to examine schizophrenia candidates premorbidly. Because of the methodological problems inherent in following groups of "at-risk" individuals over 20–30 years, other strategies may help to elucidate and explore the neurodevelopmental hypothesis and examine possible aetiological factors. Early follow-up studies have included recruits to the army or other services who were assessed at the time of enlistment and then again after developing the illness (see Rogers, chapter 2; Barber et al, chapter 4). However, the information from these studies has been limited in its value. A novel approach has been that of Walker et al (1994; Walker, 1994), who examined home movies of children which included individuals who later developed schizophrenia. Raters, who were blind to diagnosis, observed and rated each child. The study provided evidence that children who later developed schizophrenia could be differentiated from healthy siblings by behavioural observation.

Another recent and potentially exciting initiative is the assessment and follow-up of individuals with so-called "prodromal symptoms" of schizophrenia, prior to illness onset (McGorry et al, 1996; Yung & McGorry, 1996). The identification of neuropsychological and other markers premorbidly may provide further clues as to the nature of the illness, in particular, from a neurodevelopmental perspective. While this strategy has only recently evolved, some preliminary evidence from neuropsychological and structural imaging studies (Velakoulis et al, 1996; Brewer et al, 1996) provides support for the occurrence of neuropsychological impairments and brain structural changes prior to illness onset. Such studies will be important in assessing the relationship of functional deficits to structural brain changes, as indicated by Bilder and Szeszko (chapter 14).

The last decade and more has seen an emphasis on the negative symptoms of schizophrenia in neuropsychological investigations examining the relationship of cognitive deficits to both neuropsychological and structural brain abnormalities. This research has been stimulated by the early work of Crow, Johnstone and their colleagues. In particular, the notion of type I and type II schizophrenia proposed by Crow (1980) postulated that it was in those patients with a predominance of negative symptoms that the cognitive deficits and structural changes were likely to be found. However, more recent work has refocused attention on other groups of symptoms, particularly thought disorder and the positive symptoms of delusions and hallucinations. Based on factor analytic studies, Liddle (chapter 14) has extended the two-syndrome notion to include a third syndrome of "disorganisation" and has identified specific neurocognitive deficits associated with each of these syndromes. In his chapter this notion is explored further by using positron emission tomography (PET) to examine which brain regions are associated with each of these syndromes. In the chapter by Pantelis and Brewer (chapter 16), this syndrome-based approach is extended to include behavioural syndromes of schizophrenia.

The symptom of formal thought disorder is perhaps one of the most characteristic features of schizophrenia. McGrath (chapter 10) reviews the evidence for an association between thought disorder and neuropsychological deficits. He reviews the literature on thought disorder and its definitions and examines the features of this symptom from a neuropsychological perspective. He considers that the evidence supports specific deficits of executive function in the pathogenesis of thought disorder, thereby implicating prefrontal cortical function. He suggests that positive formal thought disorder is consequent on a failure in the ability to maintain set and an impaired capacity to monitor and utilise errors in speech. With regard to negative thought disorder, characterised by poverty of speech, he proposes that there is an impairment in the ability to establish set. This model implicates the various circuits of the prefrontal cortex as is also suggested by other authors in this book (see above). This model put forward by McGrath also provides testable hypotheses to examine the underlying pathophysiological mechanisms involved in thought disorder. Importantly, as he suggests in his concluding remarks, understanding the mechanisms by which the various types of thought disorder arise may help in developing treatment strategies in the rehabilitation of patients with impairments in communication. The notion of providing a template or grid to guide discourse sounds appealing as does providing strategies to assist with error monitoring and their utilisation. The ability to guide patients to structure their language is an area requiring further examination.

Two chapters are devoted to positive symptoms of delusions and hallucinations. Though the research has tended to favour an association between negative symptoms and neuropsychological deficits, Neufeld and Williamson (chapter 11) argue that the positive symptoms of schizophrenia are also associated with neuropsychological deficits. They consider that evaluation of neuropsychological tasks depends on an understanding of the component processes underlying the task and that the nature of the relationships are best examined using mathematical models. Employing such modelling, the authors are able to specify the nature of the component processes which impair performance in patients with predominantly positive symptoms. They suggest that performance deficits on tasks of executive function as well as tasks involving stimulus encoding are observed in patients with predominantly positive symptoms of delusions and hallucinations. They postulate that a number of brain regions, including the mesial temporal region, are implicated. The approach of identifying the subprocesses involved in the execution of neuropsychological tasks is also elaborated in other chapters, as already discussed.

The subject of hallucinations has received recent interest with the development of instruments which provide detailed accounts of hallucinations in patients with psychotic illness (e.g. Carter et al, 1995), a necessary first step in examining these phenomena further. In their chapter, Nayani and David (chapter 17) provide an overview and critique of a number of perspectives which attempt to understand the occurrence of hallucinations. They consider some important issues in examining the link between brain and the phenomena of the mind and suggest caution in being overly reductionist in approach. Finally, they present a model which incorporates misattribution in the context of inappropriately remembered events which are affect laden. They state that ". . . the verbal hallucination may represent the activation of memory traces by automatic, preconscious processes which are dictated by the advent of pervasive distortions of judgement caused by mood states." They propose that the connections between hippocampus and the amygdala may be relevant, as these connections are involved in processing long-term memory stores as well as emotion. Again, these ideas are consistent with the growing body of evidence for structural abnormalities in limbic structures of patients with schizophrenia (see Bilder and Szeszko, chapter 14). Nayani and David emphasise the need to focus future neuropsychological research to examine the function of these areas.

It has been suggested (e.g. Barnes, 1988; Pantelis et al, 1992) that the occurrence of abnormal involuntary movements in patients with schizophrenia is indicative of involvement of subcortical structures in this disorder. Collinson et al (chapter 12) review the evidence for a link between tardive dyskinesia and neuropsychological function. The most robust findings are with orofacial dyskinesia rather than trunk and limb dyskinesia and these authors propose some possible explanations. The evidence for global neuropsychological deficits and for more specific deficits is considered. They suggest that there is support for involvement of frontal and striatal systems. Indeed, the recent studies demonstrating that patients with tardive dyskinesia are impaired on frontal-executive tasks would support the growing evidence implicating frontal–striatal systems in schizophrenia. They hypothesise that tardive dyskinesia may result from a failure to inhibit inherent motor programs, a notion that is in keeping with possible compromise of this circuitry. Further, these authors propose that there is an interaction between age, the schizophrenic illness itself and the effects of neuroleptic medication, such that drug treatment brings forward in time the development of tardive dyskinesia. In the final section of the chapter they discuss the relevance of the "brain reserve capacity" (BRC) notion (Satz, 1993) to schizophrenia and tardive dyskinesia. The implication of this theory is that there are threshold levels which must be exceeded before clinical features are apparent. Factors which may impinge on an individual's brain reserve, such as age or the effects of the schizophrenic illness and/or neuroleptic medication, would act to reduce the BRC to threshold levels. The corollary of this is that neuronal reserve may be measurable using functional (neuropsychological) assessments or by measuring brain structures (e.g. using magnetic resonance imaging).

Evidence for eye movement abnormalities in schizophrenia and their association with neuropsychological function are reviewed by Henderson and colleagues (chapter 13). These authors provide a critical account of the work to date and examine the areas which seem most promising with regard to future studies. They examine the similarities and differences with neurological conditions where the pathology is known, such as Parkinson's disease and frontal patients. The areas of interest which emerge from these studies further implicate the frontal–striatal axis. The authors also present data which supports a prefrontal disinhibition effect which is associated with the negative symptoms of schizophrenia, a theme that emerges in other chapters also (e.g. Collinson et al, chapter 12; Liddle, chapter 15). Further, the saccadic system provides ways to examine the nature of attentional deficits in schizophrenia (see also Maruff and Currie, chapter 6). The authors make a plea for studies in this area which are methodologically rigorous, particularly as the oculomotor system provides the possibility to examine accurately the neural mechanisms involved in conditions such as schizophrenia.

While certain structural brain changes have been observed in schizophrenia, such changes are only identified in a small proportion of patients with the disorder, thereby limiting the clinical utility of such measures. Bilder and Szeszko (chapter 14) review the literature in this area and provide a possible explanation for the disparate findings together with a strategy for future research. The hypothesis proposed by Bilder and Szeszko (chapter 14) is intriguing and may provide an explanation for findings which initially appear anomalous. These authors suggest that the relationship between structural abnormalities and neuropsychological function on the one hand and the lack of such an association on the other in other groups of patients may be determined by independent processes. They consider that the lack of such an association is observed in those patients in whom cerebral specialisation is less pronounced. It is possible that a less lateralised brain, although likely to have adverse consequences including poorer language or other specialised abilities, may be less vulnerable. An example they cite is of lower degrees of manual dominance with a decreased risk for the development of persistent tardive dyskinesia. This idea is also consistent with the notion of brain reserve capacity as discussed by Collinson et al (chapter 12). Thus, greater cerebral specialisation may result in less brain reserve capacity for any particular cerebral function and, hence, a greater likelihood for both neuropsychological impairment and the development of tardive dyskinesia.

Bilder and Szeszko also provide evidence to suggest that ventricular enlargement and sulcal enlargement may be independent of each other, possibly indicative of different aetiological processes. Such dissociations are promising and suggest avenues for further study, particularly examining the different profiles of these structural deviations.

Given the complexity of examining structure–function relationships, Bilder and Szeszko recommend standardised assessment methods and data analysis to enable comparisons across research centres. Such approaches would provide the possibility of meta-analyses to achieve the adequate power necessary to address the important questions they raise. Another possibility is the multicentre study approach, which has been particularly useful in clinical trials of new medications. Such an approach combined with standardised procedures would help to clarify the often contradictory findings in this area. The need for large prospective follow-up studies is also emphasised, particularly to examine the progression of structural abnormalities within subgroups of patients. To date there have been few such longitudinal studies which examine brain structure and its relationship to neuropsychological variables.

In the final section, Bilder and Szeszko consider the development of the neocortex and how this may be important in understanding the deficits of schizophrenia from a neurodevelopmental perspective. The evidence is consistent with developmental disruption of "ventral trend" structures. These would be manifest by structural disturbances of hippocampus, cingulate or dorsal frontal cortical divisions, and may comprise a core pathological process underlying vulnerability to schizophrenia. The authors propose that further work should examine the relationship between disturbances to these structures during their development and their functional consequences.

Liddle (chapter 14) examines approaches to investigating schizophrenia using PET. He first discusses the issue of heterogeneity and summarises the work which reduces this heterogeneity using symptoms to establish syndromes of schizophrenia. The work of Crow and Liddle's own work in this area proposes the existence of at least two and probably three symptom-based syndromes, although more recently others have suggested that these three syndromes do not adequately account for the heterogeneity of the illness (Minas et al, 1992). Liddle postulates that the three syndromes he describes have differing pathophysiologies and goes on to explore the underlying neurobiology of schizophrenia using this syndrome-based approach. He first defines different patterns of functioning neuropsychologically which inform his subsequent investigations with PET. The findings thus far provide support for the three syndromes and their relationship with different prefrontal and hippocampal areas. Further confirmation of this approach will be necessary. In particular, the use of cognitive activation paradigms which tap specific prefrontal areas, using functional imaging techniques such as PET or functional magnetic resonance imaging (fMRI), will be important in future studies to examine these hypotheses further.

Liddle discusses this psychological approach, particularly focusing on the notions developed by Frith, which are elaborated by Cahill and Frith (chapter 18). The work from this group of researchers has examined psychological paradigms using PET, such as determining brain activation during internal versus external generation. Such theory-driven research is paradigmatic of the approach which is now necessary in order further to develop our understanding about schizophrenia and related functional disorders. Recent developments in fMRI will have a significant impact on such studies in the future. This technology, which visualises both structure and function, will address some of the methodological problems of PET studies.

Pantelis and Brewer (chapter 16) extend the phenomenological approach to an investigation of the behaviours as well as symptoms, arguing that the manifestations of neuropsychological impairment implicating the prefrontal areas have been characterised as disturbances of behaviour, a feature which is particularly prominent in patients with schizophrenia. Indeed, behavioural disturbance may precede other manifestations of the illness and are often the reason for referral to psychiatric services. Pantelis and Brewer describe the various syndromes of frontal dysfunction, which appear to be related to specific prefrontal areas; they characterise the neuropsychological profile of these syndromes and consider "network-specific" versus "component-specific" functions related to these prefrontal areas and their subcortical connections. They relate these prefrontal syndromes to the clinical and behavioural syndromes of schizophrenia. The implication is that independence of function in these areas may prove useful as probes to examine the integrity of the important prefrontal systems and the subcortical areas with which they connect. The parallel segregated nature of the prefrontal–striatal–thalamic circuits suggests that the functions of these circuits may be separable, that is, "network-specific". Further, the possibility that elements within a network may have different functions (i.e. "component-specific"), may provide clues to determine whether observed deficits originate in specific brain areas, such as in subcortical structures. This may help to explain the apparent inconsistencies in deficits of executive and other functions and help to identify relationships between neuropsychological impairments and other variables, including symptoms and behaviours. Interestingly, Morice and Delahunty (chapter 21) have also developed their rehabilitation programs on the basis of a notion of "circuit-specific abnormalities".

As mentioned, Cahill and Frith (chapter 18) present a sophisticated model which uses a cognitive psychological approach to understand the phenomenology of schizophrenia and to examine their pathophysiology. It is proposed that the major signs and symptoms of schizophrenia can be accounted for by three classes of cognitive dysfunction, namely, disorders of willed action, deficits in self-monitoring, and deficits in inferring the mental states of others. The authors propose that patients with "negative" symptoms, such as poverty of action and poverty of speech, have a specific deficit concerning the production of "internally generated" ("willed") action. In this instance, internally generated behaviour tends to be perseverative, whereas stimulus-driven behaviour is normal. To account for the positive symptoms of schizophrenia, such as auditory hallucinations, thought insertion and thought withdrawal, these authors propose that they share a common deficit in "self-monitoring": that is, deficits in the ability to discriminate "internally" versus "externally" generated events. Thus, it is hypothesised that misattribution of their own "willed" actions to outside agents, by patients with schizophrenia, results from a failure of self-monitoring. They propose that hallucinations result from a failure of the verbal self-monitoring system, and that delusions of control result from misattribution of internally generated action to a source outside the self. It is useful to compare this model for understanding some of the positive symptoms of schizophrenia to that proposed by Nayani and David (chapter 17) to account for hallucinations, which was mentioned earlier. To account for other sets of positive symptoms, such as paranoid delusions, delusions of reference and third person auditory hallucinations, Cahill and Frith propose that in patients with schizophrenia there is a deficit in the ability to infer and represent the mental state of others. The authors summarise the evidence which provides support for these notions, although experimental approaches to test these theories are still being developed. Further, they suggest that these functions relate to specific brain systems. They propose that the important brain systems which are likely to be implicated are the frontal–striatal circuitry. As mentioned earlier, other authors have provided evidence for involvement of these circuits in schizophrenia. The development of cognitive models, such as is proposed by Cahill and Frith, provides us with the possibility to generate testable paradigms, in particular during functional brain imaging, as exemplified by the work from Frith and his colleagues.

An intriguing chapter by Ellis and Young (chapter 19) explores the delusional misidentification syndromes in which they discuss a model for face and affect recognition in normal and pathological states. They consider that these syndromes, as well as delusions in general, reflect an interaction of deficits in which perceptual error is coupled with an impaired attributional mechanism or decision-making system. They propose that understanding the delusional misidentification syndromes may provide a model, or at least one approach, for understanding other delusions. They examine the misidentification syndromes within the context of a model they have developed of the processes underlying normal face and affect recognition. They attempt to define the various misidentification syndromes from a neuropsychological perspective, thereby delineating the target area which is dysfunctional in each. They set up a number of potentially testable hypotheses based on their approach and examine the evidence in this context. An exciting development mentioned in their chapter is the use of computerised neural networks to simulate the model put forward. Ellis and Young differ from other authors in postulating that there is a perceptual problem which is important in the genesis of the delusional misidentification syndromes. They do not, however, discount the possibility that the problem is a failure of a monitor which would act to eliminate inappropriate possibilities. The latter would be in accord with the cognitive model presented by Cahill and Frith (chapter 18). This would suggest dysfunction of frontal systems, while Ellis and Young suggest that the evidence they present would be compatible with right hemisphere dysfunction.

In the final section of the book, the effects of treatment on neurocognitive function and the possibility that treatment strategies may help to ameliorate neuropsychological deficits in schizophrenia are examined in two chapters by King and Green (chapter 20) and Morice and Delahunty (chapter 21).

There has been a great deal of speculation about the possible effects on cognitive function of various types of neuroleptic medication. In particular, the evaluation of neuropsychological studies in schizophrenia has often been complicated by possible treatment effects. King and Green (chapter 20) review the studies which examine this issue. They examine the research with regard to the effects of antipsychotic drugs, including clozapine, and anticholinergic medication; they also consider likely lateralised effects of these drugs.

King and Green conclude that the available evidence indicates that neuroleptic medication does not account for the neuropsychological deficits in schizophrenia. Further, performance on attentional tasks tends to show improvement, whereas tasks which are unpaced are not susceptible to change. Also, hemisphere asymmetries identified in schizophrenia are not explained by medication. Anticholinergic medications do appear to affect neurocognitive function, such as short-term memory. Overall, the evidence suggests that the long-term use of neuroleptic medication in patients with schizophrenia is associated with modest improvements in performance on some neuropsychological tests. However, a number of methodological issues remain which need addressing, such as practice effects and the effects of illness severity. Surprisingly, the evidence does not support a link between changes in neuropsychological functioning with parallel changes in symptomatology. This is important because, as well as improvement in symptoms, benefits to neurocognitive function may be particularly important in the successful rehabilitation of patients with schizophrenia.

King and Green suggest that further work in this area should examine the central effects of neuroleptic medications under controlled cognitive conditions. Two potentially exciting areas for future studies, which should employ cognitive activation methodologies, are intervention studies (pre- and post-treatment) using functional imaging (PET or fMRI), and receptor studies under PET.

The use of rehabilitation strategies which target cognitive impairment is a relatively uncharted area. In the final chapter, Morice and Delahunty (chapter 21) address this issue and present evidence to support the use of strategies to rehabilitate neuropsychological impairments. It has been suggested that the failure to rehabilitate these patients adequately may be governed by the degree of neuropsychological impairment (e.g. see Barber et al, chapter 4; McGrath, chapter 10). Strategies to improve such functioning may be important determinants of rehabilitation success. As Morice and Delahunty conclude: "Rehabilitation of these impairments should receive high priority in schizophrenia rehabilitation, as it seems likely that higher-level training (for example, in housekeeping, cooking, leisure activities, etc.) may be constrained by these lower-level impairments". Indeed, the successful rehabilitation of patients exhibiting the range of impairments and disabilities seen in schizophrenia requires an integrated approach which is comprehensive in targeting these impairments.

CONCLUSION

The various chapters of this book examine the nature of the disturbance(s) of brain function in schizophrenia from a neuropsychological perspective. An exciting development is the emerging consensus regarding the neurobiological underpinnings of schizophrenia, as validated by the various perspectives provided by the many contributors to this volume. Many of the chapters point to similar areas of brain being implicated in schizophrenia, in particular the frontal areas, medial temporal lobe structures and their connections with subcortex. Other evidence presented in these chapters also implicates right hemisphere involvement. However, it would seem that the anterior half of the brain is particularly relevant, this being "phylogenetically" younger and perhaps more vulnerable to the hazards of the milieu in which the brain finds itself during early development. Such convergence of evidence may reflect a focusing of the vista in our pursuit for an identifiable "schizophrenic neurobiology". It is as if we are using a magnifying glass to view similar areas from differing vantage points. However, we must tread cautiously if we are not to become locked within the constraints of a paradigm we have created; we must proceed methodically and with scientific rigour at all times, ensuring that we do not mould the evidence to suit our models. Schizophrenia has proved an elusive, yet instructive teacher. Our hypotheses must be considered with scientific objectivism and the evidence which disproves our most cherished beliefs is perhaps more important than the evidence we believe to be confirmatory.

In this "decade of the brain" there has been a re-emergence of the biological roots of psychiatry and psychology. The move from a "psychological" understanding of the cognitive deficits in schizophrenia to an appreciation that such deficits have neurobiological underpinnings has been a major step in the inexorable advance towards understanding the pathophysiological disturbance in this elusive disorder. It is likely that a condition such as schizophrenia, which is so pervasive in its devastation of that which defines our identities, emotions and thoughts, provides us with our greatest challenge in understanding the consequences of a disordered mind and brain. The initial steps have been predominantly descriptive. We are now at the stage where we can extend this work from the phenomenological to the development of models which examine the nature of the link between brain and behaviour and to test these models using a number of techniques, including neuropsychology, neurophysiology and the most recent advances in structural and functional imaging. We hope this book provides a starting point for the reader from which to explore the neurobiological roots of a complex disorder affecting our fundamental functions.

ACKNOWLEDGEMENTS

The author thanks Dr Paul Brown for helping to clarify the chronology of Kraepelin's early work and for his comments on the penultimate version of the chapter. Thanks also to Dr Hazel Nelson, Prof. Thomas Barnes and Deidre Smith for their helpful comments.

REFERENCES

Baddeley, A.D. (1986) *Working Memory*, Oxford University Press, Oxford.

Barnes, T.R.E. (1988) Tardive dyskinesia: Risk factors, pathophysiology and treatment. *Recent Advances in Clinical Psychiatry*, **6**, 185–207.

Bleuler, E. (1911/1950) Dementia Praecox oder Gruppe der Schizophrenien. In: *Handbuch der Psychiatrie, Spezieller Teil 4. Abt. 1. Hälfte.* (Ed. G. Aschaffenburg), F. Deuticke: Leipzig und Wien. (Trans. J. Zinkin, 1950, International Universities Press, Inc.: Madison, USA).

Brewer, W., Francey, S., Yung, A., Velakoulis, D., Anderson, V., McGorry, P., Copolov, D., Singh, B., Pantelis, C. (1996) Olfactory and Neuropsychological deficits in high-risk and first episode psychosis. *European Neuropsychopharmacology*, **6** (Supp 3), 136.

Carter, D.N., Mackinnon, A.J., Howard, S., Zeegers, T., Copolov, D.L. (1995) The development and reliability of the mental health research institute unusual perceptions schedule (MUPS): an instrument to record auditory hallucinatory experience. *Schizophrenia Research*, **16**, 157–165.

Crow, T.J. (1980) Molecular pathology of schizophrenia: More than one disease process? *British Medical Journal*, **280**, 66–68.

Gold J.M., Hermann B.P., Randolph C., Wyler A.R., Goldberg T.E., Weinberger D.R. (1994)

Schizophrenia and temporal lobe epilepsy: A neuropsychological analysis. *Archives of General Psychiatry*, **51**, 265–272.

Goldberg, T.E., Berman, K.F., Mohr, E., Weinberger, D.R. (1990) Regional cerebral blood flow and cognitive function in Huntington's disease and schizophrenia: A comparison of patients matched for performance on a prefrontal-type task. *Archives of Neurology*, **47**, 418–422.

Goldman-Rakic, P.S. (1987) Circuitry of primate prefrontal cortex and regulation of behaviour by representational memory. In: *Handbook of Physiology: The Nervous System*, Vol. 5 (Ed. F. Plum), pp. 373–417, American Physiological Society, Bethesda, MD.

Hanes, K.R., Andrewes, D.G., Pantelis, C. (1995) Cognitive flexibility and complex integration in Parkinson's disease, Huntington's disease and schizophrenia. *Journal of the International Neuropsychological Society*, **1**, 545–553.

Kraepelin, E. (1896) *Psychiatrie. Ein Lehrbuch für Studirende und Ärzte*, 5th edn. Barth: Leipzig.

Kraepelin, E. (1899/1904) *Lectures in Clinical Psychiatry*, 6th edn. (Translated by A.R. Diefendorf, 1904), MacMillan: New York.

Kraepelin, E. (1903–4/1918) *Lectures in Clinical Psychiatry*, 7th edn. (Translated by A.R. Diefendorf, 1918), MacMillan: New York.

Kraepelin, E. (1909–1915) 8th edn. *Vol. 1 Allgemeine Psychiatrie* (1909); *Vol. 2 Klinische Psychiatrie I* (1910); *Vol. 3 Klinische Psychiatrie II* (1913); *Vol. 4 Klinische Psychiatrie III* (1915).

McGorry, P.D., Edwards, J., Mihalopoulos, C., Harrigan, S.M., Jackson, H.J. (1996) EPPIC: An evolving system of early detection and optimal management. *Schizophrenia Bulletin*, **22**, 305–326.

Minas, I.H., Stuart, G.W., Klimidis, S. et al (1992) Positive and negative symptoms in the psychoses: Multidimensional scaling of SAPS and SANS items. *Schizophrenia Research*, **8**, 143–156.

Morel, B.A. (1857) *Traité des dégénérescences physiques, intellectuelles et morales de l'espèce humaine*. J.B. Baillière: Paris.

Pantelis, C., Barnes, T.R.E., Nelson, H.E. (1992) Is the concept of frontal–subcortical dementia relevant to schizophrenia? *British Journal of Psychiatry*, **160**, 442–460.

Satz, P. (1993) Brain reserve capacity on symptom onset after brain injury: A formulation and review of evidence for threshold theory. *Neuropsychology*, **7**, 273–295.

Torrey, E.F., Bowler, A.E., Taylor, E.H. Gottesman, I.I. (1994) *Schizophrenia and Manic-Depressive disorder: The Biological Roots Of Mental Illness As Revealed By The Landmark Study Of Identical Twins*. Basic Books, A Division of Harper Collins Publishers, Inc., NY.

Velakoulis, D., Brewer, W.J., McGorry, P., Paton, G., Yung, A., Francey, S., Pantelis, C. (1996) Hippocampal volume reduction and cognitive deficits: course from high risk to chronic schizophrenia. *European Neuropsychopharmacology*, **6 (Supp. 3)**, 100.

Walker, E. (1991) *Schizophrenia: A Life-Course Developmental Perspective*. Academic Press: San Diego, CA.

Walker, E.F., Savoie, T., Davis, D. (1994) Neuromotor precursors of schizophrenia. *Schizophrenia Bulletin*, **20**, 441–451.

Walker, E.F. (1994) Developmentally moderated expressions of the neuropathology underlying schizophrenia. *Schizophrenia Bulletin*, **20**, 453–480.

Weinberger, D.R. (1987) Implications for normal brain development for the pathogenesis of schizophrenia. *Archives of General Psychiatry*, **44**, 660–699.

Weinberger, D.R. (1991) Anteromedial temporo-prefrontal connectivity: a functional neuroanatomical system implicated in schizophrenia. In: *Psychopathology and the Brain* (Eds B.J. Carroll, J.E. Barrett), pp. 25–43, Raven Press, New York.

Weinberger, D.R., Berman, K.F., Suddath, R., Torrey, E.F. (1992) Evidence of dysfunction of a prefrontal–limbic network in schizophrenia: A magnetic resonance imaging and regional cerebral blood flow study of discordant monozygotic twins. *American Journal of Psychiatry*, **149**, 890–897.

Yung, A.R., McGorry, P.D. (1996) The prodromal phase of first-episode psychosis: past and current conceptualizations. *Schizophrenia Bulletin*, **22**, 353–370.

2

The Cognitive Disorder of Psychiatric Illness: A Historical Perspective

DANIEL G.C. ROGERS

INTRODUCTION

Cognitive disorder associated with psychiatric illness was established by the earliest studies following the introduction of standardised methods of cognitive assessment at the beginning of the century. It has been the subject of a considerable number of studies since. In this chapter a review of this literature over the last 70 years is carried out. Cross-sectional studies, longitudinal studies, the nature of the disorder, the contribution of physical treatment and the overlap with dementia and mental handicap are considered. This allows a fresh look at psychiatric disorder in the light of recent interest in their possible cerebral basis.

For a long time, the cognitive disorder of psychiatric illness was not accepted as genuine or important. For example, when Bleuler (1911) put forward his concept of schizophrenia to replace that of dementia praecox, it included the principle that associated anomalies of cognitive function were merely accidental phenomena due to the patients' negativism, indifference and reluctance to think. This remained the orthodox position for the next 50 years. This was because a psychological paradigm was the generally favoured explanation of psychiatric disorder. Cognitive disorder was equated with cerebral disorder and classically involved loss of cognitive capacity, was irreversible and associated with structural brain changes, as in dementia of the Alzheimer type. There was no neurological model appropriate for the cognitive disorder found with psychiatric disorder.

This has now changed with the evolution of the concepts of bradyphrenia, psychic akinesia and subcortical dementia, involving loss of access to cognitive capacity rather than loss of capacity, which is reversible and associated with

Schizophrenia: A Neuropsychological Perspective. Edited by C. Pantelis, H.E. Nelson and T.R.E. Barnes
© 1996 John Wiley & Sons Ltd

neurochemical rather than structural change (Rogers, 1986). In addition, there has been a recent paradigm change to a more brain-based psychiatry (Rogers, 1987). This makes a review and fresh look at the literature on the cognitive disorder of psychiatric illness over the last half-century a useful exercise.

CROSS-SECTIONAL STUDIES

The Binet–Simon Scale for measurement of intelligence first appeared in 1905 and was first used with psychiatric patients by Wender in 1915. The Stanford revision of the Binet–Simon Scale was introduced in 1916. Results on this scale were expressed in terms of mental age. Normal adult subjects had a mean mental age on the scale of 13 years 8 months, with a mean mental age on its vocabulary subtest of 13 years 2 months. Wells and Kelley (1920) set out to examine all the patients admitted to one psychiatric unit over a 12-month period with the Stanford–Binet Scale. Their findings were typical of many studies that were to follow. They only obtained the necessary cooperation in 102 patients, 60% of all the patients admitted. These patients ranged in age from 16 to 75 and included 46 with manic-depressive insanity, 22 with dementia praecox and 17 with neuro-syphilis or arteriosclerosis. The average mental age on the scale for these three groups was 13 years 3 months, 13 years 1 month and 10 years 2 months respectively. The average mental age on the vocabulary subtest for the whole group, however, was 15 years 9 months. In all three groups "superior adult" ability in vocabulary could be associated with deficiency in remaining cognitive abilities down to the upper limits of "feeble-mindedness". The authors foreshadowed ambivalent attitudes to such findings. They suggested that in functional psychotic conditions, cognitive impairment was either the result of superposed organic involvement not otherwise apparent, or indicated volitional, rather than true, cognitive disorder.

In 1941, Brody surveyed the results of intelligence tests in psychosis up to that time. In summary, most psychotic subjects showed deficiencies in perception, learning and memory. These deficiencies were more severe in organic than in functional psychoses but in both the pattern of test scores was the same with vocabulary highest, verbal test ability second and non-verbal test ability lowest. The preservation of vocabulary was such that, usually, the result on a vocabulary test could be assumed to be a reliable measure of the patient's initial ability. The average discrepancy between score on the vocabulary subtest and on the rest of the Stanford–Binet Scale in different studies of psychotic patients was about 3 mental age years. Brody's interpretation of these results was characteristic. In organic cases, a true dementia occurred. In the functional psychoses, however, test failure was the result of "pseudo-dementia", i.e. disturbance of cooperation. Different psychiatric disorders could be ranked by test performance with psychoneurosis producing the highest, manic-depressive insanity lower and schizophrenia the lowest scores. The amount of pseudo-dementia in these conditions was ranked in exactly the reverse order.

Later studies consistently confirmed the results of these early studies but recently the interpretation of the results has gradually changed. In 1970, Klonoff and colleagues, reporting the neuropsychological assessment of 66 patients with chronic schizophrenia, suggested "with the utmost caution" that these patients exhibited cerebral dysfunction. Heaton and colleagues (1978), reviewing 94 studies between 1960 and 1975 that compared test scores of psychiatric patients with scores of brain-damaged patients or established norms for organicity, agreed. For each study, they calculated the combined hit rate, i.e. the total percentage of organic and non-organic patients correctly classified by the test. Of 34 attempts to discriminate chronic schizophrenic from organic patients, the median hit rate hardly exceeded chance level prediction at 54%. In 1981, Abrams and colleagues published the results of a study very similar to that of Wells and Kelley 60 years before but now using the Wechsler Adult Intelligence Scale (WAIS). They reported the testing of 77 patients. 52 had a diagnosis of affective disorder, 17 of schizophrenia and 8 of organic brain disease. The mean full-scale IQ for these three groups was 95.39, 84.55 and 81.60. These findings were comparable to those of the 1920 study but the interpretation of the findings was different. Performance on cognitive testing in patients with schizophrenia was now, according to the authors, consistent with significant cerebral dysfunction.

Cross-sectional studies, therefore, have consistently shown that psychiatric disorder is associated with cognitive disorder, most marked in severe psychiatric disorder and notably schizophrenic illness. The interpretation of this cognitive disorder has varied significantly.

LONGITUDINAL STUDIES

The introduction of routine cognitive assessment of school children and enlisted men provided the opportunity of comparing pre- and postmorbid cognitive function in individuals later developing psychiatric illness. In 1950, Rappaport & Webb reported 10 psychotic patients who had an IQ test during their school career and who were tested again with the same IQ test and a behaviour rating scale. Their mean age was 22.4 years and mean length of hospitalisation was 22.4 months. Their mean former IQ was 97.6 and mean current IQ 63.9. There was a high correlation between current IQ and their score on the behaviour rating scale. The authors ascribed the loss of IQ to "attitudinal factors", such as inability to sustain attention, emotional disturbance and lack of motivation, which they felt were measured by the behaviour rating scale.

In 1962, three major studies were published. Lubin and colleagues (1962) reported the retesting of 385 servicemen with the Army Classification Battery, a cognitive test with five standardised subtests, which they had originally taken on US army entry (premorbidly). 159 had subsequently been hospitalised with a diagnosis of schizophrenia and 64 with brain injury, all 223 being retested within three months of admission. 162 were controls, similarly retested, with no history of brain injury or psychiatric illness. The mean age of the 385 subjects was 26 (range 18–51) and the mean interval between the two tests was 24.5 months (range 1–140) with no significant differences between the means for age and retest interval of the different groups. The control subjects showed a general increase in their scores. The schizophrenic patients had lost between 1/6 and 1/3 of a standard deviation in their scores on four of the subtests. The brain-injured patients showed a similar but more pronounced deficit. Fifty-five per cent of the schizophrenic group were on medication but none of the deficit in scores could be attributed to this.

Also in 1962, Douglas & Schwartzman reported the results of retesting 80 veterans with the Canadian Revised Examination "M", which they had all taken on enlistment in 1943, when their mean age was 22.6. By 1952, 50 had been hospitalised with a diagnosis of schizophrenia. Thirty were still in hospital and had been for at least 6 months, while 20 had been discharged for at least 1 year. A further 30 were normal controls. These groups, schizophrenic patients, schizophrenic ex-patients and controls, were matched for age, educational level, intelligence at time of enlistment and occupational status (all had returned to civilian life after enlistment). The patients and ex-patients were matched for total number of years hospitalised (mean 2.4 years). On retesting, 8 years after first testing, the control group scored significantly more (approximately 6 IQ points) and the whole schizophrenic group significantly less (approximately 6 IQ points) than on first testing. This deficit was more marked in the patient group (approximately 9 IQ points) than in the ex-patient group (approximately 3 IQ points). In 1960, 17 years after first testing, 22 of the "patient" group and 1 of the "ex-patient" group were tested with the same test a third time. Ten of these 23 were currently hospitalised. Their scores had decreased by as much again as between the first and second testing. The scores of the 13 patients who had been discharged, although lower at the time of the second test than that of the 10 still hospitalised, had increased again to almost equal their premorbid scores. There was no significant correlation between change in score over the intervals 1943–1952, 1952–1960 or 1943–1960 and length of hospitalisation. The significant factor for cognitive impairment was whether or not the patient needed to be in hospital at time of testing.

In the third study, Foulds & Dixon (1962) performed a combined cross-sectional and longitudinal study. They tested 550 hospitalised patients, drawn from the same catchment area, with two tests: Progressive Matrices (PM), a test of general cognitive ability, and the Mill Hill Vocabulary Scale (MHV). 280 had a diagnosis of neurosis and 270 were diagnosed with schizophrenia, the two groups being matched for age and sex. No patient was aged over 62 years and none had "organic complications", such as leucotomy or epilepsy. 303 schizophrenic patients were interviewed but 33 were untestable on two occasions. Of the 270 schizophrenic patients tested, 90 had been hospitalised less than one year, 90 less than 7 years and 90 over the 7 years. 186 were tested again after a 2-year interval. Compared with the neurotic group, the schizophrenic patients had a significant impairment on their PM scores but none on MHV scores. The PM score declined with age but no faster than in normals or in the neurotic group, was not related to length of hospitalisation and was reversible.

These longitudinal studies, therefore, provided strong evidence that the cognitive deficit associated with schizophrenia was confined largely to the initial impact of the illness, was not progressive and was reversible.

THE NATURE OF THE DISORDER

In 1955, Shapiro & Nelson set out to investigate the nature of cognitive impairment in cooperative psychiatric patients. They compared 20 neurotics, 20 manic-depressives, 20 schizophrenics, 20 organics and 20 normal subjects on a variety of tests. They found that the psychiatric patients appeared to be inferior in important aspects of cognitive function, including vocabulary, learning and retention. It was not possible to differentiate between chronic schizophrenic patients and the brain-damaged group; however, all types of cognitive measures differentiated between normal, neurotic and psychotic patients. Slowness was the most important of all the different variables examined because it differentiated most powerfully between normal and abnormal groups. When subjects were matched for their scores on tests of vocabulary, problem solving and memory for new word definitions, psychomotor slowness still differentiated between normal and abnormal groups. When, however, the opposite was done and relatively normal and abnormal groups were matched for scores on a psychomotor speed test, then the tests of vocabulary, problem solving and memory for the definition of new words did not differentiate significantly between the groups. Psychomotor speed tests correlated more highly and more consistently than other tests with independent subjective estimates of the severity of illness. Speed scores were calculated for heavily sedated, somewhat sedated and non-sedated patients within each psychiatric group. No trends emerged and non-sedated patients were still significantly slower than normal subjects.

In 1961, Dowis & Buchanan studied 75 consecutive psychiatric admissions to a teaching hospital who had graduated from high school and were aged between 25 and 50. Every day each patient was independently rated by two nurses on the presence or absence of 29 overt behaviours associated with psychiatric illness. Severe behavioural pathology was defined as a period of at least 3 days during which daily scores fell within the upper quarter of that patient's range of scores during hospitalisation. Minimal behavioural pathology was similarly defined but for scores falling within the lowest quarter of their range of scores. Each patient was tested with Raven's Progressive Matrices (PMT) and a Wide Range Vocabulary Test (WRVT) at least during one period of maximum and one period of minimum behavioural pathology as defined. Thirty-seven patients were tested first in the minimum period and 38 first in the maximum period. During the periods of maximum behavioural pathology, there was a significant decrease in the PMT score but not the WRVT score as compared with the periods of minimum pathology. The PMT/WRVT discrepancy increased with severity of behavioural pathology. The authors concluded that the level of cognitive efficiency was more a function of the severity of psychiatric illness than a distinguishing characteristic of any specific nosological entity.

Cognitive impairment is not restricted to schizophrenic disorder. Reviewing the literature on cognitive function in affective disorder, McAllister (1981) felt that memory, speed of performance and decision making were significantly impaired in depressive illnesses but the impairment was temporary or reversible with improvement in the depressive illness. He suggested that depression could be considered as a "treatable dementia". Kerry et al (1983) tested 27 patients with manic-depressive illness stretching back up to 65 years and with up to 100 episodes of illness and 40 years of hospitalisation and showed that complete clinical recovery could be associated with no cognitive impairment. Furthermore, this was despite frequent ECT, psychotropic medication and leucotomy. Slowing of motor and cognitive function is a prominent feature of primary depressive illness, with similarities to that found in patients with Parkinson's disease; both motor and especially cognitive slowing improving as the depressive disorder improves (Rogers et al, 1987).

As newer methods of investigating cerebral structure and function were introduced, a relation became apparent between cognitive impairment in patients with severe psychiatric illness and abnormalities on electroencephalogram and computerised axial tomography (CT) of the brain (Kennard & Levy 1952; Johnstone et al, 1978; Golden et al, 1980; Donnelly et al, 1980; Lawson et al, 1988). Recent studies have shown that cognitive deficit in severe psychiatric illness is especially related to so-called "negative" features, such as affective flattening, retardation and poverty of speech, rather than "positive" features such as hallucinations, delusions and thought disorder and, in cerebral terms, represents bilateral and diffuse disorder (Depue et al, 1975; Owens & Johnstone, 1980; Taylor & Abrams, 1984).

These studies suggest that a major component of the cognitive impairment of psychiatric illness consists of slowing of, or difficulty with access to, cognitive function. The severity of the impairment is related to the intensity of the psychiatric illness and is reversible with improvement of the illness. It is an impairment typically associated with diffuse rather than focal and functional rather than structural brain disorder.

NEUROLEPTIC MEDICATION, ECT AND LEUCOTOMY

Heaton & Crowley (1981) reviewed the literature for the possible effects of psychiatric somatic treatment on neuropsychological test performance. There was no convincing evidence that neuroleptic medication or ECT produced persistent cognitive impairment, nor that neuroleptic medication could produce improvement in cognitive functioning with improvement in psychiatric disorder. Baker (1968) had already suggested this in his review of the effect of medication on cognitive functioning. Seven studies which had used over 200 mg daily of chlorpromazine in patients with schizophrenia showed a significant increase in WAIS IQ score, or Wechsler–Bellevue IQ scores for drug groups over placebo groups under double-blind conditions. Eight studies which had used up to 200 mg daily reported no change in cognitive functioning. The only studies which showed a decrease in cognitive performance used student volunteers rather than patients.

In 1973, Templar and colleagues reported results on the WAIS in 34 patients hospitalised with a diagnosis of schizophrenia. Twenty-two had been treated with between 40 and 263 (median 58.5) electroconvulsive treatments, more than 7 years earlier. Twelve had received no ECT. The two groups were matched for age, sex, race and level of education. The ECT-treated patients' performance was inferior on the WAIS (mean full-scale IQ 65.73 as against 76.77). However, they were also found to be more psychotic on all of the 8 indices of psychosis. When the degree of psychosis was controlled for, the WAIS performances of the ECT-treated and control patients were very similar. Cutting (1979) found that the memory impairment in patients with chronic schizophrenia was worse in the 10, of the 20 patients tested, who had not received ECT.

In 1969, Hamlin reported the testing on three occasions over 14 years with the Wechsler–Bellevue of 49 patients hospitalised with a diagnosis of schizophrenia. At the outset, 16 had had psychosurgery with an orbital topectomy and 33 had been assigned at random to a control group. They were tested in 1949, 1957 and 1962. The pattern of test change over the 14 years was essentially the same in all respects for all the patients, including the 16 who had undergone the orbital topectomy. When allowances were made for aging, there was an increase in test scores, with those patients who improved on symptoms and social adequacy showing appreciable gains. Stuss and colleagues (1981) performed the WAIS and Wechsler Memory Scale as well as CT brain scans on 17 men with schizophrenia who had undergone bilateral frontal leucotomies 25 years before. The patients were divided into 3 groups: five who had shown good recovery, five moderate recovery and six with no recovery. Five schizophrenic patients with the same severity of illness who had no leucotomy acted as controls. They found a clear and obvious correlation of cognitive performance with the level of clinical recovery. Recovery level was also related to the size of leucotomy defect as measured on the CT scan. They suggested that leucotomy in these cases might have produced improved cognitive performance.

Recent studies have continued to support these findings. Owens & Johnstone (1980) examined the cognitive functioning of 510 patients with chronic schizophrenia with the Withers and Hinton series of cognitive tests and found that none of their past physical treatments were significant factors in the severe impairments found. Mathai & Gopinath (1986) examined cognitive functioning with the Mini Mental State in 80 patients with chronic schizophrenia and 16 with manic-depressive psychosis, who included outpatients, day care patients and long-stay patients in two hospitals with different amounts of social stimulation. They concluded that neither physical treatments nor long-stay hospital care but, rather, the disease process was responsible for the deficits in chronic schizophrenia.

These studies suggest that physical treatments make only a minor, if any, contribution to the cognitive impairment of patients with severe psychiatric illness and can in fact improve cognitive performance if there is improvement in the psychiatric illness (see also King and Green, chapter 20).

DEMENTIA AND MENTAL HANDICAP

Schizophrenia was previously called dementia praecox and before that primary dementia (Zelamowits, 1953). Rogers (1985) examined 100 patients with severe psychiatric illness selected by length of current admission and who were first admitted between 1907 and 1955. Ninety-two had received a diagnosis of schizophrenia at some stage after 1929. At some stage between 1922 and 1944, 54 of these patients had a previous diagnosis of dementia praecox and, before 1925, 14 of these same patients had been diagnosed as suffering with primary dementia. Twenty-two had an additional diagnosis at some stage of dementia or secondary dementia. Twenty-three had received an additional diagnosis of mental handicap, while five patients had received additional diagnoses of both dementia and mental handicap.

Abrahamson (1983) carried out a case note study of 300 long-stay inpatients with schizophrenia. These showed a surprising degree of long-term consistency. Levels of disability at the time of the survey were strikingly similar to those recorded at, or shortly after, admission even when this had been 40 or 50 years previously. In less than 10% was the final state worse than the initial and even here the deterioration had been almost entirely confined to the first third of their admission. Improvement had occurred in about 25%, predominantly in the middle or last third of their admission. One of the most striking features of schizophrenic "deterioration" was that these patients were frequently described as demented or institutionalised according to the period.

Different studies have shown that patients with severe psychiatric illness can be diagnosed as mentally handicapped in the face of a history of normal premorbid cognitive functioning, or current cognitive functioning within the normal range, especially in the absence of distinctly psychotic symptoms on admission (Richards, 1951; Raub et al, 1952–3; Chapman & Pathman 1959). Benda and colleagues (1951) forcefully criticised the rigid theoretical division between mental handicap and severe psychiatric illness in child psychiatry. They felt that the only essential difference between mental "deficiency" and mental "illness" lay in the time of onset of the disorder. This was at a time when child psychiatry was changing from a predominantly psychodynamic paradigm to a neuropsychiatric one, a generation ahead of the same change in adult psychiatry. O'Gorman (1952, 1954) argued that mental handicap was a legal and social rather than clinical concept and that schizophrenia beginning before the age of 18 could be regarded as a cause of mental handicap, the degree of handicap depending on the severity and duration of the psychiatric illness. Russell & Tanguay (1981) in a study of 193 adolescents showed that an episodic psychotic illness could be associated with transient functioning in the mild or even moderate range of mental handicap. Resolution of the psychosis could be accompanied by resolution of the cognitive deficit but severe, unremitting psychotic illness was associated with persistent cognitive impairment.

Previously, secondary diagnoses of dementia or mental handicap in patients with severe psychiatric illness with obvious cognitive impairment were needed because of prevailing concepts of psychiatric disorder, which excluded cognitive impairment as part of the psychiatric disorder. With the recent change in the prevailing paradigm in psychiatry, this is no longer necessary and the overlap between psychiatric disorder, dementia and mental handicap can be usefully explored.

CONCLUSION

Studies over the last 70 years have established, using a wide variety of standardised tests, that cognitive impairment is a frequent accompaniment of psychiatric illness. The earliest studies showed that the more severe the psychiatric illness, the more severe the cognitive impairment. At its most severe, it approached the cognitive impairment associated with known cerebral disorders, although a sharp distinction was usually drawn between the two. The pattern of the impairment suggested deterioration from a higher premorbid level. Later studies demonstrated that, typically, cognitive impairment appears with the onset of florid illness, varies in severity with other manifestations of illness, is potentially reversible and is not necessarily progressive even if persistent. It characteristically involves difficulty with access to cognitive capacity, manifested, for example, as slowness of response rather than loss of cognitive capacity. Cognitive impairment is no respecter of diagnostic boundaries except insofar as these reflect severity of illness. Treatment does not affect the impairment, except in a beneficial direction.

Since neurology and psychiatry parted conceptual company at the beginning of this century there have been developments in neurological ideas about cognitive disorder which did not make any impact on psychiatry because of its preoccupation with psychological interpretation of psychiatric disorder. Up to 25 years ago great efforts were expended in trying to distinguish schizophrenia from cerebral disorder by cognitive testing. The attempt was non-productive. The attempt continues with depression and dementia. The last 25 years have seen an increasing acceptance of the cerebral basis of at least the more severe forms of psychiatric illness. When the literature on the cognitive disorder of psychiatric illness over the last 70 years is reviewed and compared to evolving neurological concepts over this period, a coherent account emerges which points the way forward for psychiatric research in this area.

REFERENCES

Abrahamson, D. (1983) Discussion: Schizophrenic deterioration. *British Journal of Psychiatry*, **143**, 82–83.

Abrams, R., Redfield, J., Taylor, M.A. (1981) Cognitive dysfunction in schizophrenia, affective disorder and organic brain disease. *British Journal of Psychiatry*, **139**, 190–194.

Baker, R.R. (1968) The effects of psychotropic drugs on psychological testing. *Psychological Bulletin*, **69**, 377–387.

Benda, C.E., Farrell, M.J., Chipman, G.E. (1951) The inadequacy of present day concepts of mental deficiency and mental illness in child psychiatry. *American Journal of Psychiatry*, **107**, 721–729.

Bleuler, E. (1911) *Dementia Praecox or The Group of Schizophrenias*. (Transl. J. Zinkin, 1950), International Universities Press, New York.

Brody, M.B. (1941) A survey of the results of intelligence tests in psychosis. *British Journal of Medical Psychology*, **19**, 215–261.

Chapman, L.J., Pathman, J.H. (1959) Errors in the diagnosis of mental deficiency in schizophrenia. *Journal of Consulting Psychology*, **23**, 432–434.

Cutting, J. (1979) Memory in functional psychosis. *Journal of Neurology, Neurosurgery and Psychiatry*, **42**, 1031–1037.

Depue, R.A., Dubicki, M.D., Macarthy, T. (1975) Differential recovery of intellectual, associational and psychophysiological functioning in withdrawn and active schizophrenics. *Journal of Abnormal Psychology*, **84**, 325–330.

Donnelly, E.F., Weinberger, M.D., Waldman, M.S., Wyatt, R.J. (1980) Cognitive impairment associated with morphological brain abnormalities on computed tomography in chronic schizophrenic patients. *Journal of Nervous and Mental Disease*, **168**, 305–308.

Douglas, V.I., Schwartzman, A.E. (1962) Intellectual loss in schizophrenia. *Canadian Journal of Psychology*, **16**, 1–10, 161–168.

Dowis, J.L., Buchanan, E.E. (1961) Some relationships between intellectual efficiency and the severity of psychiatric illness. *Journal of Psychology*, **51**, 371–381.

Foulds, G.A., Dixon, P. (1962) The nature of intellectual deficit in schizophrenia. *British Journal of Social and Clinical Psychology*, **1**, 7–19, 141–149.

Golden, C.J., Moses, J.A., Zelazowski, R., Graber, B., Zatz, L.M., Horuath, T.B., Berger, P.A. (1980) Cerebral ventricular size and neuropsychological impairment of young chronic schizophrenics. *Archives of General Psychiatry*, **37**, 619–623.

Hamlin, R. (1969) The stability of intellectual function in chronic schizophrenia. *Journal of Nervous and Mental Disease*, **149**, 496–503.

Heaton, R.K., Crowley, T.J. (1981) Effects of psychiatric disorders and their somatic treatments on neuropsychological test results. In: *Handbook of Clinical Neuropsychology*, (Eds S.B. Filskov, T.J. Boll), pp. 481–525, Wiley, New York.

Heaton, R.K., Baade, L.E., Johnson, K.L. (1978) Neuropsychological test results associated with psychiatric disorders in adults. *Psychological Bulletin*, **85**, 141–162.

Johnstone, E.C., Crow, T.J., Frith, C.D. et al (1978) The dementia of dementia praecox. *Acta Psychiatrica Scandinavica*, **57**, 305–324.

Kennard, M.A., Levy, S. (1952) The meaning of the abnormal encephalogram in schizophrenia. *Journal of Nervous and Mental Disease*, **116**, 413–423.

Kerry, R.J., McDermott, C.M., Orme, J.E. (1983) Affective disorders and cognitive performance. *Journal of Affective Disorders*, **5**, 349–352.

Klonoff, H., Fibiger, C.H., Hutton, G.H. (1970). Neuropsychological patterns in chronic schizophrenia. *Journal of Nervous and Mental Disease*, **150**, 291–300.

Lawson, W.B., Waldman, I.N., Weinberger, D.R. (1988) Schizophrenic dementia, clinical and computed axial tomography correlates. *Journal of Nervous and Mental Disease*, **176**, 207–212.

Lubin, A., Gieseking, C.F., Williams, H.L. (1962) Direct measurement of cognitive deficit in schizophrenia. *Journal of Consulting Psychology*, **26**, 139–143.

Mathai, P.J., Gopinath, P.S. (1986) Deficits of chronic schizophrenia in relation to long-term hospitalisation. *British Journal of Psychiatry*, **148**, 509–516.

McAllister, T.W. (1981) Cognitive functioning in the affective disorders. *Comprehensive Psychiatry*, **22**, 572–586.

O'Gorman, G. (1952) Discussion: Psychoses in childhood. *Proceedings of the Royal Society of Medicine*, **45**, 800–802.

O'Gorman, G. (1954) Psychosis as a cause of mental defect? *Journal of Mental Science*, **100**, 934–943.

Owens, D.G.C., Johnstone, E.C. (1980) The disabilities of chronic schizophrenia: Their nature and the factors contributing to their development. *British Journal of Psychiatry*, **136**, 384–395.

Rappaport, S.R., Webb, W.B. (1950) An attempt to study intellectual deterioration by premorbid and psychotic testing. *Journal of Consulting Psychology*, **14**, 95–98.

Raub, E.S., Mercer, M., Hecker, A.O. (1952–3) A study of psychotic patients assumed to be mentally deficient on the basis of school progress and social adjustment. *American Journal of Mental Deficiency*, **57**, 82–88.

Richards, B.W. (1951) Childhood schizophrenia and mental deficiency. *Journal of Mental Science*, **97**, 290–312.

Rogers, D. (1985) The motor disorders of severe psychiatric illness: a conflict of paradigms. *British Journal of Psychiatry*, **147**, 221–232.

Rogers, D. (1986) Bradyphrenia in parkinsonism: a historical review. *Psychological Medicine*, **16**, 257–265.

Rogers, D. (1987) Neuropsychiatry. *British Journal of Psychiatry*, **150**, 425–427.

Rogers, D., Lees, A.J., Smith, E., Trimble, M, Stern, G.M. (1987) Bradyphrenia in Parkinson's disease and psychomotor retardation in depressive illness: An experimental study. *Brain*, **110**, 761–776.

Russell, A.T., Tanguay, P.E. (1981) Mental illness and mental retardation: Cause or coincidence? *American Journal of Mental Deficiency*, **85**, 570–574.

Shapiro, M.B., Nelson, E.H. (1955) An investigation of the nature of cognitive impairment in cooperative psychiatric patients. *British Journal of Psychiatry*, **28**, 239–256.

Stuss, D.T., Kaplan, E.F., Benson, D.F., Weir, S.F., Naeser, M.A., Levine, H.L. (1981) Long term effects of prefrontal leucotomy: An overview of neuropsychological residuals. *Journal of Clinical Neuropsychology*, **3**, 13–32.

Taylor, M.A., Abrams, R. (1984) Cognitive impairment in schizophrenia. *American Journal of Psychiatry*, **141**, 196–201.

Templar D.I., Ruff, D.F., Armstrong, G. (1973) Cognitive functioning and degree of psychosis in schizophrenics given many electroconvulsive treatments. *British Journal of Psychiatry*, **123**, 441–443.

Wells, F.L., Kelley, C.M. (1920) Intelligence and psychosis. *American Journal of Insanity*, **7**, 17–45.

Wender, L. (1915) *New York Medical Journal*, **101**, 448.

Zelamowits, J. (1953) A historical note on the simple dementing form of schizophrenia. *Proceedings of the Royal Society of Medicine*, **46**, 931–933.

3

Methodological Issues in the Neuropsychological Approach to Schizophrenia

GERALD GOLDSTEIN

INTRODUCTION: GENERAL METHODOLOGICAL ISSUES IN NEUROPSYCHOLOGY

In this chapter we will attempt to demonstrate that methodological problems related to neuropsychological research in schizophrenia are partly a matter of those issues related to neuropsychological research in general, those related to psychopathology in general and the study of schizophrenia in particular. In this section we will briefly review the area of neuropsychological methodology in general while in the next section we will provide material concerning methodology for neuropsychological research in schizophrenia.

VALIDITY IN NEUROPSYCHOLOGY

The field of human neuropsychology has been primarily concerned with assessment. There is certainly an active area of experimental human neuropsychology but the instruments used by experimental neuropsychologists are typically assessment instruments administered to patients with various brain disorders within the framework of some research design. It has become the tradition in the field to see the experimental technique of today become the clinical test of tomorrow. Therefore, the distinction between clinical and experimental human neuropsychology does not connote a major difference with regard to instrumentation.

The problem of validity is present for instruments regardless of their utilisation in research or clinical practice. Traditionally, the distinction has been made

Schizophrenia: A Neuropsychological Perspective. Edited by C. Pantelis, H.E. Nelson and T.R.E. Barnes
© 1996 John Wiley & Sons Ltd

among several forms of validity, notably predictive, concurrent, face and construct validity. The emphasis in human neuropsychology has been on concurrent validity involving validation of instruments against some external criterion available at the time the instrument is administered. The area of predictive validity in neuropsychology has been controversial having been associated with the general area of clinical judgement and prediction of outcome with behavioural measures. There are actually very few neuropsychological studies concerning the predictive validities of assessment methods. However, there have been several neuropsychologically oriented longitudinal studies, particularly in the fields of learning disability (Rourke, 1985, 1991; Spreen, 1988) and Alzheimer's disease (Kazniak et al, 1978), in which efforts have been, or are being, made to ascertain the predictive capacities of various tests. Face validity is generally considered in the design of tests and has possibly become associated with a new concept called ecological validity (Acker, 1990). Ecological validity refers to the accuracy of assessment methods in predicting behaviour in natural settings. Construct validity has been extensively studied producing a wealth of experimental literature on a wide variety of neuropsychological constructs.

The area of concurrent validity is probably the most straightforward one in neuropsychology. Traditionally, neuropsychological tests have been validated against neurological criteria. That is, the criterion was typically the presence or absence of some structural alteration of the brain that could be observed directly, generally at neurosurgery, or with radiological methods. The technology for observing the brain has increased dramatically since the beginnings of neuropsychology and so the field has had the good fortune of receiving very rapidly progressing refinement of its validation criteria.

The successful efforts made at validating neuropsychological data against neurological criteria have become associated with major advances in theorisation concerning brain function. Here we are dealing with method and not with theory but theoretical considerations have engendered the need for increasingly detailed and sophisticated validation studies. Just as examples, the theory that the frontal lobe is divided into at least two major functional regions (dorsolateral and orbitofrontal) has led to the need to develop and validate tests that can evaluate this hypothesised distinction (see Pantelis and Brewer, chapter 16, this volume). Similarly, detailed studies of the language zone in the language dominant hemisphere have required increasingly specific tests of speech and language function. This interplay between theory and validation characterises the field of neuropsychology. It would probably be fair to say that there is a general consensus concerning guidelines for the adequacy of neurological criteria. The general considerations are as follows:

1. The subject should be evaluated by a neurologist, neurosurgeon, or neuropsychiatrist with demonstrated expertise in the disorder under study.
2. Direct observation of pathology is preferable to inference or clinical judgement. Pathological data obtained at autopsy are often useful but it must be recognised that, if the individual died long after the time of neuropsycho-

logical testing, the brain may have changed substantially over that time, particularly if death was caused by brain disease or injury.

3. Laboratory or clinical procedures that allow for direct observation, such as neuroimaging, resection diagrams accomplished during surgery or brain biopsy, are preferable to secondary procedures such as the electroencephalogram (EEG) and related techniques that provide more equivocal evidence of localisation of damage and pathology.

4. Where possible, quantitative measures of the validation criteria should be used as opposed to global judgements as to normal or abnormal status.

5. The validation technology used should be as close to state-of-the-art level as possible, as long as the status of the new technology itself is not questionable. An important recent example of this process has been the change from reliance on the computerised tomographic (CT) scan to magnetic resonance imaging (MRI) (see Bilder and Szeszko, chapter 14, this volume).

6. The criterion ratings should be established blind to the neuropsychological procedure being validated.

The form of concurrent validity that has probably been of most interest to neuropsychologists is discriminative validity. Beginning with the early studies, in which efforts were made to use tests simply to discriminate between patients with or without brain damage, efforts have been made, with increasing sophistication, to use assessment instruments to distinguish among increasingly refined entities. Within that pursuit, efforts have been made to establish the sensitivity and specificity of various instruments. Sensitivity refers to the capability of an instrument to detect a condition when it is present, while specificity refers to the capability of detecting the absence of a condition when it is absent. Thus, a test with high sensitivity and low specificity would identify a condition frequently when it is present but also frequently identify it as present when it is absent; the high false-positive situation. A test with low sensitivity but high specificity would rarely identify a condition as present when it is absent but would frequently not identify the condition when it is present; the high false-negative situation.

Related to the sensitivity-specificity matter is the effort to achieve a so-called "double dissociation". In neuropsychology, a double dissociation occurs when a task is performed abnormally by one group of patients and normally by another while the reverse occurs for another task. A later refinement of this methodological concept stipulated that the two tasks be of equal difficulty. Perhaps one of the best examples of double dissociation was presented some time ago by Teuber (1959) who showed that patients with penetrating gunshot wounds of the frontal lobe performed well on a task involving estimation of the verticality of a line when presented against a diagonally striped background. However, they performed abnormally when the task was to estimate verticality of a luminous rod while seated in a tilted position in a dark room. Conversely, patients with gunshot wounds of the occipital lobe performed the first task abnormally but the second one normally. The double dissociation with tasks matched for difficulty remains the most elegant form of empirical demonstration of specific effects in neuropsychology.

In a manner of speaking, construct validity constitutes the corpus of neuro-psychological research. As in other scientific areas, there are two broad approaches to its establishment: experimental and correlational. With regard to neuropsychology, a unique feature of the experimental approach is the use of neurological parameters as independent variables. In human neuropsychology this method is the equivalent of animal research in which neurological conditions are directly induced by the experimenter, such as through the use of lesion generation. However, human neuropsychologists must depend upon accidents of nature and so typically study patients with lesions produced by trauma or disease. Recently, a trend appears to have developed away from regional locali-sation studies and more toward the study of specific disease entities. The more recent literature tends to emphasise investigation of specific disorders such as Alzheimer's disease, HIV infection, learning disability, closed head injury and multiple sclerosis. In this type of research, there appears to be an effort to determine the constructs that best epitomise the disorder. For example, there is extensive interest in the nature of the memory deficit in Alzheimer's disease and the amnesic disorders, notably Korsakoff syndrome (Carlesimo & Oscar-Berman, 1992). In general, the project is generally that of describing a disease entity in terms of neuropsychological constructs. The research is often traditionally experi-mental in nature and, except for the use of neurologically relevant independent variables, neuropsychological research shares many methodologies with experi-mental psychology.

Those involved in correlational research proceed quite differently. These inves-tigators typically use the standard, comprehensive neuropsychological test batteries or batteries constructed specifically for a particular study. Perhaps the first example of this type of research was accomplished by Halstead (1947) who performed a factor analysis based on an early version of what is now known as the Halstead–Reitan Neuropsychological Test Battery (Reitan & Wolfson, 1993). Advocates of factor analysis believe that it identifies important constructs, such as the components of intelligence. Since Halstead's early work, numerous studies have been performed in which factor analysis was applied to neuropsychological test data. Sometimes it is applied to specific populations, such as learning disabled children, and sometimes one population is compared with another to determine whether or not the factor structures differ.

Neuropsychologists interested in individual differences and classification have applied cluster analysis, a procedure that is the reverse of factor analysis in that it groups subjects rather than tests. The major application of this work has been in the field of learning disability, in which it has been shown that there are several empirically derived subtypes of this disorder (Rourke, 1985). Other correlational techniques such as multiple regression and discriminant function analysis are now widely employed in neuropsychology. These applica-tions may be purely correlational or they may be used within experimental frameworks. The basic point is that neuropsychological tests are viewed as an intercorrelated vector and become more meaningful when treated as multi-variate combinations than when they are treated individually (Goldstein & Shelly, 1973).

VALIDITY ISSUES RELEVANT TO SCHIZOPHRENIA

In this section, we will concentrate on the establishment of the concurrent validity of neuropsychological tests when they are used for the assessment of patients with schizophrenia. In doing so we will refer to the standards used for validation criteria in general neuropsychology, as outlined above, and comment on those criteria.

1. *The subject should be evaluated by a neurologist, neurosurgeon, or neuropsychiatrist with demonstrated expertise in the disorder under study.*

In this case, subjects should be evaluated by psychiatrists with particular expertise in psychiatric diagnosis and diagnosis of schizophrenia in particular. Ideally, this standard is obtainable and is now implemented in many studies.

2. *Direct observation of pathology is preferable to inference or clinical judgement.*

Here we see a substantial difference from general neuropsychology. While patients with schizophrenia may have brain pathology, that pathology is not considered to be diagnostic, regardless of whether it is identified by imaging, biopsy or autopsy data. However, such investigations are sometimes useful to rule out pathology, as in the case in which an apparent schizophrenic condition is found to be produced by some structural neurological condition, such as a brain tumour.

3. *Laboratory or clinical procedures that allow for direct observation, such as neuroimaging, resection diagrams accomplished during surgery, or brain biopsy, are preferable to secondary procedures such as the electroencephalogram (EEG) and related techniques that provide more equivocal evidence of localisation of damage and pathology.*

4. *Where possible, quantitative measures of the validation criteria should be used as opposed to global judgements as to normal or abnormal status.*

Neither direct, indirect, qualitative, nor quantitative procedures are definitively diagnostic for schizophrenia, and so we are left with the same difficulty raised under point (2). That is not to say that such procedures as the EEG, evoked potentials and related techniques have not been useful in the study of schizophrenia. We are only suggesting here that they cannot be used as adequate validity criteria.

5. *The validation technology used should be as close to state-of-the-art level as possible, as long as the status of the new technology itself is not questionable.*

This point is of particular salience because enormous efforts have been made to develop or apply new technologies that will provide definitive evidence of schizophrenia. In all likelihood, these efforts will be the ones that will ultimately provide an unequivocal valid criterion. With regard to brain function in schizophrenia there has been an application of a broad range of structural and functional imaging techniques including CT scan, MRI, nuclear magnetic resonance (NMR) spectroscopy, positron emission tomography (PET), single photon emission computerised tomography (SPECT) and cerebral blood flow (CBF) studies. Some of these studies have utilised neuropsychological tests in activation paradigms (see Liddle, chapter 15, this volume). Other studies have used a correlational approach, finding reasonably strong associations between quantitative measures of neuropsychological function and quantitative neuro-radiological indices of neuronal depletion (see Bilder & Szeszko, chapter 14, this volume). This area of investigation is still in progress and, while numerous abnormalities have been found in schizophrenic brains and indices of brain function, the findings, in and of themselves, are not diagnostic of schizophrenia. That is because the abnormalities (e.g. ventricular enlargement) are seen in other disorders and they are not seen in all patients with schizophrenia. However, based on a study of monozygotic twins discordant for schizophrenia (Suddath et al, 1990) there was some suggestion that all those with schizophrenia showed evidence of brain scan abnormalities, because the index twins showed visible evidence of brain atrophy relative to the co-twins, although the scans of the index twins may frequently have been judged as within normal limits on an absolute basis. However, the problem remains that brain atrophy lacks specificity for schizophrenia although the study by Suddath and colleagues suggests that it might have high sensitivity. In summary, while these studies of brain structure and function have not yet produced a valid criterion for schizophrenia they show some promise of ultimately doing so.

6. *The criterion ratings should be established blind to the neuropsychological procedure being validated.*

This practice can be carried out in schizophrenia research without particular difficulty. Independence of the criterion from the procedure being validated is always a crucial consideration.

In summary, the matter of obtaining concurrent validity for neuropsychological measures is problematic in the area of schizophrenia. That is, it is presently not possible to employ the traditional practice of validating neuropsychological tests against independently acquired evidence of brain pathology in schizophrenia. It may be noted that this situation is not unique to schizophrenia and even exists in certain neurological disorders. There is no definitive diagnostic indicator of multiple sclerosis and the diagnosis must be made clinically unless autopsy data are available. Alzheimer's disease is a pathological diagnosis which cannot be definitively identified in living individuals. Thus, there may be some virtue in validating tests against clinical diagnoses in the absence of objective biological criteria. That procedure is common practice in schizophrenia research and is typically accomplished through the use of structured interviews and observation procedures. It would go beyond the scope of this chapter to describe these interviews in detail but it can be said that they are structured or semi-structured procedures, administered by trained clinicians, that are designed to determine whether stated diagnostic criteria are met. With regard to schizophrenia, the criteria generally utilised are those contained in the Diagnostic and Statistical Manual of the American Psychiatric Association (DSM-IV; APA, 1994) or the research diagnostic criteria proposed by Feighner and colleagues (Feighner et al, 1972). In state-of-the-art schizophrenia research interviewers must have achieved documented reliability with other experienced interviewers and cases are reviewed by independent experts, generally by observing videotapes. Unless otherwise indicated selected cases should meet criteria only for schizophrenia and not for other psychiatric disorders.

It has also proved difficult to obtain double dissociations in schizophrenia research or to find tests with both sensitivity and specificity. Most typically, patients with schizophrenia demonstrate generalised inefficiencies in performance that lie at impairment levels between individuals with diffuse structural brain damage and normal controls. At one point it seemed that, regardless of the task given, patients with schizophrenia always did worse than normal controls. This phenomenon has become known as the "general deficit syndrome", a term devised by Chapman & Chapman (1973). Aside from the general deficit syndrome, but related to it, was the tendency of patients with schizophrenia to develop flat cognitive profiles suggesting generalised impairment (Chelune et al, 1979). Such profiles lack specificity and are seen in patients with diffuse brain dysfunction attributable to numerous pathological conditions. Thus, if schizophrenia is a brain disease, based on these currently available tests it is not associated with a particular neuropsychological profile of the types seen in conjunction with numerous other brain diseases.

Chapman & Chapman (1978) developed the method of matched tasks as a solution to the general deficit syndrome problem. Briefly, if a patient is given two tasks, matched for difficulty level in normals, one can then dissociate a specific deficit (only one of the tasks is performed poorly) from a general deficit (both tasks are performed poorly). In a later refinement, Chapman & Chapman (1989) indicated that tasks should be matched along the entire distribution of scores and not only at the mean. The matched task method has helped in identifying specific deficits in patients with schizophrenia but has not been widely employed in neuropsychological research.

Another methodological suggestion to deal with the general deficit syndrome is attributable to Sutton (1973) who suggested finding tasks that discriminate between patients with schizophrenia and normal controls but on which the patients with schizophrenia perform better than the controls. Superior performance cannot be viewed as a deficit but nevertheless may characterise schizophrenia in some instances. The problem here is that it has been difficult to find such tasks and so little success has been achieved with this method (see Maruff and Currie, chapter 6, this volume).

RELIABILITY IN NEUROPSYCHOLOGY

Unlike other areas in which psychometric methods are used relatively little attention has been paid in neuropsychology to the problem of reliability. Perhaps some of this neglect is related to practical problems having to do with the common methods of assessing reliability of tests. There is the split-half correlation or alternate forms method but many neuropsychological instruments are not itemised tests that readily lend themselves to this method. Test–retest study of the same sample is the other commonly used method but that is made difficult in neuropsychology because of the relative lack of clinical stability in target patient populations. The relatively small number of reliability studies completed with standard neuropsychological tests indicate that the tests are generally quite reliable. This is perhaps surprising given the nature of the subject populations studied (Goldstein & Watson, 1989). It is noted that test–retest reliability of many neuropsychological tests in normal individuals is quite poor because the tests are not really repeatable with normal individuals. There are "right answers" which are readily learned by normal individuals, essentially spoiling re-testing. A good example of this kind of test is the Wisconsin Card Sorting Test (Heaton, 1980). Once the point of the procedure is learned the test is not meaningfully repeatable by normal individuals who initially achieved a high performance level on the test. Recently, neuropsychologists have become increasingly aware of the "practice effects" that may occur with repeated evaluations (Chelune & Goldstein, 1991).

With regard to the study of reliability, especially when the test–retest method is used, an important distinction has been made between psychometric and clinical reliability. The reliability coefficient is really a stability coefficient, meaning that the rankings of the subjects do not change substantially across testings. Thus, actual scores may change substantially but, as long as the rankings remain stable, a high reliability coefficient will be obtained. Clinical reliability is the extent to which the assessment procedure accurately and consistently reflects the patient's condition. Some years ago, Reitan informally defined a neuropsychological test as a test that is sensitive to the condition of the brain. Thus, if the patient changes but the test does not, that would call into question the clinical reliability of the test. Since neuropsychologists are typically interested in change, either in the direction of recovery, or deterioration in the case of degenerative disorders, tests that are sensitive to such changes in either direction are particularly useful. Rather than using a stability coefficient, clinical reliability is generally assessed with sample comparison statistics. For example, a repeated measures analysis of variance may be used to assess changes in a longitudinal study.

NORMS AND DEMOGRAPHIC CONSIDERATIONS

Neuropsychological assessment shares many methodological procedures with psychological assessment and psychometrics in general. There is extensive utilisation of standardised tests and so those procedures pertinent to test development in general are pertinent to neuropsychology. Appropriate normative data must be collected, analysed and tabulated. The need for separate age, education, gender and socioethnic norms must be considered. One of the long-standing problems in the field has been that of collecting adequate normative data based upon a large random sample of the general population. In the past, most normative studies have utilised hospital patients or other restricted populations. Recently, a major contribution to the solution to this problem has been produced by Heaton and colleagues (1991) who published an extensive set of age, education and gender corrected norms for an expanded version of the Halstead–Reitan Battery (Reitan & Wolfson, 1993). Since the Halstead–Reitan battery is the most widely used of the standard comprehensive neuropsychological test batteries this contribution has major implications for neuropsychological practice and research.

While certain aspects of neuropsychological assessment began as an extension of the clinical neurological examination, neuropsychological function is not entirely dependent upon health status. It is affected by a number of non-clinical sociodemographic factors as well as by the integrity of the central nervous system. Most significantly, performance on neuropsychological tests may be influenced by age, educational level, socioeconomic status and, to some extent, gender (Heaton et al, 1991). The methodological significance of this situation cannot be overemphasised, because it is quite possible to attribute a neuropsychological test result to a neurological causation when in fact that result is entirely consistent with an individual's age, educational level, socioeconomic status, gender, or any combination thereof. Thus, the development of demographically-based norms would appear to be a crucial issue in neuropsychological assessment.

There is a somewhat controversial modification to these considerations with regard to correction for age. Neuropsychological tests are sensitive to age differences in normal individuals. Ostensibly, that is because the brain ages, with substantial neuronal depletion over the years, and that aging process has functional consequences. The procedure of "correcting" for a process that has an underlying structural basis may therefore be called into question. The question "Should we or shouldn't we use age-corrected scores in neuropsychology?" has been a substantial source of debate. Obviously, if the test in question is used for classification or selection, age norms would be needed or the test would be discriminatory. However, in clinical assessment, scores that are not age-corrected may provide a more accurate assessment of the actual condition of the brain.

A development in favour of correcting for age is the growing belief that the progressive dementias of the elderly, notably Alzheimer's disease, are actual diseases and not the end state of normal aging (Adams & Victor, 1989). Thus, dementia does not appear to be an inevitable outcome of aging and many individuals apparently will not acquire senile dementia regardless of how long they live. Thus, it is important to distinguish between dementia and normal aging in elderly individuals. Age-corrected scores are needed to accomplish that goal because there are many cognitive functions that deteriorate with normal aging. The elderly individual may produce abnormal test scores relative to the general adult population but the significance of those scores may be entirely benign and not indicative of anything other than the changes expected with normal aging. Therefore, the consensus now appears to be in favour of age-corrected scores. A remaining methodological problem, however, is that many cognitive and neuropsychological tests do not have sufficient breadth extensively to evaluate individuals across the entire adult age range. Therefore, the item base for establishing normal range scores tends to thin out in the manner of a "floor effect" as age increases.

MATCHING FOR EDUCATION[1]

The issue of matching for education in studies of schizophrenia is complicated and currently controversial. This issue is even more critical for neuropsychological studies of the schizophrenic disorders because of the significant correlations observed between neuropsychological measures and level of education (Finlayson et al, 1977; Heaton et al, 1986, 1991). As an illustration, we recently examined the relationship between educational level and performance on the Luria–Nebraska Relational Concepts Factor Scale (R2) (Golden et al, 1985) in 95 educationally-matched patients with schizophrenia, their brothers and in normal controls who were included in an earlier study (Condray et al, 1992). Level of education and number of errors on this scale were significantly correlated in these *educationally-matched* individuals ($r_{94} = -0.28$, $p < 0.01$). Thus, an association between educational level and neuropsychological performance was observed even when the educational variable was controlled. Educational level in itself is confounded by a number of factors. Among the most salient of the influences on educational success are motivation and psychiatric disturbance. A concern recently raised is that routinely matching for education may result in biases associated with additional processes, such as achievement level, that differ across patient and control groups (Resnick, 1992). For example, equivalent levels of education may be the result, at least in part, of high achievement in patients but low achievement in normal controls. Also important is the work of Dohrenwend & Dohrenwend (1969) showing that social selection (i.e. downward drift in social status) characterised the patients with schizophrenia in their sample. Thus, solutions to these difficulties will not be straightforward. As an example, use of the educational level and socioeconomic status of subjects' parents has been suggested but these pose their own difficulties due to the increased incidence of psychiatric disturbance in the family members of patients with schizophrenia (Goldberg et al, 1992; Resnick, 1992).

The chief problems in identifying a solution to the issue of educational matching include our lack of knowledge regarding how much of the variance associated with patients' educational level is due to the social selection effect documented by Dohrenwend and Dohrenwend (1969) and how much of the variance in the correlation between educational level and neuropsychological performance is due to any ameliorative or "rehabilitative" effects of the educational process in itself. Perhaps the most conservative strategy at the present time is to continue to match for education whenever the focus of an investigation concerns neuropsychological measures that are known to correlate highly with educational level in non-schizophrenic individuals. This control will reduce,

---

[1]Indebtedness is expressed to Dr Ruth Condray for her contribution to this section.

although not completely eliminate, the variability associated with the beneficial aspects of the educational process. Additionally, parents' educational level can be used to delineate sub-groups for more refined comparisons.

STANDARDISED AND FLEXIBLE BATTERIES

The battery approach is deeply embedded in neuropsychology and the use of single instruments for assessing brain dysfunction has been abandoned for some time. The rationale is basically that the complexity of brain function does not allow for assessment with a single test and that it is necessary to give a number of diverse tests to identify patterns of impaired and preserved abilities. There appears to be a reasonable consensus concerning what the major areas are and there is common usage of a basic core of tests. The term comprehensive neuropsychological assessment (Goldstein, 1990) is used when the battery contains tests of all of the major areas. The term specialised battery (Kane, 1991) is used when only one area is assessed. These major areas are typically described as abstraction and problem solving abilities, attention, memory, language, spatial abilities and perceptual and motor skills.

Beyond these points of consensus, there is a major division within the field regarding the actual conduct of assessment with one group advocating the use of comprehensive, standardised batteries and another group supporting the use of flexible batteries. A thorough exposition of this matter is contained in Kane (1991) and it will not be considered in detail here. Suffice to say that in a comprehensive, standardised battery all of the same tests are given to all patients utilising the same instructions and scoring procedures. Often, administration and scoring of these tests have been standardised to the point that these tasks can be accomplished by trained technicians. The Halstead–Reitan (Reitan & Wolfson, 1993) and Luria–Nebraska (Golden et al, 1985) are the most commonly used standardised, comprehensive batteries. Flexible batteries differ mainly in that not all tests are given to all patients. Test selection is made by the clinician on the basis of several considerations including the referral question, the presenting complaints, a review of the clinical history and an initial interview with the patient that may be supplemented by a small number of brief screening tests. The testing is typically done by the clinician, who may modify procedures for accommodation purposes (e.g. patient cannot comprehend written instructions) or to assess clinical characteristics of the patient that are not possible to evaluate with standard procedures.

We will forego any discussion of the polemics surrounding this controversy but simply point out some of the implications for methodological issues. The standardised batteries have the advantage of allowing for the collection of large databases for research purposes. All of the tests are given and scored in the same way, thereby making them amenable to large sample data analyses. In general, the extensive use of quantification, uniformity of procedure, opportunity to collect large quantities of data through the use of technicians and the possibility of providing objective interpretation of results without knowledge of the patient's clinical history, are the strong points of the standardised battery approach. The flexible approach allows for more detailing of specific disorders since extensive time and testing may be devoted to the patient's particular deficits. For example, the language function of an aphasic patient can be studied in substantially more detail with a flexible approach than would be possible for the standard batteries. Typically, advocates of the flexible approach conduct their research by recording usually non-quantitative observations of their patients and conceptualising them, as would be the case for Luria (1973), or by keeping their research studies essentially separate from their clinical assessments, as would be the case for Benton (1991). We would note that the standard and flexible battery paradigms are substantially different from each other, with clinicians and researchers in the field usually being clearly identifiable as to which model they employ. These differences have carried over to psychopathology. It is particularly interesting to note that in the section on neuropsychology in the *Handbook of Schizophrenia*, there are three chapters on the neuropsychology of schizophrenia by Benton (1991), Goldstein (1991) and Goldberg & Seidman (1991) that differ radically among themselves regarding basic paradigmatic issues.

EXPERIMENTAL PROCEDURES

There is an extensive experimental research literature in neuropsychology spanning work with brain damaged patients, normal individuals and animals. However, for our present purposes we will only elaborate briefly on work undertaken with patients. The experimental approach, as defined here, is different from studies in which standard test procedures are administered to patients and appropriate controls for test development or other psychometric purposes. Rather, we are referring to research which, while possibly based on observations made using standard tests, went on experimentally to investigate a number of alternative hypotheses. In pursuing this work, major interfaces have been developed between neuropsychology and other branches of behavioural science including linguistics and the experimental psychologies of memory, learning, perception, attention and cognition. It is clearly not our intent here to review this voluminous literature but wish to make the following methodological points. The experimental method provides the major knowledge base for theory and practice in neuropsychology. Typically, traditional and established experimental designs are used for hypothesis testing, generally using brain damaged patients as subjects. These subjects may be studied from the standpoint of the geographical localisation of their lesion (e.g. frontal lobe) or the underlying pathology (e.g. stroke). In this manner, neuropsychologists have learned a great deal about the specialised functions of different portions of the brain and about the characteristics of a number of neurobehavioural disorders.

With regard to application in assessment, caution is generally exercised with respect to the premature application of experimental procedures, that is, before appropriate standardisation has been accomplished. However, as indicated above, it is commonplace in neuropsychology for the experimental procedure of today to become the test of tomorrow after the procedure is adequately developed psychometrically. Many of the most commonly used neuropsychological tests were originally laboratory instruments. Thus, neuropsychology is an experimentally based discipline with perhaps an unusually rapid transition between laboratory findings and clinical application.

GENERAL METHODOLOGICAL ISSUES SPECIFIC TO NEUROPSYCHOLOGICAL INVESTIGATIONS OF SCHIZOPHRENIA

In this section, we will try to apply the considerations presented above to the neuropsychological investigation of schizophrenia. The investigation of a disease entity or disorder by a particular discipline suggests that the discipline has some substantive contribution to make to understanding its aetiology, pathogenesis, symptomatology, course, epidemiology, treatment, or management. However, when the cause of the disorder is unknown, as is the case for schizophrenia, there would appear to be some need to be tentative about the significance of the contribution of any particular discipline. The first discipline involved with schizophrenia was psychiatry, soon followed by psychoanalysis and clinical and abnormal psychology. For many years these two disciplines accounted for almost all of the scientific work in schizophrenia and were also responsible for leadership in patient care. More recently, however, there has emerged a proliferation of disciplines involved in schizophrenia research. An admittedly incomplete list would include neurochemistry, neuroradiology, neurophysiology, behavioural neurology, psychopharmacology, genetics, molecular biology and neuropsychology. Apparently, the growing consensus that schizophrenia is a biological disorder became associated with the gradual recruitment of the biological sciences and the neurosciences in particular.

The way in which neuropsychology fits into this development requires some historical explanation. Neuropsychologists were heavily involved in schizophrenia research long before the recent biological studies of the disorder. However, they did that work as psychiatrists, or clinical or cognitive psychologists, since the term "neuropsychology" had not yet been applied to their field. The major interests were in schizophrenic language and thought; major discoveries were made concerning such matters as the impairment of abstract thinking in schizophrenia (K. Goldstein, 1959), the development of idiosyncratic and fragmented language (Kasanin, 1946) and the disturbance of attention that appeared to characterise the disorder (Zubin, 1975). Another major interest was in the differences between patients with schizophrenia and those with structural brain damage (Goldstein, 1978). Much effort was made to develop tests and test profiles that had discriminative validity with regard to that differential diagnosis. It would probably be fair to say that the research regarding cognition and language has continued actively, while the differential diagnosis research has essentially been abandoned because of recent findings concerning brain abnormalities in patients with schizophrenia. Thus, neuropsychology's contribution to schizophrenia in recent years has been to relate ongoing work in thought and language to the evolving elucidation of the disorder from a biological standpoint and refinement of a neurobehavioural theory of the disorder.

REFERENCES

Acker, M.B. (1990) A review of the ecological validity of neuropsychological tests. In: *The Neuropsychology of Everyday Life: Assessment and Basic Competencies* (Eds D.E. Tupper, K.D. Cicerone), pp. 19–55, Kluwer, Boston.

Adams, R.D., Victor, M. (1989) *Principles of Neurology* (2nd edn), McGraw-Hill, New York.

American Psychiatric Association (1994) *Diagnostic and Statistical Manual of Mental Disorders* (4th edn), American Psychiatric Association, Washington, DC.

Benton, A.L. (1991) Basic approaches to neuropsychological assessment. In: *Handbook of Schizophrenia. Vol. 5: Neuropsychology, Psychophysiology and Information Processing* (Eds S.R. Steinhauer, J.H. Gruzelier, J. Zubin), pp. 505–523, Elsevier, London.

Carlesimo, G.A., Oscar-Berman, M. (1992) Memory deficits in Alzheimer's patients: A comprehensive review. *Neuropsychology Review*, **3**, 119–169.

Chapman, L.J., Chapman, J.P. (1973) *Disordered Thought in Schizophrenia*, Appleton-Century-Crofts, New York.

Chapman, L.J., Chapman, J.P. (1978) The measurement of differential deficit. *Journal of Psychiatric Research*, **14**, 303–311.

Chapman, L.J., Chapman, J.P. (1989) Strategies for resolving the heterogeneity of schizophrenics and their relatives using cognitive measures. *Journal of Abnormal Psychology*, **98**, 357–366.

Chelune, G.J., Goldstein, G. (1991, August) Symposium: *Interpreting Test–Retest Changes in Neuropsychological Practice.* Presented at the annual meeting of the American Psychological Association, San Francisco.

Chelune, G.J., Heaton, R.K., Lehman, R.A., Robinson, S. (1979) Level versus pattern of neuropsychological performance among schizophrenic and diffusely brain damaged patients. *Journal of Consulting and Clinical Psychology*, **47**, 155–163.

Condray, R., Steinhauer, S., Goldstein, G. (1992) Language comprehension in schizophrenics and their brothers. *Biological Psychiatry*, **32**, 790–802.

Dohrenwend, B.P., Dohrenwend, B.S. (1969) *Social Status and Psychological Disorder: A Causal Inquiry*, Wiley–Interscience, New York.

Feighner, J.P., Robins, E., Guze, S.B., Woodruff, R.A., Winokur, G., Munoz, R. (1972) Diagnostic criteria for use in psychiatric research. *Archives of General Psychiatry*, **26**, 57–63.

Finlayson, M.A.J., Johnson, K.A., Reitan, R.M. (1977) Relationship of level of education to neuropsychological measures in brain-damaged and non-brain-damaged adults. *Journal of Consulting and Clinical Psychology*, **45**, 536–542.

Goldberg, E., Seidman, L.J. (1991) Higher cortical functions in normals and in schizophrenic: A selective review. In: *Handbook of Schizophrenia. Vol. 5: Neuropsychology, Psychophysiology and Information Processing* (Eds S.R. Steinhauer, J.H. Gruzelier, J. Zubin), pp. 553–597, Elsevier, London.

Goldberg, T.E., Torrey, E.F., Weinberger, D.R. (1992) Matching for education in studies of schizophrenia. *Archives of General Psychiatry*, **49**, 246.

Golden, C.J., Purisch, A.D., Hammeke, T.A. (1985) *Luria–Nebraska Neuropsychological Battery: Manual*, Western Psychological Services, Los Angeles.

Goldstein, G. (1978) Cognitive and perceptual differences between schizophrenics and organics. *Schizophrenia Bulletin*, **4**, 160–185.

Goldstein, G. (1990) Comprehensive neuropsychological assessment batteries. In: *Handbook of Psychological Assessment* (2nd edn) (Eds G. Goldstein, M. Hersen), pp. 197–227, Pergamon Press, New York.

Goldstein, G. (1991) Comprehensive neuropsychological test batteries and research in schizophrenia. In: *Handbook of Schizophrenia. Vol. 5: Neuropsychology, Psychophysiology and Infor-*

mation Processing (Eds S.R. Steinhauer, J.H. Gruzelier, J. Zubin), pp. 525–551, Elsevier, London.

Goldstein, G., Shelly, C.H. (1973) Univariate vs. multivariate analysis in neuropsychological test assessment of lateralized brain damage. *Cortex*, **9**, 204–216.

Goldstein, G., Watson, J.R. (1989) Test–retest reliability of the Halstead–Reitan battery and the WAIS in a neuropsychiatric population. *Clinical Neuropsychologist*, **3**, 265–273.

Goldstein K. (1959) Concerning the concreteness in schizophrenia. *Journal of Abnormal and Social Psychology*, **59**, 146.

Halstead, W.C. (1947) *Brain and Intelligence*, University of Chicago Press, Chicago.

Heaton, R.K. (1980) *A Manual for the Wisconsin Card Sorting Test*, Psychological Assessment Resources, Odessa, FL.

Heaton, R.K., Grant, I., Matthews, C.G. (1986) Differences in neuropsychological test performance associated with age, education, and gender. In: *Neuropsychological Assessment of Neuropsychiatric Disorders* (Eds I. Grant, K. Adams), pp. 100–120, Oxford University Press, New York.

Heaton, R.K., Grant, I., Matthews, C.G. (1991) *Comprehensive Norms for An Expanded Halstead-Reitan Battery*, Psychological Assessment Resources, Odessa, FL.

Kane, R.L. (1991) Standardised and flexible batteries in neuropsychology: An assessment update. *Neuropsychology Review*, **2**, 281–339.

Kasanin, J.S. (Ed.) (1946) *Language and Thought in Schizophrenia*, University of California Press, Berkeley.

Kazniak, A.W., Fox, J., Gandell, D.L., Garron, D.C., Huckman, M.S., Ramsey, R.G. (1978) Predictors of mortality in presenile and senile dementia. *Annals of Neurology*, **3**, 246–252.

Luria, A.R. (1973) *The Working Brain*, Basic Books, New York.

Reitan, R.M., Wolfson, D. (1993) *The Halstead–Reitan Neuropsychological Battery: Theory and Clinical Interpretation* (2nd edn), Neuropsychology Press, Tucson.

Resnick, S.M. (1992) Matching for education in studies of schizophrenia. *Archives of General Psychiatry*, **49**, 246.

Rourke, B.P. (Ed.) (1985) *Neuropsychology of Learning Disabilities: Essentials of Subtype Analysis*, Guilford, New York.

Rourke, B.P. (Ed.) (1991) *Neuropsychological Validation of Learning Disability Subtypes*, Guilford, New York.

Spreen, O. (1988) *Learning Disabled Children Growing Up: A Follow-up into Adulthood*, Oxford University Press, London.

Suddath, R.L., Christison, G.W., Torrey, E.F., Casanova, M.F., Weinberger, D.R. (1990) Anatomical abnormalities in the brains of monozygotic twins discordant for schizophrenia. *New England Journal of Medicine*, **322**, 789-794.

Sutton, S. (1973) Fact and artifact in the psychology of schizophrenia. In: *Psychopathology: Contributions from the Biological, Behavioural and Social Sciences* (Eds M. Hammer, K. Salzinger, S. Sutton), pp. 197–213, Wiley, New York.

Teuber, H.L. (1959) Some alterations in behaviour after cerebral lesions in man. In: *Evolution of Nervous Control from Primitive Organisms to Man* (Ed. A.D. Bass), pp. 157–194, American Association for the Advancement of Science, Washington, DC.

Zubin, J. (1975) Problem of attention in schizophrenia. In: *Experimental Approaches to Psychopathology* (Eds M.L. Kietzman, S. Sutton, J. Zubin), pp. 139–166, Academic Press, New York.

Part B
SPECIFIC DEFICITS OF COGNITIVE FUNCTION IN SCHIZOPHRENIA

4

Intellectual Functioning in Schizophrenia: Natural History

FIONA BARBER, CHRISTOS PANTELIS, SUSAN BODGER
and HAZEL E. NELSON

INTRODUCTION

The subject of general intellectual impairment in schizophrenia has long been a focus of interest for neuropsychological research. While it has been established that patients with schizophrenia display greater cognitive impairment than healthy matched controls, a number of questions have been raised with respect to the characteristics of these deficits and their relevance to the aetiology and course of the illness. Specifically, research has been concerned with establishing the extent of cognitive impairment, identifying patterns of performance specific to schizophrenic populations and exploring how intellectual functioning changes across the course of the disease. With respect to these issues research has sought to discover whether deficits are progressive or static, occur before or after the onset of symptoms and if the patterns of impairment found are unique to the disorder.

Attempts to resolve these research issues have been complicated by the presence of a number of confounding variables such as medication, ageing and institutionalisation, all of which may contribute to lowered intellectual functioning. In addition, the heterogeneity of symptoms associated with the term schizophrenia may each be associated with different patterns of cognitive impairment (Liddle, chapter 15). It is not surprising, therefore, that such questions remain largely unanswered and that many studies have yielded inconclusive or contradictory results.

In this chapter we review the literature pertaining to studies of intellectual functioning in schizophrenia with reference to the specific research questions outlined above. In addition, methodological issues in the assessment of intelligence are discussed with specific reference to patients with schizophrenia.

Schizophrenia: A Neuropsychological Perspective. Edited by C. Pantelis, H.E. Nelson and T.R.E. Barnes
© 1996 John Wiley & Sons Ltd

THE ASSESSMENT OF INTELLIGENCE

Throughout the course of neuropsychological research into schizophrenia there has been overwhelming evidence that patients suffering from the disease display deficits on IQ measures. While these results have been robust and consistent, their veracity is based on the premise that the tests used are valid and reliable indices and that the IQ scores obtained accurately reflect the individual's level of global intellectual functioning.

The concept of "intelligence" encompasses a wide range of intellectual functions and abilities which are imperfectly correlated with one another, so any attempt to quantify "intelligence" in a single IQ figure is bound to involve compromise and will depend on the test items used; this is why different intelligence tests give similar but not identical test results in any one individual. Most, but not all, tests of general intelligence are a composite of different aspects of intelligence and herein lies a central problem for their use as a measure of intelligence in schizophrenia. If there are general and/or specific intellectual changes in schizophrenia then the ability of a particular intelligence test to detect these changes, and the estimated sizes of these changes, will depend on what aspects of intelligence are included in the test. Added to this is the problem that different aspects of intelligence can be differentially affected by factors such as poor motivation and concentration; these factors tend to affect intelligence test scores in a similar way to generalised intellectual decline and produce a similar pattern of results.

Another key methodological issue for research comparing different intellectual abilities and deterioration in schizophrenia is that whilst some test results are age-scaled, that is allowance is made for the deteriorating effects of ageing (e.g. the Wechsler Intelligence Scales), others are not (e.g. more specific tests such as the Card Sorting Test). Comparison of age-scaled and non age-scaled tests may give misleading results, particularly in longitudinal studies and studies including different age groups, because the latter type of test will show greater deterioration than the former because of the age differences. Some of the methodological problems in assessing cognitive functioning in patients with schizophrenia and practical ways to address them are addressed in the preceding chapter by Goldstein (chapter 3).

THE EXTENT OF GENERAL INTELLECTUAL DECLINE IN SCHIZOPHRENIA

COMPARISON WITH NORMAL POPULATIONS, MATCHED CONTROLS AND OTHER PSYCHIATRIC PATIENTS

As noted by Aylward et al (1984), the majority of studies examining intellectual functioning in schizophrenia have been directed towards identifying patterns of cognitive performance rather than the exploration of global IQ deficits. Despite this lack of interest, a review of the existing literature suggests that patients with schizophrenia display significant impairment on tasks of global intellectual functioning when compared to normal controls matched for a number of demographic variables (Pollack et al, 1970; Lehman et al, 1979).

The principal sources of information relating to this issue are the earliest studies of schizophrenia undertaken before the development of sophisticated cognitive theories and tests. Prior to 1944, the most commonly used scale was the Stanford–Binet which was developed for children. While many early investigators reported low scores for patients with schizophrenia (Roe & Shakow, 1942) on this scale, very few were able to make effective comparisons to normal subjects as the test is not standardised for adults. Despite these limitations, Hunt & Cofer (1944) reviewed the best-controlled studies and found an average intellectual deficit of 20 months for patients with schizophrenia.

Since the introduction of the Wechsler Bellevue Scale (1944), the focus of cognitive research has shifted towards analysis of patterns of impairment as measured by subtests within the overall scale. The few studies investigating global IQ deficits in schizophrenia have consistently reported performance deficits in patients with schizophrenia (Payne, 1960). More recent studies in this area using normal controls matched for socio-economic status (SES) and age have supported the conclusion that patients with schizophrenia display greater performance than verbal deficits on measures of overall intellectual functioning.

There have been relatively few studies investigating the extent of global intellectual impairment in schizophrenia as compared to patients with other psychiatric diagnoses. In a review of the existing literature Payne (1960) concluded that adult patients with schizophrenia show greater IQ deficits than patients with neurotic disorders or alcoholics and that patients suffering from personality disorders or other psychotic disorders display similar IQ deficits to those of patients with schizophrenia. Similar results were reported by Cullari (1985) in a study of patients with schizophrenic disorders, affective disorders and "other" non-psychotic psychiatric disorders. The patients with schizophrenic disorders had significantly lower full-scale IQ scores than the affective group but not the "other" group. In addition, only the patients with schizophrenia revealed significant differences between scores on the verbal and performance sections of the test.

A more recent study by Goldberg et al (1993a) compared patients with schizophrenia to those with unipolar depression and bipolar disorder. Patients with schizophrenia displayed significantly lower full-scale IQ scores than either of the other groups, as measured by the Wechsler Adult Intelligence Scale—Revised (WAIS-R; Wechsler, 1981).

While these findings have been relatively robust, they are of limited relevance to researchers unless reviewed in the context of more detailed research looking at specific patterns of cognitive impairment at different stages in the disease process. Thus, the bulk of research in this area has moved to focus on the aetiological and prognostic implications of intelligence in schizophrenia by investigating IQ at different stages of the disease. Researchers have sought to establish whether there are premorbid deficits in intellectual level as well as to investigate intellectual deterioration over the course of the disease.

THE COURSE OF INTELLECTUAL IMPAIRMENT

PREMORBID INTELLECTUAL IMPAIRMENT IN SCHIZOPHRENIA

In order to examine the role of intellectual impairments in schizophrenia it is necessary to investigate whether deficits are evident prior to the onset of symptoms or if they emerge simultaneously with the acute phase of the illness. There is growing evidence that a significant number of adult patients with schizophrenia exhibited cognitive deficits as children (Offord, 1974). Studies in this area have used a variety of control groups including peers matched for age, sex and SES as well as non-schizophrenic siblings.

In a series of retrospective studies Offord & Cross (1971; Offord, 1974) examined the school performance of adult patients with schizophrenia by comparison with both their siblings and age-matched peers. The authors reported that pre-schizophrenic children were significantly more likely than their siblings to have repeated a grade in elementary school (that is, failed to progress to the next grade due to scholastic failure) and to score lower on childhood IQ tests than both siblings and peers. A number of other interesting issues arose from their analysis: within the group of pre-schizophrenic children, those with lower IQs show an earlier onset of the disease and remain institutionalised significantly longer. This result was supported by Pollack et al (1968) who found that low IQ score at hospitalisation was related to poor adjustment after discharge. In addition, within-group analysis revealed that the school performance of pre-schizophrenic children is consistently poorer than their siblings only when the subject is male and from a low IQ sibship (that is, when both children have an IQ below 80 points). The authors concluded that, within a family which is predisposed to schizophrenia, the child with the lowest IQ is the most vulnerable to the disease. Thus, it is proposed that high IQ acts as a protective factor, preventing predisposed individuals from becoming overtly schizophrenic. In contrast, low IQ gives little protection and the child with a low IQ will break down earlier and/or more often than a child with a high IQ score.

In support of these findings, Grimes & Walker (1994) examined the relationship between pre-schizophrenic subjects' emotional expressions (from home movies), educational level and age of illness onset. The authors found a significant correlation between educational level and age of illness onset.

Goodman (1987) examined a sample of young children (0–5 years) whose mothers were suffering from either schizophrenia or a depressive illness. Children were tested on three occasions at 1-year intervals using the Bayley scales, the McCarthy scales and the Mental Development Index. The children whose mothers suffered from schizophrenia scored significantly lower on IQ measures at first testing (< 1 year) and at subsequent testing they were "over-represented in the lowest scoring group". In addition, mothers with lower IQ scores tended to have children with low IQ scores.

Overall, results from studies of pre-schizophrenic and high-risk children would suggest that cognitive deficits are evident prior to the onset of psychotic symptoms. However, a number of these studies have noted that the deficits found were not specific to pre-schizophrenic offspring; children with behavioural disturbance also displayed lower IQ scores than their peers. In addition, there is a consistent sex difference with pre-schizophrenic males scoring less well than their female counterparts.

LONGITUDINAL STUDIES

In order to evaluate the significance of premorbid IQ deficits with respect to the course and onset of schizophrenia many authors have undertaken longitudinal studies of children at high risk of developing schizophrenia, that is, children who have one or both of their parents diagnosed with schizophrenia. The majority of this research has been concerned with identifying specific areas of deficit, such as attention or memory, in an attempt to find characteristic patterns of impairment which predict disease onset and course. Overall IQ level has also been recorded in most of these studies.

Interest in neurodevelopmental aspects of schizophrenia has only recently become a focus of research and many of the subjects involved in prospective studies have not yet entered the major risk period for schizophrenia. The New York High Risk Project (Erlenmeyer-Kimling and Cornblatt, 1987) is a longitudinal, prospective study comparing high-risk children with offspring of parents with other psychiatric diagnoses and children whose parents had no mental disorder. Testing commenced in 1971 when the children were between 7 and 12 years old and has continued at 2- to 3-year intervals. Assessment on the Wechsler IQ scale (WISC) was conducted at entry to the study and approximately 6 years later. Erlenmeyer-Kimling and Cornblatt (1987) list high IQ score as a possible protective factor for children at high risk of schizophrenia. Results from the study have shown that the first five high-risk children to be hospitalised had a mean IQ of 11 points below the mean for the group as a whole. Thus, the authors suggest that low IQ may be related to early onset of psychiatric illness.

The results of a British Population Survey have also provided information relating to general intellectual functioning in childhood and later onset of schizophrenia. Jones et al (1994) reported the results of educational tests taken at ages 8, 11 and 15 years. Tests included reading ability, vocabulary, arithmetic, verbal reasoning and non-verbal skills. In all test categories, children who went on to develop schizophrenia in adulthood performed more poorly than controls. The effect became more robust with increasing age. The association between test scores and schizophrenia showed a linear trend predicting a higher frequency of the disease in those children with educational difficulties.

The most advanced longitudinal study to date is the Israeli High Risk Project which has produced data at 25 year follow-up (Mirsky et al, 1995). While full IQ tests were not performed in this study, other neuropsychological measures were employed which included subtests from the WAIS. The authors reported that children who went on to develop schizophrenia showed a significantly lower level of arithmetic proficiency and overall cognitive functioning than controls. At age 26, the high-risk group scored worse than controls on all 6 WAIS subtests used. The most striking finding was that of a consistent attentional deficit, identified in children at age 11, which was specific to high-risk subjects (for review see Wolf and Cornblatt, chapter 9).

In essence, studies of pre-schizophrenic and high-risk children have provided some evidence that IQ deficits exist prior to the onset of overt symptoms. In order to evaluate the significance of this finding it is necessary to undertake longitudinal studies which assess the importance of premorbid IQ deficits with respect to disease onset and course. While results from these studies are interesting it is unlikely that overall IQ scores will ever be used as a predictor of disease vulnerability. In isolation, an overall IQ deficit may be indicative of a number of disorders and is found in children at risk of other psychiatric illnesses as well as those with behavioural disturbance. At best, low childhood IQ may become one of a number of predictive factors to be considered when assessing susceptibility to schizophrenia. Thus, more recent research has focused on the identification of patterns of cognitive impairment, for example in attention or memory, that are specific to pre-schizophrenic subjects. These results are discussed in detail by Wolf and Cornblatt (chapter 9).

With respect to the neurodevelopmental hypothesis of schizophrenia, it has become evident that behavioural dysfunction and cognitive impairments precede the onset of overt symptomatology by a number of years. Walker and colleagues (Walker, 1994; Walker et al, 1994) for example, found that neuromotor deficits occur in pre-schizophrenic children as early as 2 years of age. In addition, specific deficits in attention have been found to occur in high-risk children who later develop the disease (Erlenmeyer-Kimling and Cornblatt, 1987). Walker (1994) cites these findings as evidence that schizophrenia originates in a congenital central nervous system (CNS) impairment which is expressed behaviourally in different ways as the CNS matures. Thus, a neurodevelopmental process underlies the different expressions of the disorder at different life stages. In this way, the onset of psychotic symptoms in early adulthood is one point in the expression of the developmentally-mediated neuropathology in the same way that neuromotor disturbances at age 2 years are a prior manifestation of the same neuropathological process.

INTELLECTUAL FUNCTIONING ACROSS THE COURSE OF THE DISEASE

The perception of schizophrenia as a degenerative disorder has been evident from the initial descriptions by Kraepelin of a dementia praecox (Kraepelin, 1913). Evidence to support this opinion has been sought from studies of intellectual functioning with the expectation that patients with chronic symptoms of the disease will show a progressive deterioration in IQ across the lifespan. Such a pattern has not been consistently identified and alternative theories have been proffered; for example, some recent descriptions of the disease observe that deficits remain relatively stable, analogous to a "static encephalopathy" (Goldberg et al, 1993b). Work in this area is, as yet, inconclusive and a number of different research paradigms have been employed to establish if and when intellectual deterioration is occurring.

Studies examining intellectual functioning across the course of schizophrenia have sought not only to establish whether there is a significant decline in IQ scores following onset of overt symptomatology but also whether deterioration is a continuing process or if a stable deficit state is reached. In addition, investigators have attempted to determine whether any apparent loss in functioning is regained as psychotic symptoms subside.

PREMORBID–POSTMORBID INTELLECTUAL CHANGES

WITHIN-PATIENT COMPARISONS

A useful strategy in assessing the degree of intellectual deterioration after the onset of illness has been to compare current IQ level with estimates of premorbid IQ. Nelson and colleagues (1990) identified intellectual deficits in a group of 62 patients with DSM-III-R (APA, 1987) schizophrenia who had been chronically hospitalised. Using the National Adult Reading Test (NART; Nelson, 1982) and the Schonell Graded Word Reading Test (Schonell, 1942) estimates of premorbid IQ were compared with current IQ as measured by the Wechsler Adult Intelligence Scale-Revised (WAIS-R; Wechsler, 1981). These patients were found to have a significant drop of about 13 IQ points from their premorbid estimates. In another recent study of a chronically hospitalised group of patients, most with a diagnosis of schizophrenia, Dunkley & Rogers (1994) used similar measures to estimate current and premorbid IQ. They found that 67% of patients completing these assessments showed a significant deterioration from estimated premorbid IQ, while a total of 65 patients were noted to have cognitive deterioration when other measures were also used to provide a cognitive impairment score. These studies suggest that those patients with chronic schizophrenia suffer a decline in general intellectual functioning from premorbid levels.

There is also evidence to suggest that patients with schizophrenia suffer a greater decline in intellectual functioning than other psychiatric groups. Goldberg et al (1993, as cited earlier) used the Wide Range Achievement Test-Revised (WRAT-R) reading test as a measure of premorbid IQ to assess cognitive functioning in patients suffering from schizophrenia, unipolar depression and bipolar disorder. The results showed that all groups had equivalent scores on the reading test indicating that premorbid intelligence was similar for all three groups. Only the patients with schizophrenia showed a deterioration from premorbid levels.

While the use of within-patient comparisons may be a convenient means of assessing deterioration in functioning it is important to note that the use of the NART and other verbal tests have not been fully validated in patients with schizophrenia. The justification for the use of the NART as an estimate of premorbid functioning is that verbal abilities are better preserved in dementia than are other intellectual functions. It has been disputed that this preservation is apparent in patients with schizophrenia and, thus, verbally based tests may not provide an accurate assessment of premorbid IQ in this population. However, if reading abilities are affected by the pathological process underlying schizophrenic illness then the use of the NART will lead to an underestimation of premorbid IQ and a consequently more conservative estimation of the extent of deterioration. In essence, studies reporting deterioration in IQ based on reading ability tasks may be underestimating the level of deterioration but will not be overestimating it. As such, these studies provide stronger evidence for postmorbid deterioration in IQ levels.

FOLLOW-UP STUDIES FROM PREMORBID STATE

A more reliable source of information regarding postmorbid decline in IQ is that derived from longitudinal follow-up studies. One of the earliest studies which compared premorbid and post-onset scores was that of Rappaport & Webb (1950), who used a group of 10 subjects who had been tested during high school prior to any hospital admissions. In contrast to most studies of patients with schizophrenia, the majority of those tested were female (90%). Those subjects who had been admitted to hospital with a diagnosis of schizophrenia were reassessed using the same battery of tests as those used in school as well as subtests of the Wechsler Bellevue scale. They found that in nine cases there had been a significant decline in IQ with the mean premorbid IQ being 97.6, while the mean present IQ was 63.9. The mean period of time that these patients had been in hospital was 22.3 months. The authors attributed the deterioration to an "operational loss" related more to attitudinal factors than an essential organic loss.

A commonly used source of information for premorbid IQ data has been the army, which routinely assesses all new recruits on entry to the forces. Lubin et al (1962) used the Army Classification Battery to assess army recruits who had later been hospitalised for schizophrenia and compared the results with assessments taken at the time of recruitment. Patients showed a drop of one-sixth to one-third of a standard deviation in their scores on four of the subtests administered, namely, Reading and Vocabulary, Army Clerical Speed, Arithmetic Reasoning Test and Mechanical Aptitudes Test. While these results are consistent with those of Rappaport and Webb the levels of deterioration were significantly greater in the earlier study. Lubin and colleagues attributed this discrepancy to the different lengths of hospitalisation between the two groups. Patients tested by Rappaport and Webb had been hospitalised for periods of up to 81 months, whereas all of the patients in Lubin et al's study were tested within 3 months of admission. It was suggested that patients with chronic schizophrenia with long hospitalisation showed more deterioration than acute, recently hospitalised patients. In addition, all patients tested by Lubin and colleagues were male while Rappaport and Webb's sample consisted almost entirely of women.

Further evidence of deterioration in cognitive ability following the onset of schizophrenia was reported in a study of conscripts to the Canadian Army, by Schwartzman & Douglas (1962). They retested 80 male veterans with the Canadian Revised Examination M, who had been given this test on recruitment in 1943. By 1952, 50 of these men had been hospitalised with a diagnosis of schizophrenia. At the time of testing, 30 of these patients with schizophrenia had been in hospital for a period of 6 months or more and the other 20 ("ex patients") had been discharged for over a year. The remaining 30 subjects served as normal controls. All subjects were well matched in terms of intelligence at the time of enlistment, age, educational level, occupational status and time interval between the two test administrations. The patients and ex patients were matched for total number of years hospitalised (mean 2.4 years). The control group scored significantly more on retesting from their original M scores (mean difference was 11.8 points, approximately equivalent to 6 IQ points) while both the patient and ex patient groups scored significantly less than on first testing (mean difference −15.2 and −5.1, respectively). Interestingly, when the patient groups were subdivided into chronic and acute groups significant differences were found between the extent of intellectual deterioration found. The chronic group lost an average of 10.5 points more than matched acute patients.

It is interesting to compare studies using premorbid IQ data from adulthood with those which assessed subjects in childhood. Albee et al (1963) extended their study of pre-schizophrenic children, cited earlier, who had been tested in second and sixth grades using the Stanford–Binet, Kuhlmann–Anderson and Cleveland Classification Test. As noted previously, the authors found that pre-schizophrenic children had lower IQs than their siblings and that these children showed a significant decline in IQ between first and second assessments. Subjects who had become schizophrenic were tested in adulthood using the Wechsler Bellevue scale. No significant differences were found between childhood and adult IQ scores and the authors hypothesised that intellectual deterioration associated with schizophrenia begins in childhood and is not initiated by the onset of symptoms.

Some inconsistencies in the above results would seem inevitable considering the widely differing methodologies used. Each of the studies used different assessment procedures and tested subjects at different ages and stages of the disease. In addition, the majority of the reported data was recorded 30–40 years ago when the neuropsychological study of schizophrenia was in its infancy. Since that time many sophisticated theories of cognitive functioning in schizophrenia have emerged and the diagnostic criteria used are more refined. In addition to concerns regarding diagnostic differences in subject selection, authors have questioned the comparability of results between studies which have used different testing procedures. The study by Albee and colleagues (1963) used different assessment batteries in adulthood to those used premorbidly. In addition, the tests they used were substantially different to those administered in the Army Batteries, specifically with regard to the number of speeded subtests. Albee et al proposed that these tests would be particularly susceptible to changes in motivation and attention, features that are integral to schizophrenic symptomatology. To counter these criticisms Schwartzman & Douglas (1962) controlled for the speed factor in their tests and found that although the patients with schizophrenia continued to manifest a deterioration from premorbid levels by comparison with controls, this decrement was reduced (see also Rogers, chapter 2).

The type of assessment used by researchers provides a vital clue to determining the extent and, possibly, the causes of post-onset intellectual deterioration. Controlling for the demands of speeded tasks has shown that large IQ decrements in patients may be accounted for by symptom factors such as decreased attention or avolition. Rappaport & Webb (1950) attempted to delineate the role of attitudinal factors in their study by using the Elgin Test Reaction Scale, an observational measure of motivation, self-confidence, effort and attention. They concluded that the significant intellectual decrement found in their sample was "closely related to attention, concentration, negativism, preoccupation and apathy". As such it is difficult to say with any certainty whether post-onset deterioration in intellectual functioning is a manifestation of organic brain changes or merely a functional deficit which is reversible following the remittance of overt symptomatology. The most effective way of resolving these issues is to look at studies which have examined changes in postmorbid intellectual functioning.

POST-ONSET INTELLECTUAL FUNCTIONING

Despite the evidence for deterioration in intellectual functioning following the onset of illness the assumption that schizophrenia inevitably involves progressive social and intellectual decline as well as worsening symptoms is true for only a proportion of patients. Even Kraepelin (1913), the originator of the term "dementia praecox", revised his initial description when 13% of his own patients showed complete recovery despite long-term hospitalisation. In terms of intellectual functioning, it is difficult to imagine that patients with schizophrenia who have shown marked post-onset deterioration in IQ are able to recover abilities and improve on test scores. This would seem particularly implausible given that deterioration in performance on certain tests is considered to be indicative of organic brain changes. The literature presented in this section offers two outcome possibilities: (1) that intellectual deterioration in patients with schizophrenia is mediated by symptom severity rather than length of illness, and (2) that patients reach a stable deficit state after which no further intellectual decline occurs. There is a large body of literature in this area which uses both cross-sectional and longitudinal designs. While the former has the potential to span all decades of life, the latter is generally understood to provide greater accuracy due to its implicit, within-subject design.

Evidence to suggest that intellectual functioning is mediated by symptom severity has come mainly from longitudinal studies. One of the most often cited, short-term, longitudinal studies reported is that by Payne (1960), who tested patients on admission to hospital and again 4–13 months later when the patients were still hospitalised. The average IQ fell by 7.6 points on the Wechsler scales. In a continuation of their Canadian Army study, cited earlier, Schwartzman et al (1962) conducted a second follow-up of 23 patients who had shown an intellectual decrement from premorbid scores. The authors tested these subjects in 1960, a total of 17 years after their original army entrance. The 10 patients who had remained in hospital for that time had suffered further intellectual decline which was equivalent to the loss they had sustained between baseline and the first assessment (that is, a total of 30 M score points or approximately 15 IQ points). The authors also noted that the range of impairments, as measured by individual subtests, increased across the time interval. Of the 13 patients who had been discharged from hospital, their assessed IQ level had improved between the second and third assessments and was not significantly different from their premorbid IQ level (that is, an improvement of between 5 and 15 M points). Thus, for those patients who had remained in hospital there had been a general decline over a 17-year period, but for those subjects who had displayed symptomatic remission functioning was restored to premorbid levels. This study would suggest that the initial loss in intellectual functioning suffered by patients with schizophrenia was not necessarily irreversible. In addition, the study raised questions concerning the possible effect of chronic hospitalisation and the effects of treatment on intellectual functioning.

More recent research has investigated the specific relationship between IQ and symptomatology. Addington et al (1991) reported significant associations between impairment on tests of general intellectual ability (e.g. WAIS) and negative symptoms. The authors also noted that improvement in positive symptoms was related to increased IQ scores while negative symptom improvements were unrelated to cognitive functioning.

Support for non-progression of intellectual decline has also been found in early, longitudinal studies. Smith (1964) assessed two groups of hospitalised patients with schizophrenia, a young group of 11 patients (mean age 34 years, mean length of hospitalisation 8 years) and an older group of 13 patients (mean age 53 years, mean length of hospitalisation 9 years). Patients were assessed using the Wechsler Bellevue scales at an 8.4 year interval. Each group showed some increase in full-scale IQ score with the younger group improving by a mean of 6 IQ points and the older group showing a lesser improvement of 2 points. This was taken as evidence against the concept of progressive deterioration in chronic schizophrenia although the authors warned that their sample was atypical (the older group were not diagnosed until after age 40 years) and their results should not be generalised across schizophrenia as a whole.

Even stronger evidence for the assertion of stability in intellectual functioning is provided by Hamlin (1969). He retested Smith's subjects after a further 6 years and found no evidence for deterioration of intellectual function. In support of Schwartzman et al (1962), Hamlin also found that in cases where the psychosis had improved so had the intellectual functioning. Hamlin stated that "the psychosis of schizophrenia would seem to be not a process that involved inevitable and continued deterioration, but rather a condition that waxes and wanes in severity". Further evidence to support an overall improvement in IQ scores over time was found by Klonoff et al (1970) in an 8-year follow-up study of World War II veterans who had been diagnosed as suffering from schizophrenia. Subjects were assessed using the WAIS as well as symptom rating scales and a neuropsychological test battery. Full-scale IQ scores improved significantly, by around 7 points, as did the psychiatric status of the group.

A more recent longitudinal study by the Scottish Schizophrenia Research Group (1988) has supported these findings. The group followed-up 49 patients after their first admission to hospital, 45% of whom had suffered no relapse and had no schizophrenic symptoms 12 months later. No evidence of intellectual decline was found on the matrices, block design and digit copying tests.

In a retrospective study, Buhrich et al (1988) examined patients with chronic schizophrenia either with or without temporal disorientation (that is, inaccurate estimation of their own age). In a previous study (Liddle & Crow, 1984) the matched groups had been given a series of cognitive tests and those with age disorientation were severely impaired on tasks of general orientation, knowledge, Raven's matrices, the digit symbol test and the mental test. In the current investigation, school attainment and past physical treatments were recorded for all subjects in order to determine whether temporally disorientated patients displayed learning difficulties prior to the onset of schizophrenia. The results showed that there were no differences between the groups based on their school records and that both groups had been treated with equivalent amounts of electroconvulsive therapy (ECT), insulin coma therapy and neuroleptic drugs. The authors concluded that premorbid intellectual dysfunction does not inevitably lead to gross cognitive deterioration following disease onset.

While these studies suggest that cognitive decline is non-progressive some studies have suggested that some patients may continue to deteriorate after illness onset. In the recent study by Dunkley & Rogers (1994), already cited above, these authors used serial measurements of IQ in the subgroup of patients where these measures were available. They found that the cognitive deterioration apparent in this chronic group of hospitalised patients occurred early after onset of illness with little evidence for cognitive decline after the first 5 years of illness in those patients completing the IQ measures. However, when the other patients were assessed using the Cognitive Impairment Scale, a smaller subgroup of patients demonstrated significant deterioration with increasing age and length of illness. The authors suggested the possibility of an interaction effect between the disease process and the decline due to ageing in a subgroup of patients.

Support for the notion of a subgroup of deteriorating patients was also found by Heinrichs & Awad (1993). The authors used four key neuropsychological tasks to identify subtypes of chronic schizophrenia on the basis of different patterns of cognitive functioning. Five clusters of patients were identified, one of which corresponded to a dementia-like multifocal disturbance. As no differences in SES or education were identified in these patients it was proposed that their global impairments were related to a deteriorative condition. The subtype consisted of 24% of a sample of chronic patients.

CROSS-SECTIONAL STUDIES

Cross-sectional research has also challenged the notion of progressive intellectual decline. Hyde et al (1994) conducted a study of five age-derived cohorts (18–29, 30–39, 40–49, 50–59 and 60–69 years of age) looking specifically at the evidence for dementia-like cognitive deterioration. Subjects were matched for age of onset and educational level. The authors found no differences across the groups on the Mini Mental State Examination (MMSE), the Dementia Rating Scale, List Learning and Semantic Fluency tasks. However, all scores were in the impaired range. It was concluded that no progressive decline in cognitive functioning occurs in chronic schizophrenia other than that which would be expected from normal ageing. Citing physiological evidence they suggest that schizophrenia should be classified as a "static encephalopathy" and not a progressive dementia. It must be noted, however, that the tests used were not intellectual assessment batteries but merely short-form screening tests which are not standardised against normative populations.

The study by Hyde and colleagues raises an important question regarding the effects of ageing on levels of cognitive functioning. In their study, performance on the Boston Naming test significantly deteriorated with increasing age. This was attributed entirely to the age of subjects and not to the duration of their illness. Heaton et al (1994) conducted a similar cross-sectional study using a more comprehensive neuropsychological test battery. They concluded that deficits are unrelated to age, age of onset and duration of illness and that they are essentially non-progressive in nature.

SUMMARY

The implications of the above findings are interesting with respect to the effects of the schizophrenic illness on global intellectual functioning. The discrepant findings of no change as opposed to variable improvement may be attributed to the different methodologies used by the research groups. Studies have employed either cross-sectional and retrospective longitudinal designs, which have advantages and disadvantages in terms of reliability and validity.

The two cross-sectional research paradigms have yielded results supporting the notion of a static encephalopathy; results provide no evidence of a dementia-like deterioration in intellectual functioning. The findings of these two studies also show that any decrement in performance is related to the effects of normal ageing and not to the duration of illness. However, this type of study presents a number of methodological difficulties principally because the same subjects cannot be used across each testing stage. While it is possible to overcome this problem with appropriate matching, this process is more error prone when subjects are taken across different age ranges. Potential criticisms of Hyde et al's study, in terms of the tests used have already been discussed. Another important factor which may affect the reliability of cross-sectional data is possible selection bias with regard to the older subjects. Subjects in this group are invariably chosen from a group of hospitalised, chronic patients while those individuals who suffer only one, or intermittent periods of psychosis are overlooked due to their higher functional capacity. In view of this bias, the "static encephalopathy" pronounced by authors such as Hyde and colleagues may be challenged. The fact that functioning across all cohorts was in the impaired range would suggest that a more appropriate conclusion is that low intellectual functioning is predictive of poor prognosis. Thus, it is not clear from the studies in their present form whether those patients who do not remain in hospital for extended periods show improvement in global IQ scores in accordance with symptom alleviation.

A similar difficulty is evident in longitudinal follow-up studies in that subjects may be "lost to follow-up" if they are too high functioning to remain in hospital for extended periods. While this criticism must be noted, it is evident that longitudinal designs present the most effective means of addressing the issue of intellectual deterioration in schizophrenia. Not only do the same patients complete all tests across each age range but the same tests may be given at each encounter. As such, longitudinal studies following children at high risk for developing schizophrenia present one of the most reliable means of assessment. The New York High Risk Project (Erlenmeyer-Kimling and Cornblatt, 1987; Wolf & Cornblatt, chapter 9) mentioned previously has not yet provided enough follow-up data to provide information about long-term deterioration. However, retrospective studies such as Schwartzman et al do have a longitudinal perspective and, at present, are the most reliable sources of information. The majority of these studies provide evidence to suggest that deficits are not necessarily stable but may fluctuate depending on the severity of the present symptoms. Thus, post-onset deterioration in scores on IQ tests may be secondary to symptom factors such as poor attention and low motivation, or it could be caused by the same pathophysiology that produces the symptoms. This proposal is supported by the finding that scores may be restored to their premorbid levels following symptom remission in some patients. It is important to note, however, that the studies also provide evidence that there is a subgroup of patients with schizophrenia who have consistently low cognitive functioning in conjunction with persistent psychotic symptoms.

An important factor which has been highlighted in these studies is that of institutionalisation and its possible effects on intellectual functioning over time. Schwartzman et al commented that discharge from hospital is not solely reliant on symptom remission, as one might hope, but is often influenced by the availability of alternative accommodation. As such, the authors proposed that the cognitive decline observed in patients who remain in hospital may not be related to the severity of their illness but to environmental factors. However, the authors note that decrements in IQ scores were related to the patient's status at the time of testing and not to the length of time spent in hospital.

Further to this work, there have been a number of more recent studies specifically investigating the effects of long-term hospitalisation on cognitive functioning. Johnstone et al (1981) compared a group of 120 patients who had been discharged 5–9 years earlier with a group of 510 inpatients with schizophrenia. It was found that the inpatients performed less well on the cognitive tests (Withers and Hinton tests) than their outpatient counterparts. However, the authors found evidence from school records that the inpatient group had poorer premorbid functioning and that, in both subject groups, scores on the cognitive tests were related to past academic records. The authors proposed that those patients who display cognitive impairment at younger ages would be less likely to be discharged. As such it is possible that pre-existing cognitive impairment has developed throughout the illness and led to long-term hospitalisation as opposed to hospitalisation being the primary causative factor.

In support of this work, Goldstein et al (1991) conducted an investigation of 245 patients using the Halstead–Reitan test battery. While they found evidence for an apparent decline in cognitive abilities associated with longer periods of hospitalisation, they concluded that this relationship was not significant when age and education were taken into account.

In summary, it would appear that many patients who have been hospitalised for long periods show cognitive deficits by comparison with patients who have spent longer in the community. However, some of these results may be accounted for by age differences between the groups and the fact that inpatients had pre-existing cognitive deficits which may have led to their continued hospitalisation.

Another important factor to consider in the context of cognitive decline is that of medication effects. A comprehensive review of this area is provided by King and Green (chapter 20, this volume). In general, findings would suggest that medication tends to improve performance on tests which are affected by symptoms "such as poor concentration, and motivation" (King, 1990). In addition, long-term medication may improve performance on tasks requiring "sustained attention and visuomotor problem solving skills" (Cassens et al 1990).

THE RELATIONSHIP OF OVERALL INTELLECTUAL ABILITY TO SPECIFIC COGNITIVE DEFICITS

While the study of global intellectual abilities in schizophrenia has been largely eclipsed by studies of specific cognitive functioning the former plays a vital role in determining the true nature of the specific deficits. In essence, researchers must establish whether a specific impairment found occurs over and above any general intellectual decline present. The standard approach to this question has been to administer large neuropsychological test batteries to patients in the hope that one specific function will be selectively impaired above and beyond a generalised deficit. This research paradigm has been subject to criticism on the basis that tests used are not psychometrically matched; for example, right hemisphere tests may have greater discriminatory power than left hemisphere tasks. In addition, variables such as age, medication, side-effects and symptomatology may also affect results differentially.

Many of these confounding factors are mentioned by Braff and colleagues (1991), in their study of chronic outpatients with schizophrenia. By comparison with healthy controls the patients with schizophrenia displayed deficits on a wide range of tests including conceptual reasoning, psychomotor speed and motor/sensory perceptual abilities. In contrast to many previous studies, performance on the Wisconsin Card Sorting Test (WCST) was relatively intact, providing little evidence for a specific frontal type deficit. The authors commented that medication, symptom differences and the alternative forms of the WCST may account for discrepant results between studies.

Saykin et al (1991) attempted to avoid the confounding affects of medication by testing unmedicated patients with schizophrenia on a battery of neuropsychological measures including many WAIS-R subtests, tests of learning and memory, attention and abstraction. Results showed that patients displayed a generalised impairment as compared to normal controls as well as specific deficits in learning and memory. These results have been challenged by Blanchard & Neale (1994), who question the statistical design of the study with relation to their use of standardised residualised scores. These authors cite Chapman and Chapman (1989), who state that this method should be interpreted with caution due to psychometric artefacts.

In contrast to Saykin et al's findings, Blanchard & Neale (1994) found no evidence for specific cognitive deficits. The study involved the administration of a comprehensive battery of tasks to 28 unmedicated patients and normal controls matched for age, education and handedness. The study analysed the results using four different methods. First, the reliability of the tests used was computed and the missing data examined. Second, a series of ANOVAs and a MANOVA were performed to measure the differences between patients with schizophrenia and controls on individual tests. Composite scores were then created which were thought to reflect global cognitive functions, for example, semantic memory, abstraction and motor ability. Finally, the clinical significance of the patients' impairments was evaluated by classifying each score obtained within either the impaired or non-impaired range for that test. The percentage of patients performing within the impaired range was calculated for each task. The patients with schizophrenia showed impairment on all the tests of both right and left hemisphere functioning regardless of the method of analysis used. The authors concluded that the results refuted claims of differential cognitive deficits in schizophrenia.

An alternative strategy to assess the significance of global deficits for specific abilities is to measure the correlations between full-scale IQ scores and performance on neuropsychological tests. Warner et al (1987) divided patients with schizophrenia into five groups on the basis of their IQ as measured by the WAIS or WAIS-R. Patients then completed the Halstead–Reitan Battery, the Wechsler Memory Scale (WMS) and the WRAT (Wide Range Achievement Test). The results showed that IQ was strongly correlated with scores on tasks of problem solving, memory measures, tactual imperceptions and academic achievement. Full-scale IQ scores were less related to motor functioning and sensory suppressions. From the results presented above it is possible to infer that tasks requiring problem solving or memory may be particularly affected by deficits in global intellectual functioning and that subjects with low FSIQ scores will perform more poorly on these tasks than those with high IQs. Thus, the discovery of specific deficits in these areas may merely be a function of a general intellectual disability and not represent an isolated impairment. As such, the above study emphasises the need for accurate matching of healthy controls and patients on the basis of IQ prior to undertaking neuropsychological tests.

An interesting study also addressing this issue is that of Smith (1964) cited earlier. In his longitudinal study, Smith found evidence for improvements in IQ scores over an 8-year period. The study also tested patients on the Weigl Sorting Test which is used to investigate set shifting ability in frontal lobe lesions. At first assessment, 10 of 48 subjects could not complete the necessary shift in sorting category. At 8-year follow-up only 16 patients were still able to complete the shift. The author concludes that global IQ measures are insensitive to deterioration in chronic patients and that more specific deficits are developing despite stable IQ scores.

It is evident that the literature in this area is plagued by statistical and psychometric difficulties. While it is unclear as to whether specific deficits exist over and above global intellectual deficits, the evidence would suggest that the use of large batteries of neuropsychological tests to achieve this end is an inadequate and error-prone procedure. Alternative procedures such as that used by Warner et al may be more useful in determining the precise effects that global intellectual impairments have on neuropsychological test scores.

COMPARISON BETWEEN PATIENTS WITH SCHIZOPHRENIA AND NEUROLOGICAL PATIENTS

In addition to comparisons with normal populations investigators have sought to establish whether patients with schizophrenia may be distinguished from those with organic brain damage on the basis of qualitative or quantitative differences in cognitive functioning. Research in this area has examined global intellectual impairments as well as patterns of performance on batteries of tests.

Studies using the Wechsler IQ scales have yielded inconsistent results with respect to this issue. Watson (1965) compared patients with schizophrenia to those with organic brain damage on the WAIS. The results showed that both groups were characterised by higher Verbal IQ scores than Performance IQ scores. This discrepancy is not found in healthy controls nor affective disorder groups (Cullari, 1985). In addition, Watson reported that scores on the digit span subtest were significantly higher for the group of patients with chronic schizophrenia than for the long-term patients with brain damage.

Similar findings were reported by DeWolfe et al (1971), who divided both groups of patients according to their age. Using the WAIS, the authors found that the patients with schizophrenia performed significantly better on the digit span subtest but more poorly on the comprehension test. In the group of older patients, the group with schizophrenia displayed significant deficits on the picture completion as compared to brain-damaged patients.

In contrast to these results, Chelune et al (1979) failed to find any significant differences between patients with schizophrenia and those with diffuse brain damage on the WAIS subtests. The results showed that the mean level of performance of patients with schizophrenia was significantly higher than that of brain-damaged patients. Pattern analysis of the subtest scores, however, revealed no significant differences between the two groups. Other authors have also failed to replicate DeWolfe et al and Watson's findings (Davis et al, 1972).

Investigations using alternative test batteries have yielded more useful results in terms of their power to discriminate between the two groups. Purisch et al (1978, as cited in Goldstein 1986) used the Luria–Nebraska Neuropsychological Test Battery (LNNB) to assess patients with chronic schizophrenia and those with brain injury. Patients with schizophrenia performed significantly better on all but four measures of the test. The authors concluded that chronic schizophrenia produced deficits on complex tasks, such as memory and intellectual processes, while simple tasks remained unaffected. In the case of brain-injured patients, however, the ability to do all tasks was impaired. In a replication of the Purisch study, Shelly and Goldstein (1983) produced similar results although the level of discrimination between the two groups was not as robust. The authors commented that this may have been due to different levels of impairment in the brain-damaged patients tested.

Results from the above studies provide a number of interesting conclusions. Patients with schizophrenia display many neuropsychological similarities with brain-damaged groups and show no specific pattern of WAIS subtest scores that can effectively discriminate them from an organic group. While the LNNB provides more evidence for distinctions between the two groups it is not yet clear whether the pattern of scores is specific to patients with schizophrenia or is of any diagnostic significance. Goldstein (1986) attributes the failure of neuropsychological tests to discriminate between schizophrenic and brain-damaged groups to the fact that there are two subtypes of schizophrenia, one of which is associated with a dementia-like organic illness. Thus, functional impairment displayed in neuropsychological tests may be associated with structural, organic damage or with attitudinal, attentional and motivational factors. As yet, neuropsychological tests cannot distinguish between these two groups because both groups perform poorly on all measures of general intellect. As a consequence, most groups of patients with schizophrenia are indistinguishable from brain-damaged patients on neuropsychological measures.

An important consideration when discussing these studies is that of appropriate matching of the brain-damaged and schizophrenia groups. In terms of levels of functioning, groups may be matched on premorbid IQ scores. This method reflects their optimum levels of functioning but is unrepresentative of the impairments existing at the time of testing. The alternative strategy would be to match groups on current global levels of functioning; however, it is unclear as to whether it is appropriate to accept these scores at face value when both groups may have suffered considerable decline in global intellectual functioning for potentially different reasons. Future studies need to take account of these issues if the nature of the neuropsychological deficits in schizophrenia are to be clarified.

SUMMARY AND CONCLUSIONS

The above review has provided an overview of studies pertaining to global intellectual impairments in patients with schizophrenia. That cognitive impairment exists in schizophrenia appears to be undisputed and the vast majority of studies have shown that patients display significantly lower scores on IQ tests than healthy control subjects. In terms of childhood markers of the disease, studies have shown that both high-risk and pre-schizophrenic children display lower educational achievement levels when compared to their siblings and peers. In addition, evidence has indicated that lower IQ scores in childhood are correlated with earlier onset of overt symptoms of the disease. While lower IQ scores are not specific to pre-schizophrenic children it has been considered that they may be one of a number of risk factors which, in combination, increase the likelihood of developing the disease early in life.

The existing literature presents an inconsistent picture of the course of intellectual impairment following disease onset. It would appear that patients show a marked deterioration in IQ scores following the onset of psychotic symptoms but that this condition remains stable or may improve following symptom remission. As such this may suggest that many of the tasks involved in standard IQ tasks are influenced by symptom variables such as poor motivation and inattention. Alternatively, it may suggest that the post-onset deterioration is caused by the same pathophysiology involved in producing the symptoms.

As is evident from the outset of this chapter, research pertaining to global IQ deficits is often out of date and suffers from a number of methodological problems in comparison with more recent studies. Often the heterogeneous nature of the disease is ignored and other issues such as medication effects and ECT treatments are not recorded. More importantly, the study of global intellectual deficits in schizophrenia has largely been replaced by more sophisticated investigations of isolated cognitive deficits which may be specific to the disease. Research in this area has produced significant advances in our understanding of the symptoms and brain areas associated with schizophrenia in a way that global IQ scores are unable to do (as is apparent from a number of the chapters in this volume).

Nevertheless, the assessment of global IQ is important, primarily because the confirmation of specific deficits, such as impairments of executive or memory function, must be considered in the context of any likely overall global impairment such that the specific deficit is confirmed to occur above and beyond any global deficit of function.

From the information recorded in this chapter it is evident that global deficits do exist in patients with schizophrenia and, as such, must be considered as one of the characteristics of the disease. While it is apparent that this overall deficit is not specific to schizophrenia, it is still important to discover the possible causes of such an impairment in this population and its implications in terms of the progress of cognitive deficits over time. The identification of global deficits early in the course of the illness or premorbidly may become useful predictors of poor outcome and continued hospitalisation.

REFERENCES

Addington, J., Addington, D., Maticka-Tyndale, E. (1991) Cognitive functioning and positive and negative symptoms in schizophrenia. *Schizophrenia Research*, **5**, 123–134.

Albee, G., Lane, E., Corcoran, C., Werneke, A. (1963) Childhood and intercurrent intellectual performance of adult schizophrenics. *Journal of Consulting Psychology*, **27**, 364–366.

American Psychiatric Association (1987) *DSM-III-R: Diagnostic Manual of Mental Disorders*, American Psychiatric Association, Washington, DC.

Aylward, E., Walker, E., Bettes, B. (1984) Intelligence in schizophrenia: meta-analysis of the research. *Schizophrenia Bulletin*, **10**, 430–459.

Blanchard, J.J., Neale, J.M. (1994) The neuropsychological signature of schizophrenia: Generalised or differential deficit? *American Journal of Psychiatry*, **151**, 40–49.

Braff, D.L., Heaton, R., Kuck, J., Cullum, M., Moranville, J., Grant, I., Zisook, S. (1991) The generalised pattern of neuropsychological deficits in outpatients with chronic schizophrenia with heterogeneous Wisconsin Card Sorting Test results. *Archives of General Psychiatry*, **48**, 891–898.

Buhrich, N., Crow, T.J., Johnstone, E.C., Owens, D.G. (1988) Age disorientation in chronic schizophrenia is not associated with pre-morbid intellectual impairment or past physical treatment. *British Journal of Psychiatry*, **152**, 466–469.

Cassens, G., Inglis, A.K., Appelbaum, P.S., Gutheil, T.G. (1990) Neuroleptics: Effects on neuropsychological function in chronic schizophrenic patients. *Schizophrenia Bulletin*, **16**, 477–499.

Chapman, L.J., Chapman, J.P. (1989) Strategies for resolving the heterogeneity of schizophrenics and their relatives using cognitive measures. *Journal of Abnormal Psychology*, **98**, 357–366.

Chelune, G., Heaton, R., Lehman, R., Robinson, A. (1979) Level versus pattern of neuropsychological performance amongst schizophrenic and diffusely brain damaged patients. *Journal of Consulting and Clinical Psychology*, **47**, 155–163.

Cullari, S. (1985) WAIS Verbal and Performance IQ for a Psychiatric Population. *Psychological Reports*, **57**, 1169–1170.

Davis, W., DeWolfe, A., Gustafson, R. (1972) Intellectual deficit in process and reactive schizophrenics and brain injury. *Journal of Consulting and Clinical Psychology*, **38**, 146.

DeWolfe, A., Barrell, R., Becker, B., Spaner, F. (1971) Intellectual deficit in chronic schizophrenia and brain damage. *Journal of Consulting and Clinical Psychology*, **36**, 197–204.

Dunkley, G., Rogers, D. (1994) The cognitive impairment of severe psychiatric illness: A clinical study. In: *The Neuropsychology of Schizophrenia* (Eds A.S. David, J.C. Cutting), pp. 181–196, Erlbaum, Hove, UK.

Erlenmeyer-Kimling, L., Cornblatt, B. (1987) The New York high-risk project: A follow up report. *Schizophrenia Bulletin*, **13**, 451–461.

Goldberg, T.E., Gold, J.M., Greenberg, R., Griffin, S., Schulz, S.C., Pickar, D., Kleinman, J.E., Weinberger, D.R. (1993a) Contrasts between patients with affective disorders and patients with schizophrenia on a neuropsychological test battery. *American Journal of Psychiatry*, **150**, 1355–1362.

Goldberg, T.E., Hyde, T.M., Kleinman, J.E., Weinberger, D.R. (1993b) Course of schizophrenia: Neuropsychological evidence for a static encephalopathy. *Schizophrenia Bulletin*, **19**, 797–804.

Goldstein, G. (1986) The neuropsychology of schizophrenia. In: *Neuropsychological Assessment of Neuropsychiatric Disorders* (Eds I. Grant, K. Adams), pp. 147–171, Oxford University Press, Oxford.

Goldstein, G., Zubin, J., Pogue-Geile, M.F. (1991) Hospitalisation and the cognitive deficits of schizophrenia, the influences of age and education. *Journal of Nervous and Mental Disease*, **179**, 202–206.

Goodman, S.H. (1987) Emory University project on children of disturbed parents. *Schizophrenia Bulletin*, **13**, 411–422.

Grimes, K., Walker, E. (1994) Childhood emotional expressions, educational attainment and age of onset of illness in schizophrenia. *Journal of Abnormal Psychology*, **103**, 784–790.

Hamlin, R. (1969) The stability of intellectual function in chronic schizophrenia. *Journal of Nervous and Mental Disease*, **149**, 495–503.

Heaton, R., Paulsen, J.S., McAdams, L.A., Kuck, J., Zisook, S., Braff, D., Harris, J., Jeste, D.V. (1994) Neuropsychological deficits in schizophrenics: Relationship to age, chronicity and dementia. *Archives of General Psychiatry*, **51**, 469–476.

Heinrichs, R.W., Awad, A.G. (1993). Neurocognitive subtypes of chronic schizophrenia. *Schizophrenia Research*, **9**, 49–58.

Hunt, J., Cofer, C.N. (1944) Psychological Deficit. In: *Personality and the Behaviour Disorders* (Ed. J. Hunt), Ronald Press, New York.

Hyde, T.M., Nawroz, S., Goldberg, T.E., Bigelow, L.B., Strong, D., Ostrem, J.L., Weinberger, D.R., Kleinman, J.E. (1994). Is there cognitive decline in schizophrenia? A cross-sectional study. *British Journal of Psychiatry*, **164**, 494–500.

Johnstone, E.C., Cunningham Owens, D.J., Gold, A., Crow, T.J., Macmillan, J.F. (1981) Institutionalisation and the defects of schizophrenia. *British Journal of Psychiatry*, **139**, 195–203.

Jones, P., Rogers, B., Murray, R., Marmot, M. (1994) Child developmental risk factors for adult schizophrenia in the British 1946 birth cohort. *Lancet*, **344**, 1398–1402.

King, D.J. (1990) The effect of neuroleptics on cognitive and psychomotor function. *British Journal of Psychiatry*, **157**, 799–811.

Klonoff, H., Fibiger, C., Hutton, G.H. (1970) Neuropsychological patterns in chronic schizophrenia. *Journal of Nervous and Mental Disease*, **150**, 291–300.

Kraepelin, E. (1913) *Dementia Praecox and Paraphrenia* (translated by R.M. Barclay, 1919), Livingstone, Edinburgh.

Lehman, R., Chelune, G., Heaton, R. (1979) Level and variability of performance on neuropsychological tests. *Journal of Clinical Psychology*, **35**, 358–363.

Lubin, A., Gieseking, C.F., Williams, H.I. (1962) Direct measurement of cognitive deficit in schizophrenia. *Journal of Consulting Psychology*, **26**, 139–143.

Liddle, P.F., Crow, T. (1984) Age disorientation in chronic schizophrenia is associated with global intellectual impairment. *British Journal of Psychiatry*, **144**, 193–199.

Mirsky, A.F., Ingraham, L.J., Kugelmass, S. (1995) Neuropsychological assessment of attention and its pathology in the Israeli cohort. *Schizophrenia Bulletin*, **21**, 193–204.

Nelson, H.E. (1982). *National Adult Reading Test (NART): Test Manual*. NFER, Nelson, Windsor, UK.

Nelson, H.E., Pantelis, C., Carruthers, K., Speller, J., Baxendale, S., Barnes, T.R.E. (1990) Cognitive functioning and symptomatology in chronic schizophrenia. *Psychological Medicine*, **20**, 357–365.

Offord, D.R. (1974) School performance of adult schizophrenics, their siblings and age mates. *British Journal of Psychiatry*, **125**, 12–19.

Offord, D.R., Cross, L.A. (1971) Adult schizophrenia with scholastic failure or low IQ in childhood: A preliminary report. *Archives of General Psychiatry*, **24**, 431–436.

Payne, R. (1960) Cognitive abnormalities. In: *Handbook of Abnormal Psychology* (Ed. H. Eysenck), Pitman Medical Publishing, London.

Pollack, M., Levenstein, S., Klein, D.F. (1968) A three-year post hospital follow up of adolescent and adult schizophrenics. *American Journal of Orthopsychiatry*, **38**, 94–109.

Pollack, M., Woerner, M.G., Klein, D.F. (1970) A comparison of childhood characteristics of schizophrenics, personality disorders and their siblings. In: *Life History Research in Psychopathology* (Eds M. Roff, A.F. Ricks), University of Minneapolis Press, Minneapolis.

Purisch, A.D., Golden, C.J., Hammecke, T.A. (1978) Discrimination of schizophrenic and brain injured patients by a standardised version of Luria's neuropsychological tests. *Journal of Consulting and Clinical Psychology*, **46**, 1266–1273.

Rappaport, S., Webb, W. (1950) An attempt to study intellectual deterioration by premorbid and psychotic testing. *Journal of Consulting Psychology*, **14**, 95–98.

Roe, A., Shakow, D. (1942) Intelligence in mental disorder. *Annals of the New York Academy of Sciences*, **42**, 361–490.

Saykin, A.J., Gur, R.C., Gur, R.E., Mozley, D., Mozley, L.H., Resnick, S.M., Kester, B., Stafiniak, P. (1991) Neuropsychological function in schizophrenia: Selective impairment in memory and learning. *Archives of General Psychiatry*, **48**, 618–624.

Schonell, F. (1942) *Backwardness in the Basic Subjects*, Oliver & Boyd, London.

Schwartzman, A.E., Douglas, V.I. (1962) Intellectual loss in schizophrenia: Part I. *Canadian Journal of Psychology*, **16**, 1–10.

Schwartzman, A.E., Douglas, V.I., Muir, W.R. (1962) Intellectual loss in schizophrenia: Part II. *Canadian Journal of Psychology*, **16**, 161–168.

Scottish Schizophrenia Research Group. (1988) The Scottish First Episode Schizophrenia Study. V. One year follow-up. *British Journal of Psychiatry*, **152**, 470–476.

Shelly, C., Goldstein, G. (1983) Discrimination of chronic schizophrenia and brain damage with the Luria–Nebraska battery: A partially successful replication. *Clinical Neuropsychology*, **5**, 82–85.

Smith, A. (1964) Mental deterioration in chronic schizophrenia. *Journal of Nervous and Mental Disease*, **139**, 479–487.

Walker, E.F. (1994) Developmentally moderated expressions of the neuropathology underlying schizophrenia. *Schizophrenia Bulletin*, **20**, 453–480.

Walker, E.F., Savoie, T., Davis, D. (1994) Neuromotor precursors of schizophrenia. *Schizophrenia Bulletin*, **20**, 441–451.

Warner, M.H., Ernst, J., Townes, B.D., Peel, J., Preston, M. (1987) Relationships between IQ and neuropsychological measures in neuropsychiatric populations: Within-laboratory and cross-cultural replications using WAIS and WAIS-R. *Journal of Clinical and Experimental Neuropsychology*, **9**, 545–562.

Watson, C. (1965) WAIS profile patterns of hospitalised brain-damaged patients. *Journal of Clinical Psychology*, **21**, 294–295.

Wechsler, D. (1994) *The Measurement of Adult Intelligence* (3rd edn), Williams & Wilkins, Baltimore.

Wechsler, D. (1981). *Wechsler Adult Intelligence Scale—Revised*, Psychological Corporation, New York.

5

Cognitive Deficits in Schizophrenia: Attention, Executive Functions, Memory and Language Processing

MONICA L. GOUROVITCH and TERRY E. GOLDBERG

INTRODUCTION

Schizophrenia is associated with a wide variety of cognitive impairments including dysfunctions of attention, memory, executive control and some aspects of language processing. Evidence has accumulated implicating several biological abnormalities of anatomic structures such as the temporal lobe and the prefrontal cortex. Recent scientific inquiry has attempted to show that the impaired cognitive operations in individuals with schizophrenia are manifestations of these underlying biological abnormalities.

In this chapter we provide an overview of some of the important areas of neurocognitive impairment identified in schizophrenia. We discuss key methodological issues that have a bearing on the interpretation of neuropsychological findings, including subtyping, medication effects and the impact of motivation and psychotic symptoms on testing behaviour (see also Goldstein, chapter 3; Liddle, chapter 15; King and Green, chapter 20). Finally, we review the neuropsychological, neuropathological, and neuroimaging evidence for understanding schizophrenia as a neuropsychiatric disease with a putative neurological pathogenesis.

Schizophrenia: A Neuropsychological Perspective. Edited by C. Pantelis, H.E. Nelson and T.R.E. Barnes
© 1996 John Wiley & Sons Ltd

METHODOLOGICAL ISSUES IN SCHIZOPHRENIA RESEARCH

SUBTYPING

In an attempt to reduce the heterogeneity of this disorder, several investigators have delineated subtypes of schizophrenia with variable success. For example, the classification of schizophrenia into disorganised, catatonic, paranoid, undifferentiated, and residual subtypes by DSM-III-R (American Psychiatric Association, 1987) has provided little insight into understanding the nature and underlying pathophysiology of cognitive impairment. Thus, while studies such as that by Goldstein & Halperin (1977) found differences in cognitive performance between paranoid and non-paranoid patients, other investigators have failed to find any differences between the two groups. Bornstein and colleagues (1990) compared paranoid, non-paranoid, and schizoaffective subtypes. They demonstrated that when the effects of symptom severity were controlled the magnitude and number of differences between the groups on measures of neuropsychological function were not significant.

More recently, the primary clinical features of schizophrenia have been classified into positive and negative features with reference to behavioural excesses and deficits. Positive symptoms generally include hallucinations, delusions and disorganised speech. Negative symptoms include apathy, blunted affect and social isolation. Although this formulation is not new, recent research has attempted to use these distinctions in refining hypotheses about pathogenesis, course and outcome variables, treatment strategies, neuropathology and genetics. For example, negative symptoms were more often correlated with ventricular enlargement (Johnstone et al, 1976; Andreasen et al, 1982), impaired cognitive performance (Crow, 1980; Andreasen et al, 1982) and poorer premorbid function and academic achievement (Andreasen et al, 1990; Kay et al, 1986). However, many of these findings have not been replicated and a few investigators have reported opposite relationships (for review: Marks & Luchins, 1990). Furthermore, factor analytic studies of symptomatology in schizophrenia have provided evidence that more than two factors may be necessary to account for the variance of symptoms in this population (Arndt et al, 1991; Bilder et al, 1985; see also: Liddle, chapter 15; Pantelis and Brewer, chapter 16). Finally, using the data from a 23-year longitudinal study, Maneros & Tsuang (1991) demonstrated that subtypes do not remain stable over the course of the schizophrenic illness.

Genetic studies also do not support a clear separation into two distinct subtypes. McGuffin et al (1991) re-evaluated the findings from previously published twin studies as well as their own data on schizophrenic families in order to explore the relationship between positive and negative symptoms. Their results supported the simple model in which positive and negative symptoms differed only in terms of their positions on the same continuum of liability, as opposed to a model in which the two clinical forms are constructed as two separate conditions.

A case can be made for neurobiological homogeneity in schizophrenia.

Evidence from recent studies of monozygotic twin pairs discordant for schizophrenia demonstrated that anatomical deviations and cerebral metabolic hypoactivity of the frontal lobe may be general characteristics of the disease, rather than being associated with only a minority of patients (Daniel & Weinberger, 1991). Suddath et al (1990), using magnetic resonance imaging (MRI) data of monozygotic twins discordant for schizophrenia, demonstrated that over 90% of the affected twins had enlargements in various components of the ventricular system, smaller areas of left anterior hippocampus and smaller areas of right anterior hippocampus when compared to their co-twins. In particular, the affected sibling had larger cerebral ventricles even when the ventricles of both siblings were small. In addition, for all twin pairs discordant for schizophrenia, prefrontal blood flow measured during performance of the Wisconsin Card Sorting Test (WCST) was lower in the twin with schizophrenia than in the unaffected twin (Berman et al, 1992).

Similarly, neuropsychological studies of twins do not support the validity of current subtype dichotomies. Goldberg et al (1990) completed a comprehensive battery of neuropsychological tests on many of these same twin pairs. They found that the affected twins consistently performed worse than their unaffected counterparts on most of the tests, irrespective of actual level of performance. Deficits were especially severe on tests of vigilance, memory and concept formation. Their results suggested that not only was neuropsychological dysfunction a frequent feature of schizophrenia but that this dysfunction does not manifest itself in a dichotomous distribution.

These recent data from the twin studies have produced consistent results in neuroanatomical, prefrontal activation and neuropsychological investigations for the majority of patients with schizophrenia, indicative of the importance of appropriate matching. Daniel & Weinberger (1991) have proposed that these consistent findings may lead to a conceptual shift back to the single entity disease concept of schizophrenia.

MEDICATION EFFECTS

The reported effects of neuroleptic drugs on cognitive and motor performance in patients with schizophrenia have been fairly consistent (see King and Green, chapter 20). Several recent reviews of the literature (King, 1990; Cassens et al, 1990; Spohn & Strauss, 1989; Medalia et al, 1988) have suggested that the effects of antipsychotic medication on specific higher cognitive functions in schizophrenia are minimal. However, antipsychotics may impair performance on tasks of motor function (Cassens et al, 1990). Medalia et al (1988) suggest that such impairments are a consequence of the blockade of dopamine. One area in which chronic neuroleptic administration appears to improve cognitive performance is on tasks requiring sustained attention and visuomotor problem solving (see Maruff and Currie, chapter 6; Cassens et al, 1990; Kornetsky, 1972).

In addition to neuroleptic medication patients with schizophrenia often receive anticholinergic medications to control extrapyramidal side effects. These drugs have been demonstrated to impair both learning and memory (Frith, 1984). Nonetheless, the severity of the memory deficit observed in schizophrenia is unlikely to be accounted for fully by these medications (Goldberg et al, 1993b). Given the advent of new drug therapies and the known effects of anticholinergic medications it would be prudent for investigators to report and continue to provide analysis of the effects of medication on behaviour.

PSYCHOTIC SYMPTOMS, MOTIVATION, OR REAL COGNITIVE DYSFUNCTION?

There has been debate in the literature as to whether cognitive impairment seen in patients with schizophrenia is "real" or simply a consequence of psychiatric symptoms and lack of motivation. Goldberg and coworkers (1993b) examined the relationship between psychiatric symptoms and cognition in patients with schizo-phrenia who received approximately 15 months treatment with clozapine. They found that despite significant improvement of psychiatric symptomatology, as measured by the Brief Psychiatric Rating Scale (BPRS), cognitive function in such areas as attention, memory and higher-level problem solving remained both impaired and essentially unchanged. Additionally, in a study contrasting neuro-psychological performance in psychiatric populations, it was found that sympto-matology had a larger impact on test performance in patients with affective disorder than in patients with schizophrenia (Goldberg et al, 1993a). These findings suggest that certain neuropsychological impairments are relatively independent of psychotic symptoms and are likely to be central and enduring features of the schizophrenic disease process.

Another line of evidence that provides support for the argument that there is a neuropathological process central to the schizophrenic disorder comes from longi-tudinal studies of children at risk for the disease (see also Wolf and Cornblatt, chapter 9). For example, Asarnow (1988), in a review of the literature, reported that neuromotor and attentional impairments assessed during middle childhood were associated with the development of schizophrenia during adolescence and early adulthood. These impairments were often found in the absence of overt behavioural symptomatology.

THE NATURE OF THE NEUROPSYCHOLOGICAL IMPAIRMENT IN SCHIZOPHRENIA

It has been found that patients with schizophrenia perform more poorly than normal controls on a wide variety of cognitive and neuropsychological tasks (Chelune et al, 1979; Goldberg & Weinberger, 1988). Furthermore, the literature suggests that these deficits emerge at the onset of diagnosable schizophrenic symptoms and remain relatively stable throughout the course of the disorder (Heaton & Drexler, 1987; Hyde et al, 1994).

There has been controversy in the literature as to whether this disorder is marked by a "generalised" deficit reflective of cognitive inefficiency, imprecision and psychomotor slowing. Alternatively, there may be specific deficits which appear to be differentially severe and central to the disease process. While current neuropsychological methodology has failed to find a specific profile of deficit from standardised tests for any psychiatric disorder (Randolph et al, 1993) four areas of cognitive impairment have been consistently implicated in studies of schizophrenia. These areas of attention, executive function, memory and language are reviewed below.

ATTENTION

Attentional dysfunction is characteristic of clinical descriptions of the schizo-phrenic disorder as well as prominent in patients' accounts of their own experi-ences (McGhie & Chapman, 1961). Cognitive research has suggested that there are many facets of the attentional system; these may include maintenance of an alert state, orienting to novel stimuli, selectively filtering relevant information, shifting from one set to another and rapidly discriminating or scanning stimuli. Moreover, recent investigations have suggested that different types of attention may be referable to different brain areas (Posner et al, 1988; Maruff and Currie, chapter 6). This section reviews selected areas of the attentional literature in schizophrenia and also includes attempts to pinpoint underlying brain areas associated with specific impairments.

Patients with schizophrenia have been shown to perform worse than normal and patient controls on immediate serial recall either with or without the presence of distracter conditions (Oltmans & Neale, 1975; Frame & Oltmans, 1982). Using a trial-by-trial analysis, Weiss et al (1988) demonstrated that vulner-ability to distraction, rather than capacity for handling information in a short term memory store, may account for impaired performance in patients with schizophrenia.

One of the most widely reported dysfunctions of attention in schizophrenia has been deficits in simple reaction time (RT) tasks (Nuechterlein, 1977). Several studies using different modifications of the RT experiment have demonstrated that patients with schizophrenia have difficulty with crossmodal cuing and benefiting from regular or preparatory warning intervals (Shakow, 1963; Nuechterlein & Dawson, 1984). With respect to the ability to process information in a timely and efficient manner, reaction time experiments have demonstrated that patients with schizophrenia have difficulty in the speed at which they can allocate attention to relevant cognitive activities due to limited processing resources.

One aspect of information processing relevant to normal and impaired attention is the ability to process several stimuli simultaneously. The span of apprehension paradigm, often employed to investigate this question, attempts to evaluate the number of items that can be attended to at one time (Woodsworth, 1948). Typical experiments involve the subject searching an array of briefly presented visual items for a particular target. Several investigators (for review: Asarnow et al, 1991) have found that schizophrenic subjects detected significantly fewer target stimuli as compared to normal controls. This pattern was further exacerbated as the complexity and number of stimuli in the array increased. Asarnow et al (1991) suggested that the major determinant of deficient performance by patients with schizophrenia is some aspect of their serial scanning process. There is still question as to whether the underlying mechanisms of this deficit are associated with an overall limited capacity of information processing resources in the early stages of attention or represent a later stage difficulty with manipulating information in short term working memory.

Several investigators have found that patients with schizophrenia have difficulty with stimulus identification in backward masking tasks (Braff & Saccuzzo, 1985). In this task a visual stimulus is presented and then "masked" or perceptually erased when a second visual stimulus is presented. In normal controls, as the time between the presentation of the target stimuli and the mask is increased the target stimulus is more easily identified. Patients with schizophrenia seem to require a particularly long time interval between the target and the "mask" in order correctly to identify the target. This pattern of performance may be associated with a dysfunction in the early stages of visual processing (Braff et al, 1991).

Patients with schizophrenia also demonstrate deficits on tasks measuring vigilance. Vigilance may be defined as "a state of readiness to detect and respond to certain small changes occurring at random intervals in the environment" (Mackworth, 1948). The most widely used measure of vigilance in clinical research is the continuous performance test (CPT). In this task patients are required to respond to predetermined targets either in the presence or absence of distracters. In comparison with control populations patients with schizophrenia make a greater number of omissions (missing targets) and commissions (false alarms) (Mirsky, 1988). This finding is associated with decreased ability to sustain attention over time and vulnerability to distraction. Buchsbaum and colleagues (1990) have recently attempted to identify brain regions activated by a degraded, more difficult version of the CPT with positron emission tomography (PET). In a study of 13 patients with schizophrenia and 37 normal controls, schizophrenic subjects were found to have relatively lower metabolic activity in bilateral prefrontal and right temperoparietal cortices but normal or higher than normal activation in the occipital and left temperoparietal regions. However, another study which used a version of the CPT which was not degraded found no differences between schizophrenic subjects and normal controls (Berman et al, 1986).

Posner et al (1988) have attempted to relate dissectible cognitive components of attention to discrete neural systems. They employed a paradigm investigating visual attention to a target appearing in right and left visual fields following valid or invalid cues. They found that patients with schizophrenia were slower to respond than normal controls on invalid-cue conditions presented to the right visual field. This result suggested that the patients had difficulty disengaging and redirecting attention to the right visual field following an invalid cue to the left visual field. This deficit is similar to that seen in patients with focal lesions to the left parietal hemisphere. However, other attempts to replicate this finding have been unsuccessful (Gold et al, 1992b; Strauss et al, 1991).

In summary, abnormalities have been described throughout various components of attention including simple vigilance, the ability to benefit from regular or preparatory warning intervals, serial scanning, the ability to sustain attention over time and perhaps the ability to disengage attention from the right visual field. Clearly, attention is an important area of deficit in patients with schizophrenia. In addition to difficulties in providing a cognitive account of the specific mechanisms it has been postulated that the neural structures implicated in the control of attention are widely distributed rather than focal (Mesulam, 1985). Future attempts to study attentional deficits in schizophrenia will require an attempt to conceptualise specific processes as well as implicate specific neural systems (see Maruff and Currie, chapter 6).

EXECUTIVE FUNCTIONS

Investigators as far back as Kraepelin in 1913 have suggested that dysfunction of the frontal cortex and "executive functions" may be responsible for the loss of integrative functions in schizophrenia. Kraepelin's descriptions of symptoms in patients with schizophrenia bear remarkable similarity to what we now consider deficits of executive function or difficulties in tasks that involve problem solving, set shifting, and response to feedback:

> . . . judgement is lost, the critical faculty, the creative gift, especially the capacity to make a higher use of the knowledge and ability . . . The patients may also exhibit volitional activity of the greatest strength and endurance, but they are wholly incapable of . . . carrying out a well considered plan.
>
> (Kraepelin, 1913, pp. 221–222)

One difficulty in neuropsychologically evaluating these deficits is a paradox described by Luria (1980); that is, although these deficits have a devastating impact on real-life functioning they are difficult to ascertain with standard psychometric techniques. One task, the WCST, which was originally used by Fey (1951) to demonstrate deficits in executive function in patients with schizophrenia, has been well studied in this population. Such patients appear to have difficulty attaining concepts and may perseverate on the incorrect response even in the face of feedback to the contrary (Stuss et al, 1983). Goldberg et al (1987) demonstrated the imperviousness of this deficit by showing that despite the fact that patient's performance could be transiently normalised following explicit card by card instruction they immediately returned to their poor baseline performance when structure was withdrawn. Recently, an analogue of the animal delayed response task (a task associated with prefrontal cortex function) with the addition of a component requiring response alternation was used to tap executive functioning (see also Pantelis and Brewer, chapter 16). Gold et al (1991) found that schizophrenic subjects were impaired in their ability to do this task as well as in their ability to perform it following explicit training and instructions.

Schizophrenic subjects also demonstrate difficulty on tests of formation of concepts and hypotheses such as the Category Test from the Halstead Reitan Battery (Heaton et al, 1978; Goldberg et al, 1988). Finally, patients with schizophrenia tend to perform more poorly than control populations on tasks measuring guided lexical search, namely word fluency (Kolb & Whishaw, 1983; Goldberg et al, 1988) and design fluency (Kolb & Whishaw, 1983).

The consistent deficits on tests assessing executive functions together with the behavioural deficits observed in schizophrenia, including poor planning abilities, impaired social judgement and insight and lack of initiative, have provided impetus for describing dysfunction of the frontal lobe in patients with schizophrenia. There has been accumulating evidence from cerebral blood flow activation studies to suggest dysfunction in areas of the prefrontal cortex. Several investigators have pointed to physiological hypofrontality in the brains of patients with schizophrenia. Ingvar & Franzen (1974) found that, while normal subjects showed relatively more blood flow to frontal areas than to other areas, patients with schizophrenia did not show this pattern. In a series of studies using various cognitive tasks, Berman and Weinberger (Berman et al, 1986, 1988; Weinberger et al, 1986, 1988, 1992) demonstrated that schizophrenic subjects were hypofrontal specifically while undertaking the WCST. The WCST was the only cognitive task they used which was an abstract problem solving task purported to assess executive cognitive processes. Other investigators have shown hypofrontality in patients with schizophrenia during tasks thought to engage the frontal lobes, including eye tracking (Volkow et al, 1987), the Continuous Performance Test (Buchsbaum et al, 1990) and auditory attention tasks (Cohen et al, 1987).

MEMORY

Memory deficits are among the most reliable findings in cognitive studies of schizophrenia (Levin et al, 1989; see also Chen and McKenna, chapter 7). Deficits have been reported from a variety of paradigms implicating all stages of memory function from initial encoding, to consolidation, retrieval and recognition (Saykin et al, 1991; Calev et al, 1983, 1984, 1987).

There has been some controversy as to whether the memory deficits in schizophrenia are primary or whether they may be secondary to other deficits, such as, dysfunction of attention or executive control. However, various studies have demonstrated consistent deficits in memory. In general, the rate of learning over trials begins and ends slower for schizophrenic subjects compared with normal controls (Goldberg et al, 1989). Additionally, patients with schizophrenia demonstrate marked deficits in their ability to recall stories or abstract designs as compared to normal control subjects (Kolb & Whishaw, 1983). Furthermore, Gold et al (1992c) have demonstrated that patients with schizophrenia perform significantly worse on the Wechsler Memory Scale—Revised than on the Wechsler Adult Intelligence Test—Revised; 30% of schizophrenic subjects had a general memory index (both verbal and visual measures) 15 or more points below their full-scale IQ.

There is not yet a clear picture as to whether specific aspects of the memory system are differentially affected in schizophrenia. McKenna and colleagues (1990) investigated 60 patients with schizophrenia with varying degrees of illness severity. They found that the pattern of memory performance in their subjects was similar to classical amnesia in that while short-term memory was intact, long-term memory and recognition performance were impaired (Tamlyn et al, 1992; McKenna et al, 1990). Gold et al (1992a), in a study of patients with schizophrenia and normal controls, documented a variety of memory abnormalities in their patient population. These included differences in recall ability, failure to use semantic cues to aid free recall, poor recognition memory, attenuated sensitivity to frequency information and the tendency to make prior list and non-list intrusions. As impairments were observed in both effortful and more automatic memory functions, the authors concluded that the data supported dysfunction of encoding of semantic information, frequency estimation, and temporal order cues.

The above evidence supports a memory disorder which involves functional compromise of neural systems involved in acquisition of new information associated with both the temporal and frontal lobe systems of the brain. Support for a primary memory deficit implicating the medial temporal lobe and hippocampus as brain sites in schizophrenia comes from neuropathologic and neuroimaging studies which have recently found evidence for diminished size of the amygdalo-hippocampal formation (e.g. Bogerts et al, 1985; Suddath et al, 1990; for review: Hyde et al, 1991; see also Bilder and Szeszko, chapter 14). In particular, the study of monozygotic twins discordant for schizophrenia (Suddath et al, 1990) found that the anterior hippocampus was smaller bilaterally in the affected twin in 14 of 15 pairs. Bogerts et al (1990) have also reported reduced hippocampal size in first-break patients who had not received chronic neuroleptic treatment. Finally, the frontal lobes have been implicated in the coding of temporal context, frequency information, semantic encoding and effortful retrieval (Schacter, 1987).

LANGUAGE

When Bleuler described the fundamental elements of symptomatology in schizophrenia he gave particular prominence to the loss of continuity of an internal associational process.

> Of the thousands of associative threads which guide our thinking, this disease seems to interrupt, quite haphazardly, sometimes single threads, sometimes a whole group . . . In this way thinking becomes illogical and often bizarre.
>
> (Bleuler, 1911)

One component of thought-disordered language is a lack of executive planning and editing of discourse together with an inability to inhibit inappropriate associations (see also McGrath, chapter 10). Several investigators have made the claim for an actual dysphasia in patients with schizophrenia (Andreasen, 1979). However, Barr and colleagues (1990) demonstrated that the majority of errors in tests of language functioning, such as perseveration of words and perseveration of prior semantic and phonemic properties of words, were related to executive dysfunction.

Models of associational disturbance in the language system have been proposed to explain the thought disorder in schizophrenia (Chapman et al, 1964; Maher, 1972). According to the network model of semantic knowledge each component of an utterance activates associated semantic units within a neuronal network of semantic nodes; these nodes then remain activated for a finite period of time (Meyer et al, 1975). Additionally, in order to prevent intrusions semantic nodes which are associated with the original utterance but unrelated to its present context must be inhibited. For example, given the sentence, "The cattle was herded in a *pen*", the associations to pen such as fence and corral would be activated while associations such as pencil and ink would be inhibited.

One type of paradigm used to assess the integrity of the activation component of the semantic network involves priming. In this task the prior presentation of a semantically associated word has been shown to facilitate the recognition of a later presented target word. For example, while prior exposure to the word "cat" will facilitate recognition to the word "dog" (as measured by reaction time), it will not facilitate recognition of the word "house". Several investigators (Manshreck et al, 1988; Chapin et al, 1989; Kwapil et al, 1990) have demonstrated normal or greater facilitation of a primed target in thought disordered patients with schizophrenia as compared to normal controls. These data support normal spread of activation within the semantic network of patients with schizophrenia.

There is evidence that in schizophrenia there is an abnormality of the inhibitory mechanism within the semantic network. As stated previously, prior to the decay of activated nodes or units of semantic activation, the speaker must call upon some mechanism to inhibit or selectively facilitate relevant words from all activated words. Bullen & Hemsley (1987) demonstrated that in a word recognition task schizophrenic performance was similar whether the target (wrist) was primed discordantly (Tree–palm–wrist) or concordantly (Hand–palm–wrist). In contrast, a normal group of subjects required a number of presentations to recognise the target in the discordant condition. This suggested that for patients with schizophrenia both alternative meanings of the word "palm" were available to consciousness.

Another paradigm which may be useful in demonstrating an abnormality of the inhibition mechanism in schizophrenic language processing is negative priming. In this paradigm, if a distracter which has been previously ignored is subsequently presented there is an increased reaction time associated with the response to that target. This increase in reaction time is said to be a consequence of prior inhibition to that target when it was previously presented as a distracter. For example, in different trials of list presentation (e.g. Stroop task), responses may include naming the ink colour of crosses, naming the ink colour of letters which spell a colour word (incongruent condition) and naming a colour which is the same as the distracting word of the preceding word in the list (e.g. naming the colour blue when the word blue was ignored in the previous trial). In this last condition, the subject must overcome the previous requirement of responding to the colour rather than the word. Beech et al (1989) found that the reaction time required to respond to a previously presented distracter was reduced in schizophrenic subjects as compared to normal controls. They concluded that this finding was a result of schizophrenic subjects' inability to inhibit distracter information from the previous trials.

Finally, Cohen & Servan-Schreiber (1992) replicated Chapman et al's (1964) finding that patients with schizophrenia tend to interpret the strong or dominant meaning of a homonym used in a sentence, even when the context provided by the sentence mediated the weaker meaning. For example, given the sentence "In warm climates palm trees are common", patients with schizophrenia would interpret the word palm to mean part of the hand more frequently than control subjects. Furthermore, they demonstrated that these types of errors only occurred when the context came before the targeted word. They concluded that patients with schizophrenia had difficulty using context to mediate word usage when the context was remote.

It is possible that some of the errors found in schizophrenic discourse are associated with this inability either to inhibit irrelevant or facilitate relevant activated units of language rather than a breakdown of the semantic system per se. One brain area which may be implicated in this lack of inhibition is the connections between the temporal cortex and prefrontal cortex which have been demonstrated to be functionally impaired in schizophrenia (Weinberger, 1991; Pantelis and Brewer, chapter 16). In future research, it may be important to examine the prevalence of disorders of speech in patients demonstrating a failure of inhibitory mechanisms in semantic activation studies.

CONCLUSIONS

Specific neuropsychological deficits, particularly in the areas of attention, executive function, memory and language processing, have been frequently demonstrated in patients with schizophrenia. Furthermore, neurocognitive impairment may represent a central feature of the disease process and not simply a consequence of non-specific deficits in motivation, cooperation or psychotic symptomatology. In addition, neuropathological and neuroimaging studies provide evidence for abnormalities in the cerebral ventricles and temporal lobe structures of the brain in schizophrenia. Together with the evidence from neuropsychological studies, these lines of investigation implicate temporal and prefrontal cortical systems.

Finally, if cognitive impairment is a central and enduring feature of the schizophrenic disorder, then it is likely to exact a cost in social and vocational functioning. This is not to say that psychiatric symptomatology does not impact on these skills but rather that symptomatology does not account for all of the variance. Neuropsychological dysfunction might therefore be considered a target symptom and, as such, be treated with cognitive enhancing drugs or cognitive rehabilitation techniques (see Morice and Delahunty, chapter 21). This approach has not often been taken and might provide an avenue to improve day-to-day functioning in this population.

REFERENCES

American Psychiatric Association. (1987) *Diagnostic and Statistical Manual of Mental Disorders, Third Edition, Revised.* APA, Washington, DC.

Andreasen, N.C. (1979) Thought, language, and communication disorders: I. Clinical assessment and evaluation of their reliability. *Archives of General Psychiatry*, **139**, 1315–1321.

Andreasen, N.C., Olson, S.A., Dennert, J.W. (1982) Ventricular enlargement in schizophrenia: Relationship to positive and negative symptoms. *American Journal of Psychiatry*, **139**, 297–302.

Andreasen, N.C., Flaum, M., Swayze, V.W., Tyrell, G., Arndt, S. (1990) Positive and negative symptoms in schizophrenia. *Archives of General Psychiatry*, **47**, 615–621.

Arndt, S., Alliger, R.J., Andreasen, N.C. (1991) The distinction of positive and negative symptoms: The failure of a two-dimensional model. *British Journal of Psychiatry*, **158**, 317–322.

Asarnow, R.F. (1988) Children at risk for schizophrenia: Converging lines of evidence. *Schizophrenia Bulletin*, **14**, 613–631.

Asarnow, R.F., Granholm, E., Sherman, T. (1991) Span of apprehension in schizophrenia. In: *Handbook of Schizophrenia. Vol. 5: Neuropsychology, Psychophysiology, and Information Processing* (Eds S.R. Steinhauer, J.H. Gruzelier, J. Zubin), Elsevier, New York.

Barr, W.B., Bilder, R.M., Goldberg, E., Kaplan. E. (1990) The neuropsychology of schizophrenic speech. *Journal of Communicative Disorders*, **22**, 327–349.

Beech, A., Powell, T., McWilliam, J., Claridge, G. (1989) Evidence of reduced cognitive inhibition in schizophrenia. *Journal of Clinical Psychology*, **28**, 109–116.

Berman, K.F., Zec, R.F., Weinberger, D.F. (1986) Physiological dysfunction of dorsolateral prefrontal cortex in schizophrenia: II. Role of neuroleptic treatment, attention, and mental effort. *Archives of General Psychiatry*, **43**, 126–135.

Berman, K.F., Illowsky, B.P., Weinberger, D.F. (1988) Physiological dysfunction of dorsolateral prefrontal cortex in schizophrenia: IV. Further evidence for regional and behavioral specificity. *Archives of General Psychiatry*, **45**, 661–622.

Berman, K.F., Torrey, E.F., Daniel, D.G., Weinberger, D.R. (1992) Regional cerebral blood flow in monozygotic twins discordant and concordant for schizophrenia. *Archives of General Psychiatry*, **49**, 927–934.

Bilder, R.M., Mukherjee, S., Rieder, R.O., Pandurangi, A.K. (1985) Symptomatic and neuropsychological components of defect states. *Schizophrenia Bulletin*, **11**, 409–417.

Bleuler, E. (1911) *Dementia Praecox, or the Group of Schizophrenias* (translated by Joseph Zinken, 1950), International Universities Press, New York.

Bogerts, B., Meertz, E., Schonfeld-Bausch, R. (1985) Basal ganglia and limbic system pathology in schizophrenia: A morphometric study. *Archives of General Psychiatry*, **42**, 784–791.

Bogerts, B., Ashtari, M., Degreef, G., Alvir, J.M. (1990) Reduced temporal limbic structure volumes on magnetic resonance images in first episode schizophrenia. *Psychiatry Research: Neuroimaging*, **35**, 1–13.

Bornstein, R., Schwarzkopf, S., Olson, S., Coffman, J., Nasrallah, H. (1990) MRI correlates of neuropsychological performance in schizophrenia. *Biological Psychiatry*, **27**, 152A.

Braff, D.L., Saccuzzo, D.P. (1985) The time course of information processing deficits in schizophrenia. *American Journal of Psychiatry*, **142**, 170–174.

Braff, D.L., Saccuzzo, D.P., Geyer, M.A. (1991) Information processing dysfunctions in schizophrenia: Studies of visual backward masking, sensorimotor gating, and habituation. In: *Handbook of Schizophrenia. Vol. 5: Neuropsychology, Psychophysiology, and Information Processing* (Eds S.R. Steinhauer, J.H. Gruzelier, J. Zubin), Elsevier, New York.

Buchsbaum, M.S., Nuechterlein, K.H., Haier, R.J., Wu, J., Sicotte, N., Hazlett, E., Asarnow, R., Potkin, S., Guich, S. (1990) Glucose metabolic rate in normals and schizophrenics during the continuous performance test assessed by positron emission tomography. *British Journal of Psychiatry*, **156**, 216–227.

Bullen, J.G., Hemsley, D.R. (1987) Schizophrenia: A failure to control the contents of consciousness. *British Journal of Clinical Psychology*, **26**, 25–33.

Calev, A., Venables, P.H., Monk, A.F. (1983) Evidence for distinct verbal memory pathologies in severely and mildly impaired schizophrenics. *Schizophrenia Bulletin*, **9**, 247–264.

Calev, A., Korin, Y., Kugelmass, S., Lerer, B. (1987) Performance of chronic schizophrenics on matched word and design recall tasks. *Biological Psychiatry*, **22**, 699–709.

Cassens, G., Inglis, A.K., Appelbaum, P.S., Gutheil, T.G. (1990) Neuroleptics: Effects on neuropsychological function in chronic schizophrenic patients. *Schizophrenia Bulletin*, **16**, 477–499.

Chapin, K., Vann, L.E., Lycaki, H., Josef, N., Meyendorff, E. (1989) Investigation of the associative network in schizophrenia using the semantic priming paradigm. *Schizophrenia Research*, **2**, 355–360.

Chapman, L.J., Chapman, J.P., Miller, G.A. (1964) A theory of verbal behavior in schizophrenia. In: *Progress in Experimental Personality Research* (Ed. B.A. Maher), Academic Press, New York.

Chelune, G.J., Heaton, R.K., Lehman, R.A., Robinson, A. (1979) Level versus pattern of neuropsychological performance among schizophrenic and diffusely brain damaged patients. *Journal of Consulting and Clinical Psychology*, **47**, 155–163.

Cohen, J.D., Servan-Schreiber, D. (1992) Context, cortex, and dopamine: A connectionist approach to behavior and biology in schizophrenia. *Psychological Review*, **99**, 45–77.

Cohen, R.M., Semple, W.E., Gross, M., Nordahl, T.E., DeLisi, L.E., Holcomb, H.H., King, A.C., Morihisa, J.M., Pickar, D. (1987) Dysfunction in a prefrontal substrate of sustained attention in schizophrenia. *Life Sciences*, **40**, 2031–2039.

Crow, T.J. (1980) Molecular pathology of schizophrenia: More than one disease process? *British Medical Journal*, **280**, 66–68.

Daniel, D.G., Weinberger, D.R. (1991) Ex multi uno: A case for neurobiological homogeneity in schizophrenia. In: *Advances in Neuropsychiatry and Psychopharmacology* (Eds C.A. Tamminga, S.C. Schultz), Raven Press, New York.

Fey, E.T. (1951) The performance of young schizophrenics and young normals on the Wisconsin card sorting test. *Journal of Consulting Psychology*, **15**, 311–319.

Frame, C.L., Oltmans, T.F. (1982) Serial recall by schizophrenic and affective patients during and after psychotic episodes. *Journal of Abnormal Psychology*, **145**, 483–486.

Frith, C.D. (1984) Schizophrenia, memory, and anticholinergic drugs. *Journal of Abnormal Psychology*, **93**, 339–341.

Gold, J.M., Berman, K.F., Randolph, C., Goldberg, T.E., Weinberger, D.R. (1991) PET validation and clinical application of a novel prefrontal task. *Journal of Experimental and Clinical Neuropsychology*, **13**, 81.

Gold, J.M., Randolph, C., Carpenter, C., Goldberg, T.E., Weinberger, D.R. (1992a) Forms of memory failure in schizophrenia. *Journal of Abnormal Psychology*, **101**, 487–494.

Gold, J.M., Randolph, C., Carpenter, C., Goldberg, T.E., Weinberger, D.R. (1992b) Visual orienting in schizophrenia. *Schizophrenia Research*, **7**, 203–209.

Gold, J.M., Randolph, C., Carpenter, C., Goldberg, T.E., Weinberger, D.R. (1992c) The performance of patients with schizophrenia on the Wechsler Memory Scale—Revised. *Clinical Neuropsychologist*, **6**, 367–373.

Goldberg, T.E., Weinberger, D.R. (1988) Probing prefrontal function in schizophrenia with neuropsychological paradigms. *Schizophrenia Bulletin*, **14**, 179–183.

Goldberg, T.E., Weinberger, D.R., Berman, K.F., Pliskin, N., Podd, M. (1987) Further evidence for dementia of the prefrontal type in schizophrenia? A controlled study of teaching the Wisconsin Card Sorting Test. *Archives of General Psychiatry*, **44**, 1008–1014.

Goldberg, T.E., Karson, C.N., Leleszi, J.P., Weinberger, D.R. (1988) Intellectual impairment in adolescent psychosis: A controlled psychometric study. *Schizophrenia Research*, **1**, 261–266.

Goldberg, T.E., Berman, K.F., Weinberger, D.R. (1989) An orientation to work on the prefrontal cortex in schizophrenia. In: *Schizophrenia: A Scientific Focus* (Eds S.C. Schultz, C.A. Tamminga), New York, Oxford University Press.

Goldberg, T.E., Ragland, D.R., Gold, J., Bigelow, L.B., Torrey, E.F., Weinberger, D.R. (1990) Neuropsychological assessment of monozygotic twins discordant for schizophrenia. *Archives of General Psychiatry*, **47**, 1066–1072.

Goldberg, T.E., Gold, J.M., Greenberg, R., Griffin, S., Schultz, S.C., Pickar, D., Kleinman, J.E., Weinberger, D.R. (1993a) Contrasts between patients with affective disorders and patients with schizophrenia on a neuropsychological test battery. *American Journal of Psychiatry*, **150**, 1355–1362.

Goldberg, T.E., Greenberg, R.D., Griffin, S.J., Gold, J.M., Kleinman, J.E., Pickar, D., Schultz, S.C., Weinberger, D.R. (1993b) The effect of clozapine on cognition and psychiatric symptoms in patients with schizophrenia. *British Journal of Psychiatry*, **162**, 43–48.

Goldstein, G., Halperin, K.M. (1977) Neuropsychological differences among subtypes of schizophrenics. *Journal of Abnormal Psychology*, **86**, 34–40.

Heaton, R.K., Drexler, M. (1987) Clinical neuropsychological findings in schizophrenia and aging. In: *Schizophrenia and Aging*. (Eds N.E. Miller, G.D. Coles), pp. 145–161, Guilford Press, New York.

Heaton, R.K., Boade, L.E., Johnson, K.L. (1978) Neuropsychological test results associated with psychiatric disorders in adults. *Psychological Bulletin*, **85**, 141–162.

Hyde, T., Cassanova, M., Kleinman, J.E., Weinberger, D.R. (1991) Neuroanatomical and neuro-chemical pathology in schizophrenia. In: *American Psychiatric Press Review of Psychiatry* (Eds A. Tasman, S.M. Goldfinger), American Psychiatric Press, Washington, DC.

Hyde, T.M., Nawroz, S., Goldberg, T.E., Bigelow, L.B., Strong, D., Ostrem, J.L., Weinberger, D.R., Kleinman, J.E. (1994) Is there cognitive decline in schizophrenia? A cross-sectional study. *British Journal of Psychiatry*, **164**, 494–500.

Ingvar, D.H., Franzen, G. (1974) Abnormalities of cerebral blood flow in patients with chronic schizophrenia. *Acta Psychiatrica Scandinavia*, **50**, 425–462.

Johnstone, E.C., Crow, T.J., Frith, C.D., Husband, J., Kreel, L. (1976) Cerebral ventricular size and cognitive impairment in chronic schizophrenia. *Lancet*, **ii**, 924–926.

Kay, S.R., Opler, L.A., Fiszbein, A. (1986) Significance of positive and negative symptoms in chronic schizophrenia. *British Journal of Psychiatry*, **149**, 439–448.

King, D.J. (1990) The effects of neuroleptics on cognitive and psychomotor function. *British Journal of Psychiatry*, **157**, 799–811.

Kolb, B., Whishaw, I.Q. (1983) Performance of schizophrenic patients on tests sensitive to left or right frontal, temporal, or parietal function in neurological patients. *Journal of Nervous and Mental Disease*, **171**, 435–443.

Kornetsky, C. (1972) The use of a simple test of attention as a measure of drug effects in schizo-phrenic patients. *Psychopharmacologia*, **24**, 99–106.

Kraepelin, E. (1913) *Dementia Praecox and Paraphrenia* (English translation by R.M. Barclay, 1919), Livingstone, Edinburgh.

Kwapil, T.R., Hegley, D.C., Chapman, L.J., Chapman, J.P. (1990) Facilitation of word recogni-tion by semantic priming in schizophrenia. *Journal of Abnormal Psychology*, **3**, 215–221.

Levin, S., Yurgelun-Todd, D., Craft, S. (1989) Contributions of clinical neuropsychology to the study of schizophrenia. *Journal of Abnormal Psychology*, **98**, 341–356.

Luria, A.R. (1980) Neuropsychology in the local diagnosis of brain damage. *Clinical Neuropsychology*, **2**, 1–7.

McGhie, A., Chapman, J. (1961) Disorders of attention and perception in early schizophrenia. *British Journal of Medical Psychology*, **34**, 103.

McGuffin, P., Harvey, L., Williams, M. (1991) The negative/positive dichotomy: Does it make sense from the perspective of the genetic researcher? In: *Negative versus Positive Schizophrenia* (Eds A. Maneros, N.C. Andreasen, M.T. Tsuang), Springer, Berlin.

McKenna, P.J., Tamlyn, D., Lund, C.E., Mortimer, A.M., Hammond, S., Baddeley, A. (1990) Amnesic syndrome in schizophrenia. *Psychological Medicine*, **20**, 967–972.

Mackworth, N.H. (1948) The breakdown of vigilance during prolonged visual search. *Quarterly Journal of Experimental Psychology*, **1**, 6.

Maher, B.A. (1972) The language of schizophrenia: A review and interpretation. *British Journal of Psychiatry*, **120**, 3–17.

Maneros, A., Tsuang, M.T. (1991) Dichotomies and other distinctions in schizophrenia. In: *Negative versus Positive Schizophrenia* (Eds A. Maneros, N.C. Andreasen, M.T. Tsuang) Springer, Berlin.

Manshreck, T.C., Maher, B., Milavetz, J.J., Ames, D., Weisstein, C.C., Schneyer, M.L. (1988) Semantic priming in thought disordered schizophrenic patients. *Schizophrenia Research*, **1**, 61–66.

Marks, R.C., Luchins, D.J. (1990) Relationship between brain imaging findings ins schizophrenia and psychopathology: A review of the literature relating to positive and negative symptoms. In: *Modern Problems of Pharmacopsychiatry: Positive and Negative Syndromes* (Ed. N.C. Andreasen), pp. 89–123, Karger, Basel.

Medalia, A., Gold, J.M., Merriam, A. (1988) The effects of neuroleptics on neuropsychological test results of schizophrenics. *Archives of Clinical Neuropsychology*, **3**, 249–271.

Mesulam, M-M. (1985) Attention confusional states, and neglect. In: *Principles of Behavioral Neurology* (Ed. M-M. Mesulam), pp. 125–168, Davis, Philadelphia.

Meyer, D., Schvaneveldt, R., Ruddy, M.G. (1975) Loci of contextual effects on visual word recognition. In: *Attention and Performance* (Eds P. Rabbit, S. Dornic), Academic Press, New York.

Mirsky, A.F. (1988) Research on schizophrenia in the NIMH laboratory of psychology and psychopathology, 1954–1987. *Schizophrenia Bulletin*, **14**, 151–156.

Nuechterlein, K.H. (1977) Reaction time and attention in schizophrenia: A critical evaluation of the data and theories. *Schizophrenia Bulletin*, **3**, 373–428.

Nuechterlein, K.H., Dawson, M.E. (1984) Informational processing and attention functioning in the developmental course of schizophrenia. *Psychological Medicine*, **10**, 160–203.

Oltmans, T.F., Neale, J.M. (1975) Schizophrenic performance when distracters are present: Attentional deficit or differential task difficulty? *Journal of Abnormal Psychology*, **84**, 205–209.

Posner, M.I., Early, T.S., Reiman, E., Pardo, P.J., Dhawan, M. (1988) Asymmetries in hemispheric control of attention in schizophrenia. *Archives of General Psychiatry*, **45**, 814–821.

Randolph, C.R., Goldberg, T.E., Weinberger, D.R. (1993) The neuropsychology of schizophrenia. In: *Clinical Neuropsychology*, 3rd edn (Eds K.M. Heilman, E. Valenstein), Oxford University Press, New York.

Saykin, A.J., Gur, R.C., Gur, R.E., Mozley, P.D., Mozley, P.H., Resnick, S.M., Kester, D.B., Stafniak, P. (1991) Selective impairment in learning and memory. *Biological Psychiatry*, **29**, 329–339.

Schacter, D.L. (1987) Implicit expressions of memory in organic amnesia: Learning of new facts and associations. *Human Neurobiology*, **6**, 107–118.

Shakow, D. (1963) Physiological deficit in schizophrenia. *Behavioral Science*, **8**, 275–305.

Spohn, H.E., Strauss, M.E. (1989) Relation of neuroleptic and anticholinergic medications to cognitive function in schizophrenia. *Journal of Abnormal Psychology*, **98**, 367–380.

Strauss, M.E., Novakovic, T., Tien, A.Y., Byslma, F., Pearlson, G.D. (1991) Disengagement of attention in schizophrenia. *Psychiatry Research*, **3**, 139–146.

Stuss, D.T., Benson, D.F., Kaplan, E.F., Weir, W.S., Naeser, M.A., Lieberman, I., Ferrill, D. (1983) The involvement of orbito-frontal cerebrum in cognitive tasks. *Neuropsychologia*, **21**, 235–249.

Suddath, R.L., Christison, G.W., Torrey, E.F., Casanova, M.F., Weinberger, D.R. (1990) Anatomical abnormalities in the brains of monozygotic twins discordant for schizophrenia. *New England Journal of Medicine*, **322**, 789–794.

Tamlyn, D., McKenna, P.J., Mortimer, A.M., Lund, C.E., Hammond, S., Baddeley, A. (1992) Memory impairment in schizophrenia: Its extent, affiliations, and neuropsychological character. *Psychological Medicine*, **22**, 101–115.

Volkow, N.D., Wolf, A.P., VanGelder, P., Brodie, J.D., Overall, J.E., Cancro, R., Gomez-Mont, F. (1987) Phenomenological correlates of metabolic activity in 18 patients with chronic schizophrenia. *American Journal of Psychiatry*, **144**, 151–158.

Weinberger D.R. (1991) Anteromedial temporal–prefrontal connectivity: A functional anatomical system implicated in schizophrenia. In: *Psychopathology and the Brain* (Eds B.J. Carrol, J.E. Barnett), pp. 25–42, Raven Press, New York.

Weinberger D.R., Berman K.F, Zec R.F. (1986) Physiologic dysfunction of dorsolateral prefrontal cortex in schizophrenia. I. Regional cerebral blood flow evidence. *Archives of General Psychiatry*, **43**, 114–124.

Weinberger, D.R., Berman, K.F., Illowsky, B.P. (1988) Physiological dysfunction of the dorso-lateral prefrontal cortex in schizophrenia. *Archives of General Psychiatry*, **45**, 609–615.

Weinberger D.R., Berman K.F., Suddath R., Torrey E.F. (1992) Evidence for dysfunction of a prefrontal–limbic network in schizophrenia: An MRI and rCBF study of discordant monozygotic twins. *American Journal of Psychiatry*, **149**, 890–897.

Weiss, K.M., Vrtunski, P.B., Simpson, D.M. (1988) Information overload disrupts digit recall performance in schizophrenics. *Schizophrenia Research*, **1**, 299–303.

Woodsworth, R.S. (1948) *Experimental Psychology*. Holt, New York.

6

Neuropsychology of Visual Attentional Deficits in Schizophrenia

PAUL MARUFF and JON CURRIE

INTRODUCTION: TOWARD A BRAIN–BEHAVIOUR MODEL OF ATTENTIONAL DEFICITS IN SCHIZOPHRENIA

The major goal of neuropsychological assessment in patients with schizophrenia is to provide evidence of disruption or disruptions to the neurocognitive networks that underlie normal cognitive performance and to help localise these disruptions to specific neural areas or neural systems. Describing the disordered thinking that characterises schizophrenia in terms of brain–behaviour models should therefore lead to increased specificity of diagnosis and improved ability to assess the efficacy of conventional and novel antipsychotic treatments. Finally, an understanding of neuropsychological deficits in schizophrenia should help to predict the difficulties that patients may have with activities of independent daily living and also provide a basis for efficient rehabilitation programs and support services.

This chapter will review studies which have attempted to link the neuropsychology of attention to the pathophysiology of schizophrenia. However, for reasons of space, the review will be limited to visual attention. Adequate brain–behaviour models of attention should seek to explain attentional processes on a number of levels. Allport (1988) recommends that attentional function should be specified within the context of the organism's normal goal-directed interactions with the world as well as in the kind of representations on which attentional processes act. To achieve this, evidence may be drawn at the cognitive level from experimental studies of normal attention, neuropsychological studies of attention in patients with focal brain lesions and from neuroimaging studies where patterns of brain activity can be investigated while individuals perform attentional tasks. This data must be considered against data from neurophysiological studies of

Schizophrenia: A Neuropsychological Perspective. Edited by C. Pantelis, H.E. Nelson and T.R.E. Barnes
© 1996 John Wiley & Sons Ltd

attention where the activity of single cells, or an animal's performance after stereotaxic brain lesions can be assessed during attentional tasks (Allport, 1988). The interaction between cognitive and neurophysiological levels of investigation provides mutual constraints for models of attention and therefore for attentional dysfunction. We discuss the literature concerned with visual attentional deficits in schizophrenia using this recommendation as a framework. A review of the relevant cognitive psychological and neuropsychological literature will show that although many theories of attention have been applied to schizophrenia only a limited number have provided heuristic brain–behaviour models that link attentional deficits and the pathophysiology of schizophrenia. The major difficulty has been in defining attention itself, as many studies simply define attention as performance on their various attentional tasks. Finally, a brain–behaviour model of directed visual spatial attention which has proven validity in describing attentional deficits in primates with stereotaxic or chemical brain lesions and in humans with focal brain lesions is discussed with reference to the pathophysiology of schizophrenia.

CLINICAL PRESENTATION

As is shown in the various chapters of this edition, careful neuropsychological examination has revealed impairments in nearly all aspects of cognition in patients with schizophrenia. However, perhaps the oldest and most commonly reported cognitive deficit in these patients is in attention. Early descriptions of the clinical phenomenology of schizophrenia emphasised disordered attention, and described patients as being unable to screen out irrelevant stimuli from the environment, as being highly distractible or as having great difficulty maintaining concentration (Bleuler, 1911; Kraepelin, 1913; McGhie & Chapman, 1961; Venables, 1960). The current clinical diagnosis of schizophrenia does not require disordered attention to be present (i.e. Diagnostic and Statistical Manual of Mental Disorders IV; DSM-IV, American Psychiatric Association, 1994), although structured scales used to rate the severity and frequency of psychotic symptoms such as the scale for Positive and Negative Symptoms (SAPS/SANS) (Andreasen, 1983) or the Brief Psychiatric Rating Scale (BPRS) (Overall & Gorham, 1962) do require ratings of patients' ability to attend to the environment. Many researchers believe the symptoms of schizophrenia such as hallucinations and delusions are manifestations of disruptions to lower level cognitive processes which include attention (McGhie & Chapman, 1961; Frith, 1979; Carr & Wale, 1986; Robbins, 1991; Gray et al, 1991; Braff, 1993). Three examples typical of this view follow. Gray et al (1991) contend that the positive symptoms of schizophrenia (hallucinations and delusions) arise because patients are unable to regulate conscious attention. This lack of control allows aspects of the environment, which are not normally perceived, to intrude into awareness. Swerdlow & Koob (1987) postulate that patients with schizophrenia are unable to segregate relevant from irrelevant cognitions or emotions due to an inappropriate filtering process and Frith (1979) states that in schizophrenia automatic cognitive processes, which usually occur without awareness, enter consciousness. Each of these three hypotheses emphasise attention as being a process of selection that underlies conscious awareness and therefore the alterations in consciousness that occur in schizophrenia are due to a failure of this selective process. The emphasis on selection is important and carries with it the assumption that the brain does not have an infinite capacity for information processing (Mesulam, 1981) and that unattended stimuli are actively hindered from gaining access to central attentional mechanisms (Broadbent, 1971). These assumptions have guided the majority of studies of attention in schizophrenia.

NEUROPSYCHOLOGICAL TESTS OF ATTENTION

The similarity between the positive and negative symptoms of schizophrenia and the behavioural changes that accompany frontal lobe lesions is frequently reported. For example, both groups of patients can show high distractibility, impulsivity, difficulty with inhibiting inappropriate behaviour, apathy, blunting of affect and decreased initiative (Levin, 1984; Mesulam, 1981; Goldman-Rakic, 1987). There are also some similarities in neuropsychological test performance between patients with lesions of the prefrontal lobe and patients with schizophrenia. The most consistently reported performance deficit of executive function has been for tests such as the Wisconsin Card Sorting Task (WCST) (for reviews: Shallice et al, 1991; Pantelis et al, 1992; Weinberger et al, 1991; Levin et al, 1989). Finally, a number of neuroimaging studies of schizophrenia using positron emission tomography (PET) have shown decreased activation of the prefrontal area while patients perform the WCST (for review: Weinberger et al, 1991). In addition to executive function deficits, patients with frontal lobe lesions also have great difficulty in directing and maintaining visual attention (for review: Fuster, 1980). Therefore, the performance deficits found in patients with schizophrenia on neuropsychological tests which involve visual attention are usually thought to reflect some aspect of frontal lobe dysfunction. A review of the neuropsychological literature indicates that although attention deficits and frontal lobe signs are considered to be hallmarks of cognitive change in schizophrenia, very few neuropsychological studies have applied well-developed models of attention to the study of schizophrenia (see Shallice et al, 1991 for an exception). Furthermore, the contribution of attentional dysfunction to the performance deficits found on tasks involving multiple component cognitive control (e.g. WCST) in patients with schizophrenia is still unclear.

Instead, deficits in attention have been inferred from patterns of performance across a number of different neuropsychological tests. For example, studies which used empirical test batteries such as the Halstead–Reitan Battery, the Luria Nebraska Neuropsychological Test Battery or the Wechsler Adult Intelligence Scale (WAIS) to compare schizophrenia to organic brain damage, found that although performance deficits could vary widely in patients with schizophrenia they became most apparent on perceptual or cognitive tasks which demanded complex information processing, maintenance of attention or rapid psychomotor speed (for reviews: Eysenck, 1968; Goldstein, 1986; Pantelis et al, 1992). In addition, studies which compared patients with schizophrenia to normal controls also found that performance deficits became most apparent whenever time limits were placed on test performance (Babcock, 1933; Watson et al, 1968; Eysenck, 1968). The slowing of performance on timed tests or low scoring on tests with time limits has become one of the most replicated findings in the neuropsychological literature concerned with schizophrenia. Performance deficits on tests such as the WAIS digit symbol subtest (Eysenck, 1968; Shapiro & Nelson, 1955; Shallice et al, 1991; Saykin et al, 1994; Heaton et al, 1994), letter and number cancellation tasks (Babcock, 1933; Shapiro & Nelson, 1955; Nelson et al, 1990), the Trail Making Test (TMT) parts A and B (Watson et al, 1968; Goldstein, 1986; Goldberg et al, 1990; Shallice et al, 1991; Gold et al, 1994; Saykin et al, 1994; Heaton et al, 1994), and simple and complex reaction time tests (Zubin, 1975; Hemsley, 1982; Goldberg et al, 1990) are continually inferred to be evidence of attentional dysfunction in schizophrenia.

A selective review of recent neuropsychological studies of schizophrenia that have specified attention as one cognitive factor under investigation gives some indication of how poor performance on these attention demanding tests can be interpreted. Saykin et al (1994) compared the neuropsychological performance of two unmedicated patient groups, one with first episode schizophrenia and one with chronic schizophrenia and a group of controls matched for age and education. They found that both schizophrenia groups performed significantly worse than controls on the TMT parts A and B and on the WAIS digit symbol subtest. They concluded that attentional deficits reflect an underlying brain disorder that is present in the earliest stages of the disease. However, as attentional performance in the chronic group was slightly worse than the first episode group the researchers inferred that exposure to antipsychotic medication increased the magnitude of impairment on neuropsychological tests of attention (Saykin et al, 1994). Gold and colleagues (1994) found that the TMT parts A and B and the WAIS digit symbol subtest together with the WCST were the only tests from an extensive neuropsychological battery to differentiate patients with chronic schizophrenia from patients with either left or right temporal lobe epilepsy. They concluded that there was a loss of attentional control in schizophrenia that could not be explained on the basis of temporal lobe abnormalities. Nelson and her colleagues (1990) suggested that cognitive slowing and negative symptoms both arose from subcortical pathology in chronic schizophrenia because performance on a cancellation task from the Adult Memory and Information Processing Battery correlated with negative symptoms in patients with chronic schizophrenia. Heaton et al (1994) compared three groups of patients with schizophrenia who differed in age and in the age of disease onset and found that they were all equally as impaired on attentional tests when compared with normal controls. Heaton and colleagues concluded that the severity of attentional (and neuropsychological) deficits did not increase with disease progression. Finally, Goldberg et al (1990) reported that chronic medicated schizophrenic subjects performed significantly worse than their monozygotic co-twin on the TMT parts A and B test. This performance, together with poor performance on the continuous performance task, was interpreted as reflecting a deficit in deployment of attention which was illness specific and not related to genetic or non-specific environmental factors.

This limited review indicates that researchers are prepared to attribute performance deficits on attention demanding tests to some underlying dysfunction to the neural areas which control attention in patients with schizophrenia. However, while attention tests such as the TMT or WAIS digit symbol may be considered as attention-demanding, they differ in the extent to which they make demands, how such demands are made and which other cognitive processes are also required for successful performance. The poor performance on attention demanding tasks is consistent with the hypothesis that there is some decrease in the limited capacity for cognitive processing in schizophrenia which becomes most evident when patients must process information rapidly. However, most neuropsychological models do not specify the nature of attention deficit in schizophrenia beyond this level. Instead researchers infer that as there is both attentional and frontal lobe dysfunction in schizophrenia, and as patients with frontal lobe lesions have deficits in attention, then attentional deficits in schizophrenia must be due to the frontal lobe dysfunction (for review: Levin et al, 1989).

One exception to this approach is found in the work of Shallice (1988) who has sought to describe the attentional deficits in schizophrenia within the context of their "supervisory attentional system" (SAS). The SAS is based on two main premises. First, there is a large but finite set of discrete and goal-directed cognitive and motor programs that are distributed throughout various neural systems. These programs may also group to form more complex goal-directed programs which will occur automatically in routine situations. Selection and activation of these programs is dependent upon: (1) the presence of an appropriate trigger, (2) strength of activation of the program, (3) presence and exclusivity of other programs which are directed to the same or higher order goals, and (4) whether the goal is achieved. This process of selection and activation is termed "contention scheduling". The second premise of the SAS is that selection of programs for non-routine situations is qualitatively different and involves a central executive system, the SAS, which modulates the operation of the rest of the system. Shallice (1988) argues that the SAS is not a central limited capacity filter through which all attentional information passes, instead most well-defined situations requiring goal directed action can be handled by the routine cognitive or motor programs, i.e. via the "contention scheduling" system. The SAS is only required for "novel" or less routine tasks where goal directed programs are insufficient to produce an appropriate response. To achieve this the SAS may alter the priorities of the contention scheduling system by activating or inhibiting particular programs. Careful neuropsychological studies indicate that integrity of the frontal lobes is essential for the operation of the SAS, while the routine cognitive and motor programs are distributed through the various neurocognitive networks which are associated with their respective sensory and higher order processes (e.g. visual; tactile; auditory perception). Attentional deficits observed in the behaviour of patients with frontal lobe lesions, such as impulsivity and distraction, occur because a dysfunctional SAS allows the activation and selection of inappropriate cognitive and motor programs in novel situations which are attention catching (Shallice, 1988). Recently, Shallice et al (1991) investigated a small group of medicated patients with chronic schizophrenia on a comprehensive battery of neuropsychological tests. They found that although levels of ability varied considerably between patients, all patients performed poorly on tests sensitive to frontal lobe function. Performance was especially impaired on the TMT part A and part B tests. Shallice and colleagues inferred that the pattern of deficits was consistent with an impairment in the SAS in schizophrenia. According to this model attentional deficits in schizophrenia may arise because the SAS fails to inhibit responses to irrelevant stimuli that are potentially attention catching. Although this model provides a useful brain–behaviour framework for neuropsychological investigation of attention in schizophrenia, more research needs to be carried out on the development of tests which are sensitive to, and diagnostic of, interruptions in the relationship between the contention scheduling system and the SAS in schizophrenia as well as in normal subjects.

INFORMATION PROCESSING MODELS OF ATTENTION

Early experimental studies found that, when compared to normal control subjects, patients with schizophrenia showed slower reaction times (RTs) to simple visual targets and were unable to use warning signals or preparatory foreperiods to benefit RT to the same extent as controls (Shakow, 1962; Kornetsky & Mirsky, 1966). The poor performance found in the schizophrenia groups was interpreted to indicate an inability to sustain the readiness to respond to task-relevant stimuli over time. Later studies of attention in schizophrenia became heavily influenced by the filter theory of Broadbent (1971). This theory conceptualised attention as a central limited processing capacity which selected information for identification or categorisation and actively excluded non-selected information from further processing. According to theorists using the attentional filter model, deficits in attention arose in schizophrenia because patients were unable to exclude irrelevant information (both internal and external) from entering conscious awareness and taking up the limited processing space, thus making it more difficult to process relevant information (for reviews: Carr & Wale, 1986). This theory still guides current information processing research, the goal of which is to identify the specific stage of attentional processing at which the defective filtering occurs. Current investigations apply more sophisticated information processing models to the examination of visual attention in schizophrenia and these generally fall into three major paradigms, the continuous performance task (CPT), the backward masking task and the span of apprehension task. The CPT requires subjects to monitor a continuous stream of stimuli (e.g. single numbers or letters) which are presented briefly at about one per second and to respond to a predetermined target or sequence of targets (e.g. "X", or "X" only when it follows "A"). Performance on the CPT is usually measured by calculating the number of correct responses (hits) and false positive responses (misses) (Rosvold et al, 1956). Compared to control subjects, patients with schizophrenia usually show lower hit rates and equal or greater false alarm rates (Orzack & Kornetsky, 1966). These performance deficits are accentuated further when the task demands of the CPT are increased. For example, when stimuli consist of degraded letters or numbers (Nuechterlein, 1983), when the rate of presentation is increased (Nuechterlein & Dawson, 1984) or when information about the previous stimuli is required to determine a target (Erlenmeyer-Kimling & Cornblatt, 1978). Performance deficits in the various CPT experiments have been interpreted as reflecting impaired signal detection performance (Cohen & Servan-Schreiber, 1992) or an impaired ability to sustain focused attention over time (Nuechterlein & Dawson, 1984).

Backward masking paradigms present a target for a short period (e.g. 20 ms) which is followed by a masking stimulus of nonsensical lines that overlap the location of the initial stimulus. This mask is capable of interfering with or erasing the conscious registration of the target stimulus thereby limiting the duration of the sensory signal itself. On each trial subjects are required to identify the target stimulus while the interval between the target and masking stimulus is varied (typically from 0 to 300 ms). Normal subjects can generally perceive the stimulus when the interstimulus interval is in the 60–240 ms range. However, in patients with schizophrenia the masking stimulus interferes with stimulus perception even when there is 100 ms between the two events (Braff, 1993). Furthermore, masking deficits, qualitatively similar to those found in schizophrenia, have been reported in patients with schizophrenia spectrum disorders (Braff, 1981) and remitted schizophrenia (Miller et al, 1979). These results have usually been interpreted as indicating that patients with schizophrenia require more time to transfer visual information from sensory registration buffers into short-term memory and that schizophrenia spectrum patients have a specific time linked vulnerability to processing rapidly presented sequential visual stimuli (Braff, 1993). A very similar test, the span of apprehension test, requires subjects to make a forced choice discrimination regarding which of two previously instructed target letters is present in a briefly presented (e.g. 50-70 msec) array. The array contains either just the target stimulus or the target stimulus in conjunction with several other irrelevant letters. Generally, patients with schizophrenia perform at similar levels to controls on target only conditions. However, performance declines markedly as the number of irrelevant letters is increased, as the arrays become more complex (Asarnow & MacCrimmon, 1978, 1981) or as the visual angle of target stimuli is increased (Asarnow et al, 1991). The decrease in performance with increase in array size found in individuals with schizophrenia or with vulnerability for schizophrenia has been interpreted to reflect the slowed processing of visual information from sensory storage (Davidson & Neale, 1974).

As with neuropsychological tests, performance deficits on the various information processing tasks are independent of the effects of antipsychotic medication. This is because similar processing deficits are found in both unmedicated and medicated patients at the acute and chronic stages of the illness (Asarnow & MacCrimmon, 1978; Braff & Sacuzzo, 1982; Nuechterlein & Dawson, 1984) and in individuals "at risk" for developing schizophrenia who are not taking any antipsychotic medication (Cornblatt et al, 1989; Sterenko and Woods, 1978; Asarnow et al, 1977). Instead, there is evidence that antipsychotic medication slightly decreases the magnitude of attentional deficits found on information processing tasks (Spohn & Strauss, 1989; Braff, 1993).

The different performance deficits found on the various information processing tasks have been difficult to equate with a specific dysfunctional stage of attention in schizophrenia. More recently, some authors have interpreted information processing performance deficits within the context of resource models of attention. These models define attentional resources as limited pools, skills, structures or processes that are available at a given moment to allow performance of cognitive tasks. Limiting task performance time or decreasing signal-to-noise ratios creates greater demands on these limited processing resources (Kahenman, 1973; Hirst & Kalmar, 1987). According to the attentional resource model, patients with schizophrenia perform poorly when attentional processing demands are high but are able to perform normally when processing loads are low. Therefore, patients with schizophrenia must either have a reduced amount of processing resources available for essential cognitive operations or reach the limits of the available resources at lower resource demands than controls (Nuechterlein & Dawson, 1984; Granholm et al, 1991; Braff, 1993).

The resource model offers a parsimonious theory within which to relate the many different types of performance deficits found in information processing studies to a general attentional deficit associated with schizophrenia. However, the assumptions of the attentional resource model have been devastatingly criticised in a number of recent reviews which conclude that attention processing resource models are generally circular in that they define attention in terms of performance on a particular attentional task (Navon, 1984; Allport, 1988). Therefore, such models do not adequately define the nature of their limited attentional processing resources, how these processing resources are limited or what the nature of any central structural bottleneck might be. Critics of the attentional resources model recommend that the focus of attentional research in general should be shifted from attempts to define a selectivity of processing to definitions which emphasise selection for action (Allport, 1988). For schizophrenia, this suggests that the attentional resource model is an inadequate explanation for the highly specific deficits found in information processing experiments. It also suggests that the emphasis on ill-defined processing resources and their limitations will be very difficult to relate to the function of specific brain systems.

ASYMMETRIES OF VISUAL SPATIAL ATTENTION IN SCHIZOPHRENIA

Neuropsychological models which define attention as the process by which visual spatial information is selected from the environment have had more success in specifying brain–behaviour hypotheses of attentional deficits in schizophrenia. In this model, the limitations on attention are most evident (and measurable) when the individual is unable to use information in the visual field contralateral to a specific brain lesion for any sort of goal-directed behaviour, for example, dressing, eating or navigation (Mesulam, 1981; Heilman et al, 1985). Experimental investigations have shown that patients with neglect fail to orient, respond to or report salient stimuli appearing in the visual field contralateral to the lesion, in the absence of any sensory or perceptual deficits and this can be accentuated if stimuli are presented to both visual fields (Mesulam, 1981; Heilman et al, 1985). This attentional neglect is most commonly seen in patients with lesions of the right parietal lobe; however, neglect can occur with unilateral lesions to other brain cortical and subcortical brain areas (for reviews: Mesulam, 1981; Heilman et al, 1985). Furthermore, single neuron recording and chemical lesion studies in primates (Robinson & Petersen, 1986; Petersen et al, 1985; Kertzman & Robinson, 1988; Colby, 1990) and PET and lesion studies in humans (Mesulam, 1981; Heilman et al, 1985; Corbetta et al, 1991, 1993; Paus et al, 1993) have found no evidence of a single brain area likely to contain a central processor which assigns processing resources or which can in some way limit the direction of attention to locations in the visual field. Instead, these studies have indicated that the control of visual spatial attention is more likely to be achieved through a distributed cortical and subcortical neural network. In such a network, the elementary cognitive operations that make up the performance of an attentional task may be localised to individual nodes within the network and the relative activation of these individual components of the network can be reconfigured depending on the task demands (for reviews: Posner, 1988; Colby 1990).

Interestingly, studies of directed visual spatial attention consistently find evidence of subtle right-sided attentional impairment in patients with schizophrenia. For example, such patients neglect the right hemispace on the face–hand test and tests for graphasthesia (Fuller-Torrey, 1980). The graphasthesia performance asymmetry was replicated by Manschreck & Ames (1984), who also demonstrated right-sided deficits on tasks of stereognosis in the same subjects with schizophrenia. The magnitude of these asymmetries correlated with measures of thought disorder. Tomer & Flor-Henry (1989) found that both unmedicated and recently medicated patients with schizophrenia omitted more right visual field (RVF) targets than left visual field (LVF) targets on letter and number cancellation tasks, while controls showed symmetrical performance. At retest, after an average of 5 weeks of antipsychotic medication, asymmetry indices were reversed in the patients with schizophrenia and they now omitted more LVF than RVF targets. However, this reversal in symmetry did not occur because the number of omissions in the RVF had decreased but because the number of omissions in the LVF had increased. Tomer (1990) also reported that in unmedicated patients with schizophrenia indices of right neglect from the cancellation task were associated with a preference for reporting RVF targets. She suggested that attentional asymmetries in schizophrenia arose from a hyper-orienting to the LVF rather than RVF neglect. Unmedicated subjects with schizophrenia also showed asymmetrical performance on an attentional filtering task (Wigal et al, 1991; LaBerge & Buchsbaum, 1990). When required to detect a target letter that appeared in the LVF or RVF, both medicated and unmedicated patients with schizophrenia, as well as controls showed symmetrical responses for all target locations. However, when a target letter appeared

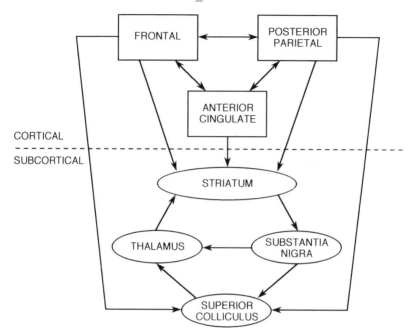

Figure 6.1. Pathways between cortical and subcortical structures involved in the neurocognitive network for directed spatial attention. Damage to any neural structure or disruption to any of the interconnections between structures will result in a change in attentional behaviour

flanked by letters of a similar appearance, the responses of the unmedicated patients to targets in the RVF were significantly slower than to targets in the LVF while performance in the medicated patients remained symmetrical (Wigal et al, 1991). Chronic medicated subjects with schizophrenia also showed evidence of a right sided neglect when required to indicate the centre of a rod while blindfolded and the extent of this neglect was positively correlated with symptom severity rated on the BPRS (Harvey et al, 1993). These findings of right sided attentional impairment in schizophrenia suggest that one neurological consequence of the disorder is an asymmetrical disruption to the neural network underlying directed visual attention.

Although lesions of the posterior parietal cortices are the most common cause of neglect (Mesulam, 1981), attempts to explain the subtle impairments in right hemispace in patients with schizophrenia have centred mainly on the role of ascending dopaminergic pathways. This probably reflects the prevailing strength of the dopamine hypothesis in the schizophrenia literature, although disruption to many different subcortical and cortical nuclei will result in a deficit in attention to contralateral visual stimuli (Posner, 1988; Colby, 1990) (see Figure 1). The dopamine hypothesis asserts that, at least in some patients with schizophrenia, there is an overactivity of mesolimbic, mesocortical or nigrostriatal dopaminergic neurones (Seeman, 1993). The normalisation of attentional asymmetries with antipsychotic medication suggests that right sided neglect found in unmedicated patients with schizophrenia may be due to lateralised dopamine dysfunction in one or more of the neural structures involved in directed attention. Tomer & Flor-Henry (1989) postulated that the right hemispace omissions in their unmedicated patients reflected lower dopamine levels in the left hemisphere. Cancellation task performance in unmedicated patients with schizophrenia is also qualitatively similar to patients with left hemi-Parkinson's disease. In hemi-Parkinson's disease the dopamine deficiency is greater in the striatum contralateral to the side of the inattentive behaviour (Miller & Beninger, 1990; Heilman et al, 1985). Tomer & Flor-Henry (1989) suggested that antipsychotic drugs reverse attentional asymmetries by suppressing right hemisphere dopamine function rather than improving left hemisphere function. Asymmetries in responses to the attentional filtering task (Wigal et al, 1991) were also attributed to left hemisphere dopaminergic dysfunction. When the same task was performed by normal subjects undergoing PET scanning, it was found that the pulvinar that was contralateral to targets presented in the flanked display showed greater glucose uptake (LaBerge & Buchsbaum, 1990). As the pulvinar has a demonstrated role in the neural network underlying directed visual attention (Petersen et al, 1985), Wigal and colleagues (1991) suggested that the slowing of responses to RVF letters reflected a dysfunction of the left pulvinar or its dopaminergic connections since performance became symmetrical after antipsychotic medication.

Other support for the relationship between attentional asymmetries and asymmetries in striatal dopamine levels in schizophrenia is derived from the rotating rodent model which has been extensively used to investigate the role of the ascending dopaminergic pathways in subcortical structures. This model is based on the finding that animals preferentially rotate toward the hemisphere with lower striatal dopaminergic activity regardless of their physical surroundings (Pycock, 1980; Miller & Beninger, 1990). This rotation is considered to be a manifestation of contralateral hemi-inattention (Heilman et al, 1985; Miller & Beninger, 1990). Dopaminergic asymmetries can also be induced by amphetamine which increases endogenous intrahemispheric asymmetries and causes animals to rotate in tight circles toward the side with the lower dopamine level (Pycock, 1980). Postsynaptic dopamine agonists produce rotation away from a nigral lesion because they most strongly affect the striatum on the lesioned side where dopamine receptors have increased in number. In unlesioned animals, only dopaminergic agonists can induce rotation while antidopaminergic drugs (i.e. antipsychotics) can block drug induced rotation in rodents (Pycock, 1980; Miller & Beninger, 1990). Circling behaviour has also been studied in patients with schizophrenia (Bracha, 1987). When measured over a single day, unmedicated subjects with schizophrenia showed significantly more 360 degree leftward than rightward turns. After a brief period of antipsychotic medication, schizophrenic subjects' turning preferences returned to normal symmetry. These results were interpreted to indicate that the subtle right sided neglect in schizophrenia arose from an imbalance in the ascending dopaminergic pathways and this imbalance occurred from an asymmetrical dopamine input to the striatum (Bracha et al, 1987).

A number of recent studies of directed visual attention in schizophrenia have further specified some aspects of the right-sided attention deficit. Posner et al (1988a) found that when targets appeared at cued locations in the RVF and LVF, schizophrenic subjects' RTs were symmetrical. This indicated that subjects could engage targets when attention was cued to the correct location. However, when the subject's attention was first cued into the LVF and the subsequent target appeared in RVF, RTs were much slower than for targets which appeared in the LVF following RVF cues. This indicated that schizophrenic subjects had difficulty disengaging attention for rightward shifts of attention. Posner and co-workers (1988a) noted the similarity between the asymmetrical disengagement deficit they found in patients with schizophrenia and that found in patients with lesions of the left parietal lobe (Posner et al, 1984). However, they also speculated that, in schizophrenia, attentional asymmetries were part of a broader range of structural and cognitive deficits that reflected the effects of reduced left striatal dopaminergic activity on the anterior attentional system through disruption of the cortico-striatal loop which involves both the anterior cingulate and the ventral striatum (Posner et al, 1988a; Early et al, 1990a, 1990b). Posner et al (1987) were also able to induce qualitatively similar attentional asymmetries to those found in schizophrenia by having normal subjects perform the covert orienting of visual attention task (COVAT) and an auditory shadowing task simultaneously. This suggested that attention to language and attention to visual spatial location share limited processing resources and that the processing of each task occurs within a single or heavily interconnected anatomical system (Posner et al, 1987; Posner et al, 1988a, 1988b). Anatomical studies have indicated that the anterior cingulate cortex has strong reciprocal connections with both frontal and parietal attentional areas (Mesulam, 1981; Goldman-Rakic, 1987) and it has been demonstrated that lesions of the anterior cingulate result in neglect in both humans and primates and also in language deficits in humans (Early et al, 1990b; Watson et al, 1973). Studies of normal subjects using PET show that activation of the anterior cingulate cortex is common to tasks that involve the selection of both visual and verbal information and that there is a positive relationship between task difficulty and activation of the anterior cingulate cortex during these attentional tasks (Pardo et al, 1990; Frith et al, 1991; Corbetta et al, 1993; Paus et al, 1993; Frackowiak, 1994).

Three subsequent studies have replicated aspects of this attentional asymmetry in schizophrenia (Potkin et al, 1989; Carter et al, 1992; Maruff et al, 1995) while several other studies have found no or very weak evidence for a RVF deficit in orienting of attention (Strauss et al, 1991, 1992; Moran et al, 1992; Nestor et al, 1992; Gold et al, 1992; Liotti et al, 1993; Maruff et al, 1995). Where studies failed to find an asymmetry in COVAT performance in schizophrenia, researchers speculated that attentional asymmetries may be specific to the acute stages of the illness (Strauss et al 1991, 1992; Nestor et al, 1992). We recently reported that attentional asymmetries were specific to the acute stages of schizophrenia (Maruff et al, 1995). In addition, we found that in the acute stages of illness, asymmetries in disengaging attention became most obvious when positive symptom levels and COVAT task demands were high. Reducing positive symptom levels with short periods of antipsychotic medication or reducing task demands in subjects with high levels of positive symptoms normalised these asymmetries. Interestingly, no asymmetrical COVAT performance was found in unmedicated subjects who were actively psychotic but who did not have schizophrenia. We interpreted the interaction between positive symptoms and attentional asymmetries as reflecting a disease specific disruption to the neural area shown to be involved in attention to both language and visual spatial attention, the anterior cingulate cortex.

Support for the involvement of striatal dopamine levels in attentional asymmetries in schizophrenia also comes from PET studies of the basal ganglia. In neuroleptic-naive patients with schizophrenia metabolic activity was increased in the left globus pallidus (Buchsbaum et al, 1987; Early et al, 1987; Early et al, 1990a; Seeman, 1993) and reduced in the right caudate and putamen (Buchsbaum et al, 1987). In addition, there was a greater binding affinity for antipsychotic medication in the right caudate and putamen (Buchsbaum et al, 1987) and Farde et al (1990) have reported greater numbers of D2 receptors in the left striatum compared to the right. Taken together, these studies provide strong support for a relationship between right sided neglect and asymmetrical dopamine function in schizophrenia. Despite this evidence, however, relatively little is known about which site(s) in the neural network underlying directed attention is responsible for the disruption to the dopamine system and whether neglect of the RVF arises from a decrease of dopaminergic input to the left hemisphere or an increase in dopaminergic input to the right hemisphere dopamine. Morphological studies of brains from patients with schizophrenia have generally failed to find abnormalities in areas rich in either dopaminergic neurones or dopaminergic terminals (Gray et al, 1991).

In addition to the striatum, converging neuropathological evidence has consistently implicated two further areas in the pathophysiology of schizophrenia, the temporal lobe and the frontal lobe (for reviews: Gray et al, 1991; Robbins, 1991; Early et al, 1990a, 1990b; Buchsbaum, 1990). Postmortem and imaging studies have revealed abnormalities in the limbic regions of the temporal lobe including enlargement of the cerebral ventricles (Crow et al, 1989) and cytoarchitectonic changes in the entorhinal cortex (Jakob & Beckman, 1986), parahippocampal gyrus (Bogerts et al, 1985) hippocampus (Bogerts et al, 1985) and cingulate gyrus (Benes & Bird, 1987; Benes, 1989). Dysfunction of the frontal lobes, particularly the dorsolateral prefrontal cortex (DLPFC) is inferred on the basis of the similarity between the behavioural symptoms of schizophrenia and those of patients with frontal lobe lesions (Goldman-Rakic, 1987), deficits on neuropsychological tasks of executive function (Shallice et al, 1991; Pantelis et al, 1992; Weinberger et al, 1991), decreased prefrontal metabolic activity during PET activation tasks (Weinberger et al, 1991) and structural abnormalities in DLPFC neurones (Benes, 1989). Although relationships between functions of the temporal lobes and directed visual spatial attention are not known, both the cingulate cortex and the frontal lobes are essential for the organism to direct visual attention to locations in the visual field (e.g. Colby, 1990).

CONCLUSION

Studies of attention have dominated the literature on neurocognitive dysfunction in schizophrenia. However, the nature of the attentional deficit and its relationship to the known pathophysiology of the disease remain unclear. Although there is some correlational evidence that suggests a relationship between the clinical symptoms of schizophrenia and performance deficits on attentional tasks, the contribution of disordered attention to the clinical phenomenology of schizophrenia is also unclear. This has occurred in part because of the difficulty in specifying an operational definition of attention itself. In schizophrenia, attempts to link disordered attention to an underlying brain change have been most successful when attention has been defined as the selection of information for a goal-directed purpose rather than as an internal limited capacity selection process. When the definition of attention is restricted to the goal-directed selection of visual spatial information there is enormous overlap between the neural systems shown to be involved in the direction of attention and the neural areas and systems consistently implicated in the pathophysiology of schizophrenia. Furthermore, both lines of research have suggested that the attentional deficit that arises in schizophrenia is unlikely to be due to disruption to a single neural area or single neurochemical system (i.e. a single central attentional processor). Instead, the attentional deficit is most probably due to a dysfunctional neurocognitive network for directed attention which is distributed across a number of cortical and subcortical brain areas and also involves a number of different neurotransmitter systems.

REFERENCES

Allport, A. (1988) Visual attention. In: *Foundations of Cognitive Science* (Ed. M.I. Posner), MIT Press, Cambridge, MA.

American Psychiatric Association (1994) *Diagnostic And Statistical Manual Of Mental Disorders (DSM-V)* (4th edn), American Psychiatric Association, Washington.

Andreasen, N.C. (1983) *The Scale For The Assessment Of Positive And Negative Symptoms*. Iowa City, Iowa.

Asarnow, R.F., MacCrimmon, D.J. (1978) Residual performance deficit in clinically remitted schizophrenics: A marker for schizophrenia? *Journal of Abnormal Psychology*, **87**, 597–608.

Asarnow, R.F., MacCrimmon, D.J. (1981) Span of apprehension deficits during postpsychotic stages of schizophrenia. *Archives of General Psychiatry*, **38**, 1006–1011.

Asarnow, R.F., Steffy, R.A., MacCrimmon, D.J., Cleghorn, J.M. (1977) An attentional assessment of foster children at risk for schizophrenia. *Journal of Abnormal Psychology*, **86**, 267–275.

Asarnow, R.F., Granholm, E., Chairman, T. (1991) Span of apprehension in schizophrenia. In: *Handbook of schizophrenia: Experimental Psychopathology, Neuropsychology and Psychophysiology*, Vol. 4 (Eds H.A. Nasrallah, J. Zubin, S. Steinhauer, J.H. Gruzelier), pp. 335–370. Elsevier, Amsterdam.

Babcock, H. (1933) *Dementia Praecox: A Psychological Study*, Science Press, New York.

Benes, F.M. (1989) Myelination of cortical–hippocampal relays during late adolescence. *Schizophrenia Bulletin*, **15**, 585–593.

Benes, F.M., Bird, E.D. (1987) An analysis of the arrangement of neurones in the cingulate cortex of schizophrenic patients. *Archives of General Psychiatry*, **44**, 608–616.

Bleuler, E. (1911) *Dementia Praecox or the Group of Schizophrenias* (translated by J. Zinkin, 1950), International Universities Press, New York.

Bogerts, B., Meetz, E., Schonfeldt-Bausch, R. (1985) Basal ganglia and limbic system pathology in schizophrenia. A morphometric study of brain volume and shrinkage. *Archives of General Psychiatry*, **42**, 784–791.

Bracha, H.S. (1987) Asymmetric rotational (circling) behaviour, a dopamine related asymmetry: Preliminary findings in unmedicated and never medicated schizophrenics. *Biological Psychiatry*, **22**, 995–1002.

Braff, D.L. (1981) Impaired speed of information processing in non-medicated schizotypal patients. *Schizophrenia Bulletin*, **7**, 499–508.

Braff, D.L. (1993) Information processing and attention dysfunctions in schizophrenia. *Schizophrenia Bulletin*, **19**, 233–259.

Braff, D.L., Saccuzzo, D.P. (1982) The effect of antipsychotic medication on speed of information processing in schizophrenia. *American Journal of Psychiatry*, **139**, 1127–1130.

Broadbent, D.E. (Ed.) (1971) *Decision And Stress*, Academic Press, London.

Buchsbaum, M.S. (1990) The frontal lobes, and temporal lobes as sites for schizophrenia. *Schizophrenia Bulletin*, **16**, 379–388.

Buchsbaum, M.S., Wu, J., DeLisi, L.E., Holcomb, H.H., Hazlett, E., Cooper-Langston, K., Kessler, R. (1987) Positron emission tomography studies of basal ganglia and somatosensory cortex neuroleptic drug effects: Differences between normal controls and schizophrenic patients. *Biological Psychiatry*, **22**, 479–494.

Carr, V., Wale, J. (1986) Schizophrenia: An information processing model. *Australian and New Zealand Journal of Psychiatry*, **20**, 136–155.

Carter, C.S., Robertson, L.C., Chanderjian, M.R., Celaya, L.J., Nordahl, T.E. (1992) Attentional asymmetries in schizophrenia. Controlled versus Automatic processing. *Biological Psychiatry*, **31**, 909–918.

Cohen, J.D., Servan-Schreiber, D. (1992) Context, cortex and dopamine: A connectionist approach to behavior and biology in schizophrenia. *Psychological Review*, **99**, 45–77.

Colby, C.L. (1990) The neuroanatomy and neurophysiology of attention. *Journal of Child Neurology*, **6**, S90–S118.

Corbetta, M., Miezen, F.M., Dobymeyer, S., Shulman, G., Petersen, S.E. (1991) Selective and divided attention during visual discriminations of shape, colour and speed. Functional anatomy by positron emission tomography. *Journal of Neuroscience*, **11**, 2383–2402.

Corbetta, M., Miezin, F.M., Shulman, G., Petersen, S.E. (1993) A PET study of visuospatial attention. *Journal of Neuroscience*, **13**, 1202–1226.

Cornblatt, B.A., Winters, L., Erlenmeyer-Kimling, L. (1989) Attentional markers of schizophrenia: Evidence from the New York high risk study. In: *Schizophrenia: Scientific Progress* (Eds S.C. Schulz, C.A. Tamminga), pp. 83–92, Oxford University Press, New York.

Crow, T.J., Ball, J., Bloom, R., Bruton, C.J., Colter, N., Frith, C.D., Johnstome, E.C., Owens, D.G., Roberts, G.W. (1989) Schizophrenia as an anomaly of the development of cerebral asymmetry. *Archives of General Psychiatry*, **46**, 1145–150.

Davidson.G.S., Neale, J.M. (1974) The effects of signal–noise similarity on visual information processing of schizophrenics. *Journal of Abnormal Psychology*, **83**, 683–686.

Early, T.S., Reiman, E.M., Raichle, M.E., Spitznagel, E.L. (1987) Left globus pallidus abnormality in never medicated patients with schizophrenia. *Proceedings of the National Academy of Science*, **84**, 561–563.

Early, T.S., Posner, M.I., Reiman, E.M., Raichle, M.E. (1990a) Hyperactivity of the left striatopallidal projection. Part 1: Lower level theory. *Psychiatric Developments*, **2**, 85–108.

Early, T.S., Posner, M.I., Reiman, E.M., Raichle, M.E. (1990b) Hyperactivity of the left striatopallidal projection. Part 2: Phenomenology and thought disorder. *Psychiatric Developments*, **2**, 109–121.

Erlenmeyer-Kimling, L., Cornblatt, B. (1978) Attentional measures in a study of children at high risk for schizophrenia. In: *Nature Of Schizophrenia: New Approaches To Research And Treatment* (Eds L.C. Wynne, R. Cromwell, S. Matthysse), pp. 359–365, Wiley, New York.

Eysenck, H.J. (Ed.) (1968) *Handbook of Abnormal Psychology: An Experimental Approach*, Pitman Medical, London.

Farde, L., Wiesel, F.A., Stone-Elander, S.S., Halldin, C., Norsdstrom, A.L., Sedvall, G. (1990) D2 dopamine receptors in neuroleptic naive schizophrenic patients. *Archives of General Psychiatry*, **47**, 213–219.

Frackowiak, S.J. (1994) Functional mapping of verbal memory and language. *Trends in Neuroscience*, **17**, 109–115.

Frith, C.D. (1979) Consciousness, information processing and schizophrenia. *British Journal of Psychiatry*, **134**, 225–235.

Frith, C.D., Friston, K.J., Liddle, P.F., Frackowiak, R.S.J. (1991) Willed action and the prefrontal cortex in man: A study with PET. *Proceedings of the Royal Society of London*, B, **244**, 241–246.

Fuller-Torrey, E.F. (1980) Neurological abnormalities in schizophrenic patients. *Biological Psychiatry*, **15**, 995–1003.

Fuster, J.M. (1980) *The Prefrontal Cortex*, Raven Press, New York.

Gold, J.M., Randolph, C., Coppola, R., Carpenter, C.J., Goldberg, T.E., Weinberger, D.R. (1992) Visual orienting in schizophrenia. *Schizophrenia Research*, **7**, 203–209.

Gold, J.M., Hermann, B.P., Randolph, C., Wyler, A.R., Goldberg, T.E., Weinberger, D.R. (1994) Schizophrenia and temporal lobe epilepsy: A neuropsychological analysis. *Archives of General Psychiatry*, **51**, 265–272.

Goldberg, T.E., Ragland, J.D., Fuller-Torrey, E., Gold, J.M., Bigelow, L.B., Weinberger, D.R. (1990) Neuropsychological assessment of monozygotic twins discordant for schizophrenia. *Archives of General Psychiatry*, **47**, 1066–1072.

Goldman-Rakic, P.S. (1987) Circuitry of primate prefrontal cortex and regulation of behavior by representational memory. In: *Higher Cortical Function. American Physiological Society Handbook of Physiology*, Vol. 5 (Eds F. Plum, V. Mountcastle), pp. 373–417, American Physiological Society, Bethesda, MD.

Goldstein, G. (1986) The neuropsychology of schizophrenia. In: *Neuropsychological Assessment Of Neuropsychiatric Disorders* (Eds I. Grant, K.H. Adams), pp. 147–171, Oxford University Press, Oxford.

Granholm, E., Asarnow, R.F., Marder, S.R. (1991) Controlled information processing resources and the development of automatic detection responses in schizophrenia. *Journal of Abnormal Psychology*, **100**, 22–30.

Gray, J.A., Feldon, J., Rawlins, J.N.P., Hemsley, D.R., Smith, A.D. (1991) The neurophysiology of schizophrenia. *Behavioural and Brain Sciences*, **14**, 1–84.

Harvey, S.A., Nelson, E., Haller, J.W., Early, T.S. (1993) Lateralized attentional abnormality in schizophrenia is correlated with severity of symptoms. *Biological Psychiatry*, **33**, 93–99.

Heaton, R., Paulsen, J., McAdams, L.A., Kuck, J., Zisook, S., Braff, D., Harris, J., Jeste, D. (1994) Neuropsychological deficits in schizophrenics. Relationship to age, chronicity and dementia. *Archives of General Psychiatry*, **51**, 469–476.

Heilman, K., Valenstein, E., Watson, R.T. (1985) Neglect and related disorders. In: *Clinical Neuropsychology* (Eds K.M. Heilman, E. Valenstein), pp. 243–293, Oxford University Press, New York.

Hemsley, D.R. (1982) Cognitive impairment in schizophrenia. In: *The Pathology And Psychology Of Cognition* (Ed. A. Burton), pp. 169–203, Methuen, London.

Hirst, W., Kalmar, D. (1987) Characterising attentional resources. *Journal of Experimental Psychology: General*, **116**, 68–81.

Jakob, H., Beckman, H. (1986) Prenatal development disturbances in the limbic allocortex in schizophrenics. *Journal of Neural Transmission*, **65**, 303–326.

Kahenman, D. (Ed.) (1973) *Attention And Effort*, Prentice-Hall, Englewood Cliffs, NJ.

Kertzman, C., Robinson, D.L. (1988) Contributions of the superior colliculus of the monkey to spatial attention. *Society for Neuroscience Abstracts*, **14**, 831.

Kornetsky, C., Mirsky, A.F. (1966) On certain psychopharmacological and physiological differences between schizophrenic patients and normal persons. *Psychopharmacologica*, **8**, 99–106.

Kraepelin, E. (1913) *Dementia Praecox And Paraphrenia* (translated by R.M. Barclay, 1919), Livingstone, Edinburgh.

LaBerge, D., Buchsbaum, M.S. (1990) Positron emission tomographic measurements of pulvinar activity during an attention task. *Journal of Neuroscience*, **10**, 613–619.

Levin, S. (1984) Frontal lobe dysfunctions in schizophrenia. I. Eye movement impairments. *Journal of Psychiatric Research*, **18**, 27–55.

Levin, S., Yugelun-Todd, D.A., Craft, S. (1989) Contributions of clinical neuropsychology to the study of schizophrenia. *Journal of Abnormal Psychology*, **98**, 341–356.

Liotti, M., Dazzi, S., Umilta, C. (1993) Deficits of the automatic orienting of attention in schizophrenic patients. *Journal of Psychiatry Research*, **27**, 119–130.

Manschreck, T.C., Ames, D. (1984) Neurologic features and psychopathology in schizophrenic disorders. *Biological Psychiatry*, **19**, 703–719.

Maruff, P., Hay, D., Malone, V., Currie, J. (1995) Asymmetries of covert attention in schizophrenia. *Neuropsychologia*, **33**, 1205–1233.

Maruff, P., Pantelis, C., Danckert, J., Smith, D., Currie, J. Deficits in the endogenous control of exogenous attention in chronic schizophrenia. *Neuropsychologia*, (in press).

McGhie, A., Chapman, J. (1961) Disorders of attention and perception in early schizophrenia. *British Journal of Medical Psychology*, **34**, 103–116.

Mesulam, M.-M. (1981) A cortical network for directed attention and unilateral neglect. *Annals of Neurology*, **10**, 309–325.

Miller, R., Beninger, R.W. (1990) On the interpretation of asymmetries of posture and locomotion produced with dopamine agonists in animals with depletion of striatal dopamine. *Progress in Neurobiology*, **36**, 229–256.

Miller, S., Saccuzzo, D., Braff, D. (1979) Information processing deficits in remitted schizophrenics. *Journal of Abnormal Psychology*, **88**, 446–449.

Moran, M.J., Thaker, G.K., Smith, D., Cassady, S., Layne-Gedge, J. (1992) Shifts of covert visual attention in schizophrenic patients and normal controls. *Biological Psychiatry*, **32**, 617–620.

Navon, D. (1984) Attentional resources—theoretical soup stone? *Psychological Review*, **91**, 216–234.

Nelson, H.E., Pantelis, C., Carruthers, K., Speller, J., Blaxendale, S., Barnes, T.R.E. (1990) Cognitive functioning and symptomatology in chronic schizophrenia. *Psychological Medicine*, **20**, 357–365.

Nestor, P., Faux, S.F., McCarley, R.W., Penhune, V., Shenton, M.E., Pollack, S., Sands, S.F. (1992) Attentional cues in chronic schizophrenia: Abnormal disengagement of attention. *Journal of Abnormal Psychology*, **101**, 682–689.

Nuechterlein, K.H. (1983) Signal detection in vigilance tasks and behavioural attributes among offspring of schizophrenic mothers and among hyperactive children. *Journal of Abnormal Psychology*, **92**, 4–28.

Nuechterlein, K.H., Dawson, M.E. (1984) Information processing and attentional functioning in the developmental course of schizophrenic disorders. *Schizophrenia Bulletin*, **10**, 160–203.

Orzack, M.H., Kornetsky, C. (1966) Attentional dysfunction in chronic schizophrenia. *Archives of General Psychiatry*, **14**, 323–326.

Overall, J.E., Gorham, D.R. (1962) Brief Psychiatric Rating Scale. *Psychological Reports*, **10**, 799–812.

Pantelis, C., Barnes, T.R.E., Nelson, H.E. (1992) Is the concept of subcortical dementia relevant to schizophrenia? *British Journal of Psychiatry*, **160**, 442–460.

Pardo, J.V., Pardo, P.J., Janer, K.W., Raichle, M.E. (1990) The anterior cingulate cortex mediates processing selection in the Stroop attentional conflict paradigm. *Proceedings of the National Academy of Science*, **87**, 256–259.

Paus, T., Petrides, M., Evans, A.C., Meyer, E. (1993) Role of the human anterior cingulate cortex in the control of oculomotor, manual and speech responses: A positron emission tomography study. *Journal of Neurophysiology*, **70**, 453–469.

Petersen, S., Fox, P.T., Posner, M.I., Mintun, M.A., Raichle, M.E. (1988) Positron emission tomographic studies of the cortical anatomy of single word processing. *Nature*, **331**, 585–589.

Petersen, S.E., Robinson, D.L., Keys, W. (1985) Pulvinar nuclei of the behaving rhesus monkey: Visual responses and their modulation. *Journal of Neurophysiology*, **54**, 867–886.

Posner, M.I. (1988) Structures and Functions of Selective Attention. In: *Structures and Functions of Selective Attention* (Ed. T. Boll), pp. 169–202, American Psychological Association.

Posner, M., Walker, J., Friedrich, F.J., Rafal, R. (1984) Effects of parietal injury on covert orienting of attention. *Journal of Neuroscience*, **4**, 1863–1874.

Posner, M.I., Inhoff, A.W., Friedrich, F.J., Cohen, A. (1987) Isolating attentional systems: A cognitive-anatomical analysis. *Psychobiology*, **15**, 107–121.

Posner, M., Early, T., Reiman, E., Pardo, P., Dhawan, M. (1988a) Asymmetries in hemispheric control of attention in schizophrenia. *Archives of General Psychiatry*, **45**, 814–841.

Posner, M.I., Sandson, J., Dhawan, M., Shulman, G.L. (1988b) Is word recognition automatic? A cognitive-anatomical approach. *Journal of Cognitive Neuroscience*, **1**, 50–59.

Potkin, S.G., Swanson, J.M., Urbanchek, M., Carreoni, D., Bravo, G. (1989) Lateralized deficits in covert shifts of visual attention in chronic and never-medicated schizophrenics compared to controls. *Schizophrenia Research*, **2**, 95.

Pycock, C.J. (1980) Commentary: Turning behaviour in animals. *Neuroscience*, **5**, 461–514.

Robbins, T.W. (1991) The case for fronto-striatal dysfunction in schizophrenia. *Schizophrenia Bulletin*, **18**, 392–402.

Robinson, D.L., Petersen, S.E. (1986) The neurobiology of attention. In: *Brain And Mind: Dialogues Between Cognitive Psychology and Neuroscience* (Eds J. Le Doux, W. Hurst), pp. 365–469, Cambridge University Press, Cambridge.

Rosvold, H.E., Mirsky, A., Sarason, I., Bransome, E.D., Beck, L.H. (1956) A continuous performance test of brain damage. *Journal of Consulting and Clinical Psychology*, **20**, 343–350.

Saykin, A., Shtasel, D.L., Gur, R., Kester, D.B., Mozley, L.H., Stafinak, P., Gur, R.C. (1994) Neuropsychological performance in first episode schizophrenia. *Archives of General Psychiatry*, **23**, 35–45.

Seeman, P. (1993) Schizophrenia as a brain disease: The dopamine receptor story. *Archives of Neurology*, **50**, 1093–1095.

Shakow, D. (1962) Segmental set: A theory of formal psychological deficit in schizophrenia. *Archives of General Psychiatry*, **6**, 1–17.

Shallice, T. (1988) *From Neuropsychology to Mental Structure*, Cambridge University Press, Cambridge.

Shallice, T., Burgess, P.W., Frith, C.D. (1991) Can the neuropsychological case-study approach be applied to schizophrenia? *Psychological Medicine*, **21**, 661–673.

Shapiro, M.B., Nelson, E.H. (1955) An investigation of the nature of cognitive impairment in co-operative psychiatric patients. *British Journal of Medical Psychology*, **28**, 239–256.

Spohn, H.E., Strauss, M.E. (1989) Relation of neuroleptic and anticholinergic medication to cognitive functions in schizophrenia. *Journal of Abnormal Psychology*, **98**, 367–380.

Sterenko, R.J., Woods, D.J. (1978) Impairment in early stages of visual information processing in non-psychotic schizotypal individuals. *Journal of Abnormal Psychology*, **87**, 481–490.

Strauss, M.E., Novakovic, T., Tien, A.Y., Bylsma, F., Pearlson, G.D. (1991) Disengagement of attention in schizophrenia. *Psychiatry Research*, **37**, 139–146.

Strauss, M.E., Alphs, L., Boekamp, J. (1992) Disengagement of attention in chronic schizophrenia. *Psychiatry Research*, **43**, 87–92.

Swerdlow, N.R., Koob, G.F. (1987) Dopamine, schizophrenia, amnia and depression: Towards a unified hypothesis of cortico-striato-pallidothalamic function. *Behavioural and Brain Sciences*, **10**, 197–245.

Tomer, R. (1990) Attention asymmetry in schizophrenia: Hemineglect or hyperorienting. *Biological Psychiatry*, **27**, 108a.

Tomer, R., Flor-Henry, P. (1989) Neuroleptics reverse attention asymmetries in schizophrenic patients. *Biological Psychiatry*, **25**, 852–860.

Venables, P.H. (1960) The effect of auditory and visual stimulation on the skin potential responses of schizophrenics. *Brain*, **83**, 77–92.

Watson, C.G., Thomas, R.W., Anderson, D., Felling, J. (1968) Differentiation of organics from schizophrenics at two chronicity levels by use of the Halstead–Reitan organic test battery. *Journal of Consulting and Clinical Psychology*, **32**, 679–684.

Watson, R.T., Heilman, K.M., Caulten, J.C., King, F.A. (1973) Neglect after cingulectomy. *Neurology*, **23**, 1003–1007.

Weinberger, D.R., Berman, K.F., Daniel, D.G. (1991) Prefrontal cortex dysfunction in schizophrenia. In: *Frontal Lobe Function And Dysfunction* (Eds H.S. Levin, H.M. Eisenberg, A. Benton), pp. 275–287, Oxford University Press, New York.

Wigal, S.B., Potkin, S.G., Raja, P., Richmond, G., LaBerge, D.L. (1991) Asymmetries in attention filtering in left and right visual fields in schizophrenic patients. *Schizophrenia Research*, **27**, 396.

Zubin, J. (1975) Problem of attention in schizophrenia. In: *Experimental Approaches To Psychopathology* (Eds M.L. Kietzman, S. Sutton, J. Zubin), pp. 139–166, Academic Press, New York.

7

Memory Dysfunction in Schizophrenia

ERIC Y.H. CHEN and PETER J. McKENNA

INTRODUCTION

Until recently memory dysfunction has not been recognised as an important aspect of schizophrenia. In their classical descriptions of schizophrenia, both Kraepelin (1913) and Bleuler (1911) considered that the memory functions of patients with schizophrenia were largely unaffected. Reviewing many subsequent studies, Cutting (1990) also expressed a similar view and concluded that memory impairment was not observed except in severely disabled chronic patients with widespread cognitive dysfunction. However, recent systematic studies of memory in schizophrenia, which have taken into account factors like premorbid intelligence and current overall cognitive performance, have reported a disproportionate degree of memory impairment in a substantial proportion of patients with both acute and chronic forms of schizophrenia. In this chapter some of these recent findings are reviewed and we evaluate the findings from this work in the light of current ideas about memory functioning.

The scientific study of human memory goes back more than 100 years. Since then memory research has developed with an emphasis on tightly controlled laboratory investigations. Theoretical frameworks have also been strongly influenced by concurrent developments in information technology (Baddeley, 1990). For example, the advent of digital computers has introduced a number of concepts such as buffer, on-line, etc., as well as the framework of the "information processing" approach. The use of parallel processing in computing is currently providing another important class of models which may yield additional insights in thinking about memory functions.

It is now clear that "memory" as such is not a homogeneous and unified function (Baddeley, 1990). It has many different aspects each characterised by a specific profile and involving different neurobiological systems. One of the more fundamental distinctions has been between long-term memory and short-term

Schizophrenia: A Neuropsychological Perspective. Edited by C. Pantelis, H.E. Nelson and T.R.E. Barnes
© 1996 John Wiley & Sons Ltd

memory. Long-term memory has an apparently limitless capacity and involves handling of information from beyond half a minute to many years. In contrast, short-term memory can hold only a small number of items for seconds. Its capacity is limited and it can be easily saturated. Long-term memory is further divided into episodic memory (memory for personal experience); semantic memory (memory for general knowledge) and procedural memory (memory for skills). These aspects of memory can be affected to different extents in different illnesses.

From a clinical point of view, the relationship between memory dysfunction and the emergence of psychiatric symptoms is an important issue. Memory is an inherent component of many everyday cognitive processes underlying conscious experience. It is conceivable that memory dysfunction could lead to distortions and aberrations in many ordinary experiences and that some of these might be related to the symptoms and disability observed in patients with schizophrenia. In the following sections, some recent studies are discussed in relation to the major subdivisions of memory function.

SHORT-TERM AND WORKING MEMORY

It is now widely accepted that human memory is partitioned into two major and distinct systems, short and long-term memory. When subjects are presented with a word list and then asked to recall as many of the words as possible, it is found that recall performance is related to the position of the word in the list: the last few words are far more likely to be recalled than earlier words (Postman & Phillips, 1965; Glanzer & Cunitz, 1966). This so-called recency effect disappears after a few seconds of delay whereas recall of earlier words is unaffected by such delay. Recall of the last few words is not dependent on factors such as concurrent task, familiarity of the word and the rate of presentation, while recall of words in the earlier part of the list is dependent on these factors (Glanzer, 1972). This, and other evidence, suggests that there is a temporary store for items which is separate from a longer-term store. The concept of this short-term store has been elaborated into that of a working memory system involving at least two "slave" subsystems (verbal phonological and visuospatial) and a "central executive system" (Baddeley, 1986). This system stores information for up to 30 seconds and has a limited capacity.

Traditionally, assessment of working memory involves evaluation of the forward digit span, that is, the maximum number of digits that can be immediately repeated by the subject after presentation at a rate of about 1 per second. It is known that in normal subjects the forward digit span is around seven (plus or minus two), unless the subject adopts a "chunking" strategy by remembering the numbers in small groups. In a more difficult version, subjects are asked to repeat the numbers in the reversed order (backward digit span). This is thought to place demands on the central executive component of working memory. Working memory for non-verbal material can also be assessed; for example, by Corsi blocks (Milner, 1971) where subjects are required to repeat a sequence by pointing at a number of blocks irregularly arranged on a board.

In schizophrenia, a number of studies have addressed working memory and most of these have focused on digit span. Recent studies include that of Gruzelier et al (1988) where 36 patients with schizophrenia were compared with 21 patients with affective disorder and 29 normal controls. In comparison with controls the patients with schizophrenia, as well as the patients with affective disorder, were found to have slightly shorter spans for both digits (mean 5.35 vs. control 6.85) and Corsi blocks (mean 4.07 vs. control 4.86). In contrast, Tamlyn et al (1992), in a study of 60 acute and chronic patients with schizophrenia, found that 86% of the patients had a digit span of at least five while the remainder had a span of four using the Middlesex Elderly Assessment of Mental State (MEAMS) (Golding, 1989). In a similar study, Duffy & O'Carroll (1994) assessed a sample of 40 patients with schizophrenia and a comparison group of Korsakoff patients. They found that both groups of patients had forward digit spans which were within normal limits. Finally, Goldberg et al (1993) studied 24 monozygotic twin pairs discordant for schizophrenia and reported that forward digit span was equal in affected and unaffected twins, whereas backward digit span showed a non-significant trend towards poorer performance in the affected co-twins.

It appears that the recent studies examining verbal working memory produced results that were consistent with most patients having a forward digit span within the normal range. Whilst performance may still be within normal limits, there are some suggestions that the mean digit span may be marginally impaired (a decrement of about one digit). This difference may be more pronounced when backward digit span is measured. Unfortunately, only a small number of studies have reported the backward span.

If a subtle working memory deficit is present in schizophrenia this does not appear to be correlated with other memory deficits. Tamlyn et al (1992) studied five patients with schizophrenia who showed a specific and substantial degree of overall impairment of long-term memory rather than short-term memory. Their digit spans were found to range from five to seven and Corsi block spans ranged from four to six (i.e. normal). This relative preservation of short-term working memory was also illustrated by the presence of a recency effect in recall tests. During a word list recall task it was found that words presented later along the list had a higher probability of being retrieved. The presence of a recency effect indicates that the short-term store holding items of information for seconds prior to retrieval (i.e. working memory) is preserved. Such a preservation of working memory in the presence of significant long-term memory impairment prompted the comparison with patients suffering from amnesic syndrome, in whom a similar profile of memory impairment is observed.

In an approach inspired by an attempt to relate psychological findings to neurobiological systems, Park & Holzman (1992) compared 12 patients with schizophrenia, 12 bipolar patients and 12 normal controls on working memory tasks in different sensory modalities. They used tests that were derived from the delay response tasks used in experimental psychology to study prefrontal cortical function (Fuster, 1991). It was found that in patients with schizophrenia, while verbal working memory was relatively preserved (measured by digit span), there was clear evidence of impairment in spatial and haptic modalities. It remains unclear, however, to what extent the differential impairment could be related to different levels of difficulty in the tasks or whether a modality specific difference is present.

LONG-TERM MEMORY

Memory for more than about 30 seconds, whether for minutes or for years, is referred to as long-term memory. Studies in cognitive psychology and neuro-psychology have provided evidence that the long-term store is not homogeneous but involves a number of separate subsystems. The first division is into memory for experiences, concepts and ideas that can be explicitly stated through language, termed "declarative" memory (e.g. remembering who was around last Christmas, or knowing the capital of France) and memory of how to perform certain tasks that are not necessarily dependent on conscious reflection, so-called "procedural" memory (e.g. knowing how to ride a bicycle). Declarative memory is further divided into episodic memory (that for personal events) and semantic memory (that related to general knowledge). The separation of declarative memory into episodic and semantic memory has been supported by a large number of observations, although there are undoubtedly interchanges of information between the two systems (Tulving, 1983). Episodic memory refers to memory for personal events which are organised around a temporal framework. The contents are experiential with associated affects and retrieval is context dependent. For example, memory of a past event is facilitated by being reminded of the locations in which it occurred. Episodic memory is typically impaired in the classic amnesic syndrome.

EPISODIC MEMORY

RETROGRADE STUDIES

Studies of episodic memory in schizophrenia fall into two general groups, retro-grade and anterograde. Retrograde studies assess memory for remote events acquired over long periods of time (years or decades) and can be used to determine the presence of a temporal gradient in episodic memory impairment (Butters & Cermak, 1986). This approach is vulnerable to certain methodological problems. For example, it is difficult with a list of famous events or personalities test to assess whether any failure is due to memory impairment or to a long-standing lack of awareness. Another question is whether famous events or person-alities tap episodic or semantic memory.

Despite these limitations several studies have reported results based on this approach. Calev et al (1987b) compared 16 patients with chronic schizophrenia and 16 normal controls on the Famous Events Questionnaire (Squire & Cohen, 1979). They found that remote episodic memory was impaired in the patients with schizophrenia. When comparing impairment in more recent and more distant memories, no temporal gradient was observed. Tamlyn et al (1992), in a detailed study of five patients, assessed knowledge of public personalities (Famous Person-alities Test; Stevens, 1979) and found that all five patients performed below the mean for normal subjects in the same age range. Standardised autobiographical memory assessment (Kopelman et al, 1990) also provided evidence for clear impairment in all time periods (recent or remote), with only an inconsistent and shallow temporal gradient.

Although few in number, these studies suggest that episodic memory is impaired in schizophrenia but, in contrast to a classical amnesic disorder, a clear temporal gradient is not observed.

ANTEROGRADE STUDIES

Anterograde studies employ tasks which involve memorising items and subse-quently testing retention of the material either by recall or by recognition tests. In this approach, memory is typically tested over a short time range (hours or days). In addition, presentation of the items to be remembered is experimentally controlled. These tasks requiring acquisition of new material are also open to a set of methodological limitations. Motivation to learn plays a crucial role and has to be carefully controlled for in patients with schizophrenia. It is also possible that "input" factors, such as attention, can affect performance.

In tasks requiring learning of new material an important objective is to produce traces of memory that are distinct from other traces. This discrimination is better examined using tests of recognition rather than recall because the latter requires additional cognitive activity to access the items. Similarity between items to be remembered will interfere with recognition but will have a variable effect on recall. On the one hand it may assist access while on the other it may interfere with discrimination (Baddeley, 1990). This probably underlies the observation that high-frequency words tend to be recalled better, whereas low-frequency words tend to be recognised better. The assessment of memory by recognition testing is also complicated by how ready the subject is to guess and answer when he cannot remember with certainty but has a vague sense of the answer.

Calev et al (1983), in a study of 10 chronic patients and 10 less severely disturbed patients, attempted to facilitate encoding with the introduction of an orienting task. This was achieved by requesting the subjects to sort the stimulus material into semantic categories prior to the learning and recall tests. However, deficits both at the encoding stage (in both chronic and mild patients) and at the post-encoding stage (chronic patients) were found. Subsequently, Calev (1984) compared 10 patients with chronic schizophrenia with 70 normal controls on recall and recognition tasks matched for level of difficulty. He found deficits in both recall and recognition in patients with schizophrenia, with recall being differ-entially more impaired. In the study described earlier, Gruzelier et al (1988) compared 36 patients with schizophrenia with 21 patients with affective disorder and 29 normal controls using a paradigm where digit and visuospatial span (Corsi blocks) were assessed with some of the stimulus sequence being presented *recurrently*, interspersed with other sequences. Stimulus sequences presented recur-rently have spans which increase over trials and reach a ceiling after several trials.

Non-repeating sequences have a constant span which corresponds to working memory capacity. Improvement in span over time for the recurrent sequences was impaired in patients with schizophrenia for digit span but not visuospatial span. The authors also investigated spatial (hand positions) and visual (colour) paired associate learning. Performance was impaired in both the patients with schizophrenia and those with affective disorder.

Goldberg et al (1989) examined the performance of 31 patients with chronic schizophrenia and 13 control subjects on the Selective Reminding Test (Buschke & Fuld, 1974). This involves learning a list of words over a number of trials. At each trial those words not recalled were given again and those recalled on two trials were considered to have entered into long-term memory. After 12 such trials subjects were tested for recognition of the words on the list. Using such a paradigm it was found that a learning curve was present in patients with schizophrenia. They initially were able to recall four words, compared with five words recalled by control subjects. After a number of trials with reminding the patients eventually achieved a recall of eight words, in comparison with controls who recalled 11 words. With regards to recall performance a group-by-trial interaction was present indicating that patients learned at a slower rate than controls.

In the study of Tamlyn et al (1992) 60 patients with acute and chronic schizophrenia completed the Rivermead Behavioural Memory Test (RBMT) (Wilson et al, 1985), which has 12 subtests covering verbal, spatial and visual recognition and recall memory as well as prospective memory (i.e. remembering to perform a task at a future time). The patients were found to be impaired on most measures of long-term memory. Only 20% of patients passed the prose recall test. Recognition performance was better, with 72% and 62% of patients passing the picture and face recognition tests respectively, while most of those who failed did so marginally. A further detailed study of five of the patients who performed poorly in the RBMT revealed that prose recall was in the impaired range in all cases. Using the Recognition Memory Test (Warrington, 1984) variable impairment was revealed in both word and face recognition. The authors concluded that not only recall but also recognition was affected in schizophrenia.

Duffy & O'Carroll (1994) replicated these findings in another study using the RBMT which involved 40 patients with schizophrenia. They showed that in a mixed group of patients with schizophrenia 25% scored in the normal range, 40% in the poor memory range, 30% had moderate memory impairment and 5% had severe memory impairment. The degree of impairment was similar to that seen in the sample investigated by Tamlyn and colleagues.

In the study of Goldberg et al (1993) 24 discordant monozygotic twin pairs were tested on paired associate learning. The twins with schizophrenia performed more poorly than their unaffected co-twins whose performance was similar to that of normal controls. There was no difference between the groups in delayed recall tasks. In an easy version of paired associate learning the twins with schizophrenia, when compared with their unaffected co-twin, failed to take advantage of semantic regularities (as seen in other groups). The presence of a learning curve over trials was considered to argue against the notion that patients with schizophrenia were similar to patients with the amnesic syndrome.

SEMANTIC MEMORY

Semantic memory refers to memory for facts, ideas and concepts that are not personal in nature. These are organised conceptually and there is little temporal coding. This system is typically spared in the classical amnesic syndrome (Baddeley, 1990). Category specific deficits are found in some patients with brain lesions (Warrington & Shallice, 1984), suggesting topographical organisation of semantic memory.

Studies of semantic memory function in schizophrenia are currently in a stage of active development. Tamlyn et al (1992) in their study of 60 patients with acute and chronic forms of schizophrenia applied the so-called "Silly Sentence Test" (Collins & Quillian, 1969) in which the subjects are asked to verify whether statements such as "rats have teeth" or "desks wear clothes" are true or false. For this task both error rate and reaction time were measured. It was observed that reaction times for sentence verification were much slower in the schizophrenic group, with two-thirds of the patients falling outside the normal range. In addition, whereas normal controls seldom made an error, 14 out of 60 patients made three or more errors, with five of them making more than 10 errors. There was a tendency for the patients with schizophrenia to misclassify statements as true and when questioned about their erroneous responses clearly irrational reasons were given. The authors suggested that the presence of semantic memory disorder distinguished patients with schizophrenia from Korsakoff patients. Duffy & O'Carroll (1994) in their replication study using 40 patients with schizophrenia also found that they were slower and made more errors in semantic memory on the "Silly Sentence Test" than Korsakoff patients.

McKenna et al (1994) further investigated the integrity of semantic memory in 41 patients with schizophrenia with mild to chronic forms of the condition using Hodges Semantic Memory Test (Hodges et al, 1992). This test assesses different aspects of semantic memory covering category fluency, naming, sorting, word to picture matching and definition. Patients with schizophrenia as a whole performed poorly in many aspects of semantic memory.

Further exploration of semantic memory structure in patients with schizophrenia has yielded preliminary results suggestive of a specific anomaly in semantic memory function in schizophrenia (Chen et al, 1994). A categorisation task was employed where subjects have to respond with "yes" or "no" to whether an exemplar such as "chair" belongs to a category such as "furniture". Exemplar and category pairs with different degrees of semantic relatedness (or typicality) were used. It was found that while internal category structures appear to be intact in patients with schizophrenia, items clearly outside the category boundary but related to the category in some attributes (e.g. "aeroplane" and category of "birds") are treated by patients as if they were actually on the category boundary; that is, considered as being within and without the category equally often. This interpretation is supported by reaction time analysis which shows that for normal controls it takes the longest to make a decision for an item along the category boundary whereas for patients with schizophrenia the longest condition is for items outside but related to the category.

Another approach to the study of semantic relationships is through the lexical decision task. In this task subjects are required to decide as quickly as possible whether a presented string of letters is a legitimate word or not. It has been observed that in normal subjects this decision is facilitated (faster reaction time) if the presentation of the word is preceded by presentation of a semantically related word; for example, decision time for "bread" is faster if the preceding word was "butter" (Meyer & Schvaneveldt, 1971). This effect, termed semantic priming, suggests that words are related to one another in the mental lexicon in an organised fashion. The lexical decision task has been used in schizophrenia in a small number of studies (e.g. Manschreck et al, 1988; Kwapil et al, 1990). The results have been inconsistent with the semantic priming effect found to be either unaffected or enhanced in patients with schizophrenia.

PROCEDURAL MEMORY

One way to subdivide long-term memory systems is to consider memory which is open to conscious reflection (declarative memory) and learning that is implicit and is not normally verbalised (procedural memory). The best evidence for this distinction comes from neuropsychological studies of patients with classical amnesic syndrome. Such patients can learn to use new tools and show a normal learning curve on a motor learning task such as the rotor pursuit task and even learn to solve the complicated Tower of Hanoi puzzle. Typically, amnesic patients improve on each subsequent trial performing the task without having the conscious memory of having encountered the task before (Baddeley, 1990).

There have been few studies investigating procedural memory in schizophrenia (see also Collinson et al, chapter 12). Huston & Shakow (1949) demonstrated that patients with schizophrenia showed improved performance on pursuit rotor type tasks over trials. This result was confirmed and elaborated in Goldberg et al's (1993) study using discordant monozygotic twins in which they found that the rate of learning on the same task was similar for the patients and their unaffected co-twins. In the pursuit rotor task, although the patient group were more impaired in their performance, they still demonstrated learning over trials and the rate of learning was comparable to normal controls.

SPECIFIC ISSUES

VERBAL AND SPATIAL MEMORY

There has been some suggestion that processing of verbal and visuospatial information is at least partially lateralised in the two cerebral hemispheres (e.g. Milner, 1971). To some extent this lateralisation applies to memory functions as well (Zaidel, 1987; Geschwind & Galaburda, 1985). A number of theoretical models of schizophrenia suggest that abnormal lateralisation of cognitive functions is important in understanding the psychopathology of the condition (e.g. Gruzelier et al, 1988; Cutting, 1990; see Gruzelier, chapter 8). This has led to an interest in the comparison between verbal and visuospatial memory function in schizophrenia. Several recent studies have addressed this issue.

Calev et al (1987a) used matched verbal and design recall tasks and found no evidence for a differential deficit. In the study by Gruzelier et al (1988), already described above, which compared *recurrent* digit and visuospatial span with *non-recurrent spans*, patients with schizophrenia were impaired in digit span performance but not in visuospatial span, suggesting a specific verbal impairment. However, it has been pointed out that laterality studies in schizophrenia are seldom constraining enough to favour one theory over another (Shallice et al, 1991). Studying their discordant monozygotic twin samples with verbal and visual memory tests from the Welsher Memory Scale, Goldberg et al (1993) reported that the affected co-twin performed worse than the unaffected co-twin in both verbal and visual memory. Duffy & O'Carroll (1994), using the Benton Visual Retention Test to assess visuospatial memory (Benton, 1974), also reported that patients with schizophrenia scored below the normal range in both verbal and visuospatial memory.

Studies in the lateralisation of memory function in schizophrenia have so far yielded inconclusive results. One serious methodological problem is that most of the studies reporting laterality differences have not employed verbal and non-verbal tasks which are matched for their levels of difficulty. This field awaits further empirical data.

COMPARISON WITH PATIENTS WITH KNOWN ORGANIC DISORDERS

The fundamental assumption of the neuropsychological approach is that comparison of the pattern of deficits between conditions with known and unknown pathologies will provide clues to lesion site in the latter. In the study of memory disorders the most obvious comparison would be with patients with a pure amnesic syndrome on the one hand (in which the focal sites of lesion are in the medial temporal or diencephalic areas) and patients with diffuse cortical lesions, such as in dementia, on the other. Several observations have been made comparing patients with schizophrenia to those with organic disease.

Tamlyn et al (1992) found that the observed pattern of episodic memory impairment without working memory impairment suggested similarity to the classical amnesic syndrome but clear evidence of semantic memory impairment is against this comparison. Duffy & O'Carroll (1994) directly tested this suggestion by comparing 40 patients with schizophrenia with 18 Korsakoff patients. It was found that the level of episodic memory impairment (RBMT) was far greater in the Korsakoff patients (5% schizophrenics vs. 100% Korsakoff in the severely impaired range), whereas semantic memory impairment was greater in the patients with schizophrenia. Regarding learning of procedural skills Goldberg et al (1993) reported the presence of a learning curve and normal motor learning in patients with schizophrenia which suggested that the impairment in performance is different from patients with striatal disease, such as Huntington's chorea.

It appears that the pattern of memory impairment in schizophrenia has unique and specific features which may eventually be related to involvement of a specific set of neural subsystems.

GENERAL OR SPECIFIC DEFICIT?

It is well recognised that in at least a proportion of patients with schizophrenia, a degree of global cognitive impairment is present (Tamlyn et al, 1992). An important question concerning memory dysfunction in schizophrenia is whether memory impairment occurs entirely in the context of a global cognitive impairment or whether such impairment can be considered as a distinct cluster of psychological deficits which stand out from the background of overall impairment (see also Barber et al, chapter 4).

Several studies have addressed this issue specifically. Braff et al (1991) in a sample of 40 outpatients reported that rather than having a specific frontal type of impairment patients with schizophrenia have a non-specific and heterogeneous pattern of neuropsychological deficit. However, this study did not employ extensive memory testing batteries.

Tamlyn et al (1992) used the MEAMS and the Mini Mental State Examination (MMSE) (Folstein et al, 1975) to assess general cognitive function in 60 patients with acute and chronic schizophrenia. Whilst the MMSE contains a number of memory related items, the MEAMS has items specifically related to memory function which can be separated out in order to isolate specific memory impairment from generalised cognitive decline. As reported in their preliminary communication (McKenna et al, 1990) the distribution of MMSE and MEAMS scores compared with RBMT scores suggested that memory impairment was disproportionate to any generalised cognitive impairment. Duffy & O'Carroll (1994) confirmed this finding that memory impairment was disproportionate to level of overall cognitive impairment.

Concerning the pattern of impairment, Gruzelier et al (1988) compared patients with schizophrenia and affective disorder with a group of normal controls. They observed that, while patients with affective disorder demonstrated spatial impairments, patients with schizophrenia had heterogeneous but specific patterns of temporal–frontal involvement which were consistent with a specific as opposed to a general deficit. The authors suggested that focal as well as general deficits co-exist in schizophrenia.

It is clear from this work, as well as that described in previous sections of this chapter, that, at least a proportion of patients with schizophrenia do have a specific pattern of memory impairment which is present over and above any global cognitive decline. However, further work is needed to establish whether and to what extent memory deficits may occur in isolation in schizophrenia.

RELATIONSHIP BETWEEN MEMORY IMPAIRMENT AND SYMPTOMS

The relationship between memory deficits and symptoms of schizophrenia is an area of considerable interest. It is tempting to speculate on the possible effect of memory dysfunction on the production of symptoms. Several authors have offered theoretical accounts (e.g. Hoffman, 1987; McKenna, 1991). Empirical data in the field is still inconclusive although several studies have reported an association with negative symptoms. Tamlyn et al (1992) found that memory impairment was associated with severity and chronicity of illness, negative symptoms and formal thought disorder. However, in a replication study with similar design, Duffy & O'Carroll (1994) found no correlation with any positive or negative symptoms. In the twin study of Goldberg et al (1993) only a modest correlation was found between negative symptoms and impairment on a procedural memory task (Tower of Hanoi). In addition, positive symptoms showed a modest correlation with episodic memory (for story) and working memory (forward digit). In an earlier investigation, Goldberg et al (1989) studied 31 patients with chronic schizophrenia using the Selective Reminding Test. It was found that all measures apart from recognition correlated with the "anergic" factor on the Brief Psychiatric Rating Scale, this factor being closely related to negative symptoms.

RELATIONSHIP BETWEEN MEMORY IMPAIRMENT AND EXECUTIVE/"FRONTAL LOBE" FUNCTION

It is increasingly recognised that executive functions, which may well be subserved by the prefrontal cortex, have a role to play in certain aspects of memory function. Particular attention has been focused on the central executive component of working memory (Baddeley, 1986) and also on the phenomenon of recollection—active searching and checking mechanisms involved in retrieval of long-term memories (Baddeley, 1990). In view of the fact that there is a body of work that implicates functional impairment of the prefrontal cortex in schizophrenia (e.g. Andreasen et al, 1992) it is important to consider whether and to what extent the memory deficits seen in schizophrenia might be secondary to executive dysfunction.

A number of authors have noted that memory impairment in schizophrenia appears to affect recall to a much greater extent than recognition and have suggested that this might reflect a prefrontal/executive pattern of impairment (Goldberg et al, 1989; Helkala et al, 1988; Jetter et al, 1986). However, it should be noted that sparing of recognition memory is not a uniform finding in schizophrenia (e.g. Tamlyn et al, 1992). Furthermore, it is not clear that patients with frontal lobe lesions invariably show a pattern of impaired recall with relatively preserved recognition memory. Indeed, Delbecq-Derousene et al (1990) have documented a patient with a clear frontal lobe syndrome due to a vascular lesion who showed a selective impairment in recognition memory. Also, a disparity between recall and recognition performance has been described in conditions without any frontal lobe pathology, such as the classical amnesic syndrome (Hirst, 1982).

A perhaps more significant issue is whether the executive deficit that has been repeatedly documented in schizophrenia (e.g. Goldberg & Weinberger, 1988; Goldberg et al, 1987; Morice, 1990; Liddle & Morris, 1991) is disproportionate to the overall level of poor intellectual performance. At present the answer to this question is uncertain. Saykin et al (1991) and Braff et al (1991) both administered wide ranging batteries of neuropsychological tests to groups of patients with schizophrenia. When the scores on these tests were statistically transformed to allow comparison across tests, it was found that the patients with schizophrenia were no more impaired on an executive test (the Wisconsin Card Sorting Test in both cases) than on the majority of the other tests. In the study by Saykin et al impairment in memory and learning was considerably more prominent than that of executive dysfunction.

In contrast, Shallice et al (1991) applied the neuropsychological case study approach to five chronically hospitalised patients with schizophrenia. Using a large battery of tests they found that the patients showed a more or less consistent pattern of severe impairment in executive function. In two of the patients this was in the context of preserved IQ level, normal performance on tests of visual perception, language and inconsistent poor performance on the memory tests. In the remaining three patients poor executive performance was part of a pattern of widespread deficits coupled with IQ decline. The authors argued that impairment of executive function is the common denominator of neuropsychological impairment in schizophrenia and that when present in relative isolation it could plausibly account for the poor performance on some, but not all, of the memory tasks.

The role of the frontal lobes in understanding or explaining the memory impairment observed in patients with schizophrenia is as yet unresolved. The corollary to these findings is that frontal processes underlying memory function need to be better understood in both normals and pathological conditions.

OTHER METHODOLOGICAL ISSUES

MEDICATION

It is generally recognised that medications, especially anti-cholinergic medication, could have a profound effect on cognitive performance and memory (Bartus et al, 1982). Most of the studies discussed considered this possibility and found that the observations could not be simply due to medication effects (see also King and Green, chapter 20). Several studies comparing patients on and off anti-cholinergic medications found no difference in memory performance (e.g. Calev, 1984; Calev et al, 1987a; Goldberg et al, 1989, 1993). Calev et al (1987b) compared groups of patients on neuroleptics with high and low anti-cholinergic activity, again finding no difference in memory performance between the groups. Gruzelier et al (1988) found that the performance of drug-free patients in their sample did not differ from patients on neuroleptics. Finally, Saykin et al (1991) in a study of 36 unmedicated acute patients found that selective memory impairment was still present.

MOTIVATION

Motivation could play a crucial role in performance especially in tasks that involve learning of new material. In studies of patients with schizophrenia the level of motivation has usually been described as surprisingly good. However, few studies have utilised standardised assessment of motivation and cooperation. McKenna et al (1990) in their study of 60 patients with schizophrenia identified 15 as showing questionable attention or cooperation at the time of testing. Exclusion of these subjects from the analysis made no great difference to the overall level of impairment found. Duffy & O'Carroll (1994), using Shakow's 5-point scale, reported that memory impairment was not attributable to poor motivation. Similarly, Goldberg et al (1993) also reported no difference in the level of cooperation between patients and controls, as measured by Shakow's scale.

ACUTE OR CHRONIC SCHIZOPHRENIA?

It has been claimed that any memory impairments observed in patients are confined only to patients with chronic schizophrenia (Cutting, 1990). To date, as described earlier in this chapter, there are many studies which included patients with acute schizophrenia and the finding of memory impairment was still apparent. In particular, the study of Saykin et al (1991) on unmedicated acute patients confirmed the finding of disproportionate memory impairment in acute schizophrenia.

CONCLUSIONS

APPROACHES TO STUDYING HUMAN MEMORY SYSTEMS

Research on memory has employed a number of testing paradigms, each with its own limitations and strengths. Cognitive psychologists have invested a great deal of effort into the refinement and critique of each testing paradigm. A full review of these would be beyond the scope of this chapter (for review see Baddeley, 1990). In addition, the use of these methods in studying patients with schizophrenia involves a further set of methodological questions. Some of these factors have been discussed above in the context of descriptions of the studies addressing the various memory systems.

Regarding the neurobiological basis of memory functions there have been a number of different approaches which have produced broadly convergent conclusions. Experimental psychologists typically apply the method of lesion studies in higher primates to observe changes in learning and memory performance after a particular part of the neural system is destroyed. The neuropsychological approach makes use of careful observation and quantitative testing of human subjects with known cerebral lesions. It also yields insights regarding the functions of particular brain structures. These two approaches are limited in that they both depend on the assumption of a relatively simple relationship between structure and function. In the ideal case a direct and specific correspondence of one structure, one function and one deficit is assumed. This is now known to be far too simplistic when applied to higher cognitive functions and brain structures.

In most instances, the notion of sets of reciprocally connected neural structures dynamically interacting with one another is more likely to provide insights into the neurological basis of psychological functions. The "basic units" of psychological functions are likewise not easily definable and, at the more empirical level, functions are best described by the actual procedures used to test them. It is likely that, at least for the current time, psychological functions such as "language" or "memory" are considered as composite functions that may have many component parts and are likely to involve overlapping sets of neural structures.

It is doubtful whether traditional neuropsychological concepts such as double dissociation will be of widespread and general use in the detailed analysis of such systems. Both the experimental psychology and the neuropsychology approaches involve the analysis of functioning of a brain structure by looking at the effect of its destruction. This is an indirect method which can have potential biases. For example, if a change of functioning is observed it is usually not possible to distinguish between the *malfunctioning* (with anomalous and aberrant outcomes) on the one hand versus *impairment* (reduction of efficiency) of a normal function on the other. Because of the nature of these approaches (i.e. destruction of structures studied) usually there is a bias in interpretation and even in observation, favouring *impairments* of normal function rather than *malfunctions* that may depart not only quantitatively but also qualitatively from normal functions. This bias is important in that it will be more difficult to derive from these ideas observations that may be relevant to understanding positive psychotic symptoms, whereas correlations with negative symptoms is expected to be found more easily.

More integrative alternatives for studying neural structures involved in memory functions are emerging with rapid advances in the field of functional imaging. Positron emission tomography (PET) and functional magnetic resonance imaging (fMRI) are promising areas that may help to delineate structure-function relationships in memory functions both in health and in disease.

NEUROANATOMICAL LOCALISATION OF MEMORY FUNCTIONS

Some initial conclusions relating to the more intensively studied memory systems are arising from a number of different approaches. In terms of working memory, the delayed response task has been a dominant method in experimental psychology and current data suggest that a network involving the dorsolateral prefrontal cortex, the parietal area and the corresponding cortico-pallido-thalamic circuit is necessary for spatial working memory functions (Goldman-Rakic & Friedman, 1991). This is consistent with neuropsychological findings of impairments in working memory when any of these interconnected structures are affected by lesions (Shimamura et al, 1991).

The laying down of new memory in the long-term store necessitates integrity of a variety of structures. It is clear that both medial temporal structures such as the hippocampus, entorhinal cortex, diencephalic structures (e.g. mamillary bodies), the anterior thalamus, dorsomedial thalamus and periventricular area are important in the laying down of new memory traces (see Dudai, 1989; Squire &

Zola-Morgan, 1991). There also appears to be a laterality difference in that dominant medial temporal structures are related to verbally mediated memory and the non-dominant medial temporal structures are related to visuospatial memory functions (Zaidel, 1987; Geschwind & Galaburda, 1985). In addition, the cholinergic projection system originating from the basal nucleus of Meynert and projecting to widespread areas in the cortex may have a modulatory function in learning and memory (Mesulam & Geula, 1988; Bartus et al, 1982).

It is of interest that a number of the areas implicated as mediating memory functions are probably affected in schizophrenia. MRI imaging studies, PET functional imaging studies and neuropathological studies suggest that in addition to non-specific cortical atrophy, medial temporal structures such as the hippocampus and the entorhinal cortex (Beckman & Jakob, 1991; Arnold et al, 1991; Jeste & Lohr, 1989; Altshuler et al, 1987; Suddath et al, 1989; Tamminga et al, 1992; Kelsoe et al, 1988), as well as the prefrontal cortex (Berman et al, 1988; Weinberger et al, 1991) may be involved either structurally or functionally in schizophrenia. Therefore, *a priori*, a degree of specific impairment in memory functions is to be expected in schizophrenia. The issue is whether a specific pattern of memory impairment could be empirically identified which corresponds to specific differential involvement of neural structures in schizophrenia.

In order to study the pattern of impairment it is necessary to employ tasks that are matched in difficulty. This avoids the pitfall of a generalised impairment giving the impression of a specific pattern of deficits (Chapman & Chapman, 1973). In practice this involves extensive preparation and relatively few studies take this into full consideration.

Memory impairment in schizophrenia has recently been recognised as an independent phenomenon apart from global cognitive impairment. Emerging data support the view that there may be a specific pattern to the memory impairment. The recent work in the field finds clearest evidence for impairments in episodic and semantic memory systems. The evidence is less clear for procedural memory due to the small number of studies. There appears to be no gross impairment in verbal working memory while there is some evidence for impairment in non-verbal working memory. The studies to date which have investigated memory have mostly adopted neuropsychological approaches with their limitations as discussed above. Further characterisation of the memory deficits associated with schizophrenia may be delineated using other methodologies (e.g. MRI and PET) together with a neuropsychological approach.

REFERENCES

Altshuler, L.L., Conrad, A., Kovelman, J.A., Scheibel, A. (1987) Hippocampal pyramidal cell orientation in schizophrenia. *Archives of General Psychiatry*, **44**, 1094–1098.

Andreasen, N.C., Rezai, K., Alliger, R., Swayze II, V.W., Flaum, M., Kirchner, P., Cohen, G., O'Leary, D.S. (1992) Hypofrontality in neuroleptic-naive patients and in patients with chronic schizophrenia: Assessment with xenon 133 single-photon emission computed tomography and the Tower of London. *Archives of General Psychiatry*, **49**, 943–958.

Arnold, S.E., Hyman, B.T., Van Hoesen, G.W., Damasio, A.R. (1991) Some cytoarchitectural abnormalities of the entorhinal cortex in schizophrenia. *Archives of General Psychiatry*, **48**, 625–632.

Baddeley, A.D. (1986) *Working Memory*, Oxford University Press, Oxford.

Baddeley, A.D. (1990) *Human Memory: Theory and Practice*, Erlbaum, Hove.

Bartus, R.T., Dean III, R.L., Beer, B., Lippa, A.S. (1982) The cholinergic hypothesis of geriatric memory dysfunction. *Science*, **217**, 408–417.

Beckmann, H., Jakob, H. (1991) Prenatal disturbance of nerve cell migration in the entorhinal region: a common vulnerability factor in functional psychosis? *Journal of Neural Transmission (Gen. Sect.)*, **4**, 155–164.

Benton, A.L. (1974) *The Revised Visual Retention Test* (4th edn), New York Psychological Cooperation, New York.

Berman, K.F., Illowsky, B.P., Weinberger, D.R. (1988) Physiological dysfunction of dorsolateral prefrontal cortex in schizophrenia: IV. Further evidence for regional and behavioral specificity. *Archives of General Psychiatry*, **45**, 616–622.

Bleuler, E. (1911) *Dementia Praecox, or the Group of Schizophrenias* (translated by J. Zinkin, 1950), International University Press, New York.

Braff, D.L., Heaton, R., Kuck, J. et al (1991) The generalised pattern of neuropsychological deficits in outpatients with chronic schizophrenia with heterogeneous Wisconsin Card Sorting Test Results. *Archives of General Psychiatry*, **48**, 891–898.

Buschke, H., Fuld, P.A. (1974) Evaluating storage, retention, and retrieval in disordered learning and memory. *Neurology*, **24**, 1019–1025.

Butters, N., Cermak, L.S. (1986) A study of the forgetting of autobiographical knowledge: Implications for the study of retrograde amnesia. In: *Autobiographical Memory*. (Ed. D. Rubin), pp. 253–272, Cambridge University Press, Cambridge.

Calev, A. (1984) Recall and recognition in chronic nondemented schizophrenics: Use of matched tasks. *Journal of Abnormal Psychology*, **93**, 172–177.

Calev, A., Venables, P.H., Monk, A.F. (1983) Evidence for distinct verbal memory pathologies in severely and mildly disturbed schizophrenics. *Schizophrenia Bulletin*, **9**, 247–264.

Calev, A., Korin, Y., Kugelmass, S., Lerer, B. (1987a) Performance of chronic schizophrenics on matched word and design recall tasks. *Biological Psychiatry*, **22**, 669–709.

Calev, A., Berlin, H., Lerer, B. (1987b) Remote and recent memory in long-hospitalised chronic schizophrenics. *Biological Psychiatry*, **22**, 79–85.

Chapman, L.J., Chapman, J.P. (1973) Problems in the measurement of cognitive deficit. *Psychological Bulletin*, **79**, 380–385.

Chen, E.Y.H., Wilkins, A.J., McKenna, P.J. (1994) Semantic memory is both impaired and anomalous in schizophrenia. *Psychological Medicine*, **24**, 193–202.

Collins, A.M., Quillian, M.R. (1969) Retrieval time from semantic memory. *Journal of Verbal Learning and Verbal Behavior*, **8**, 240–247.

Cutting, J.C. (1990) *The Right Cerebral Hemisphere and Psychiatric Disorders*, Oxford University Press, Oxford.

Delbecq-Derousene, J., Beauvois, M.F., Shallice, T. (1990) Preserved recall versus impaired recognition: a case study. *Brain*, **113**, 1045–1074.

Dudai, Y. (1989) *The Neurobiology of Memory: Concepts, Findings, Trends*, Oxford University Press, Oxford.

Duffy, L., O'Carroll, R. (1994) Memory impairment in schizophrenia: A comparison with that observed in the alcoholic Korsakoff syndrome. *Psychological Medicine*, **24**, 155–165.

Folstein, M.F., Folstein, S.E., McHugh, P.R. (1975) Mini-Mental State: A practical method for grading the cognitive state of patients for the clinician. *Journal of Psychiatric Research*, **12**, 189–198.

Fuster, J.M. (1991) Role of prefrontal cortex in delay tasks: Evidence from reversible lesion and unit recording in the monkey. In: *Frontal Lobe Function and Dysfunction*. (Eds H.S. Levin, H.M. Eisenberg, A.L. Benton), pp. 59–71, Oxford University Press, Oxford.

Geschwind, N., Galaburda, A. (1985) Cerebral lateralisation. Biological mechanisms, associations and pathology: I. A hypothesis and a program for research. *Archives of Neurology*, **42**, 428–459.

Glanzer, M. (1972) Storage mechanisms in recall. In: *The Psychology of Learning and Motivation: Advances in Research and Theory*, Vol. V (Ed. G.H. Bower), Academic Press, New York.

Glanzer, M., Cunitz, A.R. (1966) Two storage mechanisms in free recall. *Journal of Verbal Learning and Verbal Behavior*, **5**, 351–360.

Goldberg, T.E., Weinberger, D.R. (1988) Probing prefrontal function in schizophrenia with neuropsychological paradigms. *Schizophrenia Bulletin*, **14**, 179–183.

Goldberg, T.E., Weinberger, D.R., Berman, K.F., Pliskin, N.H., Podd, M.H. (1987) Further evidence for dementia of the prefrontal type in schizophrenia? A controlled study of teaching the Wisconsin Card Sorting Test. *Archives of General Psychiatry*, **44**, 1008–1014.

Goldberg, T.E., Weinberger, D.R., Pliskin, N.H., Berman, K.F., Podd, M.H. (1989) Recall memory deficit in schizophrenia: A possible manifestation of prefrontal dysfunction. *Schizophrenia Research*, **2**, 251–157.

Goldberg, T.E., Torrey, E.F., Gold, J.M., Ragland, J.D., Bigelow, L.B., Weinberger, D.R. (1993) Learning and memory in monozygotic twins discordant for schizophrenia. *Psychological Medicine*, **23**, 71–85.

Golding, E. (1989) *The Middlesex Elderly Assessment of Mental State*, Thames Valley Test Co., Tichfield, UK.

Goldman-Rakic, P.S., Friedman, H.R. (1991) The circuitry of working memory revealed by anatomy and metabolic imaging. In: *Frontal Lobe Function and Dysfunction* (Eds H.S. Levin, H.M. Eisenberg, A.L. Benton), pp. 72–91, Oxford University Press, Oxford.

Gruzelier, J., Seymour, K., Wilson, L., Jolley, A., Hirsch, S. (1988) Impairments on neuropsychologic tests of temporohippocampal and frontohippocampal functions and word fluency in remitting schizophrenia and affective disorders. *Archives of General Psychiatry*, **24**, 214–217.

Helkala, E.-L., Laurlumma, V., Soininen, H., Riekkinen, P.J. (1988) Recall and recognition memory in patients with Alzheimer's and Parkinson's disease. *Annals of Neurology*, **24**, 214–217.

Hirst, W. (1982) The amnesic syndrome: Descriptions and explanations. *Psychological Bulletin*, **91**, 435–460.

Hodges, J.R., Salmon, D.P., Butters, N. (1992) Semantic memory impairment in Alzheimer's disease: Failure of access or degraded knowledge? *Neuropsychologia*, **30**, 301–314.

Hoffman, R.E. (1987) Computer simulations of neural information processing and the schizophrenia–mania dichotomy. *Archives of General Psychiatry*, **44**, 178–188.

Huston, P.E., Shakow, D. (1949) Learning capacity in schizophrenia. *American Journal of Psychiatry*, **105**, 881–888.

Jeste, D., Lohr, J.B. (1989) Hippocampal pathologic findings in schizophrenia. *Archives of General Psychiatry*, **46**, 1019–1024.

Jetter, W., Poser, U., Freeman, R.B., Markowitsch, H.J. (1986) A verbal long term memory deficit in frontal lobe damaged patients. *Cortex*, **22**, 229–246.

Kelsoe, J.R., Cadet, J.L., Pickar, D., Weinberger, D.R. (1988) Quantitative neuroanatomy in schizophrenia. *Archives of General Psychiatry*, **45**, 533–541.

Kopelman, M.D., Wilson, B.A., Baddeley, A.D. (1990) *The Autobiographical Memory Interview*, Thames Valley Test Co, Bury St Edmunds, UK.

Kraepelin, E. (1913) *Dementia Praecox and Paraphrenia* (translated by R.M. Barclay, 1919), Livingstone, Edinburgh.

Kwapil, T.R., Hegley, D.C., Chapman, L.J., Chapman, J.P. (1990) Facilitation of word recognition by semantic priming in schizophrenia. *Journal of Abnormal Psychology*, **99**, 215–221.

Liddle, P.F., Morris, D.L. (1991) Schizophrenic syndromes and frontal lobe performance. *British Journal of Psychiatry*, **158**, 340–345.

Manschreck, T.C., Maher, B.A., Milavetz, B.A., Ames, D., Weisstein, C.C., Schneyer, M.L. (1988) Semantic priming in thought disordered schizophrenic patients. *Schizophrenia Research*, **1**, 61–66.

McKenna, P.J. (1991) Memory, knowledge and delusions. *British Journal of Psychiatry*, **159** (Suppl. 14), 36–41.

McKenna, P.J., Tamlyn, D., Lund, C.E., Mortimer, A.M., Hammond, S., Baddeley, A.D. (1990) Amnesic syndrome in schizophrenia. *Psychological Medicine*, **20**, 967–972.

McKenna, P.J., Mortimer, A.M., Hodges, J.R. (1994) Semantic memory and schizophrenia. In: *The Neuropsychology of Schizophrenia* (Eds A.S. David, J.C. Cutting), pp. 163–178, Erlbaum, Hove.

Mesulam, M.M., Geula, C. (1988) Nucleus basalis and cortical cholinergic innervation in the human brain: Observations based on the distribution of acetylcholinesterase and choline acetyltransferase. *Journal of Comparative Neurology*, **275**, 216–240.

Meyer, D.E., Schvaneveldt, R.W. (1971) Facilitation in recognizing pairs of words: Evidence for a dependence between retrieval operations. *Journal of Experimental Psychology*, **20**, 227–234.

Milner, B. (1971) Interhemispheric differences in the localisation of psychological processes in man. *British Medical Bulletin*, **27**, 272–277.

Morice, R. (1990) Cognitive inflexibility and prefrontal dysfunction in schizophrenia and mania. *British Journal of Psychiatry*, **157**, 50–54.

Park, S., Holzman, P.S. (1992) Schizophrenics show spatial working memory deficits. *Archives of General Psychiatry*, **49**, 975–982.

Postman, L., Phillips, L.W. (1965) Short-term temporal changes in free recall. *Quarterly Journal of Experimental Psychology*, **17**, 132–138.

Saykin, A.J., Gur, R.E., Mozley, P.D., Resnick, S.M., Kester, B., Stafiniak, P. (1991) Neuropsychological function in schizophrenia: Selective impairment in memory and learning. *Archives of General Psychiatry*, **48**, 618–624.

Shallice, T., Burgess, P.W., Frith, C.D. (1991) Can the neuropsychological case study approach be applied to schizophrenia? *Psychological Medicine*, **21**, 661–673.

Shimamura, A.P., Janowsky, J.S., Squire, L. (1991) What is the role of frontal lobe damage in memory disorders? In: *Frontal Lobe Function and Dysfunction* (Eds H.S. Levin, H.M. Eisenberg, A.L. Benton), pp. 173–198, Oxford University Press, Oxford.

Squire, L.R., Cohen, N. (1979) Memory and amnesia: Resistance to disruption develops. *Neuroscience*, **11**, 170–175.

Squire, L.R., Zola-Morgan, S. (1991) The medial temporal lobe memory system. *Science*, **253**, 1380–1385.

Stevens, M. (1979) The Famous Personality Test: A test for measuring remote memory. *Bulletin of the British Psychological Society*, **32**, 211–211.

Suddath, R.L., Casanova, M.F., Goldberg, T.E., Daniel, D.G., Kelsoe, J.R. Jr., Weinberger, D.R. (1989) Temporal lobe pathology in schizophrenia: A quantitative magnetic resonance imaging study. *American Journal of Psychiatry*, **146**, 464–472.

Tamlyn, D., McKenna, P.J., Mortimer, A.M., Lund, C.E., Hammond, S., Baddeley, A.D. (1992) Memory impairment in schizophrenia: Its extent, affiliations and neuropsychological character. *Psychological Medicine*, **22**, 101–115.

Tamminga, C.A., Thaker, G.K., Buchanan, R. et al (1992) Limbic system abnormalities identified in schizophrenia using positron emission tomography with fluorodeoxyglucose and neocortical alterations with deficit syndrome. *Archives of General Psychiatry*, **49**, 522–530.

Tulving, E. (1983) *Elements of Episodic Memory*, Oxford University Press, Oxford.

Warrington, E.K. (1984) *Recognition Memory Test*, NFER–Nelson, Windsor.

Warrington, E.K., Shallice, T. (1984) Category specific semantic impairments. *Brain*, **107**, 829–854.

Weinberger, D.R., Berman, K.F., Daniel, D.G. (1991) Prefrontal cortex dysfunction in schizophrenia. In: *Frontal Lobe Function and Dysfunction* (Eds H.S. Levin, H.M. Eisenberg, A.L. Benton), pp. 275–287, Oxford University Press, Oxford.

Wilson, B.A., Cockburn, J.M., Baddeley, A.D. (1985) *The Rivermead Behavioural Memory Test*, Thames Valley Test Co., Tichfield, UK.

Zaidel, D.W. (1987) Hemispheric asymmetry in long term semantic relationships. *Cognitive Neuropsychology*, **4**, 321–332.

8

Lateralised Dysfunction is Necessary but not Sufficient to Account for Neuropsychological Deficits in Schizophrenia

JOHN GRUZELIER

INTRODUCTION

Contemporary interest in lateralised dysfunction in schizophrenia had its origins in the association of schizophrenic-like symptoms in epilepsy involving the left temporal lobe (Flor-Henry, 1969). This claim was a catalyst riding on the wave of research stimulated by new discoveries about hemispheric specialisation from patients following commissurotomy. During the first decade research polarised around two, seen to be competing, views: a disorder of the left hemisphere or a disorder of the interhemispheric pathways. Much research was guided by lesion data but when results at an international symposium on the topic were reviewed (Gruzelier & Flor-Henry, 1979), structural approaches could not explain the subtle processing anomalies disclosed and the way ahead seemed to lie with functional systems: "The splitting of functions described by the term schizophrenia, but apparent in all forms of psychopathology, may plausibly have a counterpart in disordered connections among brain subsystems both within and between the hemispheres; subsystems with a working rather than anatomical unity" (Gruzelier, 1979a, p. 671).

Journal reviews quickly followed (Wexler, 1980; Gruzelier, 1981a; Newlin et al, 1981; Merrin, 1981; Marin & Tucker, 1981; Walker & McGuire, 1982), one of which documented the popularity of the concept in the 18th and 19th centuries (Harrington, 1985). Impetus was given to two further conferences (Flor-Henry &

Schizophrenia: A Neuropsychological Perspective. Edited by C. Pantelis, H.E. Nelson and T.R.E. Barnes
© 1996 John Wiley & Sons Ltd

Gruzelier, 1983; Takahashi et al, 1987) so that, by the end of the second decade of research, schizophrenia was considered of relevance to neurology and included in the *Handbook of Clinical Neurology* (Gruzelier, 1985), applications of neuropsychological tests had become widely accepted (Weinberger et al, 1986; Gruzelier et al, 1988) and clinical neuropsychological contributions warranted a review (Levin et al, 1989). In that review Levin et al reaffirmed the importance of a systems account:

> Two general models of structural and functional impairment in schizophrenia are thus evident from the review. One model proposes deficits in the cortical/subcortical processes that support attention, arousal and higher cortical functions. The second suggests an impairment in the balance of lateralised functions, which is consonant with left hemispheric overactivation. These models can be viewed in terms of a *brain systems* [author's italics] approach. Each model is based on an extended network of regions that together subserve identifiable neuropsychological processes. Functional deficits of the systems proposed, therefore reflect pathology within the neural system but not a discrete localised lesion, because any disturbance along a stream of neural connections may result in grossly similar behavioural pathology.

The organisation of this chapter will use the quote from Levin et al as a departure. First, the imbalance model will be reviewed which will show *inter alia* that the left hemisphere overactivation model cited by Levin et al cannot account for the data. Opposite states of imbalance exist and the two underpin negative and positive syndromes of schizophrenia. Second, evidence for an abnormality in interhemispheric transmission will be reviewed; this is one candidate, a strong one, for the locus of the mechanism underlying hemispheric imbalance. Third, the research on subcortical-cortical attentional asymmetry will be considered.

SYNDROME-RELATED PATTERNS OF HEMISPHERIC IMBALANCE

Gur (1978) made the first clear proposal of a dysfunction of the left hemisphere in schizophrenia due to overactivation. This was based on evidence of the coexistence of two anomalies: (1) predominantly rightward conjugate eye movements, indicative of greater left than right hemispheric activation in frontal eye fields; (2) left hemisphere deficits in the processing of linguistic information presented hemiretinally and transmitted over the direct right visual field to left hemisphere pathway. The tachistoscopic result was interpreted as a deficit which Gur attributed to left hemispheric overactivation in view of the activational bias represented by the eye movement asymmetry. Subsequent evidence of spatial deficits were explained as a consequence of a functional bias away from the right hemispheric functions due to left hemispheric over-activation (Gur, 1979). Thus, the nature of the dysfunction in schizophrenia was firmly localised to the left hemisphere (see Gur et al, 1989).

While rightward conjugate eye movements in schizophrenia were also reported by Schweitzer et al (1978) and Tomer et al (1979), Sandel and Alcorn (1980) found that non-paranoid schizophrenic and depressive patients had more leftward movements in contrast to schizoaffective and manic-depressive patients who had no consistent asymmetry. The association of rightward movements with schizophrenia was further weakened by Myslobodsky et al (1983) who noted that unmedicated patients with schizophrenia showed no consistent lateral asymmetry, whereas it was the patients on neuroleptics who showed the rightward asymmetry. The patients of Gur, Schweitzer et al and Tomer et al were medicated which suggests that the uniformity of their results may have been a function of drugs.

ELECTRODERMAL ORIENTING RESPONSE ASYMMETRIES

It was the feature of inconsistency of lateral asymmetry in a psychophysiological measure, in this instance an asymmetry in electrodermal responses to auditory orienting stimuli, which inspired the investigation of syndrome relations to asymmetry in unmedicated schizophrenic patients. This led to a new approach to cerebral asymmetry in schizophrenia (Gruzelier, 1981b, 1984; Gruzelier & Manchanda, 1982). Forty-eight patients in two consecutive samples were classified on the basis of electrodermal response asymmetry while symptoms were evaluated with the Present State Examination (PSE; Wing et al, 1974) and the modified Brief Psychiatric Rating Scale (BPRS; Overall & Gorham, 1962). Electrodermal orienting responses were recorded as a putative index of amygdaloid–hippocampal influences (Gruzelier & Venables, 1972; Gruzelier, 1983). Patients with larger left (L) than right (R) hand responses were characterised by positive symptoms of behavioural overactivity, pressure of speech, manic or grandiose ideas and exaggerated or inappropriate labile affect, while patients with the opposite pattern of asymmetry were characterised by negative symptoms of social and emotional withdrawal, blunted affect, poverty of speech and motor retardation.

The L > R and R > L asymmetry patterns were interpreted as having a counterpart in L > R and R > L hemispheric asymmetries, in keeping with the prevailing view at the time of hemispheric influences on electrodermal activity involving complementary processes of contralateral inhibition and ipsilateral excitation (Gruzelier, 1979b). This indicated that the left hemisphere was dominant in the positive syndrome and the right hemisphere dominant in the negative syndrome. This interpretation was also compatible with a neuropsychological translation of symptoms indicating a dominance of left hemisphere functions in what came to be called the "active" syndrome and a dominance of the right hemisphere with corresponding underactivation of the left hemisphere in what came to be called the "withdrawn" syndrome. The fundamental psychological features that distinguished the syndromes were consistent with social interaction/withdrawal models of left versus right hemispheric specialisation respectively (Kinsbourne, 1982; Davidson & Tomarken, 1989; Tucker & Williamson, 1984; Ehrlichman, 1987). The interpretation of lateralised influences on bilateral electrodermal recording and also the primary importance of limbic influences, has been recently confirmed by intracranial stimulation in the limbic system in neurological patients awaiting surgery. Excitatory effects were shown to be ipsilaterally transmitted and were maximal with unilateral stimulation of the amygdala, followed by the hippocampus, but were negligible with cortical stimulation (Mangina & Beuzeron-Mangina, 1994, 1996).

The syndromes did not hinge on a simple positive–negative symptom dichotomy because all patients had positive symptoms in the form of Schneiderian symptoms of first rank, which were unrelated to type or degree of asymmetry pattern. This constituted a third syndrome—the "unreality" syndrome. The three-syndrome structure is compatible with a large number of factor analytic studies of clinical ratings of schizophrenic patients which have produced a three-factor structure of one negative and two positive syndromes (Bilder, 1985; Liddle, 1987; Liddle & Barnes, 1990; Arndt et al, 1991; Gur et al, 1991). In a study of speech disorganisation in schizophrenia and mania Hoffman et al (1986) found that one-third of patients with Research Diagnostic Criteria (RDC; Spitzer et al, 1978) for schizophrenia who did not fulfil criteria for schizoaffective disorder had manic-like speech and were characterised by "elevated mood, insomnia, increased activity, grandiosity, irritability, accelerated speech and accelerated thinking", a profile which as they acknowledge is similar to the active syndrome.

FUNCTIONAL, DYNAMIC PROCESS ASYMMETRIES

Evidence of two asymmetry patterns in schizophrenia offered a possibility of unravelling some of the contradictions which were all too pervasive in the research on lateral asymmetry and schizophrenia at the time. A comprehensive review was undertaken to determine to what extent evidence of opposite asymmetries within and across studies might be resolved by the syndrome approach (Gruzelier, 1983). In many instances measures which showed either left hemisphere advantages or right hemisphere disadvantages were obtained in samples having affinities with the active syndrome such as paranoid, acute, reactive, or positive symptom, whereas right hemisphere advantages, or alternately left hemisphere losses of function, were found in patients described as non-paranoid, chronic, process or with negative symptoms, all having affinities with the withdrawn syndrome.

A main factor made apparent by that review and its updating (Gruzelier, 1987a) was that those dependent variables that most readily disclosed syndrome-related patterns of asymmetry, with few exceptions belonged to the dynamic functional class rather than the structural class of brain asymmetry. Measures included EEG power, cortical evoked potentials, the Hoffman reflex, electrodermal activity, conjugate lateral eye movements, dichotic listening, asymmetry of directed attention, dichotic and monotic shadowing, auditory thresholds, somatosensory extinction, spontaneous eye movements and eye movement patterns during visual search, visual hemi-neglect, brain metabolism and brain blood flow. Amongst measures of structure, handedness showed associations between right handedness and positive symptoms and left handedness and negative symptoms, whereas neuropsychological test batteries tended to indicate bilateral impairment (Goldstein, 1991).

ASYMMETRY PATTERNS IN LEARNING AND MEMORY

Validation of the model was undertaken with complementary left and right hemisphere experimental neuropsychological tests of learning and memory (Gruzelier et al, 1987a, 1988). These had fulfilled double dissociation criteria in distinguishing between neurological patients with unilateral lesions of temporo- and fronto-hippocampal functions: Hebb's recurring digits test, the right hemisphere analogue Corsi's blocks and spatial and non-spatial conditional associate learning (Milner, 1982). Verbal fluency was also examined. Patients with schizophrenia were classified as active and withdrawn and compared with affective psychotic patients and controls. Deficits on both temporo-hippocampal tests were found in the patients with schizophrenia, though the group as a whole only differed from controls with the verbal test, as can be seen in Figure 8.1 where learning curves for recurrent supraspan trials are plotted for digits and blocks. There it can be seen that learning across recurring trials does take place in patients with schizophrenia but the number of subjects showing this is reduced on the verbal test compared with both depressive and normal controls and on the spatial test relative to controls. As there were no group differences in non-recurrent spans the impairment in schizophrenia cannot be attributed to a gener-alised factor. The same conclusion about generalised impairment can be drawn for the spatial test.

Eighteen of the 36 patients with schizophrenia had unambiguous cognitive asymmetry with both patterns equally represented. Patients were categorised according to active and withdrawn syndromes and examined for asymmetry

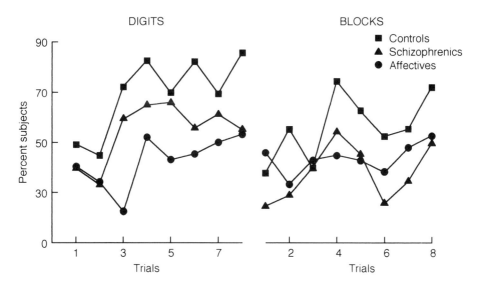

Figure 8.1. Learning curves for recurrent trials for schizophrenic and affective psychosis patients and controls

pattern. Those with the active syndrome had more deficits on the blocks test and those with the withdrawn syndrome had more deficits on the verbal test. These results showed that, in terms of hemispheric imbalance, losses of function in learning and memory corresponded with the less activated not the more activated or overactivated hemisphere.

The fronto-temporal conditional associative learning tests also provided evidence that patients with schizophrenia may manifest either pattern of asymmetry, as shown in Figure 8.2. Fifteen patients had clear asymmetry patterns. Of the nine with a spatial advantage five belonged to the predicted withdrawn syndrome and two had an active or a mixed active/withdrawn syndrome. In contrast all five patients with a non-spatial advantage belonged to the active syndrome. Thus, 10/15 patients showed results consistent with the model.

The data from the two tests were pooled and comparisons were made on those CATEGO syndromes from the PSE that contributed to the syndromes (Gruzelier & Manchanda, 1982). The 16 with an asymmetry advantaging the left hemisphere were characterised by active syndrome and non-specific factors while the 15 with left hemispheric losses of function were characterised by withdrawn syndrome features. In comparisons between patients subdivided on the basis of the frontal

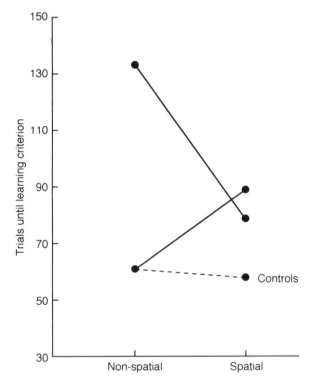

Figure 8.2. Associative learning tasks showing two asymmetry groups in patients with schizophrenia

test alone, those with a left frontal advantage were characterised by grandiose and religious delusions, that is, features of the active syndrome.

Verbal fluency deficits were present in almost one half of patients. Correlations between the tests indicated the existence of a general factor in patients with schizophrenia but not in controls. However, the two temporo-hippocampal tests did not correlate with the other tests in any of the groups suggesting a specificity of function. Twenty-eight of 36 patients had CT scans, but no relations could be found between focal memory deficits and atrophy or enlarged ventricles.

In summary, in patients with schizophrenia with patterned deficits there was consistent evidence of two cognitive asymmetry patterns associated with active or withdrawn syndromes. The impairments in learning and memory corresponded to the hemisphere with the lower level of activation, the right in the active syndrome and the left in the withdrawn syndrome. Considering the group as a whole the specific lateralised deficits were seen against a background of general impairment.

ASYMMETRY PATTERNS IN RECOGNITION MEMORY IN SCHIZOPHRENIA

The syndrome–asymmetry relations have been reexamined in a recently completed, large-scale investigation with 104 schizophrenic patients, 36 of whom were studied longitudinally across separate episodes or periods of remission (Gruzelier et al, 1996). Patients were classified as belonging to active, withdrawn and mixed syndromes and were examined for asymmetry patterns in recognition memory for words versus unfamiliar faces. The tests fulfilled double dissociation criteria in differentiating patients with unilateral lesions of the temporal and parietal lobes (Warrington, 1984), tests which have been validated with topographical mapping of electrocortical activity in normal subjects (Burgess & Gruzelier, 1996).

Male active and withdrawn patients showed opposite cognitive asymmetries, a word advantage in the active syndrome and a face advantage in both the withdrawn syndrome and the mixed syndrome. The asymmetrical impairment was on average at a level comparable to that shown in the test norms with neurological patients. Female patients as a group showed poorer memory for words (also at deficit levels) and while in withdrawn females there was a strong face advantage, in active and mixed groups no reliable asymmetry was found. Results are shown in Figure 8.3.

It follows that if asymmetry patterns constitute neurophysiological underpinnings they must be found to be stable across episodes and should the presenting symptoms change from one syndrome to another the asymmetry patterns should change correspondingly. Nine patients were tested twice in the same state in different episodes or in successive states of remission. The same cognitive asymmetry was found across sessions in eight of nine patients and the correlation between asymmetry scores was high (0.84), as it was for face scores (0.90). Only for words did the moderate correlation (0.48) not reach significance. An additional five patients belonged to different syndromes in different episodes. Asymmetry patterns varied with syndrome and were consistent with a word

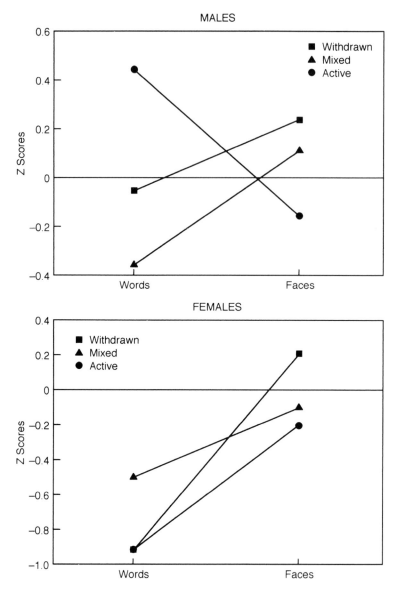

Figure 8.3. Word and face recognition memory scores for patients with schizophrenia subdivided into active, withdrawn and mixed syndromes; males, upper figure; females, lower figure

advantage when active and a face advantage when withdrawn, while in the mixed syndrome there was a face advantage or a reduced word advantage.

A functional component to impairment was disclosed by examining patients whose symptoms were in remission. Remitted patients showed better memory overall, particularly when compared with active females and withdrawn males. Longitudinal comparisons made between psychotic episodes and states of remission endorsed the functional component of the impairment. There was an improvement in memory with symptom remission; nevertheless, performance remained within the deficit range and represented a level of mild deficit.

The residual deficit may not represent structural impairment. Active syndrome patients showed a reversal in cognitive asymmetry with symptom remission such that the face disadvantage in the psychotic episode gave way to a face advantage in remission. The reversal was almost entirely due to an improvement in memory for faces. In the mixed/withdrawn syndromes there was a face advantage when psychotic and an overall improvement with symptom remission, particularly in memory for words.

Twenty-one patients were free of antipsychotic medication. The asymmetry patterns were the same as those shown in Figure 8.3. Nevertheless, when correlations were obtained between memory scores and dose of neuroleptic, expressed as the chlorpromazine equivalent, word scores fell as a function of increasing dose (median 700 mg/day, range 80–4000 mg/day); $r = -0.36$, $p < 0.002$ for words, $r = -0.11$ for faces. There is extensive evidence that neuroleptic drugs have lateralised effects and this will be referred to again in later sections (see also King and Green, chapter 20). However, correlation does not signify causation.

Some patients on neuroleptics were administered the anticholinergic drug procyclidine, to treat parkinsonian side effects. Comparisons of those with and without this drug revealed that in males on procyclidine there was a global memory impairment whereas in females on procyclidine there was an impairment in word memory and, surprisingly, superior memory for faces. The deleterious effect of the anticholinergic drug on memory is consistent with two other reports (Tune et al, 1982; Perlick et al, 1986) but this has received little systematic investigation and there is nothing to suggest an improvement in memory for faces in females. The latter effect could simply reflect underlying patient differences.

CONCLUSION

In summary, the results with recognition memory for words and faces indicate opposite asymmetry patterns in active and withdrawn syndromes in schizophrenia and in schizotypy (discussed below) in the direction of reduced performance in the hemisphere with the lower level of activation. This is consistent with the previous results with lateralised tests of learning and memory in schizophrenia (Gruzelier et al, 1987a, 1988). However, when negative symptoms were combined with active ones, as seen in the mixed syndrome, male patients had the face advantage found in the withdrawn syndrome. This was in keeping with evidence that the right hemisphere with its negative affective valence may dominate the control of emotional valence and the balance of activity between the hemispheres (Silberman & Weingartner, 1986; Heller, 1993). In this and other respects gender was a moderating variable (see below for discussion).

These data together with the psychophysiological evidence, which now includes an EEG spectrum analysis of visual evoked potentials in an augmenting/reducing paradigm (Gruzelier et al, 1993) and posterior temporal P300 asymmetries, both measured in different patient samples classified as Active and Withdrawn (Gruzelier, in press), indicate that the imbalance between the hemispheres is not unidirectional in schizophrenia. A positive, active syndrome is associated with an imbalance in the direction of higher (over)activation of the left hemisphere and underactivation of the right hemisphere, while a negative, withdrawn syndrome is associated with the opposite state of imbalance. Thus, hemispheric imbalance is associated with the expression of symptoms. It follows that the left hemisphere overactivation model first proposed by Gur (1978) is an incomplete explanation of schizophrenic dysfunction.

The nature of the underlying mechanism that gives rise to the imbalance is not known. It may be a callosal, commissural or an interhemispheric mechanism, or it may involve subcortical–cortical interactions such as brain stem/thalamocortical mechanisms that determine the topography of cortical activation (e.g. Gruzelier et al, 1993). Evidence for interhemispheric transmission anomalies, now reviewed, will be seen in many instances to show different relations with positive versus negative syndromes and with lateralised abnormalities, all suggestive of an integrated callosal transmission, lateralised dysfunction model, rather than the opposing theoretical positions that polarised the pioneering research in the field.

INTERHEMISPHERIC TRANSMISSION

CALLOSAL STRUCTURE

Interest was stimulated by postmortem findings and notions of a disconnection of conscious from unconscious processes, thought to reside in left and right hemispheres respectively (Galin, 1974; Nasrallah, 1986). Rosenthal & Bigelow (1972) reported increased width of the corpus callosum, restricted in a replication study to anterior and medial regions and to illnesses of recent onset (Bigelow et al, 1983). In the latter sample gliosis was seen in the posterior regions and was associated with late onset schizophrenic psychoses. By the end of the 1980s postmortem and magnetic resonance imaging (MRI) investigations have reported the corpus callosum to be both smaller and larger in schizophrenia (summarised by Raine et al, 1990). Of the six investigations which examined regional variation five reported anterior enlargement in females, including the study of Raine et al (1990) in which this was also characteristic of affective psychoses.

Symptom associations have been examined by Gunther et al (1991) who with MRI found that positive symptom patients had a larger callosal area than negative symptom patients. Enlargement coexisted with increased bilateral blood flow following dominant hand motor activation in those with positive symptoms, whereas there was a failure to show task-induced changes in those with negative symptoms. A review by Coger & Serafetinides (1990) came to the opposite conclusion about the relation between callosal width and positive and negative symptoms. Nevertheless, their conclusion is tempered by a slender data base for few investigators have documented symptoms. The conclusion rested on two strands of evidence. The first was the evidence of Bigelow et al (1983) above and Nasrallah et al (1983), who examined the same sample as Bigelow and colleagues, in which the distinction revolved around early versus late onset (thick versus thin callosa, respectively). Here, the inference from age of onset to symptoms is indirect and is unlikely to polarise simply around a positive/negative distinction. In the one other study which has rated symptoms, aside from the study by Gunther et al, no relation to width was found with positive/negative symptoms (Mathew et al, 1985).

Additionally, there was behavioural and psychophysiological evidence. Before considering this literature it should be noted that only one study has measured both callosal structure and callosal function with behavioural tasks (Raine et al, 1990). In this MRI study of 15 patients, no parallel was found between evidence of enlarged callosal area and deficits in interhemispheric transmission examined with verbal and non-verbal dichotic listening and intermanual transfer tasks. Nevertheless, evidence for interhemispheric transmission abnormalities does exist and this will be briefly considered; for more detailed coverage see Gruzelier (1983, 1986; see also Neufeld & Williamson, chapter 11).

AUDITORY PROCESSES

Dichotic listening studies with split brain patients have shown exaggerated right ear advantages for verbal material, suggesting that linguistic information presented to the left ear must reach the left hemisphere via the callosum after projection via the contralateral pathway to the right hemisphere (Springer & Gazzaniga, 1975). It follows that damage to the callosum should result in larger than normal right ear advantages. While not characteristic of schizophrenia in general, larger than normal right ear advantages have been shown in a subgroup of patients variously characterised as paranoid (Lerner et al, 1977; Gruzelier & Hammond, 1979, 1980), having auditory hallucinations (Colbourne & Lishman, 1979), or as electrodermally responsive to auditory stimuli (as distinct from non-responsiveness), a condition which characterises about half of the patients with schizophrenia (Gruzelier & Hammond, 1979).

While a disconnection interpretation has been offered (Walker et al, 1981), the results of this subgroup with the right ear advantage appear more in line with a functional imbalance in activity favouring the left hemisphere. This was concluded from results in the paranoid aroused group showing that if left ear recall was cued, or if stimuli were louder in the left ear, the right ear bias could largely be reversed which could not occur if there was a structural disconnection (Gruzelier & Hammond, 1979, 1980; Gruzelier, 1987b). The non-paranoid and electrodermally non-responsive subgroup showed an absence of the normal right ear advantage and a bias to the left ear–right hemisphere. It is noteworthy, in view of the confounding effects of medication that operate on lateral asymmetry, that symptom-related ear differences were found reliably across six fortnightly sessions and were not influenced by a 4-week withdrawal of medication or its reinstatement.

This same study also disclosed a subtle inhibitory deficit when instructions to attend to one ear were pitted against a 20 dB intensity advantage to the opposite ear. Thirteen of 19 patients had greater difficulty in withholding the recall of louder right ear digits in favour of quieter left ear digits than the reverse, whereas 10 of 16 controls showed the opposite asymmetry, an effect also found in an unpublished study by Bull (1972) where it characterised paranoid patients. The disability in patients was consistent with a deficit, either of left hemisphere inhibition and therefore in line with left hemispheric overactivation, or of interhemispheric transmission in a right-to-left direction.

More promising evidence of a transmission deficit has been found in the form of a disability in integrating information presented binaurally and presumed to involve interhemispheric pathways. This was found in story comprehension where there were more errors with binaural presentation (Green & Kotenko, 1980; Green et al, 1983; Kugler, 1983; Green, 1985). This disability was not true of all patients, being apparent in patients with acute schizophrenia in whom it coincided with a right ear advantage to monaural presentation. Chronic patients have shown no binaural deficit and either no ear advantage or the opposite left ear advantage (Green et al, 1983). As the right hemisphere has the auditory vocabulary of an 18-year-old it is not possible to conclude that there is an abnormal structural lateralisation of language in chronic patients, instead a functional advantage to the right hemisphere is indicated. Whether binaural deficits represent a true problem of integration or are attributable to some other parameter such as stimulus intensity has not been evaluated.

A similar subtle deficit of binaural over monaural listening has been shown in a spatial compatibility reaction time task (Gruzelier & Hammond, 1979). Reaction times were slower to the commands "left" and "right" when heard binaurally than monaurally. This was found in symptomatic patients in contrast to those with symptoms controlled by neuroleptics. The binaural deficits suggested a difficulty in integrating auditory input across interhemispheric pathways and were more apparent in acute rather than chronic patients.

In conclusion, the opposite asymmetries in dichotic listening in patients described as acute, paranoid or electrodermally responsive compared with patients described as chronic, non-paranoid and non-responsive are in keeping with the syndrome-imbalance model. The left > right hemispheric imbalance in the active, acute symptoms may also coexist with interhemispheric integration deficits.

STEREOGNOSIS

Setting aside methodological confounds of many stereognostic experiments described in previous reviews, which may have led to spurious claims for interhemispheric integration deficits, negative results (Kugler & Henley, 1979; Schrift et al, 1986; Craft et al, 1987; Raine et al, 1989, 1990) are as common as affirmative results (Green & Kotenko, 1980; Dimond et al, 1979; Carr, 1980; Hatta et al, 1984) and several studies have found support for left hemispheric impairments (Kugler & Henley, 1979; Schrift et al, 1986). There would appear to be no obvious clinical differences that would unravel the controversy, for subgroups have seldom been considered and symptoms rarely documented. Though Hatta et al (1984) specify that their patients, aside from being chronic and medicated, were hallucinated and deluded, indicating that positive symptoms (though not of the active syndrome type) are represented in patients with transfer deficits.

Experiments on the cross-localisation of touch have produced no global transfer deficit (Weller & Kugler, 1979; Raine et al, 1989, 1990; Craft et al, 1987). Asymmetrical patterns of errors in schizoaffective patients were reported in two studies in the direction of left-to-right hand localisation errors which involve right-to-left callosal transmission (Weller & Kugler, 1979; Craft et al, 1987); the last-mentioned study found the opposite pattern of errors in chronic patients.

Chronic patients with schizophrenia and schizoaffective disorder have been found to make more errors in directed movement tasks (Weller & Kugler, 1979; Craft et al, 1987), with chronic schizophrenic patients showing more mirror movements. Mirror movements are found in children and they decrease with age. This has been attributed to the development of callosal inhibitory functions and the suppression of ipsilateral pathways (Dennis, 1981).

VISUAL PROCESSES

Estimates of callosal crossing time have disclosed no evidence of interhemispheric transfer impairment in divided visual field studies (Connolly et al, 1979, 1983a; Shelton & Knight, 1984), though there has been agreement in reports of left hemispheric processing anomalies in patterns of errors (Gur, 1978; Colbourn & Lishman, 1979) or in speed of processing (Connolly et al, 1979, 1983a; Hillsberg, 1979). Left hemispheric involvement is inferred because the results have been obtained for stimuli presented to the right visual field irrespective of stimulus type, or for linguistic but not spatial stimuli.

Difficulties in matching information between hemi-fields have been reported in some (Beaumont & Dimond, 1973; Eaton et al, 1979; David, 1987) but not all studies (Magaro & Page, 1983; Wade & Taylor, 1984; Merriam & Gardner, 1987). Evidence affirming the callosal hypothesis may be confounded by the greater attentional demands of cross-matching.

May consideration of subgroups resolve the conflict of results about transfer? Reports are in conflict. David (1987) found that it was patients with currently active first rank symptoms who had a tendency to be naming colours in the left visual field, but not in matching colours within the same field. An interhemispheric deficit in transferring information from the right to the left hemisphere for linguistic expression was suggested, as found in patients with lesions of the splenium or posterior regions of the corpus callosum; though the colour naming task was not matched with a complementary right hemisphere task to allow consideration of a corresponding deficit in rightward callosal transmission. However, in another divided field investigation (David, 1993) patients with schizophrenia were distinguished from controls and affective patients but it was the recovered patients who were the more impaired. The task involved a divided-field Stroop procedure with colours and colour words presented centrally or in opposite hemi-fields in congruent or incongruent combinations. Normal controls and affective disorder patients showed both more interference and more facilitation, according to stimulus class, when stimuli were presented centrally whereas the patients with schizophrenia showed the opposite result. This was interpreted as a failure to regulate interhemispheric transmission, signifying functional hyperconnection.

Hyperconnection has previously been reported in patients with schizophrenia and schizoaffective disorder in studies of the interocular transfer of movement after-effects involving monocular viewing of a rotating pattern (Tress et al, 1979; Craft et al, 1987). Contrary to the impaired transfer model (the effect is absent in acallosals) the results indicated that, in those patients who showed reliable after-effects, the difference between contralateral and ipsilateral conditions was unexpectedly smaller, suggesting increased callosal connectivity and/or a deficit in transcallosal inhibition. However, the shorter after-effect duration raises the question of whether attentional factors may have interfered with the results; measurement of psychophysical ogives of stimulus duration would add to the reliability of the findings (Gruzelier, 1979a).

CORTICAL EVOKED POTENTIALS

Evoked potential studies have suggested abnormal ipsilateral–contralateral relationships in somatosensory (Tress et al, 1979, 1983; Jones & Miller, 1981; Shagass et al, 1983; Cooper et al, 1985; Andrews et al, 1986, 1987) and auditory (Connolly et al, 1983b, 1985) modalities. A possible callosal abnormality was indicated by the report of an unusual symmetry of latency or response amplitude to unilateral stimulation of the finger (Jones & Miller, 1981: Tress et al, 1979; Cooper et al, 1985; Andrews et al, 1986). This research has been subject to methodological criticism and uncertainty as to whether the distal extremities have callosal representation. Accordingly, abnormally short ipsilateral latencies and apparent bilateral symmetry of amplitude may indicate the abnormal development of ipsilateral pathways, perhaps secondary to developmental callosal abnormalities.

Andrews et al (1986, 1987) examined the phenomenon in association with the active and withdrawn syndromes of Gruzelier & Manchanda (1982). The abnormal symmetry was found to be associated with the withdrawn syndrome. A subgroup of patients were examined on a selection of lateralised and interhemispheric tasks, including verbal and non-verbal dichotic listening, finger sequence repetition, block design, auditory thresholds and the stereognosis cross-matching task used by Hatta et al (1984) and including an assessment of whether task strategy was verbal or spatial. While patients as a group did not differ from patient controls, those with the symmetrical evoked potential pattern ($N = 5$) showed slower right hand crossed matching relative to uncrossed matching, poorer right ear auditory thresholds and used right hemispheric strategies on the stereognostic task. Consistent with the association of these abnormalities with the withdrawn syndrome, poorer right ear thresholds have been found in patients with the BPRS item "motor retardation" (Mathew et al, 1993), which is one feature of the withdrawn syndrome.

Two somatosensory studies have employed stimulation to the arm or wrist, areas which do have callosal representation and are therefore not subject to uncertainties over callosal transmission in the genesis of ipsilateral evoked potentials. With median nerve stimulation the normal asymmetrical effects were found only when callosal transmission proceeded from left to right and this characterised patients described as actively psychotic. Transmission time was shorter, not longer, in patients and was more reliable in male patients (Gulmann et al, 1982). Tress et al (1983), with an apparatus that tapped the forearm, found slower evoked potential latencies on the ipsilateral than contralateral hand in controls, an asymmetry not found in patients with schizophrenia. They concluded that in patients there appears a more rapid spread of activity from the ipsilateral primary receiving areas. The abnormal pattern was reduced with symptom improvement (BPRS total scores).

In the visual modality evoked potentials have been recorded to two flash intensities with hemi-retinal stimulation in the peripheral visual field during attend (count repetitions of a pattern) and ignore (mental arithmetic) conditions (Buchsbaum et al, 1979). Patients with schizophrenia were compared with temporal lobe epilepsy patients, patients with affective psychosis and normal controls. Electrodes were located over the temporoparietal and occipital regions. Response amplitudes (N120) were larger in the attend condition. The same N120 component was smaller in patients with schizophrenia than controls when stimuli were transmitted over indirect pathways (responses ipsilateral to the visual field), whereas contralateral evoked potentials were of normal amplitude. In the lower intensity condition this tendency was asymmetrical and occurred only with left visual field stimuli, that is, when transmission across the callosum was from right to left. These results were like those of the left temporal lobe epileptic patients who showed reduced amplitudes for indirect pathway responses. Interestingly, right temporal lobe patients showed augmented direct pathway responses as did the affective patient group, interpreted as a right hemispheric inhibitory deficit.

CONCLUSION

Studies of callosal structure have disclosed a heterogeneity of findings implicating attributes such as length (longer versus shorter), width (thicker/thinner), the rostral–caudal dimension and gender. In the one small study which sought both structural and behavioural evidence no parallel was found between structural abnormalities and interhemispheric transfer deficits (Raine et al, 1990). While symptoms have also been implicated the data base is so sketchy that opposite conclusions have been drawn (Gunther et al, 1991; Coger & Serafetinides, 1990).

These limitations notwithstanding, the answer may lie in syndrome differences. In support of this conjecture the interhemispheric transmission deficit has been shown to be subject to lateral asymmetry; an abnormality of transmission in one direction coexisting with normal transmission in the other. Furthermore, these asymmetries have been found in both directions of transmission. The majority of evidence supports a dominance of left hemispheric influences or a difficulty in transmitting information across the callosum from the right to the left hemisphere. This has been documented in patients described as acute (Green et al, 1983; Green, 1985), paranoid (Bull, 1972; Gruzelier & Hammond, 1979, 1980), autonomically responsive (Gruzelier & Hammond, 1979, 1980), actively psychotic

(Buchsbaum et al 1979; Gruzelier & Hammond, 1979; Gulmann et al, 1982), schizoaffective (Weller & Kugler, 1979; Craft et al, 1987) or with first rank symptoms (David, 1987). The opposite pattern of asymmetry depicting a dominance of right hemispheric influences, or a difficulty in transmitting information in a rightward direction, has been described in non-paranoid and electrodermally hyporesponsive patients (Gruzelier & Hammond, 1979, 1980) and in chronic patients (Craft et al, 1987).

Accordingly, syndromes and syndrome-related lateral asymmetries may also be associated with hyper versus hypoconnection. In support of Gunther et al (1991) it is proposed that functional and structural hyperconnection is associated with positive syndrome features. Gunther et al (1991) found that patients with purely positive symptoms had a thicker callosum than those with negative symptoms. In addition to this is the evidence that abnormalities of movement after-effects, suggestive of too much callosal transmission, have been reported in patients with case note evidence of first rank symptoms. Furthermore, there is consistent evidence of a thicker callosum in anterior regions of female patients with schizophrenia, a result shared with affective disorder patients (Raine et al, 1990). This finding may also support the hypothesis if one considers that female patients with schizophrenia have more positive symptoms of an affective type than males (Lewine, 1981; Goldstein & Link, 1988) and that the expression of affect is underpinned by anterior cortical regions (Heller, 1993). The binaural integration impairments may also support the hypothesis of callosal hyperconnection, with or without a lateralised deficit, as all the experiments have required the integration of verbal material. The integration deficit was described in patients who were actively psychotic or acute, in whom the deficit has been associated with lateral asymmetry in the form of a right ear advantage. In other words, this represents a left lateralised deficit in conjunction with a difficulty of transmission interhemispherically in a leftward direction.

Callosal hypoconnection may be associated with chronic, negative and withdrawn syndrome schizophrenia. The somatosensory evoked potential abnormality, manifested in augmented ipsilateral responses which has been interpreted as suggesting an absence of callosal transfer, has been associated with the withdrawn syndrome (Andrews et al, 1987). Chronic patients have disclosed mirror movements which characterise the immature nervous system due to motor overflow and which have been attributed to delayed callosal maturation. Lastly, the binaural interhemispheric integration dysfunction is absent in chronic patients and they showed either no ear advantage or a left ear advantage, the opposite to the asymmetry seen in acute patients. Together these results suggest an association of negative symptoms or maturational deficit with a callosal hypoconnection.

The evoked potential results indicate that in addition to the apparent absence of callosal transmission there is an abnormal facilitation of subcortical–cortical transmission (Tress et al, 1983). Abnormal subcortical–cortical relationships were the focus of research before the interest in lateralised dysfunction arose towards the end of the 1960s (Venables, 1967). The emphasis then was on disturbances in arousal, attention and input dysfunction and consideration was given to abnormal interactions between the brain stem reticular activating system and the cortex. Some of these interests have reemerged in another contemporary systems model based around asymmetry of attention.

ATTENTIONAL ASYMMETRY

HEMI-NEGLECT

In schizophrenia subtle forms of hemi-neglect have been reported. Scarone et al (1981, 1983, 1987) found evidence of neglect of either side of space with a double simultaneous haptic extinction test. Chronicity appeared to influence lateral asymmetry; left neglect was found in acute patients and right neglect in chronic patients. Kawazoe et al (1987) measured eye movements during the Benton visual retention test in patients with schizophrenia who were described as mostly in remission with blunted affect and social withdrawal. More errors of recall were found in the right visual field and eye movement recording disclosed a relative neglect of the right visual field. The neuropsychological results were replicated in the same type of patients (Tsuru & Fujiwara, 1987) and were examined in unilateral temporal lobe epileptic patients who also showed asymmetrical patterns of errors; more right-sided errors in the left foci group and left-sided errors in the right foci group.

These studies are consistent with the syndrome-lateral imbalance model. Left extinction (right-sided loss of function) was found in acute patients, while right extinction (loss of left-sided function) was found in chronic patients, as were more errors of recall and less time spent looking in the right hemi-field reported in patients with social withdrawal and blunted affect.

The same model is applicable to results reflecting overactivation. Bracha (1985) reported visual hallucinations as occurring either bilaterally or more frequently on the right side of space in patients with schizophrenia who were left hemispheric on tests of motor dominance. The opposite asymmetry was found in those who were inconsistently lateralised. They reviewed evidence that lateralisation of visual hallucinations occurs in migraineurs in the hemisphere opposite to the laterality of pain, in epileptic patients contralateral to occipital or parietal foci and in neurosurgical patients contralateral to electrical stimulation of the visual association cortex. Attention to the contralateral side of space will be favoured by electrical stimulation, an irritative focus in epilepsy and the laterality of pain in migraineurs, which has been found to correspond with the more activated hemisphere (Crisp et al, 1985; Gruzelier et al, 1987b). These results suggest greater activation of the left than right hemisphere in the strongly left dominant patients with schizophrenia at the time of visual hallucinations.

Neuroleptic influences on hemi-neglect in schizophrenia have been reported by Tomer & Flor-Henry (1989). In an open study, unmedicated patients made more errors in a cancellation test on the right side of space yet, on retest when medicated, they made more errors on the left side of space. When subdividing patients according to the length of time on neuroleptics only those treated for more than 3 weeks showed the subtle left hemi-space neglect. They note the results were consistent with asymmetry differences in lateral eye movements and in visual evoked potentials in schizophrenic patients with and without neuroleptic medication. Harvey et al (1993) measured hemi-neglect with a tactile–kinaesthetic task involving the centring of a rod while blindfolded. The more severe the symptoms on the BPRS and the higher the chlorpromazine equivalent the greater was the right-sided neglect.

COVERT SPATIAL ORIENTING WITH EXOGENOUS VERSUS ENDOGENOUS CUES

Particular consideration has been given to the role of dopamine in attentional asymmetry utilising spatial orienting procedures. One influential paradigm was devised by Posner and colleagues involving covert visuospatial orienting (Posner et al, 1988). If a cue stimulus is presented at a target location, such as an illuminated ground against which a target will appear, the cue will automatically engage attention at the target location and facilitate speed of detection for up to 300 ms. This slows disengagement of attention should attention be required in another location. Because it occurs automatically this cueing is referred to as "exogenous". "Endogenous" cueing is where a cue presented centrally has symbolic predictive value, such as an arrow pointing, or the word "left" or "right", referring to the probable location of the target. The symbolic cue may be compatible (valid) with target location, may be neutral, or may be incompatible (invalid), such as where the cue points to the left and the target is presented to the right. Symbolic cueing is said to involve effortful or controlled processing. Controlled (endogenous) cueing has been shown to involve cortical functions whereas automatic (exogenous) cueing is subcortical.

Posner et al (1988) examined 12 patients with schizophrenia with positive symptoms (four with withdrawal), with an exogenous cue spatial orienting task and described a slowing of responses in the right visual field when there was no cue or where the cue was invalid. This asymmetry had some affinities with the one found in left parietal stroke patients, yet at the same time was distinguished by an absence of the left-sided attentional bias found in left stroke patients. Informally observing that patients with auditory hallucinations had the more extreme asymmetry and reasoning that hallucinations may contribute to divided attention, they went on to show that the effects in schizophrenia were mimicked to some extent by normal subjects who were submitted to a divided attention shadowing procedure. A third experiment with endogenous cues drew on evidence of verbal versus spatial deficits in left and right hemisphere stroke patients. While six medicated patients with schizophrenia showed no difference between the linguistic and spatial target conditions, four never-medicated patients performed like left stroke patients. Retesting the patients on medication their spatial performance was impaired and their word performance improved.

Potkin et al (1989) replicated the results and, in addition to inattention, reported fewer eye fixations on the right side of space. However, Strauss et al (1991) using an exogenous cue paradigm found no asymmetry in 10 schizophrenic and six bipolar affective disorder patients who were in remission and on stable medication. This suggests that the deficits are related to active symptomatology and that antipsychotic medication modifies the effects. The importance of the endogenous or exogenous nature of the cue was emphasised by Carter et al (1992) who in 14 unmedicated outpatients with schizophrenia found a slowing in the right visual field to all exogenous cue conditions. However, when cues were endogenous there was a slowing to the left visual field target when the arrow cue was invalid. Left visual field anomalies have also interested Coppola and Gold (1990) who have argued that because the slowing of responses in the right visual field was not found in the valid cue condition, this indicated that patients with schizophrenia could take advantage of cue compatibility in the right visual field, as was the case in the normal controls for both visual fields. What was of greater interest to these authors was the absence of a cue effect in the left visual field in the patients with schizophrenia. This result was akin to the well documented disability in making use of preparatory cues in schizophrenia, especially in non-paranoid and process patients (Rist & Cohen, 1991).

In general results with the exogenous cue paradigm, thought to tap subcortical lateralised mechanisms, provide support for subtle right visual field impairments. These take the form of slower responses on no cue or invalid cue (but not valid cue) trials (Posner et al, 1988), or of a generalised slowing (Carter et al, 1992), an anomaly which may coexist with fewer eye fixations (Potkin et al, 1989) and with anomalies in the opposite, left visual field (Coppola & Gold, 1990). These occur in unmedicated patients or in those with predominantly positive symptoms uncontrolled by medication. The use of endogenous cues, tapping lateralised cortical processes, has produced less consistent results. These include response patterns like left hemisphere stroke patients (Posner et al, 1988) and, more confusingly, a left visual field deficit in the same patients who showed the generalised right visual field slowness to endogenous cues (Carter et al, 1992). Such results cannot be reconciled straightforwardly with gross lesion models. Additionally, the lateral asymmetry is masked by antipsychotic medication, which in turn may produce asymmetrical effects.

DOPAMINE AND OVERT ATTENTIONAL ASYMMETRY

In animals asymmetric circling behaviour in the form of behavioural orienting and rotational or turning preferences has been related to an asymmetry in dopaminergic activity in the subcortex and frontal cortex (but not posterior cortex). Animals rotate towards the hemisphere with the lower dopaminergic activity, termed ipsilateral turning. Bracha et al (1987) developed a belt-mounted rotameter and has shown individual differences in rotational asymmetry in normals, uninfluenced by handedness. Nine of 10 unmedicated patients with schizophrenia were found prone to turn to the left (Bracha, 1987) as were right-sided hemi-parkinsonian patients (Bracha et al, 1987), an asymmetry that signified a right > left imbalance in dopamine.

Bracha (1989) has marshalled evidence to interpret this asymmetry as right-sided dopaminergic hyperactivity in preference to left-sided hypoactivity and has stressed that the imbalance is likely to be true only of a subgroup of patients.

One source of evidence concerned asymmetrical neuroleptic-induced parkinsonism, interpreted as reflecting asymmetrical dopaminergic hyperactivity. Tomer et al (1987) also had reported this condition in six of 12 patients with schizophrenia and observed that the five with predominantly right limb pathology were all paranoid (positive syndrome) while the one with the opposite asymmetry was disorganised. According to Bracha the asymmetry in paranoid patients signified lower responsivity of the right striatum to dopamine blockade, such that right limb parkinsonism was due to the effects of the neuroleptic on the left striatum. Another condition is tardive dyskinesia which has been reported predominantly on the left side in patients with schizophrenia (Waziri, 1980; Altshuler et al, 1988). Tardive dyskinesia is thought to reflect hyperactivity of the contralateral nigrostriatal system which implicates the right subcortex in schizophrenia. A final source of evidence concerned kindling of the left amygdala which resulted in left turning behaviour in animals, greatest in those with an increase in D2 receptors in the right caudate. The evidence, discussed earlier, of relative neglect contralateral to the focus in temporal lobe epileptic patients (Tsuru & Fujiwara, 1987) is consistent with the laterality of inattention produced by amygdala kindling. Bracha's thesis is also supported by evidence of asymmetrical neuroleptic-induced muscle stiffness in the upper extremities (Caligiuri et al, 1989).

In addition, unilateral cortical lesions in animals have shown that whereas the acute post-lesion effect was one of ipsilateral turning and contralateral neglect, in all but those with occipital lesions the asymmetry reversed after about a fortnight, a delay attributed to denervation supersensitivity of the subcortical nigrostriatal system (Pycock et al, 1980). In support of this Bracha et al (1989) found in stroke patients that old ischaemic lesions of the frontal and inferior parietal cortices resulted in asymmetric turning tendencies contralateral to the lesion. Thus, Bracha concluded that both left amygdala kindling and right frontoparietal lesions (left > right imbalance) result in left turning and "In both cases the final common pathway seems to be unilateral right striatal hyper-dopaminergia."

Right hemi-neglect may also occur as a result of generalised dopamine depletion, as shown in children with phenylketonuria in whom there is a developmental depletion of dopamine along with noradrenaline and serotonin. Craft et al (1992) applied Posner's spatial orienting test with exogenous cueing and a 100 versus 800 ms delay between the cue and target. Male phenylketonuric children showed a significant slowing in reaction times, with a particular difficulty when the target was presented in the right hemi-field and in the incompatible cue condition (100 ms delay), an effect similar to that reported by Posner et al (1988) in schizophrenia. Other effects with the 800 ms delay are difficult to interpret because of complex influences on controlled, endogenous processes that occur when delays between cue and target are as long as 800 ms. The main result is in keeping with an asymmetry of dopamine pathways in the brain, one which favours the left hemisphere (Tucker & Williamson, 1984).

An opposing interpretation to right subcortical dopamine overactivity was put forward by Early et al (1989) who prefers the role of reduced dopamine activity in the left ventral striatum and its influence on an anterior attentional system. This was based on the demonstration of left globus pallidus hypermetabolism and blood flow in neuroleptic-naive patients with schizophrenia; a region known to be hypermetabolic bilaterally in Parkinson's disease. The hypermetabolism was interpreted as reflecting enhanced firing to the pallidum from the striatum. However, Early et al (1989) noted that this proposal is apparently at odds with the dopaminergic theory of schizophrenia which proposes increased not decreased dopamine.

The systems interpretation placed upon the visual attention asymmetries involves connections between the ventral striatum and the medial frontal lobe. This is a system which contains dopaminergic neurons and which has been shown, in blood flow studies, to be activated when subjects look or listen to words. The anterior cingulate, which is part of the anterior medial system, is associated with a network implicated in directed attention and unilateral neglect and which involves the posterior parietal lobe as well as the lateral prefrontal cortex involved in semantic processing (Posner et al, 1988).

In summary, dopamine does seem inextricably involved in overt motoric orienting and in covert visual orienting. Reversals of asymmetry may occur in either direction. The right hemi-neglect appears to characterise patients with positive symptoms though patient numbers in the various investigations are small and no one has examined contrasting subgroups for opposite asymmetries. Consideration of evidence of attentional asymmetries in the auditory modality, overlooked in spatial orienting model building, serves to reinforce these conclusions.

AUDITORY ATTENTIONAL ASYMMETRIES

In the only controlled study of neuroleptic influences on attentional asymmetries systematic influences were reported in the auditory modality in a chlorpromazine withdrawal/reinstatement study (Hammond & Gruzelier, 1978; Gruzelier, 1978). This involved the ability of patients with chronic schizophrenia to shift attention between the ears in order to detect longer target tones which shifted from ear to ear at two rates of switching and two speeds of presentation. Patients were examined six times at fortnightly intervals, the first two sessions after being stabilised on chlorpromazine, sessions three and four on placebo and the final two sessions after chlorpromazine reinstatement. While overall performance was not influenced by drug withdrawal, the longer the time on drug the greater was the right ear advantage and the longer the drug withdrawal the greater was the reduction in the right ear advantage. These effects were confirmed by correlations between dose and ear asymmetry where there was a progressive reversal of sign as shown in Figure 8.4 where sessions are ranked from the maximum time off drug to the maximum time on drug. Thus there was a progressive shift in attention from a left ear advantage off drug (right > left hemisphere asymmetry) to a right ear advantage on drug (left > right asymmetry).

The asymmetries in detection did not vary with speed of presentation and importantly, because they were independent of rate of switching, they were not a function of disabilities in attentional disengagement. The asymmetry was dynamic and may represent an attentional bias or may denote a dysfunction in later stages of processing, as suggested by the patients' greater frequency of commission

John Gruzelier

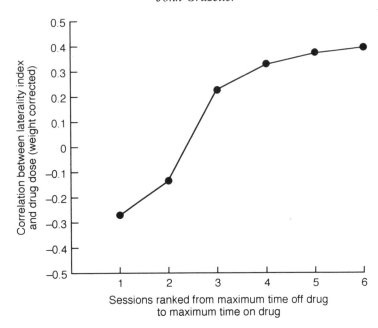

Figure 8.4. Auditory discrimination asymmetry as a function of chlorpromazine dose

errors. Overactivation may also be a contributory factor as it was the electroder-mally responsive patients who were the more impaired by presentation rate, were poorer in discriminating differences in temporal duration and made more commission errors (Gruzelier & Hammond, 1979).

Results from dichotic listening measures in the same patients (Gruzelier & Hammond, 1979, 1980) also suggested no impairment in disengaging attention. Patterns of recall were examined for left–right alternations and comparisons were made between compatible trials (where the ear cued corresponded to the ear with the louder digits) and incompatible trials (where cueing and intensity were in conflict). Patients were more influenced by physical intensity (an automatic as distinct from a controlled process) and were more likely to recall first a louder, non-cued digit. There was also more evidence of switching in patients on incompatible trials irrespective of ear, though more so when attention was directed to the left ear and the louder digits were presented to the right ear. This was greater in paranoid than non-paranoid patients and was in contrast to the opposite asymmetry in controls. The asymmetry in paranoid patients denotes a primacy of intensity, an exogenous parameter, facilitating attention switching when the louder digit was presented to the left hemisphere and when attention was directed (a controlled process) to the right hemisphere. This evidence in paranoid patients is compatible with evidence that it is their left hemisphere that is more activated (as also discussed earlier).

Hemi-space orienting advantages have been examined with a spatial compatibility paradigm (Simon, 1969) where manual reaction times are faster to the word "left" or "right" presented to either ear when there is spatial correspondence between ear and hand. This well-replicated effect is also found in the visual modality, occurs with symbolic commands (high versus low tones) instead of verbal commands and has been shown to be dependent on hemi-space rather than hand because it is retained when the arms are crossed. Schizophrenic patients were examined in three studies (Gruzelier & Hammond, 1979). In the two that involved normal controls and recovered patients, these groups showed spatial compatibility but, whereas controls showed a left hemi-space advantage (perhaps due to the right hemispheric specialisation for attention and spatial processing), recovered patients showed a right hemi-space advantage in one study and a trend to faster responses of the right hand in the other study. Patterns of response differed in the two studies of symptomatic patients. In both there were disadvantages to the left hemisphere and no reliable evidence of spatial compatibility. In one study both commands in the right ear were responded to more slowly than left ear commands, as were binaural commands (see above). While in a study of patients refractory to drug treatment, tested on two occasions on different antipsychotic medications, there was an asymmetry in the direction of slower responses of the right hand. The results with the symptomatic patients were indicative of a neurophysiological right > left hemispheric imbalance disadvantaging the left hemisphere rather than an attentional asymmetry to one side of space. With recovery on medication this asymmetry was reversed.

CONCLUSION

The pervasive feature of all approaches to attentional asymmetry including overt and covert visual and auditory attention was the evidence of drug influences, dopamine in particular. Medication had a consistent effect of producing an asymmetry favouring the right side of space, particularly when it was efficacious in controlling symptoms. The drug influence on asymmetry appeared to be progressive within a month of the introduction of the drug (Hammond & Gruzelier, 1978; Mintz et al, 1982) and it was dose related.

However, the drug influence was more than an attentional bias and represented a neurophysiological influence as shown by advantages to anatomical lateralisation (ear and hand) in the spatial compatibility experiments (Gruzelier & Hammond, 1979) and asymmetrical influences on electrophysiological (Serafetinides, 1972; Gruzelier et al, 1981; Tomer & Flor-Henry, 1989; Myslobodsky et al, 1983) and cognitive measures (Gruzelier et al, 1996). These asymmetrical influences may depend on normal left > right asymmetries in dopamine transmission (Tucker & Williamson, 1984). While most drug influences were compatible with an attentional bias to the right side of space and/or advantages to left hemispheric function and performance, this parsimonious interpretation was complicated by some evidence of reciprocal drug influences on the two hemispheres leading to right hemispheric impairment and, at high doses, deleterious effects on left-sided functions (Harvey et al, 1993; Gruzelier et al, 1996).

The asymmetries of attention operate at both subcortical and cortical levels. As yet the significance of the attentional asymmetries for lateralised subcortical mechanisms have not been resolved. Symptom correlates have only been reported by Tomer et al (1987) in the form of an association of a right > left imbalance in dopamine with paranoid patients. At a cortical level hemi-space inattention varied with symptom picture and/or chronicity. Inattention to the right side of space (as in left lesioned patients) was associated with blunted affect and emotional withdrawal (Kawazoe et al, 1987; Tsuru & Fujiwara, 1987), chronicity (Scarone et al, 1987) and severity of symptoms on the BPRS which in the case of high total scores presumably involve negative and positive symptoms (Harvey et al, 1993). The counterpart of this asymmetry—an attentional bias to the right side of space—was reported in patients with visual hallucinations (Bracha, 1985) and in paranoid patients (Hammond & Gruzelier, 1978). The opposite asymmetry of inattention to the left side of space was associated with acute as distinct from chronic patients (Scarone et al, 1987) and chronic symptomatic and drug refractory patients (Gruzelier & Hammond, 1979).

NEURODEVELOPMENTAL INFLUENCES ON CEREBRAL ASYMMETRY AND SYNDROMES IN SCHIZOPHRENIA

CEREBRAL ASYMMETRY AND A 3-SYNDROME STRUCTURE OF SCHIZOTYPAL PERSONALITY

The recognition memory tasks used in the more recent and substantive test of the imbalance-syndrome model (Gruzelier et al, 1996) have been applied to investigations of the schizotypal personality in university students (Gruzelier & Richardson, 1994; Gruzelier et al, 1995; Gruzelier & Doig, 1996). A link between schizophrenia and schizotypal personality follows evidence of a genetic association between schizophrenia and DSM-IV schizotypy. This has contributed to a dimensional view which posits a continuity between the signs and symptoms of schizophrenia and both clinical schizotypal personality and a subclinical predisposition in the normal population called schizotypy, psychoticism or psychosis proneness (Eysenck & Eysenck, 1975; Claridge, 1985). Subtle lateralised anomalies have been associated with schizotypy, but the pattern of asymmetries has been inconsistent from study to study (for review: Gruzelier, 1991a). In three investigations the three-syndrome model of schizophrenia was applied to factor analytic approaches to schizotypy in university students, with the prediction that opposite patterns of asymmetry would be associated with active and withdrawn schizotypy factors but not with the third unreality syndrome. Three factor solutions were obtained. Word > face advantages were found associated with active or impulsive nonconformity factors/subscales while face > word advantages were associated with withdrawn or introvertive-anhedonia factors/subscales, especially in males. In one male subject who subsequently had two psychotic episodes characterised by withdrawn and unreality syndromes, the extreme face > word asymmetry obtained premorbidly was predictive of the presenting withdrawn syndrome. Thus, the associations between cognitive asymmetry and syndromes found in schizophrenia had a parallel with active and withdrawn personality features of schizotypy. In both schizophrenia and schizotypy these features appear at opposite poles of an arousal/activity dimension, an interpretation reinforced in schizotypy with self report activation scales. In summary, syndromes and asymmetry patterns arise out of normal developmental processes (see also Gruzelier & Kaiser, 1996).

GENDER AND CEREBRAL ASYMMETRY IN SCHIZOPHRENIA

Sexual dimorphism in brain structure and function has been associated with cerebral laterality both through genetic and hormonal influences (Kimura, 1992). It is not surprising, therefore, that gender was a moderating factor in the relationships between syndrome and cerebral asymmetry. Female patients did not always share the word deficit shown by active syndrome males (Gruzelier et al, 1996) as was the case in one of the schizotypy investigations (Gruzelier & Doig, 1996). Two reasons may be suggested for this. The first concerns bilateral representation of abilities in females. Hemispheric specialisation is less clear cut in females, possibly due to a greater bilateral representation of cognitive abilities (McGlone, 1980). It has been speculated that this may be because females possess a thicker corpus callosum in the region that interconnects the plana temporali, the regions associated with sexually dimorphic cognitive specialisation (Witelson, 1991). This same reasoning could be applied to the finding that female patients with schizophrenia have been shown to have a thicker anterior callosum region than males (see above) and memory storage involves frontal regions (Shimamura, 1995). Further, it was female patients with a mixed syndrome who did not show a consistent asymmetry (Gruzelier et al, 1996), a feature that may also stem from interhemispheric hyperconnection in anterior regions as the frontal regions are involved in the expression of emotions (Davidson & Tomarken, 1989; Heller, 1993). The second reason for the absence of a word deficit in active syndrome females may lie with anxiety. Females have higher levels of anxiety than males (Feingold, 1994), a feature also reported in schizophrenia (Lewine, 1981; Goldstein & Link, 1988). Anxiety is another factor that moderates functional asymmetry (Tucker, 1981; Gruzelier & Phelan, 1991) and has been shown to advantage right hemispheric processing at the expense of the left hemisphere (Gruzelier & Phelan, 1991). High anxiety in females may account for the absence of a word asymmetry in many active syndrome female patients.

Crow (1988) has theorised that there is a single locus on the X chromosome, namely the autosomal region in which there is exchange between X and Y chromosomes, where variation accounts for the varieties of psychosis. He speculates that the mechanism that determines cerebral laterality is also located in the pseudo-autosomal region. The sex chromosome disorders show affinities between symptoms and neuropsychological profiles having a strong correspondence with the hemisphere-imbalance syndrome model and hormones influence the course of development of cerebral functions asymmetrically (Gruzelier, 1991a, 1991b, 1994). Saugstad (1989, 1994) has theorised that sex differences in rate of maturation at puberty may be causally related to syndrome differences.

STRUCTURAL ASYMMETRY

Structural asymmetries in schizophrenia have been associated with syndromes and gender. Evidence of structural asymmetries will be reviewed in other chapters (see Bilder & Szeszko, chapter 14) and only one phenomenon will be mentioned which has several bearings on neuropsychological issues. In first-episode, positive-symptom patients with schizophrenia there has been found a significant deviation in the normal pattern of morphological asymmetries characterised by what has been termed torque (Bilder et al, 1994). Torque describes larger right-sided anterior regions encompassing premotor, prefrontal and temporal regions and larger left-sided posterior regions encompassing occipitoparietal and sensorimotor areas. Patients with schizophrenia as a group lacked asymmetries in the premotor and prefrontal region and occipitoparietal region. When subgroups were examined it was those patients with the undifferentiated subtype that had the absence of normal asymmetry in comparison with the paranoid subtype, in particular dextral males with negative symptoms including alogia, avolition/apathy and anhedonia.

These results are compatible with those obtained with recognition memory for words and faces in patients with schizophrenia and in schizotypal students. It was dextral males who showed the predicted patterns of cognitive asymmetry and it was the withdrawn syndrome group who showed the impairment in left hemispheric functions that might be predicted on the basis of a reduction in left posterior regions. An association with left hemispheric impairment and symmetry or reversed asymmetry was reported earlier in the form of lower verbal than performance IQ (Luchins et al, 1979). The structural anomaly has also been associated with negative symptoms by Luchins & Meltzer (1983) insofar as the asymmetry in the occipital regions belonged to patients with an interview of poor quality, suggestive of social withdrawal. Thus, there is some evidence that the nature of the associations correspond to the pattern of asymmetry associated with the withdrawn syndrome.

The other feature of the structural findings is anomalous lateralisation. As reviewed before (Gruzelier, 1981a, 1983), there is no consistent evidence that schizophrenia is associated with an excess of sinistrality; however, there is growing interest in the possibility that ambiguous handedness is over represented in schizophrenia as has also been observed in autism (Green et al, 1989; Soper et al, 1986). An association has been shown between ambiguous handedness and thought disorder (Manoach, 1994). Abnormal or arrested prenatal maturation may contribute to impaired left hemispheric functions (Best, 1985) and children with a schizophrenic parent have been shown to have reduced verbal compared with performance IQ (Gruzelier et al, 1979; see Wolf & Cornblatt, chapter 9).

CONCLUSION

Evidence has been reviewed showing that lateralised dysfunction of both left and right hemispheres has an extensive data base in neuropsychological investigations of schizophrenia. The development has been charted of a three-syndrome model of schizophrenia in which two syndromes are related to opposite patterns of cerebral asymmetry suggestive of functional imbalances between the hemispheres, relations best seen in male, right-handed patients. Associations between lateralised deficits and symptom patterns or subtypes has been a common theme running through the chapter and has been shown to have a bearing on interhemispheric transmission deficit as well as on attentional asymmetry models. An attempt has been made to integrate the lateralised imbalance and interhemispheric transfer models of schizophrenia, with both the direction of abnormal transmission (leftward or rightward) and the nature of the transmission abnormality (hyper- or hypoconnection). The data base for attentional asymmetry in schizophrenia is more limited with most studies having small sample sizes and little consideration for individual differences. The interplay of subcortical–cortical influences, instrumental in attentional asymmetry, will be necessary not only for a comprehensive model of lateralised dysfunction but is likely to elucidate the mechanisms creating functional hemispheric imbalance. The way forward in elucidating the importance of lateralised dysfunction in schizophrenia will require careful characterisation of patients in terms of symptoms and syndromes and subclassification on the basis of gender and handedness. This must be combined with an awareness that antipsychotic and antiparkinsonian medication both have an impact on functional asymmetries. The drug issue, rather than being considered a nuisance variable, may go to the heart of the aetiology of schizophrenia. The importance of antipsychotic drugs on both cortical and subcortically mediated attentional asymmetries may resurrect the dopamine theory of schizophrenia which is just as theoretically tenable as it ever was, but which has waned through lack of evidence. What may be of more importance than abnormalities in brain dopamine concentrations are the influences of neurotransmitters on syndrome differences in functional brain activity.

In essence the thesis has been developed that hemispheric imbalance contributes to the expression of symptoms in schizophrenia, results consistent with a neuropsychological translation of active and withdrawn symptoms based on hemispheric specialisation. However, the third syndrome consisting of hallucinations and delusions, or of unreality experiences in schizotypy in the normal population, has shown no consistent relations with functional asymmetry (Gruzelier, 1994). This syndrome may represent a more generalised dysfunction of the nervous system, a basis for which we are currently exploring in magnocellular function and maturation extremes (Stein, 1994; Richardson & Gruzelier, 1994; Gruzelier & Kaiser, 1996). Generalised impairment has been commonly reported in schizophrenia (see Barber et al, chapter 4) and associated with enlarged ventricles and cortical atrophy (Crow, 1980). General impairment was in evidence in acute patients in the study of lateralised tests in conjunction with active and withdrawn syndromes; specific deficits were disclosed against a background of generalised impairment (Gruzelier et al, 1988). This leads us to the conclusion that functional cerebral asymmetry is a necessary but not sufficient factor in understanding the nature of schizophrenia.

REFERENCES

Altshuler, L.L., Cummings, J.L., Bartzokis, G., Hill, M.A., May, P.R.A. (1988) Lateral asymmetries of tardive dyskinesia in schizophrenia. *Biological Psychiatry*, **24**, 83.

Andrews, H.B., House, A.O., Cooper, J.E., Barber, C. (1986) The prediction of abnormal evoked potentials in schizophrenic patients by means of symptom pattern. *British Journal of Psychiatry*, **149**, 46–50.

Andrews, H.B., Cooper, J.E., Barber, C., Raine, A. (1987) Early somatosensory evoked potentials in schizophrenia: Symptom pattern, clinical outcomes and interhemispheric functioning. In: *Cerebral Dynamics, Laterality and Psychopathology* (Eds R. Takahashi, P. Flor-Henry, J. Gruzelier, S. Niwa), pp. 175–186, Elsevier, Amsterdam.

Arndt, S., Alliger, R.J., Andreasen, N.C. (1991) The distinction of positive and negative symptoms: The failure of a two-dimensional model. *British Journal of Psychiatry*, **158**, 317–322.

Beaumont, J.G., Dimond, S. (1973) Brain disconnection and schizophrenia. *British Journal of Psychiatry*, **123**, 661–662.

Best, C. (1985) *Hemispheric Function and Collaboration in the Child*, Academic Press, London.

Bigelow, L.B., Nasrallah, H.A., Rauscher, F.P. (1983) Corpus callosum thickness in chronic schizophrenia. *British Journal of Psychiatry*, **141**, 284–287.

Bilder, R.M. (1985) *Subtyping in Chronic Schizophrenia: Clinical, Neuropsychological and Structural Indices of Deterioration*. University microfilms, Ann Arbor.

Bilder, R.M., Wu, H., Bogerts, B., Degreef, G., Ashtari, M., Alvir, J.M.J., Synder, P.J., Leiberman, J.A. (1994) Regional hemispheric volume asymmetries are absent in first episode schizophrenia. *American Journal of Psychiatry*, **151**, 1437–1447.

Bogerts, B., Ashtari, M., Degreef, G., Alvir, J.M., Bilder, R.M., Lieberman, A. (1990) Reduced temporal limbic structure volumes on magnetic resonance images in first episode schizophrenia. *Psychiatry Research*, **35**, 1–13.

Bracha, H.S. (1985) Lateralization of visual hallucinations in chronic schizophrenia. *Biological Psychiatry*, **20**, 1132–1136.

Bracha, H.S. (1987) Asymmetric rotational (circling) behaviour, a dopamine-related asymmetry: preliminary findings in unmedicated and never-medicated schizophrenic patients. *Biological Psychiatry*, **22**, 995–1003.

Bracha, H.S. (1989) Is there a right hemi-hyper-dopaminergic psychosis? *Schizophrenia Research*, **2**, 317–324.

Bracha, H.S., Schults, C., Glick, S.D., Kleinman, J.E. (1987) Spontaneous asymmetric circling behaviour in hemi-parkinsonism: A human equivalent of the lesioned-circling rodent behaviour. *Life Sciences*, **40**, 1127–1130.

Bracha, H.S., Lyden, P.D., Khansarinia, S. (1989) Delayed emergence of striatal dopaminergic hyperactivity after anterolateral ischaemic cortical lesions in humans: Evidence from turning behaviour. *Biological Psychiatry*, **25**, 265–274.

Buchsbaum, M.S., Carpenter, W.T., Fedio, P., Goodwin, F.M., Murphy, D.L., Post, E.M. (1979) Hemispheric differences in evoked potential enhancement by selective attention to hemiretinally presented stimuli in schizophrenic, affective and post-temporal lobectomy patients. In: *Hemispheric Asymmetries of Function in Psychopathology*, Vol. 3 (Eds J.H. Gruzelier, P. Flor-Henry), pp. 317–328, Elsevier/North-Holland, Amsterdam.

Bull, H.O. (1972) *Speech Perception and Short Term Memory in Schizophrenia*, PhD thesis, University of London.

Burgess, A., Gruzelier, J. (1996) Localisation of word and face recognition memory using topographical EEG. *Psychophysiology*, in press.

Caligiuri, M.P., Bracha, H.S., Lohr, J.B. (1989) Asymmetry of neuroleptic-induced rigidity: Development of quantitative methods and clinical correlates. *Psychiatry Research*, **30**, 275–284.

Carr, S.A. (1980) Interhemispheric transfer of stereognostic information in chronic schizophrenics. *British Journal of Psychiatry*, **136**, 53–58.

Carter, C.S., Robertson, L.C., Chaderjian, M.R., Celaya, L.J., Nordahl, T.E. (1992) Attentional asymmetry in schizophrenia: Controlled and automatic processes. *Biological Psychiatry*, **31**, 909–918.

Claridge, G.S. (1985) *Origins of Mental Illness*, Blackwell, Oxford.

Coger, R.W., Serafetinides, E.A. (1990) Schizophrenia, corpus callosum, and interhemispheric communication. A review. *Biological Psychiatry*, **34**, 163–184.

Colbourn, C.J., Lishman, W.A. (1979) Lateralisation of function and psychotic illness: A left hemispheric deficit? In: *Hemispheric Asymmetries of Function in Psychopathology*, Vol. 3 (Eds J.H. Gruzelier, P. Flor-Henry), pp. 539–560, Elsevier/North-Holland, Amsterdam.

Connolly, J.F., Gruzelier, J.H., Kleinman, K.M., Hirsch, S.R. (1979) Lateralised abnormalities in hemisphere-specific tachistoscopic tasks in psychiatric patients and controls. In: *Hemispheric Asymmetries of Function in Psychopathology*, Vol. 3 (Eds J.H. Gruzelier, P. Flor-Henry), pp. 491–510, Elsevier/North-Holland, Amsterdam.

Connolly, J.F., Gruzelier, J.H., Manchanda, R. (1983a) Electrocortical and perceptual asymmetries in schizophrenia. In: *Developments in Psychiatry. Vol 6: Laterality and Psychopathology* (Eds P. Flor-Henry, J.H. Gruzelier), pp. 363–378, Elsevier/North-Holland, Amsterdam.

Connolly, J.F., Manchanda, R., Gruzelier, J.H., Hirsch, S.R. (1983b) Auditory event-related potentials in schizophrenic patients. In: *Advances in Biological Psychiatry: Neurophysiological Correlates of Normal Cognition and Psychopathology* (Eds E. Perris, D. Kemali, M. Koukkou-Lehmann), pp. 93–97, Karger, Basel.

Connolly, J.F., Manchanda, R., Gruzelier, J.H., Hirsch, S.R. (1985) Pathway and hemispheric differences in the event-related potential (ERP) to monaural stimulation: A comparison of schizophrenic patients with normal controls. *Biological Psychiatry*, **20**, 293–303.

Cooper, J.E., Andrews, H.B., Barber, C. (1985) Stable abnormalities in the lateralisation of early cortical evoked somato-sensory responses in schizophrenic patients. *British Journal of Psychiatry*, **146**, 585–593.

Coppola, R., Gold, J. (1990) What is left of attention in schizophrenia? *Archives of General Psychiatry*, **47**, 393–395.

Craft, S., Willerman, L., Bigler, E.D. (1987) Callosal dysfunction in schizophrenia and schizo-affective disorder. *Journal of Abnormal Psychology*, **96**, 205–213.

Craft, S., Gourovitch, M.L., Dowton, B., Swanson, J.M., Bonforte, S. (1992) Lateralized deficits in visual attention in males with developmental dopamine depletion. *Neuropsychologia*, **30**, 341–351.

Crisp, A.H., Karmen, J., Potamianos, G., Bhat, A.V. (1985) Cerebral hemisphere function and laterality of migraine, *Psychotherapy and Psychosomatics*, **43**, 49–55.

Crow, T.J. (1980) Molecular pathology of schizophrenia: More than one disease process? *British Medical Journal*, **280**, 66–68.

Crow, T.J. (1988) Sex chromosomes and psychosis: The case for a pseudoautosomal locus. *British Journal of Psychiatry*, **153**, 675–683.

David, A.S. (1987) Tachistoscopic tests of colour naming and matching in schizophrenia: Evidence for posterior callosum dysfunction? *Psychological Medicine*, **17**, 621–630.

David, A.S. (1993) Callosal transfer in schizophrenia: Too much or too little? *Journal of Abnormal Psychology*, **102**, 573–579.

Davidson, R.J., Tomarken, A.J. (1989) Laterality and emotion: An electrophysiological approach. In: *Handbook of Neuropsychology* (Eds L. Squire, G. Gainotti), pp. 419–442, Elsevier, Amsterdam.

Dennis, M. (1981) Language in a congenitally acallosal brain. *Brain and Language*, **12**, 33–53.

Dimond, S.J., Scammell, R.E., Pryce, J.Q., Huss, D., Gray, C. (1979) Callosal transfer and left-handed anomia in schizophrenia. *Biological Psychiatry*, **14**, 735–739.

Early, T.S., Posner, M.I., Reiman, E.M., Raichle, M.E. (1989) Hyperactivity of the left striato-pallidal projection: Part I. Lower level theory. *Psychiatric Developments*, **84**, 561–563.

Eaton, E.M., Busk, J., Maloney, M.P., Sloane, R.B., Whipple, K., White, K. (1979) Hemisphere dysfunction in schizophrenia. *Psychiatry Research*, **1**, 325–332.

Ehrlichman, H. (1987) Hemispheric asymmetry and positive–negative affect. In: *Duality and Unity of the Brain: Unified Functioning and Specialisation of the Hemispheres* (Ed. D. Ottoson), pp. 194–206, Macmillan, Basingstoke.

Eysenck, H.J., Eysenck, S.B.G. (1975) *Manual of the Eysenck Personality Questionnaire (Junior and Adult)*, Hodder & Stoughton, London.

Feingold, A. (1994) Gender differences in personality: A meta analysis. *Psychological Bulletin*, **116**, 429–456.

Flor-Henry, P. (1969) Psychosis and temporal lobe epilepsy: A controlled investigation. *Epilepsia*, **10**, 365–395.

Flor-Henry, P., Gruzelier, J.H. (1983) (Eds) *Developments in Psychiatry. Vol 6: Laterality and Psychopathology*, Elsevier/North-Holland, Amsterdam.

Galin, D. (1974) Implications for psychiatry of left and right cerebral specialization: A neuropsychological context for unconscious processes. *Archives of General Psychiatry*, **31**, 572–583.

Goldstein, G. (1991) Comprehensive neuropsychological test batteries and research in schizophrenia. In: *Handbook of Schizophrenia. Vol. 5: Neuropsychology, Psychophysiology and Information Processing* (Eds S.R. Steinhauer, J.H. Gruzelier, J. Zubin), pp. 525–551, Elsevier, Amsterdam.

Goldstein, J.M., Link, B.G. (1988) Gender and the expression of schizophrenia. *Journal of Psychiatric Research*, **22**, 141–155.

Green, E. (1985) Interhemispheric coordination and focused attention in chronic and acute schizophrenia. *British Journal of Clinical Psychology*, **24**, 197–204.

Green, M.F., Satz, P., Smith, C., Nelson, L. (1989) Is there atypical handedness in schizophrenia? *Journal of Abnormal Psychology*, **98**, 57–61.

Green, P., Kotenko, V. (1980) Superior speech comprehension in schizophrenics under monaural versus binaural listening conditions. *Journal of Abnormal Psychology*, **89**, 399–408.

Green, P., Hallet, S., Hunter, H. (1983) Abnormal interhemispheric integration and hemispheric specialisation in schizophrenics and high-risk children. In: *Developments in Psychiatry. Vol 6: Laterality and Psychopathology* (Eds P. Flor-Henry, J.H. Gruzelier), pp. 443–470, Elsevier/North-Holland, Amsterdam.

Gruzelier, J.H. (1978) Bimodal states of arousal and lateralised dysfunction in schizophrenia: The effect of chlorpromazine. In: *The Nature of Schizophrenia: New Approaches to Research and Treatment* (Eds L. Wynne, R. Cromwell, S. Matthysse), pp. 167–187, Wiley, New York.

Gruzelier, J.H. (1979a) Synthesis and critical review of the evidence for hemisphere asymmetries of function in psychopathology. In: *Hemispheric Asymmetries of Function in Psychopathology*, Vol. 3 (Eds J.H. Gruzelier, P. Flor-Henry), pp. 647–672, Elsevier/North-Holland, Amsterdam.

Gruzelier, J.H. (1979b) Lateral asymmetries in electrodermal activity and psychosis. In: *Hemispheric Asymmetries of Function in Psychopathology*, Vol. 3 (Eds J.H. Gruzelier, P. Flor-Henry), pp. 149–168, Elsevier/North-Holland, Amsterdam.

Gruzelier, J. (1981a) Cerebral laterality and psychopathology: Fact or fiction. *Psychological Medicine*, **11**, 93–108.

Gruzelier, J.H. (1981b) Hemispheric imbalances masquerading as paranoid and non-paranoid syndromes. *Schizophrenia Bulletin*, **7**, 662–673.

Gruzelier, J.H. (1983) A critical assessment and integration of lateral asymmetries in schizophrenia. In: *Hemisyndromes: Psychobiology, Neurology, Psychiatry* (Ed. M.S. Myslobodsky), pp. 265–326, Academic Press, New York.

Gruzelier, J. (1984) Hemispheric imbalances in schizophrenia. *International Journal of Psychophysiology*, **1**, 227–240.

Gruzelier, J. (1985) Central nervous system signs in schizophrenia. In: *Neurobehavioural Disorders. Vol. 46: Handbook of Clinical Neurology* (Eds J.A.M. Frederiks), pp. 481–521, Elsevier, Amsterdam.

Gruzelier, J. (1986) Theories of lateralised and interhemispheric dysfunction in syndromes of schizophrenia. In: *Handbook of Studies on Schizophrenia. Part 2: Management and Research* (Eds G. Burrows, T. Norman, T. Rubinstein), pp. 175–196, Elsevier, Amsterdam.

Gruzelier, J.H. (1987a) Commentary on neuropsychological and information processing deficits in psychosis and neuropsychophysiological syndrome-relationships in schizophrenia. In: *Cerebral Dynamics, Laterality and Psychopathology* (Eds R. Takahashi, P. Flor-Henry, J. Gruzelier, S. Niwa), pp. 23–54, Elsevier, Amsterdam.

Gruzelier, J.H. (1987b) Cerebral laterality and schizophrenia: A review of the interhemispheric disconnection hypothesis. In: *Individual Differences in Hemispheric Specialisation* (Ed. A. Glass), pp. 357–376, Plenum, London.

Gruzelier, J.H. (1991a) Hemispheric imbalance: Syndromes of schizophrenia, premorbid personality and neurodevelopmental influences. In: *Handbook of Schizophrenia. Vol. 5: Neuropsychology, Psychophysiology and Information Processing* (Eds S.R. Steinhauer, J.H. Gruzelier, J. Zubin), pp. 599–650, Elsevier, Amsterdam.

Gruzelier, J. (1991b) Brain localisation and neuropsychology in schizophrenia: Implications for syndromes, sex differences and genetics. In: *Searches for the Causes of Schizophrenia* (Eds H. Hafner, W.F. Gattaz), pp. 301–320, Springer Verlag, Bern.

Gruzelier, J.H. (1994) Syndromes of schizophrenia and schizotypy, hemispheric imbalance and sex differences: Implications for developmental psychopathology. *International Journal of Psychophysiology*, **18**, 167–178.

Gruzelier, J.H. A review and synthesis of neuro-psychophysiological lateral asymmetry in schizophrenia. *Schizophrenia Bulletin* (in press).

Gruzelier, J., Doig, A. (1996) Syndromes of schizotypy: Patterns of cognitive asymmetry, arousal and gender. *Schizophrenia Bulletin*, in press.

Gruzelier, J.H., Flor-Henry, P. (Eds) (1979) *Hemispheric Asymmetries of Function in Psychopathology*, Elsevier/North-Holland, Amsterdam.

Gruzelier, J.H., Hammond, N.V. (1979) Lateralised auditory processing in medicated and unmedicated schizophrenic patients. In: *Hemispheric Asymmetries of Function in Psychopathology*, Vol. 3 (Eds J.H. Gruzelier, P. Flor-Henry), pp. 603–638, Elsevier/North-Holland, Amsterdam.

Gruzelier, J.H., Hammond, N.V. (1980) Lateralised deficits and drug influences in the dichotic listening of schizophrenic patients. *Biological Psychiatry*, **15**, 759–779.

Gruzelier, J., Kaiser, J. (1996) Syndromes of schizotypy and timing of puberty. *Schizophrenia Research* (in press).

Gruzelier, J.H., Manchanda, R. (1982) The syndrome of schizophrenia: Relations between electrodermal response lateral asymmetries and clinical ratings. *British Journal of Psychiatry*, **141**, 488–495.

Gruzelier, J., Phelan, M. (1991) Laterality-reversal in a lexical divided visual field task under stress. *International Journal of Psychophysiology*, **11**, 267–276.

Gruzelier, J., Richardson, A. (1994) Patterns of cognitive asymmetry and psychosis proneness. *International Journal of Psychophysiology*, **18**, 217–226.

Gruzelier, J.H., Richardson, A. (1996) Lateralised dysfunction and the psychophysiology of schizophrenia. *Schizophrenia Bulletin*, Special issue on Lateralisation and Schizophrenia (in press).

Gruzelier, J.H., Venables, P.H. (1972) Skin conductance orienting activity in a heterogeneous sample of schizophrenics: Possible evidence of limbic dysfunction. *Journal of Nervous and Mental Disease*, **155**, 277–287.

Gruzelier, J.H., Mednick, S., Schulsinger, F. (1979) Lateralised impairments in the WISC profiles of children at genetic risk for psychopathology. In: *Hemispheric Asymmetries of Function in Psychopathology*, Vol. 3 (Eds J.H. Gruzelier, P. Flor-Henry), pp. 105–110, Elsevier/North-Holland, Amsterdam.

Gruzelier, J.H., Connolly, J.C., Eves, F.F., Hirsch, S.R., Zaki, S.A., Weller, M.F., Yorkston, N.J. (1981) Effect of propranolol and phenothiazines on electrodermal orienting and habituation in schizophrenia. *Psychological Medicine*, **11**, 93–108.

Gruzelier, J.H., Nikolau, T., Connolly, J.F., Peatfield, R.C., Davies, P.T.G., Clifford-Rose, F. (1987b) Laterality of pain in migraine distinguished by interictal rates habituation of electrodermal responses to visual and auditory stimuli. *Journal of Neurology, Neurosurgery and Psychiatry*, **50**, 410–422.

Gruzelier, J., Seymour, K., Haynes, R., Wilson, L., Jolley, T., Flynn, M., Hirsch, S. (1987a) Neuropsychological evidence of hippocampal and frontal impairments in schizophrenia, mania and depression. In: *Cerebral Dynamics, Laterality and Psychopathology* (Eds R. Takahashi, P. Flor-Henry, J. Gruzelier, S. Niwa), pp. 273–286, Elsevier, Amsterdam.

Gruzelier, J., Seymour, K., Wilson, L., Jolley, T., Hirsch, S. (1988) Impairments on neuropsychological tests of temporo-hippocampal and fronto-hippocampal functions and word fluency in remitting schizophrenia and affective disorders. *Archives of General Psychiatry*, **45**, 623–629.

Gruzelier, J., Jutai, J., Connolly, J. (1993) Cerebral asymmetry in EEG spectra in unmedicated schizophrenic patients: Relationship with active and withdrawn syndromes. *International Journal of Psychophysiology*, **15**, 239–246.

Gruzelier, J.H, Stygall, J., Irving, G., Raine, A. (1995) Patterns of cognitive asymmetry and syndromes of schizotypal personality. *Psychiatry Research*, **56**, 71–79.

Gruzelier, J., Wilson, L., Dennis, P., Liddiard, D., Richardson, A., Peters, E., Pusavat, L. (1996) Cognitive asymmetry patterns in schizophrenia: Syndrome specificity of reversible recognition memory impairments. (Submitted).

Gulmann, N.C., Wildschiodtz, G., Orbaek, K. (1982) Alteration of interhemisphere conduction through corpus callosum in chronic schizophrenia. *Biological Psychiatry*, **17**, 585–594.

Gunther, W., Petsch, R., Steinberg, R., Moser, E., Streck, P., Heller, H., Kurtz, G., Hippius, H. (1991) Brain dysfunction during motor activation and corpus callosum alterations in schizophrenia measured by cerebral blood flow and magnetic resonance imaging. *Biological Psychiatry*, **29**, 535–555.

Gur, R.E. (1978) Left hemisphere dysfunction and left hemispheric overactivation in schizophrenia. *Journal of Abnormal Psychiatry*, **87**, 226–238.

Gur, R.E. (1979) Cognitive concomitants of hemispheric dysfunction in schizophrenia. *Archives of General Psychiatry*, **36**, 269–274.

Gur, R.E., Resnick, S.M., Ruben, C.G. (1989) Laterality and frontality of cerebral blood flow and metabolism in schizophrenia: Relationship to symptom specificity. *Psychiatry Research*, **27**, 325–334.

Gur, R.E., Mozley, P.D., Resnick, S.M., Levick, S., Erwin, R., Saykin, A.J., Gur, R.C. (1991) Relationships among clinical scales in schizophrenia. *American Journal of Psychiatry*, **148**, 472–478.

Hammond, N.V., Gruzelier, J.H. (1978) Laterality, attention and rate effects in the auditory temporal discrimination of chronic schizophrenics: The effects of treatment with chlorpromazine. *Quarterly Journal of Experimental Psychology*, **30**, 91–103.

Harrington, A. (1985) Nineteenth-century ideas on hemisphere differences and "duality of mind". *Behavioural and Brain Sciences*, **8**, 617–660.

Harvey, S.A., Nelson, E., Haller, J.W., Early, T.S. (1993) Lateralised attentional abnormality in schizophrenia is correlated with severity of symptoms. *Biological Psychiatry*, **33**, 93–99.

Hatta, T., Yamamoto, M., Kawabata, Y. (1984) Functional hemispheric differences in schizophrenia: Interhemispheric transfer deficit or selective hemisphere dysfunction? *Biological Psychiatry*, **19** 1027–1036.

Heller, W. (1993) Neuropsychological mechanisms of individual differences in emotion, personality and arousal. *Neuropsychology*, **7**, 476–489.

Hillsberg, B. (1979) A comparison of visual discrimination performance of the dominant and nondominant hemispheres in schizophrenia. In: *Hemispheric Asymmetries of Function in Psychopathology*, Vol. 3 (Eds J.H. Gruzelier, P. Flor-Henry), pp. 527–538, Elsevier/North-Holland, Amsterdam.

Hoffman, R.E., Stopek, S., Andreasen, N.C. (1986) A comparative study of manic vs schizophrenic speech disorganisation. *Archives of General Psychiatry*, **43**, 831–838.

Jones, G.H., Miller, J.J. (1981) Functional tests of the corpus callosum in schizophrenia. *British Journal of Psychiatry*, **139**, 553–557.

Kawazoe, S., Fujiwara, M., Tsuru, N. (1987) Eye movements and the Benton Visual Retention Test in Schizophrenics. In: *Cerebral Dynamics, Laterality and Psychopathology* (Eds R. Takahashi, P. Flor-Henry, J. Gruzelier, S. Niwa), pp. 157–172, Elsevier, Amsterdam.

Kimura, D. (1992) Sex differences in the brain. *Scientific American*, **267**, 119–125.

Kinsbourne, M. (1982) Hemispheric specialisation and the growth of human understanding. *American Psychologist*, **37**, 411.

Kugler, B.T. (1983) Auditory processing in schizophrenic patients. In: *Laterality and Psychopathology* (Eds P. Flor-Henry, J.H. Gruzelier), pp. 471–506, Elsevier/North-Holland, Amsterdam.

Kugler, B.T., Henley, S.H.A. (1979) Laterality effects in the tactile modality in schizophrenia. In: *Hemispheric Asymmetries of Function in Psychopathology*, Vol. 3 (Eds J.H. Gruzelier, P. Flor-Henry), pp. 475–489, Elsevier/North-Holland, Amsterdam.

Lerner. J., Nachshon, I., Carmon, A. (1977) Responses of paranoid and non-paranoid schizophrenics in a dichotic listening task. *Journal of Nervous and Mental Disease*, **164**, 247–252.

Levin, S., Yurgelun-Todd, D., Craft, S. (1989) Contributions of clinical neuropsychology to the study of schizophrenia. *Journal of Abnormal Psychology*, **98**, 341–356.

Lewine, R.J. (1981) Sex differences in schizophrenia—timing or subtypes? *Psychological Bulletin*, **90**, 432–444.

Liddle, P.F. (1987) The symptoms of chronic schizophrenia: A re-examination of the positive–negative dichotomy. *British Journal of Psychiatry*, **151**, 145–151.

Liddle, P.F., Barnes, T.R.E. (1990) Syndromes of chronic schizophrenia. *British Journal of Psychiatry*, **157**, 558–561.

Luchins, D.J., Meltzer, H.Y. (1983) A blind, controlled study of occipital asymmetry in schizophrenia. *Psychiatry Research*, **10**, 87–95.

Luchins, D.J., Weinberger, D.R., Wyatt, R.J. (1979) Schizophrenia: Evidence of a subgroup with reversed cerebral asymmetry. *Archives of General Psychiatry*, **36**, 1309–1311.

Magaro, P.A., Page, J. (1983) Brain disconnection, schizophrenia and paranoia. *Journal of Nervous and Mental Disease*, **171**, 133–140.

Mangina, C.A., Beuzeron-Mangina, J.H. (1994) Electrical stimulation of the human brain and bilateral electrodermal activity. *International Journal of Psychophysiology*, **18**, 124.

Manoach, D.S. (1994) Handedness is related to formal thought disorder and language dysfunction in schizophrenia. *Journal of Clinical and Experimental Neuropsychology*, **16**, 3–13.

Marin, R.S., Tucker, G.J. (1981) Psychopathology and hemisphere dysfunction. *Journal of Nervous and Mental Disease*, **169**, 546–557.

Mathew, R.J., Partain, C.L., Prakash, R., Kulkarin, M.V., Logan, T.P., Wilson, W.H. (1985) A study of septum pellucidum and corpus callosum in schizophrenia with MR imaging. *Acta Psychiatrica Scandinavica*, **72**, 414–421.

Mathew, V.M., Gruzelier, J.H., Liddle, P.F. (1993) Lateral asymmetries in auditory acuity distinguish hallucinating from non-hallucinating schizophrenic patients. *Psychiatry Research*, **46**, 127–138.

McGlone, J. (1980) Sex differences in human brain asymmetry: A critical survey. *Behavioural and Brain Sciences*, **3**, 215–263.

Merriam, A.E., Gardner, E.B. (1987) Corpus callosum function in schizophrenia: A neuropsychological assessment of interhemispheric information processing. *Neuropsychologia*, **25**, 185–193.

Merrin, E.L. (1981) Schizophrenia and brain asymmetry. *Journal of Nervous and Mental Disease*, **169**, 405–416.

Milner, B. (1982) Some cognitive effects of frontal-lobe lesions in man. In: *The Neuropsychology of Cognitive Function* (Eds D.E. Broadbent, L. Weiskrantz), pp. 211–266, Royal Society, London.

Mintz, M., Tomer, R., Myslobodsky, M. (1982) Neuroleptic-induced lateral asymmetry of visual evoked potentials in schizophrenia. *Biological Psychiatry*, **17**, 815–828.

Myslobodsky, M.S., Mintz, M., Tomer, R. (1983) Neuroleptic effects and the site of abnormality in schizophrenia. In: *Hemisyndromes: Psychobiology, Neurology, Psychiatry* (Ed. M.S. Myslobodsky), pp. 347–388, Academic Press, New York.

Nasrallah, H.A. (1986) Cerebral hemisphere asymmetries and interhemispheric integration in schizophrenia. In: *Handbook of Schizophrenia. Vol. 1: The Neurology of Schizophrenia* (Eds H.A. Nasrallah, D.R. Weinberger), pp. 157–167, Elsevier, Amsterdam.

Nasrallah, H.A., Andreasen, N.C., Coffman, J.A., Olson, S.C., Dunn, V.D., Erhardt, J.C., Chapman, S.M. (1986) A controlled magnetic resonance imaging study of corpus callosum thickness in schizophrenia. *Biological Psychiatry*, **21**, 274–282.

Nasrallah, H.A., McCalley-Witters, M., Bigelow, L.B., Rauscher, F.P. (1983) A histological study of the corpus callosum in chronic schizophrenia. *Psychiatry Research*, **8**, 251–260.

Newlin, D.B., Carpenter, B., Golden, C.J. (1981) Hemispheric asymmetries in schizophrenia. *Biological Psychiatry*, **16**, 561–582.

Overall, V.E., Gorham D.R. (1962) The Brief Psychiatric Rating Scale. *Psychological Reports*, **10**, 799–812.

Perlick, D., Stastny, P., Katz, I., Mayer, M., Mattis, S. (1986) Memory deficits and anticholinergic levels in chronic schizophrenia. *American Journal of Psychiatry*, **143**, 230–232.

Posner, M.E., Early, T.S., Reiman, E., Pardo, P.J., Dhawan, M. (1988) Asymmetries in hemispheric control of attention in schizophrenia. *Archives of General Psychiatry*, **45**, 814–821.

Potkin, S.G., Swanson, J.M., Urvanchek, M., Carreon, D., Bravo, G. (1989) Lateralised deficits in covert shifts of visual attention in chronic and never-medicated schizophrenics compared to normal controls. *Schizophrenia Research*, **2**, 95.

Pycock, C.G., Kerwin, R.W., Carter C.J. (1980) The effect of lesion of cortical dopamine terminals on sub-cortical dopamine receptors in rats. *Nature*, **286**, 74–77.

Raine, A., Andrews, H., Sheard, C., Walder, C., Manders, D. (1989) Interhemispheric transfer in schizophrenics, depressives and normal with schizoid tendencies. *Journal of Abnormal Psychology*, **98**, 35–41.

Raine, A., Harrison, G.N., Reynolds, G.P., Sheard, C., Cooper, J.E., Medley, I. (1990) Structural and functional characteristics of the corpus callosum in schizophrenics, psychiatric controls and normal controls. *Archives of General Psychiatry*, **47**, 1060–1064.

Richardson, A.J., Gruzelier, J. (1994) Visual processing, lateralization and syndromes of schizotypy. *International Journal of Psychophysiology*, **18**, 227–241.

Rist, F., Cohen, R. (1991) Sequential effects in the reaction times of schizophrenics: crossover and modality shift effects. In: *Handbook of Schizophrenia. Vol. 5: Neuropsychology, Psychophysiology and Information Processing* (Eds S.R. Steinhauer, J.H. Gruzelier, J. Zubin), pp. 241–271, Elsevier, Amsterdam.

Rosenthal, R., Bigelow, L.B. (1972) Quantitative brain measurement in chronic schizophrenia. *British Journal of Psychiatry*, **121**, 259–294.

Sandel, A., Alcorn, J.D. (1980) Individual hemisphericity and maladaptive behaviours. *Journal of Abnormal Psychology*, **89**, 514–517.

Saugstad, L.F. (1989) Age at puberty and mental illness: Towards a neuro-developmental aetiology of Kraepelin's endogenous psychoses. *British Journal of Psychiatry*, **155**, 536–544.

Saugstad, L.F. (1994) The maturational theory of brain development and cerebral excitability in the multifactorially manic-depressive psychosis and schizophrenia. *International Journal of Psychophysiology*, **18**, 189–204.

Scarone, S., Garvaglia, P.F., Cazzulo, C.L. (1981) Further evidence of dominance hemisphere dysfunction in chronic schizophrenia. *British Journal of Psychiatry*, **140**, 354–355.

Scarone, S., Gambini, O., Pieri, E. (1983) Dominant hemisphere dysfunction in chronic schizophrenia. Schwartz Test and Short Aphasia Screening Test. In: *Developments in Psychiatry. Vol 6: Laterality and Psychopathology* (Eds P. Flor-Henry, J.H. Gruzelier), pp. 129–142, Elsevier/North-Holland, Amsterdam.

Scarone, S., Cazzullo, C.L., Gambini, O. (1987) Asymmetry of lateralised hemispheric functions in schizophrenia: Influence of clinical and epidemiological characteristics on quality extinction test performance. *British Journal of Psychiatry*, **151**, 15–17.

Schrift, M.J., Bandla, H., Shah, P., Taylor, M.A. (1986) Interhemispheric transfer in major psychoses. *Journal of Nervous and Mental Disease*, **174**, 203–207.

Schweitzer, L., Becker, E., Walsh, H. (1978) Abnormalities of cerebral lateralisation in schizophrenic patients. *Archives of General Psychiatry*, **35**, 982–985.

Serafetinides, E.A. (1972) Laterality and voltage in the EEG of psychiatric patients. *Diseases of the Nervous System*, **33**, 622–630.

Shagass, C., Josiassen, R.C., Roemer, R.A., Straumanis, J.J., Slepner, S.M. (1983) Failure to replicate evoked potential observations suggesting corpus callosum dysfunction in schizophrenia. *British Journal of Psychiatry*, **142**, 471–476.

Shelton, E.J., Knight, R.G. (1984) Inter-hemispheric transmission times in schizophrenics. *British Journal of Clinical Psychology*, **23**, 375–383.

Shimamura, A.P. (1995) Memory and frontal lobe function. In: *The Cognitive Neurosciences* (Ed. M. Gazzaniga), pp. 803–814, MIT Press, London.

Silberman, E.K., Weingartner, H, (1986) Hemispheric lateralization of functions related to emotion. *Brain and Cognition*, **5**, 322–353.

Simon, J.R. (1969) Reactions toward the source of Stimulation. *Journal of Experimental Psychology*, **81**, 174–176.

Soper, H.V., Satz, P., Orsini, D.L., Henry, R.R., Zvi, J.C., Schulman, M. (1986) Handedness patterns in autism suggest subtypes. *Journal of Autism and Developmental Disorders*, **16**, 155–167.

Spitzer, R.L., Endicott, J., Robins, E. (1978) *Research Diagnostic Criteria for A Selected Group of Functional Disorders* (3rd edn). New York Psychiatric Institute, New York.

Springer, S.P., Gazzaninga, M.S. (1975) Dichotic listening in partial and complete split-brain patients. *Neuropsychologia*, **13**, 341–346.

Stein, J.F. (1994) Developmental dyslexia, neural timing and hemispheric lateralisation. *International Journal of Psychophysiology*, **18**, 241–251.

Strauss, M.E., Novakovic, T., Tien, A.Y., Bylsma, F., Pearlson, G.D. (1991) Disengagement of Attention in Schizophrenia. *Psychiatry Research*, **37**, 139–146.

Takahashi, R., Flor-Henry, P., Gruzelier, J.H., Niwa, I. (1987) *Cerebral Dynamics, Laterality and Psychopathology*. Elsevier, Amsterdam.

Tomer, R., Flor-Henry, P. (1989) Neuroleptics reverse attention asymmetries in schizophrenic patients. *Biological Psychiatry*, **25**, 852–860.

Tomer, R., Mintz, M., Levy, A., Myslobodsky, M. (1979) Reactive gaze laterality in schizophrenic patients. *Biological Psychiatry*, **9**, 115–122.

Tomer, R., Mintz, M., Kempler, S., Sigal, M. (1987) Lateralised neuroleptic-induced side effects are associated with asymmetric visual evoked potentials. *Psychiatry Research*, **22**, 311–318.

Tress, K.H., Kugler, B.T., Caudrey, D.J. (1979) Interhemispheric integration in schizophrenia. In: *Hemispheric Asymmetries of Function in Psychopathology*, Vol. 3 (Eds J.H. Gruzelier, P. Flor-Henry), pp. 449–462, Elsevier/North-Holland, Amsterdam.

Tress, K.H., Caudrey, D.J., Mehta, B. (1983) Tactile-evoked potentials in schizophrenia: Interhemispheric transfer and drug effects. *British Journal of Psychiatry*, **143**, 156–164.

Tsuru, N., Fujiwara, M. (1987) Neuropsychological studies and somatosensory evoked potentials in schizophrenics. In: *Cerebral Dynamics, Laterality and Psychopathology* (Eds R. Takahashi, P. Flor-Henry, J. Gruzelier, S. Niwa), pp. 187–197, Elsevier, Amsterdam.

Tucker, D.M. (1981) Lateral brain function, emotion, and conceptualisation. *Psychological Bulletin*, **89**, 19–46.

Tucker, D.M., Williamson, P.A. (1984) Asymmetric neural control systems in human self-regulation. *Psychological Review*, **91**, 185–215.

Tune, L.E., Strauss, M.E., Lew, M.F., Breitlinger, E., Coyle, J.T. (1982) Serum levels of anticholinergic drugs and impaired recent memory in chronic schizophrenic patients. *American Journal of Psychiatry*, **139**, 1460–1461.

Venables, P.H. (1967) Partial failure of cortical–subcortical integration as a factor underlying schizophrenic behaviour. In: *The Origins of Schizophrenia* (Ed. J. Romano), Excerpta Medica, Amsterdam.

Wade, J.B., Taylor, M.A. (1984) Interhemispheric transfer in schizophrenia and affective disorder. *Biological Psychiatry*, **19**, 107–111.

Walker, E., McGuire, S. (1982) Intra- and inter-hemispheric information processing in schizophrenia. *Psychological Bulletin*, **92**, 701–725.

Walker, E., Hoppes, E., Emory, E. (1981) A reinterpretation of findings on hemispheric dysfunction in schizophrenia. *Journal of Nervous and Mental Disorder*, **169**, 378–380.

Warrington, E.K. (1984) *Recognition Memory Test Manual*. NFER–Nelson, Windsor.

Waziri, R. (1980) Lateralisation of neuroleptic-induced dyskinesia indicates pharmacologic asymmetry in the brain. *Psychopharmacology*, **68**, 51–53.

Weinberger, D.R., Berman, K.F., Zec, R.F. (1986) Physiologic dysfunction of dorsolateral prefrontal cortex in schizophrenia. I. Regional cerebral blood flow evidence. *Archives of General Psychiatry*, **43**, 114–124.

Weller, M., Kugler, B.T. (1979) Tactile discrimination in schizophrenia and affective psychoses. In: *Hemispheric Asymmetries of Function in Psychopathology*, Vol. 3 (Eds J.H. Gruzelier, P. Flor-Henry), pp. 463–474, Elsevier/North-Holland, Amsterdam.

Wexler, B.E. (1980) Cerebral laterality and psychiatry: A review of the literature. *American Journal of Psychiatry*, **137**, 285–292.

Wing, J.K., Cooper, J.E., Sartorius, H. (1974) *Measurement and Classification of Psychiatric Symptoms*, Cambridge University Press, London.

Witelson, S.F. (1991) Neural sexual mosaicism: Sexual differentiation of the human temporo-parietal region for functional asymmetry. *Psychoneuroendocrinology*, **16**, 131–153.

9

Neuropsychological Functioning in Children at Risk for Schizophrenia

LORRAINE E. WOLF and BARBARA A. CORNBLATT

INTRODUCTION

Interest in the neuropsychological dysfunctions associated with schizophrenia has rapidly increased over the past decade. Most recently, research concerned with neuropsychological functioning has been stimulated by neuroimaging findings linking brain abnormalities to chronic schizophrenia (for review: Bilder, 1992; Bilder & Szeszko, chapter 14). However, little is yet known about the role of neuropsychological deficits in the aetiology of the illness and the extent to which they can serve as genetic markers or indicators of schizophrenia.

A major source of such information can be found in studies of children at risk for schizophrenia. Empirical evidence indicates that children of schizophrenic parents are at much higher risk for developing schizophrenia as adults than are children in the general population. The risk is considered to be about 7–10 times higher if one parent has schizophrenia and closer to 50 times greater if both parents have the disorder (Gottesman & Shields, 1984). By studying high-risk children many years before onset of the clinical symptoms, deficits that are likely to be causes rather than consequences of the disorder can be identified and their potential as predictors of future illness validated.

Because of the advantages of studying the young offspring of schizophrenic patients in research seeking predictors of illness, a number of high-risk studies were initiated in the United States, Europe and Israel in the late 1960s and early 1970s. Many of these were interested in clinical precursors of illness while others focused on childhood cognitive predictors, especially in the area of attention (for review: Watt et al, 1984; Nuechterlein & Dawson, 1984). Since the field of neuropsychology was only in its infancy at the time that these studies were designed, few neuropsychological measures were included. Nevertheless, in several studies a

Schizophrenia: A Neuropsychological Perspective. Edited by C. Pantelis, H.E. Nelson and T.R.E. Barnes
© 1996 John Wiley & Sons Ltd

variety of neuropsychological functions were indirectly examined. In this chapter we evaluate the evidence from high-risk studies that, in combination with more direct findings from the adult literature, suggest specific neuropsychological abnormalities may be potential indicators or predictors of schizophrenia. Our discussion will not include impaired attention since this is the only neuropsychological abnormality that has been thoroughly examined in previous reviews and has already been established as a highly promising candidate genetic marker (Cornblatt & Keilp, 1994).

As conceptualised in this paper, an indicator or marker is an abnormality that indicates a biological susceptibility to schizophrenia. Based on the criteria specified by other researchers (e.g. Cloninger, 1987; Gershon & Goldin, 1986; Spring & Zubin, 1978), to be considered a biological marker or indicator, a given deficit should be: (1) associated with schizophrenia in the population (i.e. patients differ from normal controls); (2) specific to schizophrenia; (3) independent of clinical state; (4) predate the illness; (5) heritable, and (6) co-segregate with the illness (see Cornblatt et al, 1995, for more details about marker criteria).

In the discussion to follow, we have selected neuropsychological abnormalities that fulfil the first of these criteria. We will then establish the extent to which these potential indicators fulfil the fourth requirement by being detectable in children at risk for schizophrenia.

POTENTIAL NEUROPSYCHOLOGICAL MARKERS

Three domains of candidate abnormalities have been selected for review as these are considered to be most relevant to schizophrenia from a neuropsychological and neuroanatomical framework. These are: (1) executive (frontal lobe) deficits, (2) verbal memory and language (dominant temporal lobe and temporolimbic) abnormalities, and (3) neuromotor (subcortical) dysfunctions.

EXECUTIVE FUNCTIONING

Definition and Measurement

Executive control generally refers to the ability to establish, maintain and shift response set in order to achieve a goal, involving anticipation, planning and response flexibility (Luria, 1973; Mesulam, 1986; Stuss & Benson, 1986). Related domains of executive behaviour include concept formation, mental tracking and perseveration. Brain regions thought to be involved include the frontal lobes, particularly the prefrontal cortex (Luria, 1973; Stuss & Benson, 1986).

As with most neuropsychological functions, measurement of executive and frontal lobe behaviour is multidimensional. Thus, each related domain may be measured by a wide range of tasks, only some of which have been validated in neurological patients (Milner, 1963; Nelson, 1976; Robinson et al, 1980). Two of the most widely used tests of executive function are the Wisconsin Card Sorting Test (WCST) (Grant & Berg, 1948; Heaton, 1981) and the Trail Making Test

Part B (Reitan, 1979). Both tasks have been extensively used in research with schizophrenic patients (Fey, 1951; also see Goldberg & Weinberger, 1988).

Conceptual Sorting Tasks

The WCST (Heaton, 1981; Heaton et al, 1993) and the Object Sort Test (OST) (Goldstein & Scheerer, 1953) both measure concept formation as the ability to sort cards, objects or pictures and involve categorising material according to conceptual as well as procedural rules (Lezak, 1995). For example, the WCST requires a series of shifts in sorting strategy (e.g. sorting by colour to sorting by shape) in response to performance feedback (subject informed whether sort is correct or incorrect). Adequate performance therefore places demands on concept formation (deducing the correct strategy), maintaining set (sticking with what works) and response flexibility (shifting set and abandoning incorrect or previously correct strategies). Poor performance might include failure to establish or maintain a correct set or, more interestingly from the perspective of schizophrenia research, failure to switch between sets (perseverative responding). The OST (Neale et al, 1984; Weintraub, 1987) requires subjects to group pictures of common objects into various conceptual categories depending on a number of shared attributes (e.g. "all tools", "things you can hold", etc.).

Relevance to Schizophrenia

Executive deficits assessed by the WCST and comparable measures have been reported in adults with schizophrenia (Braff et al, 1991; Fey, 1951; Goldberg & Weinberger, 1988; Liddle & Morris, 1991). Neuroimaging studies suggest that frontal lobe dysfunctions underlie sorting deficits in these subjects (Weinberger et al, 1986; Robbins, 1990; for reviews: Levin, 1984; Goldberg & Seidman, 1991). From the perspective of genetic indicators, sorting deficits have been found in the clinically unimpaired parents and siblings of patients with schizophrenia (Franke et al, 1992; Seidman et al, 1992; Steinhauer et al, 1991).

High-risk Findings

Compared to research with affected adults with schizophrenia, few studies of executive functioning have involved children at risk for schizophrenia. This is due in part to the fact that developmental investigations of pre-adolescent executive functioning have only recently been initiated (Levin et al, 1991; Welsh et al, 1991). For example, the WCST, the measure of executive functioning most often used with schizophrenic adults has, to date, been included in only one high-risk study, the Israeli high-risk project conducted by Mirsky and colleagues (e.g. Mirsky et al, 1995). In a recent round of follow-up testing, these investigators reported that young adult high-risk subjects performed more poorly than normal controls on the WCST. However, the differences are not significant and are difficult to interpret as none of the subjects had been tested on comparable tasks during childhood.

Nevertheless, deficits in concept formation and abstraction have been demonstrated on other sorting tasks (Asarnow et al, 1978; Neale et al, 1984; Weintraub & Neale, 1984). Using the OST, Neale and colleagues found that children at risk for schizophrenia (HRSz) made more "complexive" sorts (i.e. sorts without an obvious unifying theme) than normal controls (NCs) or children at risk for affective disorder (HRAff), even after controlling for differences in IQ (Winters et al, 1981; Neale et al, 1984).

Similarly, Asarnow et al (1978) reported sorting deficits in HRSz children using a somewhat different measure, the Concept Attainment Task (CAT) (Walker & Bourne, 1961). Although conceptualised by Asarnow and colleagues as an attentional measure (Asarnow et al, 1978), the CAT integrates features of both the WCST and OST tasks and is thus also likely to measure executive functions. It resembles the WCST in that card sorting involves response to performance feedback and the OST in that the sorting categories are based on concept formation and abstraction (cards may be sorted on the basis of relevant or irrelevant stimulus dimensions). Foster home reared HRSz children were found to make more errors than either foster reared control children or NCs on all but the most difficult condition of the CAT (Asarnow et al, 1978).

Thus, at least three groups of investigators suggest that HRSz offspring may have deficits in concept formation, even though no two studies used the same methodology and only the Israeli study was explicitly designed to investigate executive skills (Mirsky et al, 1995). However, concept formation deficits in HRSz subjects are supported by studies that have measured other aspects of executive function, as discussed below.

Mental Tracking Tasks

A few studies have examined mental tracking and set-switching in HRSz. Tracking is a process of active attention to either an external stimulus or direct train of thought and is often measured with either the Stroop or Trail Making tasks. Both tasks require perceptual shifts in the face of changing task demands and have thus often been conceptualised as executive measures (Lezak, 1995). The Stroop task (Stroop, 1935) is a classic measure of response competition. Subjects are first required to name colours and read colour names then asked to inhibit reading while naming the colour ink in which the words are printed (e.g. the word "red" printed in blue ink). The Trail Making task is part of the Halstead–Reitan neuropsychological battery (Reitan, 1979). Trails Part A requires simple perceptual search and scanning; the more difficult Trails Part B requires shifting between different response sets (e.g. number sequences and letter sequences). Thus, both Trails B and the Stroop task require cognitive and behavioural flexibility in response to changing task demands and consequently tap executive functioning.

High-risk Findings

Studies using versions of Trail Making Part B have provided some evidence of tracking and set shifting difficulties in HRSz offspring. In a study by Asarnow et al (1978), HRSz children were reported to show deficits relative to foster controls using the "Spokes Test" version of Part B. More recently, Mirsky et al (Mirsky et al, 1992, 1995) reported similar deficits in HRSz subjects as compared to NCs on the standard Trail Making Part B task. These findings support the results of studies of executive function using sorting tasks discussed above, indicating that HRSz offspring have difficulties with cognitive flexibility.

Few studies have included more than one or two measures of executive functioning at the same time, thus examination of interrelationships among different executive skills in HRSz subjects is difficult. The early study by Asarnow et al (1978) is one of the few utilising multiple measures, permitting some speculation about a possible relationship between tracking and shifting in HRSz subjects. While finding differences on the Spokes task Part B between HRSz and controls, he did not detect deficits on the Stroop Test. These results suggest that difficulties on the Spokes task may not be related to a general shifting deficit in HRSz subjects. This is further indicated by Nuechterlein et al (1980), who did not find shifting deficits in HRSz compared either to NCs or to several psychiatric control groups using a cross-modality reaction time paradigm. Thus, while some HRSz offspring show deficits in Trail Making performance, it is unclear if this is related to dysfunctional shifting of response set or to other performance factors such as perceptual motor speed or visual attention.

Asarnow et al (1978) detected both tracking (as measured by the Spokes Task) and conceptual sorting (as measured by the CAT) deficits in their HRSz sample. However, correlations between the Spokes Test Part B and the CAT (two of the most discriminating tests in that study) were reportedly low. Mirsky et al (1995) used both the Wisconsin and Trail Making tasks in the same study and were similarly unable to relate Trail Making Part B to WCST deficits. However, they did find that Trails B, in association with several other tests of perceptual motor speed and visual attention, best discriminated among HRSz, NCs and adult patients with schizophrenia (Mirsky et al, 1995). Thus, while there is evidence for both sorting and tracking difficulties in HRSz, the relationship between these executive functions remains unclear.

Overview of Executive Functioning

To summarise, when tasks are grouped according to different executive functions, the preliminary evidence suggests that subjects at risk for schizophrenia have difficulties in conceptual sorting and mental tracking or set-shifting compared to controls. This is consistent with the findings reported in patients with schizophrenia (Braff et al, 1991; Liddle & Morris, 1991) and their adult relatives (Franke et al, 1992; Keefe et al, 1994; Seidman et al, 1992; Steinhauer et al, 1991). However, while most of the adult studies have the advantage of using the same task, such as the WCST or Trails B, the high-risk studies use a variety of different measures which may not be directly comparable. This methodological flaw leads to the question of whether concept formation and set-shifting are related in HRSz. If they are not related then it will be necessary to determine which is the more promising genetic indicator. Alternatively, there may be a predictive advantage involved in combining them into a composite category representing multiple functions.

VERBAL MEMORY

Definition and Measurement

Verbal memory may be more familiar and thus more easily defined than executive functioning. A general definition of verbal memory would include an acquisition stage (perceptual or sensory), encoding or storage (learning) and retrieval (recall) of language-based information (see Squire, 1982, 1987; see Chen and McKenna, chapter 7).

Verbal memory is often measured by such tasks as serial digit or list learning and recall of stories or paragraphs which are either read to or by the subject. Many tasks measure both encoding (recognition that material has been learned) as well as retrieval (recall of learned information) processes. In general, recognition tasks do not require active rehearsal or effortful encoding strategies, while recall tasks place additional emphasis on organisation of information (Calev, 1984; Squire, 1987). Both verbal recognition and recall are thought to involve mesial temporal and temporolimbic areas in the left hemisphere, as lesions in these areas commonly produce deficits in verbal memory (Squire, 1987).

Relevance to Schizophrenia

Current findings of structural abnormalities in the left temporal lobe of adults with schizophrenia (Bogerts et al, 1990; Shenton et al, 1992) are consistent with deficits of verbal memory which implicate these areas (for review of neuro-imaging and neuropsychological findings: Bilder, 1992; Bilder and Szeszko, chapter 14).

Deficits in short-term verbal memory have consistently been found in adult patients with schizophrenia (Goldberg et al, 1989; Saykin et al, 1991). Typical findings are of impairment in recall but not recognition memory (Gold et al, 1992; Goldberg et al, 1989; Koh, 1978), although this has been attributed to recall tasks being generally more difficult and requiring greater effort than recognition tasks (Calev, 1984). Furthermore, preliminary evidence of verbal recall deficits in the adult relatives of patients with schizophrenia have been reported (Seidman et al, 1992).

High-risk Findings

Memory function has not been extensively tested in high-risk populations, thus evidence for memory impairment is weaker than for adult patients. For clarity, the evidence that does exist will be discussed separately for recognition versus retrieval deficits.

Verbal Recognition Tasks

Evidence linking deficits in verbal recognition with risk for schizophrenia is tentative and contradictory. As part of the New York High Risk Project (NYHRP), Rutschmann et al (1980) demonstrated impairment in recognition of verbally presented words and trigrams in the HRSz adolescents compared to both normal and psychiatric controls. However, Driscoll (1984) failed to find deficits in verbal recognition in HRSz subjects which is in keeping with the findings in adults with schizophrenia (see Chen and McKenna, chapter 7; Gourovitch and Goldberg, chapter 5).

Verbal Recall Tasks

In contrast with the findings for adult patients with schizophrenia, indicating a general deficit in verbal recall (see Chen and McKenna, chapter 7; Gourovitch and Goldberg, chapter 5), retrieval deficits have not typically been reported in HRSz offspring unless memory tasks include a distraction condition. Most often this has involved tasks of digit and/or word recall. While these tasks are often considered tests of auditory attention, both have also been used as indices of short-term memory for auditory material in high-risk studies. Typical findings are that HRSz do not manifest deficits in absolute word or digit span. However, subtle difficulties are apparent in the presence of distraction, for example, when words or digits are read with competing voices in the background.

In the studies by Lifschitz et al (1985) and Winters et al (1981) HRSz children did not differ from NCs in recall of digit strings. Similarly, Hallet et al (1986) found no differences between age and IQ matched HRSz and NC children in absolute memory units recalled from stories presented verbally. In contrast, Cornblatt and Erlenmeyer-Kimling (1984, 1985) reported that young HRSz children performed significantly more poorly than NCs on the most demanding test condition, involving five letters and a fast presentation rate, of a letter recall test administered during the early rounds of the NYHRP. It is possible that memory impairments in clinically unaffected, at-risk children are only detectable on highly demanding tasks.

The importance of difficulty level is further supported by more consistent findings on recall tasks when auditory distraction is added. Deficits become more apparent in subjects at risk for schizophrenia on tasks which incorporate distraction conditions, such as story recall (Lifschitz et al, 1985), letter recall (Cornblatt & Erlenmeyer-Kimling, 1984, 1985) and memory for digit strings (Erlenmeyer-Kimling & Cornblatt, 1992; Harvey et al, 1981; Winters et al, 1981). In the study by Harvey et al (1981), all subjects recalled fewer digits in the presence of auditory distraction; however, HRSz children were differentially impaired in recall of digits presented early in the list (primacy effects). The investigators concluded that the deficit was not related to the general effects of distraction but reflected a deficit of memory and that the encoding stages of verbal memory may be especially vulnerable in HRSz children. This is similar to the conclusions of Rutschmann et al (1980), who interpreted the findings in their verbal recognition task as indicating deficits at the input stage of memory, thus implicating encoding rather than retrieval mechanisms (Squire, 1987). It is possible that the memory deficit, indicating a vulnerability to schizophrenia, is better conceptualised by stage of information processing (early versus late) rather than type (recognition versus recall) of process. This possibility has not been systematically investigated in HRSz children.

Overview of Memory Functioning

In summary, there are potential deficits in short-term verbal memory in HRSz children. However, the findings of recognition deficits are contradictory and recall deficits are consistent only when task difficulty is increased or distraction is added to the central task. This suggests that other brain systems, such as frontal lobe, may interact with left temporolimbic areas in producing verbal memory deficits in schizophrenia.

LANGUAGE

Definition and Measurement

Comprehensive language assessment in adults (Benton & Hamsher, 1983; Goodglass & Kaplan, 1987) and children (Crary et al, 1988; Semel & Wiig, 1980) requires detailed descriptions of both receptive and expressive processes. Receptive processes include auditory perception of speech sounds (phoneme and word discrimination), receptive vocabulary (word knowledge) and understanding of complex syntax. Expressive processes are associated with production of language ranging from naming common objects through to use of syntactically complex speech. As with verbal memory, language processing is associated with the temporal lobe of the dominant hemisphere (for recent review: Alexander & Benson, 1992).

Relevance to Schizophrenia

Language deficits in adults with schizophrenia have been related to left hemisphere dysfunction (Flor-Henry & Yeudall, 1979), thought disorder (Brown, 1973) and to dysfunction in information processing (Frith, 1987). Language difficulties which resemble those of aphasic patients with left hemisphere disease have been described in adults with schizophrenia. These include expressive disturbances (Andreasen, 1979; Barr et al, 1989) and difficulties in the comprehension of spoken language (Condray et al, 1992; Morice & McNicol, 1985). In addition, deficient comprehension of complex syntax has been reported in the first-degree adult relatives of patients with schizophrenia (Condray et al, 1992; Condray & Steinhauer, 1992).

High-risk Findings

Few studies have conducted comprehensive assessments of language skills in high-risk subjects. A number of alternate strategies have been used ranging from an examination of global patterns of intelligence to the study of more specific areas of language function.

Verbal Intelligence

One language-oriented approach examines relative differences between overall verbal and non-verbal skills (see also Gourovitch & Goldberg, chapter 5; Barber et al, chapter 4). Since formal measures of intelligence (IQ) were widely used in high-risk research a substantial number of studies have reported relevant data. The primary findings suggest a subtle or mild verbal dysfunction to be characteristic of subjects at risk for schizophrenia.

Lower Verbal IQ (VIQ) scores on the Wechsler Intelligence Scale for Children (WISC) (Wechsler, 1974) have been consistently found in HRSz children and adolescents compared to NCs (Erlenmeyer-Kimling et al, 1984; Gruzelier et al, 1979; Mednick & Schulsinger, 1968; Neale et al, 1984; Schreiber et al, 1992; Worland & Hesselbrock, 1980; Worland et al, 1984). In addition, a number of studies have found greater variability in verbal subtests as compared to performance measures (Greenwald et al, 1982; Gruzelier et al, 1979; Wynne et al, 1987). In the general population this pattern typically reflects an underlying language weakness (Kaufman, 1979); however, the implications of these findings in studies of HRSz children have not been fully explored.

Receptive Language

Although receptive deficits have been described in HRSz children, it is unclear whether there are any overall deficiencies in language comprehension. For example, while Hallet & Green (1983) reported that HRSz children made more errors than NCs in basic phonemic discrimination, Gamer et al (1977) did not find deficits in the receptive vocabulary of three year old HRSz children relative to controls. However, few high-risk studies have completed comprehensive assessments of language skills. Thus, the impact of deficits in discrimination of speech sounds on later acquisition of receptive vocabulary has not yet been established.

Expressive Language

There is considerably more evidence in favour of expressive language problems in high-risk youngsters, partly due to the greater number of studies. Deficits associated with language expression in HRSz children include word communication (e.g. the ability to provide relevant narrative cues to listeners) (Winters et al, 1981), speech output, productivity and narrative cohesion (Harvey et al, 1982), deviant communication patterns and thought disorder (Arboleda & Holzman, 1985; Neale et al, 1984; Parnas et al, 1986; Sohlberg, 1985; Worland et al, 1979). Furthermore, the impaired VIQ performance of HRSz children on the WISC has been attributed in part to poor scores for the comprehension subtest (Asarnow,

1988; Fish, 1984; Rieder & Nichols, 1979; Schreiber et al, 1992). This result may be explained by the high demand for oral expression as compared to the other verbal subtests (Kaufman, 1979).

Despite evidence suggesting that HRSz children may have language deficits, it is difficult to relate difficulties in communication directly with language abilities. For example, core deficits in language may not be separable from thought disorder, rendering the results difficult to interpret from a linguistic point of view. Interpretive confusion is compounded because linguistic parameters are not clearly defined from a neuropsychological perspective, nor do most studies speculate about underlying brain mechanisms. More neuropsychologically based language research, such as studies of cerebral asymmetry would help to clarify these findings.

Language Lateralisation

Neuropsychological investigations of patients with schizophrenia have suggested that deficits are lateralised (see Gruzelier, chapter 8). Clues to laterality are provided by observations of unusual patterns of handedness as well as more direct laboratory measures such as dichotic listening. Abnormal patterns of lateralisation have been described in adult patients with schizophrenia (for review: Nasrallah, 1986; see Gruzelier, chapter 8) as well as in HRSz. With reference to language, left hemisphere dysfunction may be inferred indirectly by the presence of language abnormality.

The first study to examine differences between left and right hemisphere functioning in HRSz children was that by Gruzelier et al (1979), who found that HRSz children had lower verbal than non-verbal IQ scores relative to children at genetic risk for other psychiatric disorders and to normal control children. The findings indicated an abnormal pattern of lateralisation and a dysfunction in the left hemisphere, similar to that displayed by adults with schizophrenia (Gruzelier et al, 1979).

Consistency of lateral hand preference has been interpreted as an outward expression of hemispheric dominance (Dean, 1984). Deviations from the pattern expected in the general population have been hypothesised to reflect abnormalities in cerebral lateralisation of language (Orton, 1937). Some authors have suggested that left handedness reflects subtle damage or dysfunction in the left hemisphere (Nasrallah, 1986).

Hallet and colleagues (Hallet & Green, 1983; Hallet et al, 1986) found a disproportionate number of age and gender-matched HRSz children to be left handed (38% and 23% of HRSz in the original study and the replication, as compared to 0% and 8% of NCs). As the distribution of the normal controls (less than 10% in both studies) is close to the expectation of left handedness in the general population, these results suggest anomalous cerebral lateralisation in the HRSz children. However, the relationship between hand preference and underlying brain organisation may be indirect (Dean, 1982) and further support from linguistic studies is necessary before concluding that HRSz have abnormal patterns of language lateralisation.

The above studies (Hallet & Green, 1983; Hallet et al, 1986) also examined speech comprehension and recall of verbal material under binaural and monaural conditions. In both studies, HRSz children had relative difficulty understanding speech presented to both ears as compared to comprehension in either ear alone. This was interpreted as reflecting poor integration between the left and right hemispheres.

Further differences were found when stimuli were presented under verbal dichotic conditions. Although often used in attentional research with high-risk subjects, dichotic listening tasks can also serve as a tool for investigating parameters such as language dominance. In normal adults (Kimura, 1961) and children (Hynd & Obrzut, 1977) there is typically an advantage for verbal material presented dichotically to the right ear (left hemisphere), presumably reflecting unilateral specialisation for language. However, HRSz children do not display a right ear advantage for speech even after controlling for the effects of handedness (Hallet et al, 1986). Hallet and colleagues interpreted this atypical lateralisation pattern as evidence of bilateral, rather than normal unilateral, representation of language in some HRSz children. It was suggested that this may be secondary to immaturity in the development of the corpus callosum (Hallet et al, 1986).

Overview of Language Functioning

In their original and replication studies, Hallet and colleagues (Hallet & Green, 1983; Hallet et al, 1986) reported evidence of disturbed lateralisation on both hand preference and linguistic measures in HRSz children as compared to NCs. They found an excess of left-handed HRSz children and reported atypical patterns of language lateralisation (Hallet & Green, 1983; Hallet et al, 1986). These findings provide support for the hypothesis that children at risk for schizophrenia are characterised by left hemisphere dysfunction. This may underlie the language problems characteristic of adults with schizophrenia which are also detected in HRSz children.

NEUROMOTOR SOFT SIGNS

Neuromotor "soft signs" represent an additional category of potential markers or indicators of biological susceptibility to schizophrenia. Although a somewhat different domain than the neuropsychological deficits, soft signs have been included in this review because they meet marker criteria number one and number four (see above) in that they are frequently found in HRSz children compared to a variety of controls.

Definition and Measurement

Neuromotor "soft signs" are defined as non-localising signs of neurological delay or damage, such as clumsiness, poor balance and motor impersistence. Diffuse subcortical systems are proposed to underlie such functions since no specific lesion has been found to account for these dysfunctions (Fish et al, 1992; Kennard, 1960).

Relevance to Schizophrenia

Motor soft signs are found in adult patients with schizophrenia and in their clinically unaffected first-degree relatives (Kinney et al, 1986; Rossi et al, 1990; Walker & Shaye, 1982).

High-risk Findings

Neuromotor signs are thought to characterise HRSz children, although neither simple motor slowness (Asarnow et al, 1978; Phipps-Yonas, 1984) nor motor perseveration (Schreiber et al, 1992) have differentiated HRSz from controls. It is the more subtle deviations in sensorimotor development that appear to have the potential to serve as markers of illness vulnerability.

Fish and colleagues (Fish & Alpert, 1963; Fish, 1987; Fish et al, 1992) described a syndrome of non-focal temporal delays (e.g. lags in development which are not pathological *per se*) and inconsistencies in motor development, sensorimotor integration and physical growth (termed "pandysmaturation" or PDM) in about half of HRSz infants compared to normal controls. PDM in infancy has been associated with attentional dysfunctions at age 10 and is thought to be stable through adolescence and early adulthood (Fish, 1984; Fish et al, 1992). Findings of neuromotor delay in HRSz children have been well replicated (Marcus et al, 1984, 1987), with motor findings somewhat more consistent than sensory delays (Orvaschel et al, 1979; Erlenmeyer-Kimling & Cornblatt, 1987).

The relationship between neurodevelopmental delay and later psychiatric symptoms in HRSz has been described by several groups (Erlenmeyer-Kimling et al, 1984; Asarnow & Goldstein, 1986; Rinaldi et al, 1991). In the NYHRP, Erlenmeyer-Kimling et al (1984) reported the worst motor performance in those HRSz children who later developed behaviour problems.

Several studies have related early neuromotor deficits to adolescent behavioural difficulties. A recent study from the NYHRP found that childhood neuromotor deficit predicted affective disturbances (flat affect) in adolescence in HRSz but not children at risk for bipolar disorder or NCs (Dworkin et al, 1993). In addition, Silverton et al (1988) related motor impairments during infancy to the emergence of antisocial behaviours during adolescence in HRSz but not NC subjects.

Overview of Neuromotor Functions

It appears that some delay in motor development is present in at least a subset of HRSz children. The possibility that neuromotor dysfunction may serve as a marker of genetic vulnerability to schizophrenia is suggested by the finding that these abnormalities may be especially severe in those HRSz offspring who eventually develop the disease (Erlenmeyer-Kimling et al, 1984).

CONCLUSIONS AND FUTURE DIRECTIONS

Preliminary evidence from a number of high-risk studies suggests that some subtle neuropsychological deficits are potential genetic markers of schizophrenia. Several candidate indicators satisfying the first criterion, that is, detected in patients with schizophrenia, were reviewed. These included executive functions, verbal memory, language and neuromotor soft signs. A number of these also appear to satisfy the fourth criterion of predating illness onset in that they are detectable in the HRSz.

Based on the evidence reviewed in this chapter we conclude that conceptual sorting, verbal retrieval, language processing and neuromotor soft signs have the greatest potential to be neuropsychological markers of a biological susceptibility to schizophrenia. Several other functions including mental tracking, verbal recognition and language lateralisation appear promising, but are not as well supported by the literature.

Overall, the evidence above suggests that dysfunction in the frontal lobe, dominant temporal lobe and subcortical systems may play a role in the pathophysiology of schizophrenia and underlie the neuropsychological dysfunctions observed. Future research needs to investigate at what point in the development of the disorder these neuroanatomical abnormalities are expressed.

We have proposed that several neuropsychological dysfunctions are potential indicators of genetic risk for schizophrenia; however, four of our original six criteria have yet to be examined. For example, for a neuropsychological deficit to be a potential genetic marker it must be specific to schizophrenia (criterion 2). That is, not only must the deficit discriminate between patients with schizophrenia and NCs but it must also discriminate patients with schizophrenia from patients with other psychiatric disorders. Specificity of neuropsychological deficits for the functions discussed above has not been consistently demonstrated in adult patients (Hoff et al, 1990; Morice, 1990; Flor-Henry & Yeudall, 1979). In addition, the issue of specificity has not been adequately addressed in many early high-risk studies. Only a few groups, such as the NYHRP (Erlenmeyer-Kimling & Cornblatt, 1992) and Stony Brook (Weintraub & Neale, 1984) studies, directly compared HRSz offspring to another psychiatric risk group.

Among the potential markers discussed, specificity was only directly established for three: a lack of a primacy effect in memory function in the Stony Brook high-risk studies (Harvey et al, 1981), diminished verbal IQ in the Danish study (Gruzelier et al, 1979) and deficits of sustained attention in the NYHRP (Erlenmeyer-Kimling & Cornblatt, 1992). Therefore, a logical progression to establish which neurocognitive deficits are specific markers of schizophrenia requires the comparison of HRSz offspring with children at risk for other psychiatric disorders. Once specificity has been established the remaining criteria, that is, genetic transmission, independence of clinical state and co-segregation with illness, can be investigated.

Moreover, future studies of young at-risk populations require the use of neuropsychological instruments comparable to those used in the adult patient populations. Assessment of children requires that developmentally appropriate instruments be utilised and that principles of cognitive development underlie comparisons between adults and children. This approach was not always explicit in the earlier studies and consequently we have few direct comparisons between at-risk children and adult patients on these potential markers.

SUMMARY

We have listed six criteria for evaluating whether a behaviourally observable deficit has potential as a genetic indicator or marker of schizophrenia. An array of neuropsychological deficits was accordingly selected that fulfilled the first of the criteria, that patients differ from normal controls. We then evaluated the extent to which each candidate deficit fulfilled a second criterion on our list (criterion number four), which is to predate illness. We concluded that of our original list of potential markers, four deficits are strong candidates (conceptual sorting, verbal recall, language processing and neuromotor soft signs) with an additional three (mental tracking, verbal recognition and lateralisation pattern) as possible candidates.

We suggest that future research more conclusively validate these markers by examining the remaining criteria using age-appropriate and standard instruments. Of these, establishing specificity appears to be the most logical next step at this stage of neuropsychological research in schizophrenia.

REFERENCES

Alexander, M.P., Benson, D.F. (1992) The aphasias and related disturbances. In: *Clinical Neurology* (Ed. R.J. Joynt), pp. 1–58, Lippincott, Philadelphia.

Andreasen, N.C. (1979) The relationship between schizophrenic language and the aphasias. In: *Schizophrenia as a Brain Disease* (Eds F.A. Henn, H.A. Nasrallah), pp. 99–111, Oxford University Press, New York.

Arboleda, C., Holzman, P.S. (1985) Thought disorder in children at risk for psychosis. *Archives of General Psychiatry*, **42**, 1004–1013.

Asarnow, J.R. (1988) Children at risk for schizophrenia: Converging lines of evidence. *Schizophrenia Bulletin*, **14**, 613–631.

Asarnow, J.R., Goldstein, M.J. (1986) Schizophrenia during adolescence and early adulthood: A developmental perspective on risk research. *Clinical Psychology Review*, **6**, 211–235.

Asarnow, R.F., Steffy, R.A., MacCrimmon, D.J., Cleghorn, J.M. (1978) An attentional assessment of foster children at risk for schizophrenia. In: *The Nature of Schizophrenia: New Approaches to Research and Treatment,* (Eds L.C. Wynne, R.L. Cromwell, S. Matthysse), pp. 339–358, Wiley, New York.

Barr, W.B., Bilder, R.M., Goldberg, E., Kaplan, E., Mukherjee, S. (1989) The neuropsychology of schizophrenic speech. *Journal of Communication Disorders*, **22**, 327–349.

Benton, A.L., Hamsher, K. de S. (1983) *Multilingual Aphasia Examination*, University of Iowa, Iowa City.

Bilder, R.M. (1992) Structure–function relations in schizophrenia: Brain morphology and neuropsychology. In: *Experimental Personality and Psychopathology Research* (Eds E.F. Walker, R.H. Dworkin, B.A. Cornblatt), pp. 183–251, Springer, New York.

Bogerts, B., Ashtari, M., Degreef, G., Alvir, J., Bilder, R.M., Lieberman, J.A. (1990) Reduced temporal limbic structure volumes on magnetic resonance images in first episode schizophrenia. *Psychiatry Research: Neuroimaging*, **35**, 1–13.

Braff, D.L., Heaton, R., Kuck, J., Cullum, M., Moranville, J., Grant, I., Zisook, S. (1991) The generalized pattern of neuropsychological deficits in outpatients with chronic schizophrenia with heterogeneous Wisconsin Card Sorting Test results. *Archives of General Psychiatry*, **48**, 891–898.

Brown, R. (1973), Schizophrenia, language, reality. *American Psychologist*, **28**, 395–403.

Calev, A. (1984) Recall and recognition in mildly disturbed schizophrenics: The use of matched tasks. *Psychological Medicine*, **14**, 425–429.

Cloninger, C.R. (1987) Genetic principles and methods in high-risk studies of schizophrenia. *Schizophrenia Research*, **13**, 515–523.

Condray, R.C., Steinhauer, S.R. (1992) Schizotypal personality disorder in individuals with and without schizophrenic relatives: Similarities and contrasts in neurocognitive and clinical functioning. *Schizophrenia Research*, **7**, 33–41.

Condray, R.C., Steinhauer, S.R., Goldstein, G. (1992) Language comprehension in schizophrenics and their brothers. *Biological Psychiatry*, **32**, 790–802.

Cornblatt, B.A., Erlenmeyer-Kimling, L. (1984) Early attentional predictors of adolescent behavioural disturbances in children at risk for schizophrenia. In: *Children at Risk for Schizophrenia: A Longitudinal Perspective,* (Eds N.F. Watt, E.J. Anthony, L.C. Wynne, J.E. Rolf), pp. 198–211, Cambridge University Press, New York.

Cornblatt, B.A., Erlenmeyer-Kimling, L. (1985) Global attentional deviance as a marker of risk for schizophrenia: Specificity and predictive validity. *Journal of Abnormal Psychology*, **94**, 470–486.

Cornblatt, B.A., Keilp, J.G. (1994) Impaired attention: A trait indicator of the schizophrenia genotype and contributor to the clinical phenotype. *Schizophrenia Bulletin*, **20**, 31–46.

Cornblatt, B.A., Dworkin, R.A., Wolf, L.E., Erlenmeyer-Kimling, L. (1995) Markers, developmental process & schizophrenia. In: *Frontiers of Developmental Psychopathology* (Eds M. Lenzenweger, J. Haugaard), Oxford University Press, New York.

Crary, M.A., Voeller, K.S., Haak, N.J. (1988) Questions of developmental neurolinguistic assessment. In: *Assessment Issues in Child Neuropsychology* (Eds M.G. Tramontana, S.R. Hooper), pp. 249–280, Plenum Press, New York.

Dean, R.S. (1982) Assessing patterns of lateral preference. *Journal of Clinical Neuropsychology*, **4**, 124–128.

Dean, R.S. (1984) Functional lateralisation of the brain. *Journal of Special Education*, **18**, 240–256.

Driscoll, R.M. (1984) Intentional and incidental learning in children vulnerable to psychopathology. In: *Children at Risk for Schizophrenia: A Longitudinal Perspective* (Eds N. F. Watt, E.F. Anthony, L.C. Wynne,, J.E. Rolf), pp. 320–333, Cambridge University Press, New York.

Dworkin, R.H., Cornblatt, B.A., Friedmann, L.M., Kaplansky, L.M., Lewis, J.A., Rinaldi, A., Shilliday, C., Erlenmeyer-Kimling, L. (1993) Childhood neuromotor and attentional precursors of affective versus social deficits in adolescents at risk for schizophrenia. *Schizophrenia Bulletin*, **19**, 563–577.

Erlenmeyer-Kimling, L., Cornblatt, B. (1987) The New York High-Risk Project: A follow-up report. *Schizophrenia Bulletin*, **13**, 451–460.

Erlenmeyer-Kimling, L., Cornblatt, B.A. (1992) A summary of attentional findings in the New York High-Risk Project. *Journal of Psychiatric Research*, **26**, 405–426.

Erlenmeyer-Kimling, L., Kestenbaum, C., Bird, H., Hildoff, U. (1984) Assessment of the New York High-Risk Project subjects in Sample A who are now clinically deviant. In: *Children at Risk for Schizophrenia: A Longitudinal Perspective* (Eds N.F. Watt, J.E. Anthony, L.C. Wynne, J.E. Rolf), pp. 227–239, Cambridge University Press, New York.

Fey, E.T. (1951) The performance of young schizophrenics and young normals on the Wisconsin Card Sorting Test. *Journal of Consulting Psychology*, **15**, 311–319.

Fish, B. (1984) Characteristics and sequelae of the neurointegrative disorder in infants at risk for schizophrenia: 1952–1982. In: *Children at High Risk for Schizophrenia: A Longitudinal Perspective* (Eds F. Watt, E.J. Anthony, L.C. Wynne, J.E. Rolf), pp. 422–439, Cambridge University Press, New York.

Fish, B. (1987) Infant predictors of the longitudinal course of schizophrenic development. *Schizophrenia Bulletin*, **13**, 395–409.

Fish, B., Alpert, M. (1963) Patterns of neurological development in infants born to schizophrenic mothers. In: *Recent Advances in Biological Psychology*, Vol. 5 (Ed. J. Wortis), Plenum Press, New York.

Fish, B., Marcus, J., Hans, S.L., Auerbach, J.G., Perdue, S. (1992) Infants at risk for schizophrenia: Sequelae of a genetic neurointegrative defect. *Archives of General Psychiatry*, 49, 221–235.

Flor-Henry, P. (1979) Laterality, shifts of cerebral dominance, sinistrality and psychosis. In: *Hemisphere Asymmetries of Function in Psychopathology* (Eds J. Gruzelier, P. Flor-Henry), Elsevier, Amsterdam.

Flor-Henry, P., Yeudall, L.T. (1979) Neuropsychological investigation of schizophrenia and manic-depressive psychosis. In: *Hemisphere Asymmetries of Function in Psychopathology* (Eds J. Gruzelier, P. Flor-Henry), pp. 341–362, Elsevier, Amsterdam.

Franke, P., Maier, W., Hain, C., Klinger, T. (1992) Wisconsin Card Sorting Test: An indicator of vulnerability to schizophrenia? *Schizophrenia Research*, 6, 243–249.

Frith, C.D. (1987) The positive and negative symptoms of schizophrenia reflect impairments in the perception and initiation of action. *Psychological Medicine*, 17, 631–648.

Gamer, E., Gallant, D., Grunebaum, H.U, Cohler, B.J. (1977) Children of psychotic mothers: Performance of 3-year old children on tests of attention. *Archives of General Psychiatry*, 34, 592–597.

Gershon, E.S., Goldin, L.R. (1986) Clinical methods in psychiatric genetics I. Robustness of genetic marker investigative strategies. *Acta Psychiatrica Scandinavica*, 74, 113–118.

Gold, J.M., Randolph, C., Carpenter, C.J., Goldberg, T.E., Weinberger, D.R. (1992) Forms of memory failure in schizophrenia. *Journal of Abnormal Psychology*, 10, 487–494.

Goldberg, E., Seidman, L.J. (1991) Higher cortical functions in normals and in schizophrenia: A selective review. In: *Neuropsychology, Psychophysiology and Information Processing* (Eds S.R. Steinhauer, J.H. Gruzelier, J. Zubin), pp. 553–597, Elsevier, Amsterdam.

Goldberg, T.E., Weinberger, D.R. (1988) Probing prefrontal function in schizophrenia with neuropsychological paradigms. *Schizophrenia Bulletin*, 14, 179–183.

Goldberg, T.E., Weinberger, D.R., Pliskin, N.H., Berman, K.F., Podd, M.H. (1989) Recall memory deficit in schizophrenia: a possible manifestation of prefrontal dysfunction. *Schizophrenia Research*, 2, 251–257.

Goldstein, K.H., Scheerer, M. (1953) Tests of abstract and concrete behaviour. In: *Contributions to Medical Psychology*, Vol. 2 (Ed. A. Weider), Ronald Press, New York.

Goodglass, H., Kaplan, E. (1987) *The Assessment of Aphasia and Related Disturbances*, Lea & Febinger, Philadelphia.

Gottesman, I.I., Shields, J. (1984) *Schizophrenia: The Epigenetic Puzzle*, Cambridge University Press, Cambridge.

Grant, D.A., Berg, E.A. (1948) A behavioural analysis of degree of reinforcement and ease of shifting to new responses in a Weigl-type card sorting problem. *Journal of Experimental Psychology*, 38, 404–411.

Greenwald, D., Harder, D., Fisher, L. (1982) WISC scatter and behavioural competence in high risk children. *Journal of Psychology*, 38, 397–401.

Gruzelier, J.H., Mednick, S., Schulsinger, F. (1979) Lateralized impairments in the WISC profiles of children at risk for psychopathology. In: *Hemisphere Asymmetries of Function in Psychopathology* (Eds J. Gruzelier, P. Flor-Henry), Elsevier, Amsterdam.

Hallet, S., Green, P. (1983) Possible defects in interhemispheric integration in children of schizophrenics. *Journal of Nervous and Mental Disease*, 171, 421–425.

Hallet, S., Quinn, D., Hewitt, J. (1986) Defective interhemispheric integration and anomalous language lateralisation in children at risk for schizophrenia. *Journal of Nervous and Mental Disease*, 174, 418–427.

Harvey, P.D., Winters, K., Weintraub, S., Neale, J.M. (1981) Distractibility in children vulnerable to psychopathology. *Journal of Abnormal Psychology*, 90, 298–304.

Harvey, P.D., Weintraub, S., Neale, J.M. (1982) Speech competence of children vulnerable to psychopathology. *Journal of Abnormal Child Psychology*, 10, 373–388.

Heaton, R.K. (1981) *The Wisconsin Card Sorting Test Manual*, Psychological Assessment Resources, Odessa, FL.

Heaton, R.K., Chelune, G.J., Talley, J., Kay, G.G.,, Curtiss, G. (1993) *Wisconsin Card Sorting Test Manual, Revised and Expanded*, Psychological Assessment Resources, Odessa, FL.

Hoff. A.S., Shukla, S., Aronson, T., Cook, B., Ollo, C., Baruch, S., Jandorf, L., Schwartz, J. (1990) Failure to differentiate bipolar disorder from schizophrenia on measures of neuropsychological functioning. *Schizophrenia Research*, **3**, 253–260.

Hynd, G.W., Obrzut, J.E. (1977) Effects of grade level and sex on the magnitude of the right ear advantage. *Neuropsychologia*, **15**, 689–692.

Kaufman, A.S. (1979) *Intelligent Testing with the WISC-R in Children*, Raven Press, New York.

Keefe, R.S.E., Silverman, J.M., Lees, S.E., Harvey, P.D., Duncan, A.M., Alroy, D., Siever, L.J., Davis, K.L., Mohs, R.C. (1994) Performance of nonpsychotic relatives of schizophrenic patients on cognitive tests. *Psychiatry Research*, **53**, 1–12.

Kennard, K. (1960) Value of equivocal signs in neurological diagnosis. *Neurology*, **10**, 753–764.

Kimura, D. (1961) Cerebral dominance and the perception of verbal stimuli. *Canadian Journal of Psychology*, **15**, 166–171.

Kinney, D.K., Woods, B.T., Yurgelun-Todd, D. (1986) Neurologic abnormalities in schizophrenic patients and their families. II. Neurologic and psychiatric findings in relatives. *Archives of General Psychiatry*, **43**, 665–668.

Koh, S.D. (1978) Remembering of verbal material by schizophrenic young adults. In: *Language and Cognition in Schizophrenia* (Ed. S. Schwartz), pp. 55–99, Erlbaum, Hillsdale, NJ.

Levin, S. (1984) Frontal lobe dysfunctions in schizophrenia II: Impairments of psychological and brain functions. *Journal of Psychiatric Research*, **18**, 57–72.

Levin, H.S., Culhane, K.A., Hartman, J., Evankovich, K., Mattson, A.J., Harward, H., Ringholz, G., Ewings-Cobbs, L., Fletcher, J.M. (1991) Developmental changes in performance on tests of purported frontal lobe functioning. *Developmental Neuropsychology*, **7**, 377–396.

Lezak, M. (1995) *Neuropsychological Assessment* (3rd edn), Oxford University Press, New York.

Liddle, P.F., Morris, D.L. (1991) Schizophrenic syndromes and frontal lobe performance. *British Journal of Psychiatry*, **158**, 340–345.

Lifschitz, M., Kugelmas, S., Karov, C. (1985) Perceptual-motor and memory performance of high-risk children. *Schizophrenia Bulletin*, **11**, 74–84.

Luria, A.R. (1973) *The Working Brain*, Basic Books, New York.

Marcus, J., Auerbach, J., Wilkinson, L., Burack, C. (1984) Infants at risk for schizophrenia: The Jerusalem Infant Development Study. In: *Children at Risk for Schizophrenia* (Eds N. Watt, E. Anthony, L. Wynne, J. Rolf), pp. 444–464, Cambridge University Press, New York.

Marcus, J., Hans, S.L., Nagler, S., Auerbach, J.G., Mirsky, A.F., Aubrey, A. (1987) Review of the NIMH Israeli Kibbutz-City Study and the Jerusalem Infant Developmental Study. *Schizophrenia Bulletin*, **13**, 425–438.

Mednick, S., Schulsinger, F. (1968) Some premorbid characteristics related to breakdown in children with schizophrenic mothers. In: *The Transmission of Schizophrenia* (Eds D. Rosenthal, S. Kety), pp. 267–291, Pergamon Press, Oxford.

Mesulam, M.M. (1986) Frontal cortex and behaviour. *Annals of Neurology*, **19**, 320–325.

Milner, B. (1963) Effects of different brain lesions on card sorting. *Archives of Neurology*, **9**, 90–100.

Mirsky, A.F., Lochhead, S.J., Jones, B.P., Kugelmas, S., Walsh,, Kendler, K.S. (1992) On familial factors in the attentional deficit in schizophrenia: A review and report of two new subject samples. *Journal of Psychiatric Research*, **26**, 383–403.

Mirsky, A.F., Ingraham, L.J., Kugelmas, S. (1995) Neuropsychological assessment of attention and its pathology in the Israeli cohort. *Schizophrenia Bulletin*, **21**, 193–204.

Morice, R. (1990) Cognitive inflexibility and pre-frontal dysfunction in schizophrenia and mania. *British Journal of Psychiatry*, **157**, 50–54.

Morice, R., McNicol, D. (1985) The comprehension and production of complex syntax in schizophrenia. *Cortex*, **21**, 567–580.

Nasrallah, H.A. (1986) Cerebral asymmetries and interhemispheric integration in schizophrenia. In: *Handbook of Schizophrenia, Vol. 1: The Neurology of Schizophrenia* (Eds H.A. Nasrallah, D.R. Weinberger), pp. 157–174, Elsevier, New York.

Neale, J.M., Winters, K.C., Weintraub, S. (1984) Information processing deficits in children at high risk for schizophrenia. In: *Children at Risk for Schizophrenia: A Longitudinal Perspective* (Eds N.F. Watt, E.J. Anthony, L.C. Wynne, J.E. Rolf), pp. 264–279, Cambridge University Press, New York.

Nelson, H. (1976) A modified card sorting test sensitive to frontal lobe deficits. *Cortex*, **12**, 313–324.

Nuechterlein, K.H., Dawson, M.E. (1984) Information processing and attentional functioning in the developmental course of schizophrenic disorders. *Schizophrenia Bulletin*, **10**, 160–203.

Nuechterlein, K.H., Phipps-Yonas, S., Driscoll, R.M., Garmezy, N. (1980) The role of different components of attention to children vulnerable to schizophrenia. In: *Preventive Intervention in Schizophrenia: Are We Ready?* (Ed. M.J. Goldstein), pp. 54–77, US Department of Health and Human Services, Rockville.

Orton, S.T. (1937) Specific reading disability—strephosymbolia. *Journal of the American Medical Association*, **90**, 1095–1099.

Orvaschel, H., Mednick, S.A., Schulsinger, F., Rock, D. (1979) The children on psychiatrically disturbed parents: Differences as a function of the sex of the sick parent. *Archives of General Psychiatry*, **36**, 691–695.

Parnas, J., Mednick, S.A., Schulsinger, F. (1986) *An Interactionist View of Schizophrenia*, presented at the World Psychiatric Association Regional Symposium, Copenhagen.

Phipps-Yonas, S. (1984) Visual and auditory reaction time in children vulnerable to psychopathology. In: *Children at Risk for Schizophrenia: A Longitudinal Perspective* (Eds N. F. Watt, E.J. Anthony, L.C. Wynne, J.E. Rolf), pp. 313–319, Cambridge University Press, New York.

Reitan, R.M. (1979) *Manual for Administration of Neuropsychological Test Batteries for Adults and Children*, R.M. Reitan, Arizona.

Rieder, R.O., Nichols, P.L. (1979) Offspring of schizophrenics III: Hyperactivity and neurological soft signs. *Archives of General Psychiatry*, **36**, 665–674.

Rinaldi, A., Dworkin, R.H., Cornblatt, B.A., Erlenmeyer-Kimling, L. (1991) *Neuromotor Deficits and Positive and Negative Symptoms in Children at Risk for Schizophrenia and Affective Disorder*, presented at the Annual Meeting of the Society for Research in Psychopathology, Cambridge, MA.

Robbins, R.W. (1990) The case for frontostriatal dysfunction in schizophrenia. *Schizophrenia Bulletin*, **16**, 391–402.

Robinson, A.L., Heaton, R.K., Lehman, R.W., Stilson, D.W. (1980) The utility of the Wisconsin Card Sorting Test in detecting and localizing frontal lobe lesions. *Journal of Consulting and Clinical Psychology*, **48**, 605–614.

Rossi, A., De Cataldo, S., Di Michele, V., Manna, V., Ceccoli, S., Stratta, P., Casacchia, M. (1990) Neurological soft signs in schizophrenia. *British Journal of Psychiatry*, **157**, 735–739.

Rutschmann, J., Cornblatt, B.A., Erlenmeyer-Kimling, L. (1980) Auditory recognition memory in adolescents at risk for schizophrenia: Report on a verbal continuous recognition task. *Psychiatry Research*, **3**, 151–161.

Saykin, A.J., Gur, R.C., Gur, R.E., Mozley, P.D., Mozley, L.H., Resnick, S.M., Kester, B., Stafniak, P. (1991) Neuropsychological function in schizophrenia: Selective impairment in memory and learning. *Archives of General Psychiatry*, **8**, 618–624.

Schreiber, H., Stolz-Born, G., Heinrich, H., Kornhuber, H.H., Born, J. (1992) Attention, cognition and motor perseveration in adolescents at genetic risk for schizophrenia and control subjects. *Psychiatry Research*, **44**, 125–140.

Seidman, L.J., Kremen, W.S., Faraone, S.V., Pepple, J.R., Lyons, M.J., Tsuang, M.T. (1992) *Vulnerability Indicators for Schizophrenia: Neuropsychological Profiles of First-degree Relatives*, presented at the Annual Meeting of the New York Neuropsychology Group (joint meeting with the New York Academy of Science, Psychology Section), New York.

Semel, E., Wiig, E.H. (1980) *Clinical Evaluation of Language Functions*, Merril, Columbus, OH.

Shenton, M.E., Kikinis, R., Jolesz, F.A., Pollack, S.D., LeMay, M., Wible, C.G., Hokama, H., Martin, J., Metcalf, D., Coleman, M., McCarley, R.W. (1992) Abnormalities of the left temporal lobe and thought disorder in schizophrenia. *New England Journal of Medicine*, **327**, 614–612.

Silverton, L., Harrington, M.,, Mednick, S. (1988) Motor impairment and antisocial behaviour in adolescent males at high risk for schizophrenia. *Journal of Abnormal Psychology*, **16**, 177–186.

Sohlberg, S.C. (1985) Personality and neuropsychological performance of high-risk children. *Schizophrenia Bulletin*, **11**, 48–60.

Spring, B.J., Zubin, J. (1978) Attention and information processing as indicators of vulnerability to schizophrenic episodes. *Journal of Psychiatric Research*, **14**, 289–302.

Squire, L.R. (1982) The neuropsychology of human memory. *Annual Review of Neuroscience*, **5**, 241–273.

Squire, L.R. (1987) *Memory and the Brain*, Oxford University Press, New York.

Steinhauer, S.R., Zubin, J., Condray, R., Shaw, D.B., Peters, J.L., van Kammen, D.P. (1991) Electrophysiological and behavioural signs of attentional disturbance in schizophrenics and their siblings. In: *Advances in Neuropsychiatry & Psychopharmacology, Vol. I: Schizophrenia Research* (Eds C. Tamminga, S.C. Schulz), pp. 169–178, Raven Press, New York.

Stroop, J.R. (1935) Studies of interference in serial verbal reaction. *Journal of Experimental Psychology*, **18**, 643–662.

Stuss, D.T., Benson, D.F. (1986) *The Frontal Lobes*, Wiley, New York.

Walker, C.M., Bourne, I.C. (1961) The identification of concepts as a function of amounts of relevant and irrelevant information. *American Journal of Psychology*, **16**, 410–417.

Walker, E., Shaye, J. (1982) A predictor of neuromotor and attentional abnormalities in schizophrenia. *Archives of General Psychiatry*, **39**, 1153–1156.

Watt, N.F., Anthony, E.J., Wynne, L.C., Rolf, J.E. (Eds) (1984) *Children at Risk for Schizophrenia: A Longitudinal Perspective*, Cambridge University Press, New York.

Wechsler, D. (1974) *The Wechsler Intelligence Scale for Children—Revised*, Psychological Corporation, New York.

Weinberger, D.R., Berman, K.F., Zec, R.F. (1986) Physiological dysfunction of dorsolateral prefrontal cortex in schizophrenia I. Regional cerebral blood flow evidence. *Archives of General Psychiatry*, **43**, 114–124.

Weintraub, S. (1987) Risk factors in schizophrenia: The Stony Brook High-Risk Project. *Schizophrenia Bulletin*, **13**, 439–450.

Weintraub, S., Neale, J. (1984) The Stony Brook High Risk Project. In: *Children at Risk for Schizophrenia: A Longitudinal Perspective* (Eds F. Watt, E. Anthony, L. Wynne, J. Rolf), pp. 212–226, Cambridge University Press, New York.

Welsh, M., Pennington, B., Grozier, D. (1991) A normative developmental study of executive function: A window or prefrontal function in children. *Developmental Neuropsychology*, **7**, 131–149.

Winters, K.C., Stone, A.A., Weintraub, S., Neale, J.M. (1981) Cognitive and attentional deficits in children vulnerable to psychopathology. *Journal of Abnormal Child Psychology*, **9**, 435–453.

Worland, J., Hesselbrock, V. (1980) The intelligence of children and their parents with schizophrenia and affective illness. *Journal of Child Psychology and Psychiatry*, **21**, 191–201.

Worland, J., Lander, H., Hesselbrock, V. (1979) Psychological evaluation of clinical disturbance in children at risk for psychopathology. *Journal of Abnormal Psychology*, **88**, 13–26.

Worland, J., Edenhart-Pepe, R., Weeks, D., Konen, P.M. (1984) Cognitive evaluation of children at risk: IQ, differentiation, and egocentricity. In: *Children at Risk for Schizophrenia: A Longitudinal Perspective* (Eds N.F. Watt, E.J. Anthony, L.C. Wynne, J.E. Rolf), pp. 149–159, Cambridge University Press, New York.

Wynne, L.C., Cole, R.E., Perkins, P. (1987) University of Rochester Child and Family Study: Risk research in process. *Schizophrenia Bulletin*, **13**, 463–484.

Part C

COGNITIVE IMPAIRMENTS IN SCHIZOPHRENIA AND THEIR CORRELATES

10

The Pathogenesis of Thought Disorder

JOHN McGRATH

The potential payoff of success in understanding schizophrenic thought disorder is great. Schizophrenia is the most massive unsolved puzzle in the whole field of psychopathology, and thought disorder is schizophrenia's most prominent symptom. A true understanding of the nature of thought disorder might illuminate the nature of schizophrenia itself.

(Chapman & Chapman, 1973, p. ix)

INTRODUCTION

Schizophrenia is almost certainly an aetiologically heterogeneous group of disorders that just happen to share certain neurological symptoms. In contrast to neurodevelopmental syndromes such as cerebral palsy that have prominent motor and sensory impairments, schizophrenia is a syndrome that primarily affects higher level (i.e. integrative) cognitive, perceptual, affective and language functions. The measurement of these functions is considerably more challenging than the assessment of motor strength and reflexes. Not only are the symptoms of schizophrenia more subtle, they can emerge and fade across the lifespan in parallel with the development and involution of the central nervous system. As well, the symptoms of schizophrenia fluctuate within and between acute episodes.

Another level of complexity is introduced by the fact that the symptoms that characterise schizophrenia can also be found in a range of other disorders. When diagnostic boundaries result in heterogeneity at the symptom level, then grouping data by diagnosis may be misleading. Faced with such challenges, one solution is to restrict the research focus to a particular symptom. By examining a symptom in diverse diagnostic groups, it may be possible to delineate a generic pathogenesis for the symptom. Presumably, at some level, the cognitive mechanisms involved in the genesis of a symptom are shared across diagnostic boundaries. For these

Schizophrenia: A Neuropsychological Perspective. Edited by C. Pantelis, H.E. Nelson and T.R.E. Barnes
© 1996 John Wiley & Sons Ltd

reasons, there is a strong case to focus research at the level of the symptom rather than the level of the syndrome (Neale et al, 1985; Persons, 1986; Costello, 1992).

The aim of this chapter is to examine one symptom, thought disorder. Data from studies that have examined this symptom in schizophrenia, mania and in healthy controls are presented. A range of cognitive, neuropsychological and linguistic measures have been correlated with thought disorder in an attempt to unravel factors that may be involved in the pathogenesis of this interesting symptom. Finally, one model of pathogenesis of thought disorder will be presented that incorporates results from past experimental and neuropsychological research.

DEFINITIONS

The term "thought disorder" has accumulated many layers of meaning over the decades. Even from the beginning, this term was used to describe a range of features that were really epiphenomena of "thought". One can never be sure what another person is really thinking, although communication (oral, written, non-verbal) provides the closest approximation to knowing another's thoughts. Andreasen (1982a) points out that thought disorder describes aspects of language, thought and communication. Because the term thought disorder is so imprecise, the task of collating literature on this topic requires a degree of caution.

For the purposes of this chapter, the term thought disorder will be used interchangeably with the term *formal thought disorder*. Formal thought disorder refers to a disturbance in the form of thought. It describes the manner in which thoughts, as reflected in speech, are linked. The judgement that someone is thought disordered rests on a certain level and quality of confusion induced by the speaker in the mind of the listener. Formal thought disorder comprises a heterogeneous group of disturbances of thought, language and communication, which is distinct from disorders in the content of thought, such as delusions. It is crucial to distinguish these two concepts when attempting to investigate the pathogenesis of thought disorder (Simpson & Davis, 1985).

Broader definitions of thought disorder can encompass performance on tasks such as object sorting, word association and so called tests of abstract thinking. These definitions have focused predominantly on thinking and cognition rather than language and communication. Allusive thinking, described by McConaghy (1960, 1961, 1989) is an example of research based on a broad definition of thought disorder. This research has provided measures that correlate with evoked response potentials (Ward et al, 1992) and has identified conceptual loosening in the unaffected relatives of patients with schizophrenia (Romney, 1990). Research based on the broader definitions of thought disorder will not be further addressed in this chapter.

Several scales have been devised that allow thought disorder to be reliably measured (Marengo et al, 1986; Johnston & Holzman, 1986; Andreasen, 1986). Each scale brings different subtleties to the field of study. The most widely used instrument to measure thought disorder is Andreasen's Scale for the Assessment of Thought, Language and Communication (TLC) (Andreasen, 1979a, 1979b,

1986). This instrument has 20 items which describe features such as *derailment*, *tangentiality*, *loss of goal*, *perseveration*, and *poverty of speech*. Definitions, anchor points and examples are provided. Many of the items included in this instrument have achieved widespread use in the research community via other instruments developed by the same author such as the Scale for the Assessment of Negative Symptoms (SANS) (Andreasen, 1982b) and the Scale for the Assessment of Positive Symptoms (SAPS) (Andreasen, 1982c). As a result of publication of these scales, a degree of consistency has been introduced into the field of thought disorder research. For the remainder of the chapter, references to TLC items are italicised (e.g. *derailment*).

THOUGHT DISORDER AND ISSUES OF RESEARCH DESIGN

Because of the influential work of Bleuler and Kraepelin, thought disorder and schizophrenia became closely linked. Bleuler included associative disturbances among his list of fundamental symptoms and postulated that thought disorder resulted because of "disconnecting of associative threads" (Bleuler, 1911, p. 21). However, not all patients with schizophrenia have thought disorder and thought disorder is found in a range of psychiatric conditions apart from schizophrenia. For example, patients with mania have high levels of thought disorder (Andreasen, 1979b; Harvey et al, 1984; Holzman et al, 1986; Jampala et al, 1989). Behaviour rated as "mild" on TLC items such as *derailment, loss of goal, circumstantiality*, and *pressure of speech* can be found in people without a major psychiatric disorder (Andreasen & Grove, 1986).

Another key feature of thought disorder is that people with thought disorder do not have this symptom continuously. Levels of thought disorder can vary as a result of many factors such as the structure of the dialogue, the complexity of the topic, the concentration of the speaker and the amount of background noise and distraction. This symptom can vary markedly both within an episode of illness and between episodes (Harvey et al, 1984; Harrow et al, 1986; Earle-Boyer et al, 1986; Docherty et al, 1988). These two cardinal features of thought disorder warrant repeating. Thought disorder is not specific to one diagnosis and can fluctuate in severity over time within an individual. Both of these features must be taken into account when designing research investigating thought disorder.

THE PATHOGENESIS OF THOUGHT DISORDER: A REVIEW OF SELECTED LITERATURE

Several commentators have noted that the large quantity of thought disorder research to date has not been balanced by a similar quantity of productive theories or models. Blaney (1978), wondering why we had so few answers about thought disorder, observed that "a huge but relatively fruitless literature exits" (p. 101). Rochester noted the same problem in her review (1980) and commented that the various theories of thought disorder had been unsuccessful "because they have not led to theories which are both testable and relevant to the confusing productions of the schizophrenic speaker" (p. 18). Despite the above comments not all of the research has been fruitless. This section will not attempt to present all of the experimental literature on the topic (see reviews by: Reed, 1970; Maher, 1972; Schwartz, 1978; Harvey & Neale, 1983; Marengo & Harrow, 1988; Chaika, 1990; Neale & Oltmanns, 1980; Chapman & Chapman, 1973; Cozolino, 1983; Morice, 1986a). The aim of the following section is to review several of the more influential theoretical models that have been proposed to explain thought disorder.

Behavioural psychology influenced the early word-level thought disorder research. From this perspective, words were linked in complex webs of strong and weak associations. Research involved behaviour that could be observed (in this case speech output) and internal events such as thoughts and feelings were outside the field of inquiry. This research was influenced by a key feature of the early descriptions of schizophrenia; that patients had problems with associations of ideas and of words (Bleuler, 1911). The patterns of communication in thought disorder were considered to be due to the loosening of associations between ideas and between words. Speech output was less goal driven because of these deviant associations. Studies examined the word associations of patients with schizophrenia. These were generally thought to be bizarre in comparison to the word associations of well controls. Whether on not the patients had clinical thought disorder was considered irrelevant. The area has been critically reviewed by Schwartz (1982) who details several major problems in research methodology and contends that the best-controlled studies show no differences in word association between patients and controls.

Chapman and colleagues (Chapman et al, 1964) proposed that patients had a tendency to choose an association (a response bias) that is governed by the individual word rather than the overall context. With particular attention to issues of research design, this group found that patients with schizophrenia were more prone to biases towards strong responses. It was proposed that these response biases reduced communication efficiency as the speaker would be diverted by non-topic relevant "strong" word associations. Salzinger's "Immediacy Hypothesis", which details how verbal behaviour could be captured by stimuli in the immediate environment, drew attention to the importance of distractibility and its impact on efficient communication (Salzinger et al, 1978).

Cohen and colleagues (1974) examined the ability of the speaker to take into account the needs of the listener by using words as stimuli. The "referent communication" task requires the subject to provide clues to a listener in order to aid the listener to make a choice between two stimuli (the referents). To do well on this task the subject has to assess the stimuli and assess possible clues that will aid the listener. In essence, the speaker must make an assessment of what will be of most assistance to the listener and has to resist the internal associations triggered by the clues. The role of speaker and listener can be swapped. Cohen et al (1974) found that patients with schizophrenia were adequate listeners (clue receivers) but poor speakers (clue givers). Cohen (1976) refined his theory with the "perseverative speaker model" in which he suggests that the speaker is editing output and attempting to reject inappropriate material. However, the speaker is unable to access alternate, appropriate material and resampling of the rejected material results in perseveration. The "disattention deficit" theory described by Cromwell & Dockecki (1968) has features in common with Cohen's theory.

All of the above work relies essentially on the word as the unit of observation. The problems in attempting to understand thought disorder from analyses performed at the word level have been well described by Schwartz (1982). The total amount of information conveyed within a sentence or within a discourse far exceeds the sum of the information conveyed by the constituent words. When the problem of thought disorder revolves around efficiency of communication, the choice of category for investigation should be at the appropriate level. Words and their associations are a convenient unit for investigation but do not reflect the complexity of thought disorder.

Recent research has been influenced by advances in our understanding of attention and information processing, linguistics, aphasiology and neuro-psychology. The role of attention has always been central to our understanding of schizophrenia (Kraepelin, 1913; Bleuler, 1911). Subjective reports highlight the central role of this variable in the phenomenology of schizophrenia and several theories implicating attention and information processing in the pathogenesis of thought disorder have been proposed (McGhie & Chapman, 1961; Chapman, 1966; Freedman & Chapman, 1973).

This field is reviewed by Maruff and Currie (chapter 6) but the early work of Broadbent (1958, 1971) should be mentioned briefly. Broadbent proposed a model that highlighted two forms of selective attention. He considered that information was first filtered at a perceptual level and was then "pigeonholed". This latter term referred to the adoption of a response set or a predisposition to respond to certain stimuli. Filtering allows a degree of processing of the stimuli while "pigeonholing" determines the likelihood of responses to selected stimuli. After critically reviewing past research, Schwartz (1982) proposed that the features of thought disorder, including increased distractibility, bias towards strong meanings and sensitivity to a limited quantity of verbal context, can be economically explained by a defect in "pigeonholing".

More recently, Harvey and colleagues postulated that capacity limited mechanisms of attention (mediated by arousal) may be linked to positive thought disorder. Using tasks of auditory and visual distraction and of short-term memory, this model has received consistent support (Harvey, 1983; Harvey & Neale, 1983; Harvey et al, 1984; Harvey, 1985; Neale et al, 1985; Earle-Boyer et al, 1986; Harvey et al, 1986; Harvey & Brault, 1986; Harvey et al, 1990; Hotchkiss & Harvey, 1990; Walker & Harvey, 1986; Docherty et al, 1988; Harvey et al, 1988; Wielgus & Harvey, 1988; Harvey & Neale, 1989; Harvey & Pedley, 1989; Harvey & Serper, 1990; Moskowitz et al, 1991). Aspects of these studies will be described below.

In a further elaboration of the model, Harvey and colleagues have proposed that thought disorder involved confusion in the mind of the speaker between what has been said (spoken out loud) and what has been thought (not spoken out loud). This group used a task in which the subject is shown two lists of words, one to be spoken out loud, the other to read only. When presented with words from one of the two lists the thought-disordered speaker was less capable of correctly remembering whether the word was actually spoken or only read. It is proposed that the end result of such a deficit might be discourse that cannot be accurately monitored and edited. Research to date has supported this model (Harvey, 1985; Matthysse, 1987; Harvey et al, 1990). The importance of error monitoring and error utilisation is discussed further below.

Advances in linguistics have informed recent thought disorder research. Hoffman & Sledge (1984) described several levels of organisation from the basic articulation of phonemes to the highest level of concept formation. They suggest that patients with thought disorder are impaired on the level that is required for the planning and editing of discourse. Efficient discourse relies on an orderly sequence of propositions. In order to test this model Hoffman and colleagues (Hoffman et al, 1982, 1986; Hoffman, 1986) deconstructed discourse into constituent elements. Results from these studies suggested that thought disorder in schizophrenia was a result of the inability to generate coherent patterns of discourse, while that observed in mania resulted from rapid shifts from one coherent pattern to another.

The work of Morice has linked the study of linguistics with that of cognitive psychology, neuropsychology and aphasiology. Morice and co-workers have demonstrated that patients with schizophrenia use less complex sentences (Morice & Ingram, 1982, 1983; Morice & McNicol, 1985; Morice & McNicol, 1986). The construction of complex sentences requires the speaker to plan out the linear sequence of several clauses within the overall discourse structure. A model was proposed that involved dysfunction of the prefrontal cortex leading to impaired executive planning. Thought disorder was postulated to be one consequence of this impaired executive planning (Morice, 1986b). However, this innovative work relates to the performance of the patient groups as a whole and does not provide details of sentence complexity for thought-disordered versus non-thought-disordered patients. If the finding of reduced sentence complexity had been associated with those patients with *poverty of speech* or *derailment,* for example, then more refined interpretations could have been offered.

Disillusioned with existing frameworks, Andreasen developed a reliable instrument (Scale for the Assessment of Thought, Language and Communication; TLC) to measure thought disorder (1979a, 1979b). The work led on to research involving comprehension in schizophrenia (Groves & Andreasen, 1985), the construction of discourse (Hoffman et al, 1986) (detailed above) and, more recently, studies examining the underlying neurological and anatomical correlates of schizophrenia (Andreasen et al, 1985; Yates et al, 1990; Andreasen et al, 1990). This research has suggested that patients with thought disorder are inefficient at planning complex discourse and that this may be related to dysfunction of the frontal, subcortical or left hemisphere language systems (Andreasen et al, 1985).

It should be noted that the various models of thought disorder need not be mutually exclusive. Language and communication are exceedingly complex systems and thought disorder is one of the most perplexing disturbances of these systems. It would be simplistic to think that one model could encompass all the features of thought disorder. Disparate philosophies, methodologies and results need not discredit competing research. Instead they can serve to highlight the complexity of the area.

CORTICAL LESIONS AND THOUGHT DISORDER

In this section the links between cortical lesions and thought disorder are briefly examined, as this will be relevant to a subsequent model of the pathogenesis of thought disorder. It is of interest to read the occasional case reports in the aphasiology literature describing the "language of confusion" (Halpern et al, 1973; Drummond, 1986) which phenotypically resemble thought disorder (Chaika, 1974). It is apparent that the various disciplines of psychiatry, neurology and aphasiology have developed lexical conventions that can improve intra-discipline communication at the expense of inter-discipline communication. Cross-fertilisation between these disciplines would be of benefit as language disturbance associated with cortical lesions may provide clues to the pathogenesis of thought disorder. For example, Daniels et al (1988) examined patients with schizophrenia and mania and compared them with a group of patients with various types of right cortical damage. All three groups showed similar total scores on the Thought Disorder Index (Johnston & Holzman, 1986); however, differences on subscores were found between the groups which suggested differences in the quality of disturbance.

Transcribed speech samples from patients with schizophrenia and from a heterogeneous group of patients with aphasia were reviewed by Faber et al (1983). They concluded that, while some features were shared, the schizophrenic group did not approximate any of the classic aphasia syndromes. Gerson et al (1977) compared the language of a group of patients with schizophrenia to a heterogeneous group of neurological patients with posterior aphasia. The language of patients with schizophrenia was characterised by more bizarre themes in response to open-ended questions (e.g. "Tell me about your favourite hobby"), while the posterior aphasia group had shorter responses, were more aware of communication problems and made more substitution errors.

Kaczmarek (1984) compared the utterances of patients with various cortical lesions to those of normal controls. He found that the left dorsolateral frontal region was crucial in the planning and sequential organisation of linguistic information. Those subjects with prefrontal damage had perseveration of speech and had difficulty maintaining set due to distractibility. A later study (Kaczmarek, 1987), which specifically investigated the utterances of patients with prefrontal lesions, found that patients with lesions of the dorsolateral prefrontal cortex perseverated, used simple sentences (similar to the findings of Morice and colleagues in schizophrenia) and had poverty of speech. The group of patients with left orbitofrontal lesions digressed frequently and did not monitor for errors.

Novoa & Ardila (1987) also investigated language in patients with prefrontal lesions. When compared to a group of age and education matched controls they found that the utterances of the patient group were characterised by higher rates of perseveration, free association of ideas, apathy and adynamia. They concluded that while language was formally preserved in patients with prefrontal lesions, functions that require complex or conceptual verbal activities were impaired.

Based on their own cases and the aphasiology literature, Alexander et al (1989) provided a review of the role of the prefrontal region in language. They highlighted the role of the left cingulate and supplementary motor areas in activating speech. Lesions in these regions lead to reduced verbal output. They suggested that left anterior frontal regions are involved in the organisation and overall control of language. The non-dominant prefrontal region also has a crucial role in the organisation of language, particularly in a social context. The authors describe the clinical manifestations of right frontal communication disorders as including "tangentiality, unanticipated changes of topic, socially inappropriate discourse and humour and, in severe cases, frankly confabulatory or delusional content in a clear sensorium" (p. 684).

It can be seen from the available literature that patients with known lesions of prefrontal systems display a range of language and communication problems similar to that observed in patients with thought disorder. Morice (1986a) noted the links between the prefrontal cortex and thought disorder in a seminal review that examined converging data from neuroimaging, linguistics and psychology. He presented evidence to suggest that the prefrontal systems were involved in the pathogenesis of certain types of thought disorder.

This more recent research echoes the early writings of Karl Kleist (1930/1987):

> [Thought disorder] can also be seen with damage to the left forebrain and is characterised by a lack of productivity of thought and by an incapacity to carry through a chain of thought. Such patients show poverty of thought and are incapable of producing coherent thoughts from single ideas or perceptions . . . The "thought formulae" of ordinary thinking operations seems to have disappeared. (p. 77)

If the classic neuropsychological features associated with prefrontal system dysfunction are applied to language then one would predict, *a priori*, communication characterised by the inability to establish, maintain and change sets, an inability to handle the planning of sequential behaviour and an inability to monitor and utilise errors (McGrath, 1991).

CORRELATES OF THOUGHT DISORDER: COGNITIVE, LINGUISTIC AND NEUROPSYCHOLOGICAL MEASURES

In this section the performance of patients with and without thought disorder on tests that measure behaviours relevant to the prefrontal system are examined. Performance on various measures of information processing and linguistics are also reviewed.

One of the defining characteristics of late twentieth-century schizophrenia research has been the subgrouping of patients according to positive, negative and mixed symptomatology clusters. Positive symptoms include hallucinations, delusions and types of formal thought disorder such as *tangentiality, derailment, loss of goal, distractible speech* and *incoherence*. Negative symptoms include blunted affect, lack of motivation, poor hygiene and *poverty of speech*. Unfortunately, the allocation of certain symptoms to either positive or negative is not always straightforward. For example, *poverty of content of thought* has been included as a type of negative thought disorder by some researchers (Harvey et al, 1988), despite the fact that it tends to cluster with positive symptoms (Liddle, 1987a, 1987b; Liddle & Morris, 1991; Harvey & Serper, 1990; Pogue-Geile & Harrow, 1984; Harvey et al, 1992; Peralta et al, 1992; Minas et al, 1992). Attentional impairment is included in the Schedule for the Assessment of Negative Symptoms (SANS) (Andreasen, 1982b), while some would argue that a certain type of attentional impairment is involved in the pathogenesis of positive thought disorder (Green & Walker, 1986).

Allen (1983, 1984) tested the hypothesis that positive symptoms reflect loss of cognitive control, while negative symptoms reflect restriction of cognitive processing. Using various methods of linguistic analysis, Allen has systematically explored language production in patients with schizophrenia. Using a picture description task to elicit speech samples, Allen (1984) measured a range of variables including the type–token ratio (see below), a measure of speech disruption and measures pertaining to "ideas" in speech. The finding that both positive and negative groups displayed fewer and shorter "ideas" and had lower speech variability, prompted Allen to reject the hypothesis being examined. In a follow-up paper Allen & Allen (1985) extended the research by analysing the cohesion between ideas. The results of this study suggested that within and between idea organisation did not differentiate positive or negative schizophrenia from normal controls. However, the group with positive syndrome schizophrenia failed to plan out and connect ideas in the discourse. This failure results in confusion for the listener, leading to the listener labelling the speaker "thought disordered".

Thomas et al (1987) examined syntax in schizophrenia by re-analysing earlier data with respect to positive versus negative symptoms. Those with positive symptoms were reported as having more serious errors of syntax and semantics. Green & Walker (1985, 1986) examined a range of variables in positive and negative symptom schizophrenia. Both studies used a schizophrenic group (subdivided into positive, negative and mixed symptomatology), a manic group and a normal control group. Using a range of tasks drawn from neuropsychology, Green and Walker (1985) commented that positive symptoms, which included positive thought disorder, were associated with poor verbal memory performance. The same authors tested this further by using a digit span task with and without distraction (Green & Walker, 1986). The positive symptom patients with schizophrenia showed significant deficits on the digit span test when compared with normals. The distraction condition worsened performance only in the group with positive symptoms. These results support the link between positive symptoms (including positive thought disorder) and increased distractibility. In a replication study, Walker & Harvey (1986) found an association between distractibility and thought disorder in both thought-disordered patients with schizophrenia and mania. However, these studies did not separate thought disorder from other positive symptoms.

In recent years a three-syndrome concept has been detailed by Liddle and co-workers (Liddle, 1987a, 1987b; Liddle & Barnes, 1990; Liddle & Morris, 1991; see also Liddle, chapter 15). Liddle and Morris (1991) examined these syndromes with respect to tests sensitive to prefrontal lobe function. The Disorganisation syndrome, consisting of inappropriate affect, poverty of content of speech and positive thought disorder, was associated with impairment of the ability to inhibit inappropriate responses. These findings support an association between impaired set maintenance and positive thought disorder. The Psychomotor Poverty syndrome, which includes blunting of affect, poverty of speech and decreased spontaneous movement, was associated with slowness in mental activity and the inability to generate set as measured on a verbal fluency task.

Harvey et al (1988) reported an association between increased thought disorder and increased distractibility in both schizophrenia and mania. In a later study of schizophrenia only, Harvey & Pedley (1989) used auditory and visual tasks with and without distraction conditions. A further refinement was made by including medicated and unmedicated patients. Positive thought disorder predicted greater auditory distraction regardless of medication status. Oltmanns et al (1978) also reported an association between greater distractibility and the presence of positive thought disorder using a digit span task with and without distraction. Wielgus & Harvey (1988) reported a study using a dichotic listening task with and without shadowing. An association between increased positive thought disorder and inefficient performance on the shadowing task was found. The authors proposed that the monitoring process is vulnerable to overload, such that the system breaks down if too much information competes for the limited attentional capacity. The speaker's discourse plan becomes confused leading to inefficient, thought-disordered output.

The links between distraction and thought disorder have been examined from another perspective. Hotchkiss & Harvey (1990) recorded speech samples in the presence and absence of distracting information. Reference failures (poorly connected clauses and sentences) were prominent in the schizophrenic group during the distraction condition. In a follow-up study, Moskowitz et al (1991) examined the links between medication and vulnerability to distraction-induced reference failure. The unmedicated schizophrenic group displayed a substantial increase in reference failures during distraction. In their investigation of aspects of verbal memory, Harvey & Brault (1986) found that thought disorder was associated with impaired recall performance, while registration was less affected.

Manschreck and his group (Manschreck et al, 1979, 1981, 1985, 1988) have also specifically looked for associations between thought disorder and performance on a variety of tests. Measures of thought disorder generated from the Schedule for Affective Disorders and Schizophrenia (SADS) (Spitzer et al, 1978) were used to divide their patients with schizophrenia into "positive thought disorder present" and "positive thought disorder absent" groups. The measures were for positive thought disorder and included features of understandability, derailment, logic, poverty of information conveyed and neologisms. Using this approach several interesting associations emerged. It was found that "type–token ratios", which are an objective measure of the variability of word usage calculated by dividing the total word count by the number of different words used, and measures of phrase repetition could differentiate the two groups (Manschreck et al, 1981; Manschreck et al, 1985). The Cloze analysis, which is a semi-objective measure of predictability that assesses the ability of a "rater" to predict every fourth or fifth word in a transcript of a subject's speech, could also differentiate thought-disordered patients with schizophrenia from those without thought disorder (Manschreck et al, 1979).

Two other interesting findings also emerged from this group's research. One study found an association between scores on the type–token ratio and disruptions in motor behaviour (Manschreck et al, 1981). The authors suggested that attentional deficits may underpin both speech and movement disorders. In another study, using a semantic priming paradigm, Manschreck et al (1988) demonstrated significantly greater facilitation in recognition speed with semantic primes in the thought-disordered patients with schizophrenia. The notion of an uninhibited "spreading activation" of semantic networks was introduced to explain this finding, with attentional factors once again implicated in the dysfunction.

Persons & Baron (1985) found a significant correlation between poor performance on a Stroop-like test of attention and increased positive thought disorder. This result supports the theory that impaired ability to maintain set in the face of distraction is associated with positive thought disorder.

Barr et al (1989) used a confrontation naming task to assess perseveration and its possible role in thought disorder. They found that perseverative errors accounted for 20% of the total errors on this task and suggest that this dysfunction is due to faulty monitoring of language output by the prefrontal systems. The ability to change sets, which underlies perseveration, may also play a role in the pathogenesis of thought disorder.

SET ABILITY, ERROR MONITORING, ERROR UTILISATION AND THOUGHT DISORDER

In order to be an efficient communicator the speaker must be able to establish set to guide the topic focus, must be able to maintain this set in the face of external or internal distractions and must be able to change set at the appropriate juncture. Patients with thought disorder display verbal behaviour congruent with disturbances of the three central tenets of set ability. First, inability to establish communication results in *poverty of speech*. Second, inability to maintain set impairs the ability to hold a focus on a topic, resulting in *tangentiality*, *derailment*, *loss of goal* and *distractible speech*. Third, the inability to change set results in *perseveration*.

However, impaired set ability is not sufficient to explain thought disorder, as evidenced by the many efficient communicators who do poorly on tests sensitive to set ability. For example, most patients with frontal lobe lesions do not have impaired communication. Other factors must also be relevant. Apart from the ability to establish, maintain and change sets, the production of efficient communication requires error monitoring and error utilisation. An internal process of monitoring speech output for errors is required, followed by active monitoring of the needs of the listener for apparent confusion and evidence of communication failures. An efficient speaker will utilise errors and dynamically reprogram speech output in order to improve communication. In other words, the speaker must monitor and correct errors in order to meet the needs of the listener.

McGrath (1991) has proposed that thought disorder is related to impaired executive functioning. It was proposed that impaired set ability and impaired error utilisation and monitoring are the crucial elements in the pathogenesis of thought disorder. Also, it was suggested that dysfunction of the cortical–subcortical loops that project to the prefrontal cortex may be involved in thought disorder. In the following section the strands of evidence that support this theory are discussed.

THE PATHOGENESIS OF POVERTY OF SPEECH

It is proposed that the impaired ability to establish a set underlies negative thought disorder. Patients with poverty of speech do poorly on verbal fluency tasks which, *inter alia*, assess the ability to establish set (Liddle, 1987a). Patients with known lesions of the dorsolateral prefrontal cortex have poverty of speech (Walsh, 1985; Kaczmarek, 1987; Alexander et al, 1989). This finding coincides with the body of evidence that points to decreased metabolism over this region in patients with schizophrenia (Weinberger et al, 1986; Weinberger & Berman, 1988; Weinberger, 1988).

Studies utilising PET scans in well control subjects provide insights into the neural mechanisms of normal mental phenomena. Subjects required to self-generate words, as opposed to merely repeating given words, have increased metabolism over the dorsolateral prefrontal cortex (Sheremata et al, 1985; Parks et al, 1988; Warkentin et al, 1991; Damasio & Damasio, 1992; Petersen et al, 1988). For example, Frith et al (1991) used regional cerebral blood flow in well controls to compare the different patterns of blood flow between two experimental conditions. The subjects were first required to repeat words out loud that had been given to them by the examiner and then to self-generate new words to be spoken out loud. The greatest difference in cerebral blood flow between the two conditions was recorded over the left dorsolateral prefrontal cortex, with increased metabolism observed when subjects had to generate words themselves. The ability to self-generate words taps the more general ability to establish set. In summary, impaired ability to establish set, perhaps secondary to dysfunction of the prefrontal systems, may underlie *poverty of speech*.

THE PATHOGENESIS OF *TANGENTIALITY, DERAILMENT, LOSS OF GOAL* AND *DISTRACTIBLE SPEECH*

It is proposed that the impaired ability to maintain a set underlies many aspects of positive thought disorder. Four TLC items, namely *tangentiality, derailment, loss of goal* and *distractible speech*, measure features related to the ability to maintain set in communication. The above review of the literature demonstrates a relatively consistent association between positive thought disorder and impaired set maintenance as demonstrated by impaired ability to inhibit inappropriate responses (Liddle & Morris, 1991) and increased distractibility (Harvey et al, 1988; Oltmanns et al, 1978; Wielgus & Harvey, 1988; Hotchkiss & Harvey, 1990; Moskowitz et al, 1991; Persons & Baron, 1985).

The neural mechanisms that are associated with the ability to maintain set have been explored with functional neuroimaging. Pardo et al (1990) used PET scans to determine the areas of increased metabolism in well controls performing a Stroop task. This task requires the subject to maintain set (e.g. name the colour of the ink used to print a word) in the face of strong, competing stimuli (e.g. reading the word "red" instead of naming the colour blue when the word RED is printed in blue ink). The competing tendency to report the word rather than the colour of the ink requires the subject to inhibit the distracting influence in order to maintain set. In brief, Pardo's group compared simple and demanding elements of the Stroop task and reported that increased metabolism in the right cingulate area occurred during the demanding element of the task that requires set maintenance.

Liddle et al (1992) reported that, in patients with schizophrenia who had the disorganisation syndrome, which includes positive thought disorder, increased cerebral blood flow was found in the right anterior cingulate cortex. There was also a decrease in regional cerebral blood flow in the right ventral prefrontal cortex extending back to the insula and a decrease in blood flow to both parietal cortices.

Based on the evidence from these PET findings and the evidence for an association between performance on the Stroop test and the presence of positive thought disorder, it is proposed that dysfunction of the right anterior cingulate region and its associated prefrontal and parietal systems may be related to the pathogenesis of *tangentiality*, *derailment*, *loss of goal* and *distractible speech*.

THE PATHOGENESIS OF PERSEVERATION

It is proposed that the impaired ability to change a set underlies *perseveration*. Little data are available on the correlates between the ability to change set and functional neuroimaging in well controls. However, using regional cerebral blood flow studies, Weinberger et al (1986) reported a significant negative correlation between percent perseverative error and prefrontal blood flow.

ERROR MONITORING, ERROR UTILISATION AND THE NEEDS OF THE LISTENER

Errors in speech production are common (Deese, 1978). If a topic is novel or complex, or if the speaker is fatigued, anxious, or cognitively impaired, then the error rate can rise. However, the efficient speaker copes with a modest increase in the error rate by actively monitoring output, identifying errors in discourse and correcting output. Error monitoring can include issues to do with the form of speech such as false starts, faulty word selection, syntactical errors and topic shifts without adequate linkage or warning to the listener. The correction of identified errors (error utilisation) can occur between planning and execution (internal monitoring), as well as during or after execution (external monitoring). There is an important secondary level of error monitoring that involves the speaker taking into account the needs of the listener; for example, does the listener have sufficient background knowledge to follow the discourse development; is the listener confused; do segments of discourse need to be repeated with improvements, etc.

Impairments of set ability may be necessary but not sufficient "causes" of positive thought disorder. The loss of error monitoring and/or error utilisation may be the additional elements that precipitate positive thought disorder. In other words, impairment of both set ability and error correction may be necessary and sufficient steps in the pathogenesis of thought disorder. Future research would need to examine if these variables are truly independent or if they form a continuum of prefrontal system impairment.

Such a model builds on the work of Frith & Done (1988) and their contribution to the neuropsychology of schizophrenia. They postulate that many symptoms in schizophrenia result from either a failure to initiate spontaneous action (e.g. negative symptoms) or a failure of internal monitoring (e.g. thought alienation, hallucinations). Their theory could be extended to include the internal monitoring of language production. If the speaker does not check speech outcome against speech plans, then errors will accumulate and communication efficiency will suffer.

The work of Harvey and colleagues on "reality monitoring" and efficient discourse construction also highlights the need of the speaker accurately to monitor speech output and recall the difference between what has been said and what has been thought (Harvey et al, 1988, 1990; Harvey & Serper, 1990; Harvey, 1985). The impaired ability of the speaker to self-monitor and to make an assessment of world knowledge has also been commented on by Harrow and colleagues (1989).

Recently, McGrath et al (1994) have reported on the subjective awareness of deficit in thought disorder. Using a scale designed to assess awareness of the frequency of communication inefficiency this group found that, within the thought-disordered group, there was a statistically significant correlation between increased awareness and higher levels of positive thought disorder. In other words, the patients seemed to be monitoring their increased errors accurately but seemed unable to utilise the information subsequently to improve the efficiency of their output.

Patients with lesions of the prefrontal systems can have both impaired error monitoring and utilisation and occasionally demonstrate impaired error utilisation in the presence of intact error monitoring (Stuss & Benson, 1984). Patients with a dissociation between these functions can be aware of errors on psychometric tasks, but appear incapable of utilising this knowledge to improve their performance on the tasks. This is often cited as a "curious dissociation between knowing and doing" (Konow & Pribram, 1970).

In summary, a "two-hit" hypothesis of positive thought disorder is proposed. The first "hit" relates to impaired set ability which results in an increase in the background error rate of communication. In the case of positive thought disorder, failure of set maintenance and change contribute to the increased error rate. The second "hit" relates to the capacity of the impaired speaker to monitor and utilise errors. This second step incorporates the complex processes involved in the speaker making an assessment of the needs of the listener and contributes to a variable threshold beyond which "breakthrough" thought disorder occurs. In other words, error monitoring and utilisation are important, rate-limiting steps in the pathogenesis of thought disorder. The proposed model of negative thought disorder is less complex, implicating impairment in the ability to establish set as the crucial factor underlying *poverty of speech*. Mindful of David's (1992) caveats about indiscriminate "frontal lobology", the factors proposed as critical in the pathogenesis of thought disorder (set ability, error monitoring and utilisation) are associated with dysfunction of the prefrontal systems. However, one needs to be cautious when extrapolating a neurocognitive model derived from classical neuro-psychology, based largely on lesion studies, to a neurodevelopmental disorder such as schizophrenia (Strauss & Summerfelt, 1994).

As mentioned above, functional neuroimaging can provide insights into the pattern of activation in healthy controls when faced with cognitive tasks. If symptoms show robust associations with impairment of certain cognitive tasks, for example, the association between positive thought disorder and impaired performance on the Stroop task, then the neuroanatomical systems involved in the performance of the cognitive task may provide clues to neuroanatomical correlates of that particular symptom. Of course, an association does not prove causality and evidence from a range of other sources is also required. One strategy is to examine functional neuroimaging correlates of individual symptoms, as has recently been demonstrated for auditory hallucinations (McGuire et al, 1993). Differences in patterns of cerebral metabolism could be examined in patients who were scanned while thought disordered and again when this symptom had settled. The development of functional neuroimaging paradigms for thought disorder needs attention. To complement this technology, activation tasks that can reliably precipitate the symptom in the thought disorder-prone patients require development (McGrath, 1991). Structural neuroimaging, using magnetic resonance imaging (MRI), has found correlations between measurements of temporal lobe structures and the presence of thought disorder in schizophrenia (Shenton et al, 1992; Rossi et al, 1994). The correlations of both functional and structural neuroimaging with thought disorder may invite attempts to map neuro-cognitive models of thought disorder onto anatomical substrates. However, this area requires particularly careful attention to research design because of the many potential uncontrolled confounding variables and biases that can occur. As well, hypotheses should be proposed *a priori* and should have a degree of coherence and plausibility as judged by genera! neuroscience. As Serper & Harvey (1994) have pointed out, the task for the researcher will be to develop comprehensive and integrative models that build on diverse sources such as experimental, neuro-psychological and neuroimaging research.

FUTURE DIRECTIONS: "SPEECH THERAPY" FOR THOUGHT DISORDER?

A clear understanding of the pathogenesis of thought disorder could provide the foundation for a rational rehabilitation program for this symptom. Just as speech therapy can assist with the reduction of disability after stroke or head injury, the thought-disordered speaker may be able to maximise function and use prompts and aids to assist in the production of coherent speech. For example, set maintenance is affected by increased distractibility. For distractible patients, clinicians should endeavour to reduce distractions to maximise set maintenance at times when clear communication is important. If set establishment is impaired then speech output might be facilitated by providing the speaker with a template or grid to guide discourse. The caregivers could be provided with education about direct and close-ended questioning in order to assist the impaired speaker to generate topics, thus helping the flow of communication. Similarly, these templates may also help the speaker refocus on the topic after *derailment* and *distractible speech*, or assist the speaker to "break away" from a topic that has captured the cognitive set resulting in *perseveration*.

Interventions may assist the speaker who has impaired error monitoring and utilisation. For example, cognitive rehabilitation techniques can assist some neurological patients who are unaware of their deficit (McGlynn, 1990). Thought-disordered patients who are aware of their deficit may benefit from interventions that reduce the planning load on the speaker and maximise available error utilisation capacities. Thought-disordered patients who are not aware of their deficit may benefit from social skills training, prompting them occasionally to check on the listener's needs. It remains to be seen whether thought-disordered patients could benefit from such cognitive rehabilitation techniques and other types of "speech therapy".

REFERENCES

Alexander, M.P., Benson, D.F., Stuss, D.T. (1989) Frontal lobes and language. *Brain and Language*, **37**, 656–691.

Allen, H. (1983) Do positive symptoms and negative symptom subtypes of schizophrenia show qualitative differences in language production? *Psychological Medicine*, **13**, 787–797.

Allen, H. (1984) Positive and negative symptoms and the thematic organization of schizophrenic speech. *British Journal of Psychiatry*, **144**, 611–617.

Allen, H.A., Allen, D.S. (1985) Positive symptoms and the organization within and between ideas in schizophrenic speech. *Psychological Medicine*, **15**, 71–80.

Andreasen, N. (1979a) Language, thought, and communication disorders: I. Clinical assessment, definition of terms, and evaluation of their reliability. *Archives of General Psychiatry*, **36**, 1315–1321.

Andreasen, N. (1979b) Thought, language, and communication disorders: II. Diagnostic significance. *Archives of General Psychiatry*, **36**, 1325–1330.

Andreasen, N.C. (1982a) Should the term "thought disorder" be revised? *Comprehensive Psychiatry*, **23**, 291–299.

Andreasen, N.C. (1982b) Negative symptoms in schizophrenia: Definition and reliability. *Archives of General Psychiatry*, **39**, 784–788.

Andreasen, N.C. (1982c) *Scale for the Assessment of Positive Symptoms*, unpublished rating manual, University of Iowa.

Andreasen, N.C. (1986) Scale for the assessment of thought, language, and communication (TLC). *Schizophrenia Bulletin*, **12**, 473–482.

Andreasen, N.C., Grove, W.M. (1986) Thought, language, and communication in schizophrenia: Diagnosis and prognosis. *Schizophrenia Bulletin*, **12**, 348–359.

Andreasen, N.C., Hoffman, R.E., Grove, W.M. (1985) Mapping abnormalities in language and schizophrenia. In: *Controversies in Schizophrenia. Changes and Constancies* (Ed. M. Alpert), pp. 199–226, Guilford Press, New York.

Andreasen, N.C., Ehrhardt, J.C., Swayze, V.W., Alliger, R.J., Yuh, W.T.C., Cohen, G., Ziebell, S. (1990) Magnetic resonance imaging of the brain in schizophrenia: The pathophysiologic significance of structural abnormalities. *Archives of General Psychiatry*, **47**, 35–44.

Barr, W.B., Bilder, R.M., Goldberg, E., Kaplan, E., Murherjee, S. (1989) The neuropsychology of schizophrenic speech. *Journal of Communication Disorders*, **22**, 327–349.

Blaney, P.H. (1978) Schizophrenic thought disorder: Why the lack of answers? In: *Language and Cognition in Schizophrenia* (Ed. S. Schwartz), pp. 101–116, Erlbaum, Hillsdale, NJ.

Bleuler, E. (1911) *Dementia Praecox: Or the Group of Schizophrenias* (translated by S.M. Clemens, 1950), International Universities Press, New York.

Broadbent, D.E. (1958) *Perception and Communication*, Pergamon Press, Oxford.

Broadbent, D.E. (1971) *Decision and Stress*, Academic Press, New York.

Chaika, E. (1974) A linguist looks at "schizophrenic" language. *Brain and Language*, **1**, 257–276.

Chaika, E.O. (1990) *Understanding Psychotic Speech: Beyond Freud and Chomsky*, Thomas, Springfield, IL.

Chapman, J. (1966) The early symptoms of schizophrenia. *British Journal of Psychiatry*, **112**, 225–251.

Chapman, L.J., Chapman, J.P. (1973) *Disordered Thought in Schizophrenia*, Appleton, New York.

Chapman, L.J., Chapman, J.P., Miller, G.A. (1964) A theory of verbal behaviour in schizophrenia. In: *Progress in Experimental Personality Research*, Vol. 1 (Ed. B.A. Maher), Academic Press, New York.

Cohen, B.D. (1976) Referent communication in schizophrenia: The perseverative-chaining model. *Annals of the New York Academy of Sciences*, **270**, 124–140.

Cohen, B.D., Nachmani, G., Rosenberg, S. (1974) Referant communication disturbances in acute schizophrenia. *Journal of Abnormal Psychology*, **83**, 1–13.

Costello, C.G. (1992) Research on symptoms versus research on syndromes. Arguments in favour of allocating more research time to the study of symptoms. *British Journal of Psychiatry*, **160**, 304–308.

Cozolino, L.J. (1983) The oral and written productions of schizophrenic patients. *Progress in Experimental Research*, **12**, 101–152.

Cromwell, R.L., Dockecki, P.R. (1968) Schizophrenic language: A disattention interpretation. In: *Developments in Applied Psycholinguistic Research* (Eds S. Rosenberg, J.H. Koplin), Macmillan, New York.

Damasio, A.R., Damasio, H. (1992) Brain and Language. *Scientific American*, **267**, 88–95.

Daniels, E.K., Shenton, M.E., Holzman, P.S., Benowitz, L.I., Coleman, M., Levin, S., Levine, D. (1988) Patterns of thought disorder associated with right cortical damage, schizophrenia, and mania. *American Journal of Psychiatry*, **145**, 944–949.

David, A.S. (1992) Frontal lobology—psychiatry's new pseudoscience. *British Journal of Psychiatry*, **161**, 244–248.

Deese, J. (1978) Thought into speech. *American Scientist*, **66**, 314–321.

Docherty, N., Schnur, M., Harvey, P.D. (1988) Reference performance and positive and negative thought disorder: A follow-up study of manics and schizophrenics. *Journal of Abnormal Psychology*, **97**, 437–442.

Drummond, S.S. (1986) Characterization of irrelevant speech: A case study. *Journal of Communication Disorders*, **19**, 175–183.

Earle-Boyer, E.A., Levinson, J.C., Grant, R., Harvey, P.D. (1986) The consistency of thought disorder in mania and schizophrenia. II. An assessment at consecutive admissions. *Journal of Nervous and Mental Disease*, **174**, 443–447.

Faber, R., Abrams, R., Taylor, M.A., Kasprison, A., Morris, C., Weisz, R. (1983) Comparison of schizophrenic patients with formal thought disorder and neurologically impaired patients with aphasia. *American Journal of Psychiatry*, **140**, 1348–1351.

Freedman, B., Chapman, L.J. (1973) Early subjective experiences in schizophrenic episodes. *Journal of Abnormal Psychology*, **82**, 46–54.

Frith, C.D., Done, D.J. (1988) Towards a neuropsychology of schizophrenia. *British Journal of Psychiatry*, **153**, 437–443.

Frith, C.D., Friston, K.J., Liddle, P.F., Frackowiak, R.S.J. (1991) Willed action and the prefrontal cortex in man: a study with PET. *Proceedings of the Royal Society B*, **244**, 241–246.

Gerson, S.N., Benson, D.F., Frazier, S.H. (1977) Diagnosis: Schizophrenia versus posterior aphasia. *American Journal of Psychiatry*, **134**, 966–969.

Green, M., Walker, E. (1985) Neuropsychological performance and positive and negative symptoms in schizophrenia. *Journal of Abnormal Psychology*, **94**, 460–469.

Green, M., Walker, E. (1986) Attentional performance in positive- and negative-symptom schizophrenia. *Journal of Nervous and Mental Disease*, **174**, 208–213.

Groves, W.M., Andreasen, N.C. (1985) Language and thinking in psychosis: Is there an input abnormality? *Archives of General Psychiatry*, **42**, 26–32.

Halpern, H., Darley, F.L., Brown, J.R. (1973) Differential language and neurologic characteristics in cerebral involvement. *Journal of Speech and Hearing Disorders*, **38**, 162–173.

Harrow, M., Marengo, J., McDonald, C. (1986) The early course of schizophrenic thought disorder. *Schizophrenia Bulletin*, **12**, 208–224.

Harrow, M., Lanin-Kettering, I., Miller, J.G. (1989) Impaired perspective and thought disorder pathology in schizophrenic and psychotic disorders. *Schizophrenia Bulletin*, **15**, 605–623.

Harvey, P.D. (1983) Speech competence in manic and schizophrenic psychoses: The association between clinically rated thought disorder and cohesion and reference performance. *Journal of Abnormal Psychology*, **92**, 368–377.

Harvey, P.D. (1985) Reality monitoring in mania and schizophrenia: The association of thought disorder and performance. *Journal of Nervous and Mental Disease*, **173**, 67–73.

Harvey, P.D., Brault, J. (1986) Speech performance in mania and schizophrenia: The association of positive and negative thought disorders and reference failures. *Journal of Communication Disorders*, **19**, 161–173.

Harvey, P.D., Neale, J.M. (1983) The specificity of thought disorder to schizophrenia: Research methods in their historical perspective. In: *Progress in Experimental Personality Research*, Vol. 12 (Ed. B. Maher), pp. 153–180, Academic Press, New York.

Harvey, P.D., Neale, J.M. (1989) Comments on innovations in the assessment of thought disorder. *Schizophrenia Bulletin*, **15**, 2–3.

Harvey, P.D., Pedley, M. (1989) Auditory and visual distractibility in schizophrenia. Clinical and medication status correlations. *Schizophrenia Research*, **2**, 295–300.

Harvey, P.D., Serper, M.R. (1990) Linguistic and cognitive failures in schizophrenia: A multivariate analysis. *Journal of Nervous and Mental Disease*, **178**, 487–493.

Harvey, P.D., Earle-Boyer, E.A., Wielgus, M.S. (1984) The consistency of thought disorder in mania and schizophrenia: An assessment of acute psychotics. *Journal of Nervous and Mental Disease*, **172**, 458–463.

Harvey, P.D., Earle-Boyer, E.A., Wielgus, M.S., Levinson, J.C. (1986) Encoding, memory, and thought disorder in schizophrenia and mania. *Schizophrenia Bulletin*, **12**, 252–261.

Harvey, P.D., Earle-Boyer, E.A., Levinson, J.C. (1988) Cognitive deficits and thought disorder: A retest study. *Schizophrenia Bulletin*, **14**, 57–66.

Harvey, P.D., Docherty, N.M., Serper, M.R., Rasmussen, M. (1990) Cognitive deficits and thought disorder: II. An 8-month follow-up study. *Schizophrenia Bulletin*, **16**, 147–156.

Harvey, P.D., Lenzenweger, M.F., Keefe, R.S.E., Pogge, D.L., Serper, M.R., Mohs, R.C. (1992) Empirical assessment of the factorial structure of clinical symptoms in schizophrenic patients: Formal thought disorder. *Psychiatry Research*, **44**, 141–151.

Hoffman, R.E. (1986) Tree structure, the work of listening, and schizophrenic discourse: A reply to Beveridge and Brown. *Brain and Language*, **27**, 385–392.

Hoffman, R., Sledge, W. (1984) A microgenetic model of paragrammatisms produced by a schizophrenic speaker. *Brain and Language*, **21**, 147–173.

Hoffman, R.E., Kirstein, L., Stopek, S., Cicchetti, D. (1982) Apprehending schizophrenic discourse: A structural analysis of the listener's task. *Brain and Language*, **15**, 207–233.

Hoffman, R.E., Stopek, S., Andreasen, N.C. (1986) A comparative study of manic vs schizophrenic speech disorganization. *Archives of General Psychiatry*, **43**, 831–838.

Holzman, P.S., Shenton, M.E., Solovay, M.R. (1986) Quality of thought disorder in differential diagnosis. *Schizophrenia Bulletin*, **12**, 360–372.

Hotchkiss, A.P., Harvey, P.D. (1990) Effect of distraction on communication failures in schizophrenic patients. *American Journal of Psychiatry*, **147**, 513–515.

Jampala, V.C., Taylor, M.A., Abrams, R. (1989) The diagnostic implications of formal thought disorder in mania and schizophrenia: A reassessment. *American Journal of Psychiatry*, **146**, 459–463.

Johnston, M.H., Holzman, P.S. (1986) Scoring manual for the Thought Disorder Index. *Schizophrenia Bulletin*, **12**, 483–496.

Kaczmarek, B.L.J. (1984) Neurolinguistic analysis of verbal utterances in patients with focal lesions of the frontal lobes. *Brain and Language*, **21**, 52–58.

Kaczmarek, B.L.J. (1987) Regulatory function of the frontal lobes: A neurolinguistic perspective. In: *The Frontal Lobes Revisited*, (Ed. E. Perecman), pp. 225–240, IRBN Press, New York.

Kleist, K. (1930/1987) Alogical thought disorder: an organic manifestation of the schizophrenic psychological deficit. In: *The Clinical Roots of the Schizophrenia Concept. Translations of Seminal European Contributions on Schizophrenia* (Eds J. Cutting, M. Shepherd), pp. 75–78, Cambridge University Press, Cambridge.

Konow, A., Pribram, K.H. (1970) Error recognition and utilization produced by injury to the frontal cortex in man. *Neuropsychologia*, **8**, 489–491.

Kraepelin, E. (1913) *Dementia Praecox and Paraphrenia* (translated by R.M. Barclay, 1919), Livingstone, Edinburgh.

Liddle, P.F. (1987a) Schizophrenic syndromes, cognitive performance and neurological dysfunction. *Psychological Medicine*, **17**, 49–57.

Liddle, P.F. (1987b) The symptoms of chronic schizophrenia: A re-examination of the positive–negative dichotomy. *British Journal of Psychiatry*, **151**, 145–151.

Liddle, P.F., Barnes, T.R.E. (1990) Syndromes of chronic schizophrenia. *British Journal of Psychiatry*, **157**, 558–561.

Liddle, P.F., Morris, D.L. (1991) Schizophrenic symptoms and frontal lobe performance. *British Journal of Psychiatry*, **158**, 340–345.

Liddle, P.F., Friston, K.J., Frith, C.D., Hirsch, S.R., Jones, T., Frackowiak, R.S.J. (1992) Patterns of cerebral blood flow in schizophrenia. *British Journal of Psychiatry*, **160**, 179–186.

Maher, B.A. (1972) The language of schizophrenia: A review and reinterpretation. *British Journal of Psychiatry*, **120**, 3–17.

Manschreck, T.C., Maher, B.A., Rucklos, M.E., White, M.T. (1979) The predictability of thought disordered speech in schizophrenic patients. *British Journal of Psychiatry*, **134**, 595–601.

Manschreck, T.C., Maher, B.A., Ader, D.N. (1981) Formal thought disorder, the type–token ratio, and disturbed voluntary motor movement in schizophrenia. *British Journal of Psychiatry*, **139**, 7–15.

Manschreck, T.C., Maher, B.A., Hoover, T.M., Ames, D. (1985) Repetition in schizophrenic speech. *Language and Speech*, **28**, 255–268.

Manschreck, T.C., Maher, B.A., Milavetz, J.J., Ames, D., Weisstein, C.C., Schneyer, M.L. (1988) Semantic priming in thought disordered schizophrenic patients. *Schizophrenia Research*, **1**, 61–66.

Marengo, J.T., Harrow, M. (1988) Thought disorder in schizophrenia. In: *Handbook of Schizophrenia, Vol. 3: Nosology, Epidemiology and Genetics* (Eds M.T. Tsuang, J.C. Simpson), pp. 85–115, Elsevier, Amsterdam.

Marengo, J.T., Harrow, M., Lanin-Kettering, I., Wilson, A. (1986) Evaluating bizarre idiosyncratic thinking: A comprehensive index of positive thought disorder. *Schizophrenia Bulletin*, **12**, 497–511.

Matthysse, S. (1987) Schizophrenic thought disorder: A model-theoretic perspective. *Schizophrenia Bulletin*, **13**, 173–184.

McConaghy, N. (1960) Modes of abstract thinking and psychosis. *American Journal of Psychiatry*, **117**, 106–110.

McConaghy, N. (1961) The measurement of an inhibitory process in human higher nervous activity: Its relation to allusive thinking and fatigue. *American Journal of Psychiatry*, **118**, 125–132.

McConaghy, N. (1989) Thought disorder or allusive thinking in the relatives of schizophrenics? A response to Callahan, Madsen, Saccuzzo and Romney. *Journal of Nervous and Mental Disease*, **177**, 729–734.

McGhie, A., Chapman, J. (1961) Disorders of attention and perception in early schizophrenia. *British Journal of Medical Psychology*, **34**, 103–116.

McGlynn, S.M. (1990) Behavioral approaches to neuropsychological rehabilitation. *Psychological Bulletin*, **108**, 420–441.

McGrath, J. (1991) Ordering thoughts on thought disorder. *British Journal of Psychiatry*, **158**, 307–316.

McGrath, J.J., Kerr,R., Dark, F.L. (1994) Are patients with thought disorder aware of their deficit? *Schizophrenia Research*, **11**, 156–157.

McGuire, P.K., Shah, G.M.S., Murray, R.M. (1993) Increased blood flow in Broca's area during auditory hallucinations in schizophrenia. *Lancet*, **342**, 703–706.

Minas, I.H., Stuart, G.W., Klimidis, S., Jackson, H.J., Singh, B.S., Copolov, D.L. (1992) Positive and negative symptoms in the psychoses: Multidimensional scaling of SAPS and SANS items. *Schizophrenia Research*, **8**, 143–156.

Morice, R. (1986a) The structure, organization, and use of language in schizophrenia. In: *Handbook of Studies on Schizophrenia. Part 1: Epidemiology, Aetiology and Clinical Features* (Eds G.D. Burrows, T.R. Norman,, G. Rubinstein), pp. 131–144, Elsevier, Amsterdam.

Morice, R. (1986b) Beyond language: Speculation on the prefrontal cortex and schizophrenia. *Australian and New Zealand Journal of Psychiatry*, **20**, 7–10.

Morice, R.D., Ingram, J.C.L. (1982) Language analysis in schizophrenia: Diagnostic implications. *Australian and New Zealand Journal of Psychiatry*, **16**, 11–21.

Morice, R.D., Ingram, J.C.L. (1983) Language complexity and age of onset of schizophrenia. *Psychiatry Research*, **9**, 233–242.

Morice, R., McNicol, D. (1985) The comprehension and production of complex syntax in schizophrenia. *Cortex*, **21**, 567–580.

Morice, R., McNicol, D. (1986) Language change in schizophrenia: A limited replication. *Schizophrenia Bulletin*, **12**, 239–251.

Moskowitz, J., Davidson, M., Harvey, P.D. (1991) Effect of concurrent distraction on communication failures in schizophrenic patients. II. Medication status correlations. *Schizophrenia Research*, **5**, 153–159.

Neale, J.M., Oltmanns, T.F. (1980) *Schizophrenia*. Wiley, New York.

Neale, J.M., Oltmanns, T.F., Harvey, P.D. (1985) The need to relate cognitive deficits to specific behavioural referents of schizophrenia. *Schizophrenia Bulletin*, **11**, 286–291.

Novoa, O.P., Ardila, A. (1987) Linguistic abilities in patients with prefrontal damage. *Brain and Language*, **30**, 206–225.

Oltmanns, T.F., Ohayon, J., Neale, J.M. (1978) The effect of anti-psychotic medication and diagnostic criteria on distractibility in schizophrenia. *Journal of Psychiatric Research*, **14**, 81–91.

Pardo, J.V., Pardo, P.J., Janer, K.W., Raichle, M.E. (1990) The anterior cingulate mediates processing selection in the Stroop attentional conflict paradigm. *Proceedings of the National Academy of Science*, **87**, 256–259.

Parks, R.W., Loewenstein, D.A., Dodrill, K.L., Barker, W.W., Yoshii, F., Chang, J.Y., Emran, A., Apicella, A., Sheramata, W.A., Duara, R. (1988) Cerebral metabolic effects of a verbal fluency test: A PET scan study. *Journal of Clinical and Experimental Neuropsychology*, **10**, 565–575.

Peralta, V., de Leon, J., Cuesta, M.J. (1992) Are there more than two syndromes in schizophrenia? A critique of the positive–negative dichotomy. *British Journal of Psychiatry*, **161**, 335–343.

Persons, J.B. (1986) The advantages of studying psychological phenomena rather than psychiatric diagnoses. *American Psychologist*, **41**, 1252–1260.

Persons, J.B., Baron, J. (1985) Processes underlying formal thought disorder in psychiatric inpatients. *Journal of Nervous and Mental Disease*, **173**, 667–676.

Petersen, S.E., Fox, P.T., Posner, M.I., Mintun, M., Raichle, M.E. (1988) Positron emission tomographic studies of the cortical anatomy of single-word processing. *Nature*, **331**, 585–589.

Pogue-Geile, M.F., Harrow, M. (1984) Negative and positive symptoms in schizophrenia and depression: a follow-up. *Schizophrenia Bulletin*, **10**, 371–387.

Reed, J.L. (1970) Schizophrenic thought disorder: A review and hypothesis. *Comprehensive Psychiatry*, **11**, 403–432.

Rochester, S. (1980) Thought disorder and language use in schizophrenia. In: *Applied Psycholinguistics and Mental Health* (Ed. R.W. Rieber), pp. 11–67, Plenum Press, New York.

Romney, D.M. (1990) Thought disorder in the relatives of schizophrenics: A meta-analytic review of selected published studies. *Journal of Nervous and Mental Disease*, **178**, 481–486.

Rossi, A., Serio, A., Stratta, P., Petruzzi, C., Schiazza, G., Mancini, F., Casacchia, M. (1994) Planum temporale asymmetry and thought disorder in schizophrenia. *Schizophrenia Research*, **12**, 1–7.

Salzinger, K., Portnoy, S., Feldman, R.S. (1978) Communicability deficit in schizophrenics resulting from a more general defect. In: *Language and Cognition in Schizophrenia* (Ed. S. Schwartz), pp. 35–53, Erlbaum, Hillsdale, NJ.

Schwartz, S. (1978) Language and cognition in schizophrenia: A review and hypothesis. In: *Language and Cognition in Schizophrenia* (Ed. S. Schwartz), pp. 237–276, Erlbaum, Hillsdale, NJ.

Schwartz, S. (1982) Is there a schizophrenic language? *Behavioral and Brain Sciences*, **5**, 579–626.

Serper, M.R., Harvey, P.D. (1994) The need to integrate neuropsychological and experimental schizophrenia research. *Schizophrenia Bulletin*, **20**, 1–11.

Shenton, M.E., Kinis, R., Jolesz, F.A., Pollak, S.D., LeMay, M., Wible, C.G., Hokama, H., Martin, J., Metcalf, D., Coleman, M., McCarley, R.W. (1992) Left-lateralized temporal lobe abnormality and their relationship to thought disorder: A computerized, quantitative MRI study. *New England Journal of Medicine*, **327**, 604–612.

Sheremata, W.A., Siddharten, R., Duara, R., Heilman, K.M. (1985) Activation of frontal cortex by the verbal fluency task: A positron emission tomographic (PET) study. *Neurology*, **35**, 97.

Simpson, D.M., Davis, G.C. (1985) Measuring thought disorder with clinical rating scales in schizophrenic and nonschizophrenic patients. *Psychiatry Research*, **15**, 313–318.

Spitzer, R., Endicott, J., Robins, L. (1978) *The Schedule for Affective Disorders and Schizophrenia*, Biometrics Research, New York.

Strauss, M.E., Summerfelt, A. (1994) Response to Serper and Harvey. *Schizophrenia Bulletin*, **20**, 13–21.

Stuss, D.T., Benson, D.F. (1984) Neuropsychological studies of the frontal lobes. *Psychological Bulletin*, **95**, 3–28.

Thomas, P., King, K., Fraser, W.I. (1987) Positive and negative symptoms of schizophrenia and linguistic performance. *Acta Psychiatrica Scandinavica*, **76**, 144–151.

Walker, E., Harvey, P. (1986) Positive and negative symptoms in schizophrenia: Attentional performance correlates. *Psychopathology*, **19**, 294–302.

Walsh, K.W. (1985) *Understanding Brain Damage. A Primer of Neuropsychological Evaluation*, Churchill Livingstone, Edinburgh.

Ward, P.B., Catts, S.V., McConaghy, N. (1992) P300 and conceptual thinking in normals: An event-related potential correlate of "thought disorder"? *Biological Psychiatry*, **31**, 650–660.

Warkentin, S., Risberg, J., Nilsson, A., Karlson, S., Graae, E. (1991) Cortical activity during speech production: A study of regional cerebral blood flow in normal subjects performing a word fluency task. *Neuropsychiatry, Neuropsychology and Behavioural Neurology*, **4**, 305–316.

Weinberger, D.R. (1988) Schizophrenia and the frontal lobes. *Trends in Neurosciences*, **11**, 367–370.

Weinberger, D.R., Berman, K.F. (1988) Speculation on the meaning of cerebral hypofrontality in schizophrenia. *Schizophrenia Bulletin*, **14**, 157–168.

Weinberger, D.R., Berman, K.F., Zec, R.F. (1986) Physiologic dysfunction of the dorsolateral prefrontal cortex in schizophrenia. I Regional cerebral blood flow evidence. *Archives of General Psychiatry*, **43**, 114–124.

Wielgus, M.S., Harvey, P.D. (1988) Dichotic listening and recall in schizophrenia and mania. *Schizophrenia Bulletin*, **14**, 689–700.

Yates, W.R., Swayze, V.W., Andreasen, N.C. (1990) Neuropsychological effects of global and focal cerebral atrophy in schizophrenia. *Neuropsychiatry, Neuropsychology and Behavioural Neurology*, **3**, 98–106.

11

Neuropsychological Correlates of Positive Symptoms: Delusions and Hallucinations

RICHARD W.J. NEUFELD and PETER C. WILLIAMSON

INTRODUCTION

The distinction between positive and negative symptoms in schizophrenia has been made since the later part of the 19th century. Hughlings Jackson, who is generally given credit for popularising the terms, saw negative symptoms as arising from a loss of inhibition from higher cortical regions caused by a disease process (Taylor, 1932). A similar distinction can be seen in Bleuler's (1911) fundamental versus accessory symptoms.

The more recent interest in positive and negative symptoms comes from the suggestions that each might characterise a syndrome with a different pathophysiology (Crow, 1980). Crow suggested that Type I syndrome was associated with positive symptoms (delusions, hallucinations and thought disorder) and is related to a change in dopaminergic transmission and more likely to respond to neuroleptic treatment. Type II was associated with negative symptoms (affective blunting, alogia, apathy, avolition and asociality) and likely was related to structural changes in the brain (Crow, 1980). Patients with the Type II syndrome were less likely to respond to neuroleptics and more likely to show intellectual deterioration. Type I syndrome, on the other hand, was usually not associated with intellectual deterioration. This typology has stimulated considerable research over the past decade (Kay & Opler, 1987; Walker & Lewine, 1988; Marks & Luchins, 1990; Pickar et al, 1990).

It might seem contradictory to discuss the neuropsychology of positive symptoms when at least clinical lore in some circles has it that these symptoms are associated with little intellectual deterioration. However, there is reason to believe that the phenomenology of schizophrenia is not so neatly divided into two syndromes. Most patients seem to demonstrate a mixture of symptoms which

Schizophrenia: A Neuropsychological Perspective. Edited by C. Pantelis, H.E. Nelson and T.R.E. Barnes
© 1996 John Wiley & Sons Ltd

might be better characterised by a three or four factor model, detailed further below (Liddle et al, 1989; Kay, 1990; Arndt et al, 1991). Even the assumption that negative symptoms early in illness indicate a poor prognosis has been questioned by some (Kay, 1991). Consequently, it might be also worthwhile to re-examine the relationship between neuropsychological tests and positive symptoms (see also in this volume: Liddle, chapter 15; Pantelis and Brewer, chapter 16; Nayani and David, chapter 17; Cahill and Frith, chapter 18).

A number of problems are inherent to such a discussion. First of all, there are several types of positive symptoms. For the purposes of this chapter, we will limit our review to studies of delusions and hallucinations. Included in this category are symptoms of paranoid schizophrenia, specifically, delusions and (thematic) hallucinations (Burack & Zigler, 1989; Strauss et al, 1974). Thought disorder will be addressed by others in this volume (see McGrath, chapter 10). Second, both positive and negative symptoms usually change over time with a general tendency to increasing negative and decreasing positive symptoms (Fenton & McGlashan, 1991; McGlashan & Fenton, 1992). Thus, the relationship between neuropsychological tests and positive symptoms may be quite different depending on the stage at which the assessments were made. It is also very difficult to characterise any one patient as having a positive "syndrome", as an enduring trait in this dynamic nature of the syndrome. Third, most studies are conducted on patients who are being treated with neuroleptics. The persistence of positive symptoms in these patients may suggest a degree of treatment resistance. The assumption is made then that these patients are the same as those who respond to medication. Even if this assumption is correct, the medications may influence several cognitive variables independently (Spohn & Strauss, 1989). Finally, there is reason to believe that schizophrenia is a progressive illness (Miller, 1989). Measurements of cognitive functioning in patients early in their illness are not necessarily comparable to those completed later in the illness. In view of these limitations, our discussion will be selective and by and large limited to those studies which at least noted these variables.

We will first address studies employing neuropsychological tests which can be localised to frontal regions. This will be followed by those examining less localised functions such as memory and information processing. Finally, neuropsychological studies addressing the relationship between lateralised neuropsychological function and the addressed positive symptoms will be considered.

DELUSIONS AND HALLUCINATIONS DEFINE A SYMPTOMATOLOGICAL SUBTYPE

It is especially fitting that the volume editors have asked us to address neuropsychological correlates of the positive symptoms, delusions and hallucinations. Several sources of data endorse the presence of prominent delusions, often combined with hallucinations, as defining a prevalent subtype of schizophrenia (Nicholson et al, 1995; Nicholson & Neufeld, submitted).

The positive association between delusions and hallucinations, and their negative or weak association with other symptomatology, is readily apparent in a correlation matrix presented by Andreasen and Olson (Andreasen, 1982; Andreasen & Olson, 1982). Scales for the assessment of positive and negative symptoms were administered to 52 inpatients. Our secondary analyses indicate that the positive correlation between delusions and hallucinations of 0.47 significantly exceeds the next highest positive correlation of 0.20, between delusions and positive formal thought disorder ($z = 1.67$, $p < 0.05$, one-tailed). Similar results are obtained from analysis of the correlation matrix of positive and negative symptoms across 302 monozygotic probands and their co-twins, presented by Lenzenweger et al (1989). The correlation between delusion and hallucination scales is 0.385, significantly higher than the next highest positive correlation involving delusions, with bizarre behaviour ($r = 0.260$, $p < 0.05$, one-tailed), although lower, but not significantly so, than the correlation between hallucinations and catatonic motor behaviour ($r = 0.405$). A similar set of associations is apparent in related data, reported by these same authors (Lenzenweger et al, 1991). The first correlation increased to 0.410, however, and the second two were reduced to 0.234 and 0.389, respectively. The increased spread between the first and second correlations reduces the p-value for the test on their comparison to less than 0.004. Such a configuration is accordant with a confirmatory factor analysis of symptom distribution among a sample of 207 patients, employing maximum-likelihood estimation of factor loadings and associated tests of goodness of fit (Arndt et al, 1991). A three-factor model was a significantly better fit for the observed pattern of correlations than a two-factor model; for two of three subsamples, the three factors represented a sufficiently complex structure for an adequate fit ($p \geqslant 0.28$, for the test on departure of observed data from model predictions). Principal components analysis, followed by simple-structure rotation indicated a separate factor of delusions and hallucinations (loadings of 0.83 and 0.78, in contrast to the next highest loading of 0.18). Results from a principal components analysis of intercorrelations among positive and negative symptoms, reported by Schuldberg et al (1990), are compatible with those of the foregoing multivariate analysis.

Apropos these observations, reference can be made to the findings of Liddle (1987). Interrelations among positive and negative symptoms were analysed using principal factor analysis, followed by oblique rotation. Liddle's "reality distortion factor", representing delusions of reference and persecution and auditory hallucinations, correlated essentially zero with the "psychomotor poverty" and "disorganisation syndrome" factors; the latter two factors, in turn, correlated 0.25. Again, a separate covariation between delusions and hallucinations was indicated.

An obvious tack to examining neuropsychological correlates of delusions and hallucinations is to focus on data from samples of patients with paranoid schizophrenia. In DSM-IV (American Psychiatric Association, 1994) and ICD-X (World Health Organization, 1994), delusions and thematic hallucinations are the defining symptoms of the paranoid subtype, just as formal positive thought disorder, bizarre behaviour, and flat or grossly inappropriate affect are contraindications (DSM-IV), or are stated to be generally dissociated from the subtype (ICD-X). Items from psychometric scales designed to distinguish paranoid from non-paranoid varieties of schizophrenia, as well, are accordant with our target symptom picture being present among paranoid patients (Gordon & Gregson, 1970; Magaro et al, 1981).

Moreover, the paranoid subtype is considered to be the most common form of schizophrenia, at least according to ICD-X (e.g. World Health Organization, 1994). Finally, considerable clinical and experimental data indicate that the paranoid subtype represents a less severe form of disorder than non-paranoid schizophrenia, in terms of onset and course of illness, and level of functioning on several variables during active phases (Nicholson & Neufeld, 1993).

It is difficult to overstate the methodological importance of making allowances as much as possible, for symptomatological subgroups in experimental psycho-pathology. Inferential risks of not doing so include the following. Data comprising an amalgam of non-parallel response patterns generated by a sample made up of heterogeneous subsamples, may be unrepresentative of any one of the enclaves composing the sample (a technical review of contemporary and several historical issues concerning data aggregation can be found in Neufeld & Gardner, 1990). On this note, identification of subgroups as paranoid schizophrenic even may be preferable to simply verifying within a sample the presence of delusions and hallucinations. Paranoid and non-paranoid symptoms tend to be mutually exclusive, if classificatory schemata such as DSM-IV and ICD-X are employed. Conversely, high factor scores on a factor of delusions/hallucinations (e.g. Arndt et al, 1991) may co-exist with or without high scores on the remaining symptom factors, to the degree that the factors are orthogonal. The task of identifying neurological and neurochemical substrata of symptomatology probably will become more complicated in the company of unwarranted symptom diffuseness.

By way of caveat, inferences drawn from samples of patients with paranoid schizophrenia may apply to prominent systematic delusions, thematic hallucina-tions, or both. In other words, some residual heterogeneity inevitably remains. In keeping with the above moderate correlations, cluster analyses of clinical-data protocols indicate that delusions and hallucinations (thematic and otherwise) can be separated from one another in defining symptom-demographic profiles (Farmer et al, 1983; Zemlan et al, 1986).

SPECIFICITY OF FUNCTIONS TAPPED BY COGNITIVE TASKS

The argument for specificity extends, of course, to the measurement of cognitive functions. Tasks involving information processing, or cognition, have been used in several ways in the neuropsychology of schizophrenia. They have been employed to draw inferences regarding functions subserved by given neuroana-tomical structures or systems: according to performance deficits accompanying injury or lesions, according to patterns of regional activation during task perfor-mance, and according to performance correlates of structural or neurochemical deviations as detected by magnetic resonance imaging techniques. More often than not, the rigour of exploring neuroanatomical and neurochemical substrata of cognitive/behavioural functions exceeds that of specifying the functions themselves

(Levin et al, 1989; Miller, 1984). Tasks employed in much of cognitive neuropsychology involve (inferred) composites of functions (see, for example, comments on the Wisconsin Card Sorting Test by Levin et al, 1989) and formal models of performance usually are lacking. Such formal models specify the cognitive architecture of task performance, with respect to requisite processes such as stimulus encoding, referral of the encoded product to memory-held information, response organisation, and so on (e.g. Fisher & Goldstein, 1983; Schweikert, 1989). Whether or not formal models of reaction time and error rate are invoked, there is apt to be more progress accruing to efforts at uncovering neuropsychological correlates of rigorously circumscribed cognitive/behavioural functions, than to those guided by task performance embodying informally inferred multiple functions (cf. Vanderwolf & Robinson, 1981). We hope to maximise available precision in this respect, recruiting the axiomatic arguments of quantitative developments where appropriate. Doing so should sharpen interpretation of existing findings and enhance suggestions concerning future work.

FRONTAL–POSTERIOR CONSIDERATIONS

FRONTAL LOBE FUNCTIONING

Do patients with delusions and hallucinations show evidence of inferior prefrontal lobe functioning? Findings indicate that, although frontal dysfunction may not be as pronounced as that of other patients with schizophrenia, it certainly is far from absent; indeed, as indicated below, there are instances where it appears to be more pronounced.

We consider first a study by Bornstein et al (1990). These investigators gave the Wisconsin Card Sorting Test (WCST) (Heaton, 1981) to paranoid, undifferentiated and disorganised non-paranoid schizophrenic patients, to schizoaffective patients, and to non-patient controls. Integrity of the prefrontal area, specifically the dorsolateral prefrontal cortex, is considered to be essential to efficient performance of the WCST (e.g. Weinberger et al, 1991).

With respect to the question at hand, our secondary analysis of the presented data indicated that the performance of paranoid patients ($n = 28$) was significantly inferior to the controls ($n = 52$) on each of the two "frontal measures". The measures tapped frontally located functions in as much as scores had been found to suffer with the presence of frontal lesions. For WCST perseverative errors (sorting according to an earlier stimulus dimension, despite negative feedback), $F(1/121) = 5.60$, $p < 0.03$; for the Verbal Concept Formation Test (VCAT) (Bornstein & Leason, 1985), $F(1/121) = 7.54$, $p < 0.01$, and for the mean of the (standardised) scores on the two tests, $F(1/121) = 16.807$, $p < 0.001$ (note that the latter result could be viewed as exaggerating the relevant group differences regarding observed frontal test performance, due to inflationary effects of score aggregation on statistical significance; Neufeld & Gardner, 1990).

The following additional analyses were undertaken by Bornstein et al (1990). Total "symptom severity" had been monitored according to the average global severity ratings on the respective subscales of the Scale for the Assessment of Negative Symptoms (SANS) (Andreasen, 1982) and the Scale for the Assessment of Positive Symptoms (SAPS) (Andreasen & Olson, 1982). The paranoid subgroup scored significantly lower than the non-paranoid patients on the sum of the average ratings from the two scales; this observation led the investigators to use symptom severity as a covariate, in an ensuing analysis, below. In addition, our secondary analyses of their data indicated that the paranoid patients were older than the controls ($p < 0.05$) and had significantly less education ($p < 0.01$). Thus, the significant differences on the frontal tests between the paranoid schizophrenic sample and controls may have been attributable to differences in one or both of these variables (e.g. Goldstein et al, 1991). Bornstein et al (1990) re-examined test performance scores after statistically adjusting them for several covariates, specifically chlorpromazine-equivalence drug dosage (CPZ equivalence), symptom severity and education (analysis of multiple covariance, ANMCOVA).

Consideration of the post-adjusted results should be prefaced by stating the interpretational risks incurred by such statistical control. It is possible inadvertently to misrepresent authentic differences, especially if, as in the present case, the covariate measure contributes to the make-up of the independent-variable measure (Cochran, 1957). Bornstein et al (1990) employed DSM-III-R criteria for subgroup composition. Doing so implies that seven of the nine symptom subscales of the SAPS and SANS by and large represent *exclusion* criteria for diagnosis of the paranoid subtype. Hence, adjustment for symptom severity, as measured here, risks distortion of *bona fide* independent-variable effects. On the other hand, it can be shown that underadjustment also is possible, given significant group differences on the covariate and imperfectly reliable covariate measurement (e.g. drug effect estimates; estimates of educational benefits on test performance; e.g. Humphreys, 1978). In addition, the psychometric structure of the dependent variable is altered from that of its original structure, following adjustment (Winne, 1983). Finally, within-group estimates of covariate–dependent-variable relations necessarily would be zero for the non-patient control group, with respect to drug dosage and presumably symptom severity. Consequently, applicability of the within-group regression estimates to the control subjects, at least for these variables, would be dubious at best.

Nevertheless, following statistical adjustment, the group differences on WCST perseverative errors evidently remained intact ($p < 0.001$), unlike those of the VCAT ($p < 0.50$). Apparently, the group means on the WCST perseverative errors underwent less adjustment for "drug dosage" than did the VCAT, owing to considerably less within-group association ($p = 0.90$ versus 0.06). Accordingly, the aggregate frontal index made up of these two measures also was somewhat attenuated but remained significant ($p < 0.03$). It would seem, then, that elevation in WCST perseverative errors among the paranoid schizophrenic subsample was especially robust. The robustness, however, may have stemmed in part from "underadjustment" for differences in the covariates of drug dosage and/or education, mentioned above. Also, the psychometric composition of the adjusted measure, meaning the functions variously to which it is sensitive, is not interchangeable with that of its non-residualised format. Perseverative errors on the WCST, for example, are known to covary with symptoms displayed by frontal lobe patients. These symptoms, in turn, resemble some of those on the SAPS and SANS. Removal from variance in WCST perseverative errors of the within-groups covariance with SAPS and SANS global severity values will leave a residualised measure potentially much less related, or unrelated, to frontal symptoms. In other words, the original measure validity data no longer apply (Winne, 1983; Lees & Neufeld, 1994).

A somewhat more straightforward investigation of paranoid and non-paranoid subtypes has been presented by Rosse et al (1991). Patients were classified as chronic, unlike those of Bornstein et al (1990). However, subgroups approximately were matched at the outset on several demographic variables, including age and education. When perseverative-error rate was compared to that of norms for age-matched controls, the paranoid subgroup was significantly higher, $t(13) = 1.92$, $p < 0.05$ (one-tailed; based on pooled normative- and patient-group variances, $F_{max}(13) = 1.82$, n.s.). Similar results were obtained by Paulman et al (1990) for total WCST sorting errors and for the number of sorting categories achieved.

Rosse et al (1991) reported findings also from computerised tomography (CT) scans and related them to WCST performance. A moderate correlation between frontal right sulcus enlargement and perseverative errors was obtained ($r = 0.526$). Paranoid–non-paranoid differences in frontal sulcus measures, however, were non-significant, even though non-paranoid patients produced significantly more perseverative errors than did paranoid patients ($p < 0.027$, one-tailed). Taken at face value, then, the most parsimonious conclusion from these results is that differences between paranoid and non-paranoid schizophrenic subgroups on perseverative errors of the WCST are attributable to variables other than right frontal sulcus enlargement. As Levin et al (1989) have pointed out, the WCST is a multi-process/cognitive-function test. Therefore, orthogonal processes potentially can contribute to poorer WCST performance. The associated functions, in turn, may have different neurological sites and substrata. They may interact with the frontal cortex in augmenting the latter's effective workings (Suddath et al, 1989). Also, they may reflect frontal cortex physiological dysfunction distinct from the type of structural abnormality identified by the present CT scan procedure (cf. Zec & Weinberger, 1986).

Taking a different tack to the investigation of neuropsychological deficits in schizophrenia, Shallice et al (1991) administered an extensive battery of neuropsychological tests to each of five schizophrenic patients, and examined in considerable detail each patient's individual profile. All patients were found to be impaired on tests where performance has been shown to suffer with frontal lobe lesions, including a modified WCST. Of the five patients studied, two displayed symptomatology clearly indicative of paranoid schizophrenia, and the remaining three at least had delusions. Convergently, seven frontal lobe tumour cases studied by Avery (1971) gave evidence that delusions clearly were part of their symptom picture.

In their study of eye tracking and other behaviours among diagnostically mixed patients with schizophrenia, Bartfai et al (1985) employed the Trail Making Test and finger tapping speed task, among other tests. The Trail Making Test involves the joining of digits and letters in a given sequence, a task considered to depend on frontally hosted functions. The finger tapping test is considered specifically to be a posterior frontal lobe task (see, for example, Katsanis & Iacono, 1991). Performance on both tasks suffered as patients displayed higher scores on the symptoms, "delusional mood", referring in part to a ". . . sudden conviction that trivial events or things have a profound and bizarre significance" (p. 19), and "commenting voices" (Asberg et al, 1978). Similar findings for finger tapping among paranoid schizophrenic subjects were reported by Paulman et al (1990).

As mentioned above, results from certain studies have suggested the possibility of greater dysfunction of the frontal cortex among paranoid than among non-paranoid schizophrenic subgroups. Paulman et al (1990) investigated regional cerebral blood flow (rCBF) among 40 medicated and unmedicated male patients with chronic schizophrenia and 31 age- and sex-matched controls, employing single-photon emission computerised tomography (SPECT) scans. Frontal flow deficits were greatest among the 21 DSM-III diagnosed patients with paranoid schizophrenia. Neuropsychological tests also were administered to all patients and controls. Paranoid and non-paranoid subgroups were equally deficient on WCST error and categories-achieved scores, as well as on finger tapping scores. Moreover, WCST errors significantly decreased and left-hand finger tapping increased as the ratio of left frontal to left hemisphere flow increased (following our Bonferroni adjustment for 12, one-tailed tests on correlations of frontal flow and cognitive test, family-wise alpha = 0.10; no other correlations were significant, following simultaneous alpha adjustment for tests applied to non-frontal areas).

Morrison-Stewart et al (1992) found significant correlations between WCST performance scores and total SAPS scores. A value of -0.42 ($p < 0.005$, one-tailed) was obtained for categories completed, and a value of 0.31 ($p = 0.024$, one-tailed) occurred for perseverative errors. No significant correlations were obtained for the total SANS scores. The correlations with the SAPS scores are noteworthy because the delusion and hallucination subscales figured prominently in these total scores, accounting for 79% of the total SAPS variance among unmedicated patients, independently of all other scales (i.e. ignoring their additional contributions through covariance between themselves and with the other subscales). In the case of medicated patients, the two subscales accounted for 49% of the total SAPS variance. It is noteworthy, as a side observation, that the *net* correlation among the subscales of the SAPS essentially was zero, unlike that for the SANS for each group, and the SAPS subscales among the unmedicated group.

More indirect evidence of at least equal, if not more pronounced frontal lobe dysfunction among paranoid schizophrenic patients, has to do with eye movements during oculomotor tracking of a continuously moving target. The occurrence of saccadic eye movements during target pursuit categorically has been linked by some investigators to frontal lobe dysfunction (e.g. Levin, 1984; see Henderson et al, chapter 13). Of paranoid and non-paranoid subgroups, affective disorder patients, and non-patient controls, paranoid patients have exhibited the highest rates of saccades, especially to slower moving targets (11 degrees/s and 22 degrees/s; Mather et al, 1992). The smooth-pursuit eye tracking disruption of saccadic movements has been interpreted as reflecting cognitive-perceptual deficits, especially among paranoid patients (Neufeld et al, 1995). In particular, the excessive saccades have been considered to reflect inefficiency in encoding of the spatial stimulus properties necessary for effective tracking.

Interestingly, eye movements are involved in two aspects of task transaction. One is the appropriation from presenting stimulation data relevant to updating target location and movement dynamics, as gauged against momentary gaze location. From this information presumably is "computed" the continuing requisite tracking response, the second aspect of eye movement involved in task transaction. Undoubtedly, one cannot come to grips with the dynamics of these rapid functional interactions, nor with the complexities of the computational processing involved, without appealing to the differential equations of servocybernetic systems (Staddon, 1984) nor, with respect to information processing, to stochastic and/or connectionist models (e.g. McClelland & Rummelhart, 1986; Townsend & Ashby, 1983). What can be said in the interim is that the morphology of the two aspects of eye behaviours involved in the overall tracking task are not necessarily compatible. The "response" facilitating external-stimulus encoding has been shown to be one of fixation, according to relevant observations from the field of experimental cognitive psychology (e.g. Just & Carpenter, 1976, 1987); that comprising execution of the prescribed "tracking response" is considered to be one of "smooth pursuit".

It is perhaps not surprising then, that saccades and smooth pursuit have been considered to reflect two separate "eye movement systems" (Levin, 1984; Mather et al, 1992; see also Henderson et al, chapter 13). Subjects experiencing difficulties in encoding immediate stimulation into its task facilitative format may display apparent difficulties in the coordination of these forms of movement. In effect, those subjects who are less efficient in negotiating the encoding process may be expected to have encoding-related movements as more prominent features of their oculomotor profile during the tracking task.

Accordingly, cognitive psychological correlates of paranoid schizophrenia have included, most notably, increased latency for encoding-process completion (for review: Neufeld, 1991; Neufeld et al, 1993). Second, multivariate analysis of the structure of eye movement dysfunction, as defined by concomitant measures, has aligned saccade disruption of smooth pursuit with other tasks rich in spatial encoding requirements (Neufeld et al, 1995).

Regarding tendered neurological substrata, first we would note an informal parallel between the task demands of oculomotor pursuit and other frontal lobe tasks, such as the WCST, and the Delayed Response Task (e.g. Goldman-Rakic, 1987). Each task requires the encoding of presenting stimulus properties into a format permitting the assessment of immediate events with respect to memory-held ongoing task constraints. Depending on task composition and duration of retention, the structural hosts of the latter information may be temporal (Weinberger et al, 1991) and/or hippocampal (Goldman-Rakic, 1987). In any event, the specific area that appears to be the seat of "working memory", mediating the stimulation at hand to the task-defined status of the stimulation, is Walker's frontal area 46 (Goldman-Rakic, 1987). Functions associated with area 46, then, putatively are served by eye movements facilitating stimulus encoding; execution of such movements are considered to implicate the interaction between this area and that of the frontal eye field (area 8; Goldman-Rakic, 1987).

The above interpretation of saccade production among paranoid subgroups can be viewed in the light of the influential analysis of eye movement dysfunction put forth by Levin (1984):

> Taken together, the studies of eye movement impairments suggest that these impairments are limited to conditions of tracking a slow moving or a stationary visual target. Furthermore, the data suggest that the impaired eye movement patterns, particularly the disruption of pursuit by saccadic intrusions, are not related to specific impairments of the dynamic characteristics of smooth pursuit (e.g. gain and velocity) or saccades (e.g. velocity or duration as a function of saccade size). Rather, they are related to a *functional* impairment of the mechanisms that regulate smooth pursuit and saccades. Whereas impairments of dynamic characteristics reflect specific oculomotor dysfunctions, functional impairments are related to visual attention. (p. 48)

Other investigators (e.g. Khurana & Kowler, 1987; Kowler et al, 1984; Steinman, 1986) also have pointed to the possible overlap between the visual "attentional components" of oculomotor tracking and those of more or less traditional visual search tasks (e.g. Townsend & Ashby, 1983, chapter 6).

A microanalysis of the parameters of smooth pursuit among paranoid subgroups and others, superimposed on the frequency of saccadic disruption (Mather et al, 1992), has endorsed Levin's suggestion, that there appears to be a functional impairment (encoding deficit), rather than a dynamic impairment (deficit in the mechanics of pursuit), among the paranoid subjects. This functional impairment may well reside with selected sites within the frontal cortex and/or with those of other structures interacting with and augmenting the workings of these sites.

THE STRUCTURE OF STIMULUS ENCODING DEFICIT

Reference has been made above to the apparent difficulties encountered by patients with schizophrenia, especially those with paranoid schizophrenia, in the encoding of stimulus properties into a task-facilitative format. In this section, the structure of this deficit is examined employing data on the performance of tasks adopted from the fields of experimental cognitive psychology and neuropsychology (Neufeld, 1990b; Neufeld et al, 1993). The analysis then is drawn out with respect to the way in which dysfunctional stimulus encoding may evince inferior performance on more molar tasks, such as the WCST.

Patients with paranoid schizophrenia have displayed increased latency for completion of the encoding components of a variety of information processing tasks. Such tasks have included the extraction of linguistic properties relevant to the verification of simple statements (Neufeld, 1977, 1978), the implementation of stimulus features required for template matching in memory search tasks

(Wishner et al, 1978; Broga & Neufeld, 1981a; George & Neufeld, 1987), the accessing of memory-held physical magnitudes of stimuli and of phonemic stimulus properties, for purposes of mental comparison (George & Neufeld, 1984; Highgate-Maynard & Neufeld, 1986), and the positioning of stimulus dimensions for purposes of sorting-rule identification in card sorting tasks (Dobson & Neufeld, 1982). The above enumeration, while not exhaustive, has emphasised those studies where the deficits of paranoid patients have been separated out from those of non-paranoid patients and have tended to be more pronounced. Additional studies suggesting encoding deficits among mixed samples have been discussed elsewhere (e.g. Broga & Neufeld, 1981b).

As mentioned, the specific form of deficit being referred to comprises a delayed latency for encoding-process completion. This observation occurs primarily under conditions where a time limit is not imposed and where the subject is asked to respond as quickly and accurately as possible. Error rates generally are similar, and relatively low, across groups and are not correlated with reaction time in any confounding way (Townsend & Ashby, 1983, chapter 9). It may be anticipated, however, that error rates would reflect the encoding process retardation, should a time limit be imposed (see section on Lateralisation Abnormalities, below, and Appendix B).

The route to elucidation of this deficit takes the following form. Response time data from studies where encoding demands, or load, systematically have been varied across one or more diagnostic groups are scrutinised. The simplest form of this design is a 2 (encoding load) by 2 (more versus less target symptomatology) factorial combination, one commonly used to delineate processing structures (e.g. Schweikert, 1989; Townsend, 1994). Response time quantities of principal interest are those of distribution lower-order moments, in part because of their explicit relations to other response-time distribution properties (Townsend, 1990), their relative stability and their familiarity. Specifically, interest is focused on mean latency values, $E(T)$, and variance in response times, across trials, within subjects, $Var(T)$. The configuration of these values then is examined in the light of seemingly relevant mathematical models of information processing. Of special interest are the structures of those models accommodating the configuration of the latency means and variances and also the parameters that must be adjusted for modelled configurations of means and variances to conform to the class of those observed across the groups and task conditions (Neufeld et al, 1993). Such parameter changes are considered potentially to implicate the nature of changes in processing associated with psychopathology.

Values for $E(T)$ and $Var(T)$, averaged over subjects within groups (e.g. Townsend, 1984), were available from two studies meeting at least the minimal 2×2 factorial requirements, above (Highgate-Maynard, 1984; George, 1985; Highgate-Maynard & Neufeld, 1986; George & Neufeld, 1987). In each case, differences in mean $E(T)$ values occurred between encoding load, and between paranoid schizophrenic patients and non-patient controls. These effects were highly additive, however, in that the differences between task conditions were almost identical between groups (each of the above statements confirmed by corresponding analysis-of-variance results).

Turning to average values of $Var(T)$, group and task-demand differences were in the same directions as those of $E(T)$. However, in the study by Highgate-Maynard (1984; Highgate-Maynard & Neufeld, 1986), $Var(T)$ under the higher load condition exceeded the lower-load condition counterpart more for the paranoid subjects than for the controls (Neufeld, 1990a; a case of "subadditivity" of variances; see, e.g. Townsend, 1984; Townsend & Thomas, 1994). In George's study, non-additivity of $Var(T)$ was much less in evidence (Neufeld, 1990b).

Two mathematical models, representing a class accommodating additivity of $E(T)$, and subadditivity of $Var(T)$, are presented in Appendix A; a third has been discussed elsewhere, in sources cited in the appendix. Two models representing a class of those predicting additivity both of means and variances are presented in Appendix A, also. Augmenting analyses of the "goodness of model fit" are available elsewhere (Neufeld, 1994; Vollick, 1994).

Inferences from these formal analyses converge on the same conclusion in each instance. Component steps, or stages (subprocesses) of the covert encoding process are transacted at the same rate by each group; the number of subprocesses for the modelled paranoid schizophrenic performance, however, exceeds that of the controls. In other words, processing capacity, specified as the rate parameter of the respective models (see e.g. Townsend & Ashby, 1978) remains intact; application, however, is less efficient, where efficiency is identified with the subprocess parameter.

Note that the subprocesses referred to are considered to be covert steps in completing the encoding process. These events, at least for the time being, quite legitimately may exist as a mathematical variable within a formal logical system (Braithwaite, 1968). At the same time, suggestive stimulus correlates come to the fore. Levin et al (1989; see also Neufeld & Mothersill, 1980), for example, have made note of two forms of processing dysfunction potentially relevant to the findings at hand: (a) implementation of stimulus features which, although relevant to the given process, are unnecessary (see also, Cromwell & Dokecki, 1968); and, (b) failure to unitise stimulus features which ordinarily might form a "natural Gestalt" (see also, Snodgrass & Townsend, 1980, for a formal operationalisation of this point). Added to these possibilities, is that of a "priming of the system" (e.g. Russell & Knight, 1977) to perform the processing requirements, resulting in an added preliminary set of subprocesses.

The line of reasoning underlying the presented fabric of the encoding deficit is sketched out in Appendix A. More elaborate developments are cited, as are references to relevant background material.

How might the above encoding dysfunction be expressed on more molar neuropsychological tests, such as the WCST? Efficient performance on the latter test, as with other card sorting tests (Bourne, 1970), can be broken down into component requirements (Goldman-Rakic, 1987; see also Kolb & Whishaw, 1980). The goal of the task is to employ that dimension of the key card (figure shape, colour, number of figures) to be shared by target cards during a particular phase of the task. The subject, then, is faced with a sequence of sorting responses and their attendant positive/negative feedback from the experimenter. Benefits to performance of feedback attending one's sorting responses should be enhanced by the classification of target cards into four classes (cf. Bourne, 1970): those sharing one or more of the three attributes with the key card, and those sharing none. More valuable would be an awareness that only cards sharing one or two attributes have any diagnostic value regarding the key card's critical attribute. Identification of the organising principle, then, would be served by associating the stimuli having diagnostic value with their positive and negative feedback. In other words, an array of stimulus properties must be processed into an arrangement compatible with the memory-held task goal.

Assume that the arrangement of the stimulus constellation comprises a number of component processes whereby the diagnostic significance of the respective stimulus properties are encoded. Encoded material completed earlier in the sequence of completions, stands a greater chance of being lost, if the subsequent completions are delayed; such delay is risked with additional encoding subprocesses (cf. Townsend, 1984; Chechile, 1987; Neufeld, 1991). When it comes to responding, earlier encoded material may be less available, undermining the full complement of external stimulus information bearing specifically on the task goal (Broga & Neufeld, 1981b). Results from other card sorting tasks (Dobson & Neufeld, 1982) and from the analysis of multidimensional judgements among paranoid schizophrenic samples (Neufeld, 1975, 1976) are congruent with the above suggestion. Furthermore, the tendered association between delayed completion of encoding, and undermining of existing encoding–product traces, recently has been translated into a formal model of deficits in multidimensional judgements (Carter, 1994; Carter & Neufeld, in submission). The model has been subjected to several tests of goodness of fit to empirical data, the data being made up of encoding latencies and multidimensional judgements obtained from schizophrenic subgroups and controls. Results have been supportive of the tenability of the stated model.

Possible physiological substrata of diminished encoding efficiency can be tendered, although speculatively at best. It has been suggested by Weinberger et al (1991) that information-processing difficulties may arise from dysfunctional communication between the prefrontal cortex and anterior–medial temporal lobe structures (cf., Frith & Done, 1988; Liddle & Morris, 1991; Liddle et al, 1992). The latter structures appear to be part and parcel of the memorial maintenance of task constraints. Reduced access to these constraints may precipitate less efficient deployment of otherwise intact attentional resources. Weinberger et al (1991) view diminished temporal–prefrontal communication basically as being in agreement with findings of diminished prefrontal rCBF, glucose metabolism, and electroencephalograph (EEG) coherence. More recently, patients reporting hallucinations have been shown to activate prefrontal, subcortical, and temporal regions compared to the non-hallucinating state on PET (Silbersweig et al, 1995).

Finally, we return to the rate parameter of formal processing models, referred to above. This parameter can be considered to vary with the "amount of cognitive work done" during a given time interval of processing (Townsend & Ashby, 1978). As mentioned, patients studied do not display diminished values on this specific parameter, as it participates in the models employed to examine performance.

Similarly, to the value of the cognitive rate parameter, the above indexes of cerebral activation have been considered to be indirect measures of cognitive work performed (Weinberger & Berman, 1988). Frontal areas stand both to take part directly in encoding transactions, as well as to "coordinate" the differential activation of other structures leading to the efficient undertaking of these transactions. Measures of total activation are not necessarily lower for (mixed) schizophrenic samples (Buchsbaum et al, 1990; Paulman et al, 1990; Mattes et al, 1991). The topography of activation across multiply measured brain areas, however, has been found not to parallel that of controls (Buchsbaum et al, 1990). Overall, it can be said only that the above configuration of findings is not incompatible with the cognitive behavioural concept of reduced efficiency in the implementation of processing capacity. In this spirit, and in a related context, Buchsbaum et al (1990) have stated, "Poor organization of task performance and activation of less appropriate, efficient, or capable brain areas might be a consequence of diminished frontal lobe functioning" (p. 225).

NON-FRONTAL AREAS

From the foregoing, the neuropsychology of delusions and hallucinations evidently implicates selected regions of the frontal cortex. Other areas also have been mentioned and it is to non-frontal areas that we now turn our attention.

The study by Bornstein et al (1990), cited above, reported findings on a "posterior index". This index consisted of an aggregate of measures, variously found to indicate the presence of posterior, non-frontal lesions. Secondary analyses indicated that paranoid patients scored significantly higher on this index than controls ($F(1/121) = 13.6$, $p < 0.001$). Following the authors' covariance adjustment, described in the preceding section, the among-group differences on the posterior index were attenuated and its component measures (e.g. finger agnosia, and graphaesthesia) either became non-significant, or at least were highly attenuated from their unadjusted values. As detailed earlier, statistical adjustment of this nature presents substantial interpretative difficulties. The initial unadjusted results suggest the possibility of deficit in functions identified with heterogeneous non-frontal areas.

What might these areas be? To address this question, we identify as much as possible the intersection between documented deficits among patients with the target symptomatology and those with known lesions or damage. To minimise unknowns, we restrict our focus by and large to performance under relatively similar experimental conditions; even so, some compromises remain, a point returned to later.

First, observe that paranoid schizophrenic subgroups appear to be less efficient than others in their mnemonic organisation of categorical word lists (Broga & Neufeld, 1981a). Their recall performance has been found to be inferior both to that of non-patient control subjects and closely matched non-paranoid patients. Additionally, evidence of categorising, according to quantitative clustering indexes, have been deflated. Neuropsychological studies of memory among patients with frontal lobe damage, on the other hand, do not indicate such deficits under similar performance conditions (Jetter et al, 1986).

A survey of other structures that may be implicated presents no unequivocal picture. Patients with left temporal lobe lesions, for example, have shown reduced clustering of categorical word lists, as well as high susceptibility to intrusions (production of words not previously presented), during recall (Hiatt, 1978). Patients with paranoid schizophrenia too have emitted increased intrusions, although during consonant trigram recall trials (Broga & Neufeld, 1981a). On the other hand, on serial position recall curves, left temporal patients also have shown evidence of a reduced "primacy effect "(the tendency for items to be better recalled when presented earlier in a list); such deficit has not been in evidence among paranoid patients (Broga & Neufeld, 1981a). Indeed, though not specifically in the form of serial position differences, non-paranoid patients have evinced heightened susceptibility to retroactive inhibition (Sengel et al, 1985). Furthermore, evidence of diminished rCBF among paranoid patients has been associated with the right rather than the left temporal region (Paulman et al, 1990).

Consideration might be given also to hippocampal functioning, as follows. Performance has been examined on a spatial memory task, slightly modified from one shown by Smith & Milner (1981) to be especially problematic for patients with ablations of portions of the hippocampus. Paranoid patients significantly have fallen behind controls in their performance of this task (Neufeld et al, 1995). Yet evidence presented by Hiatt (1978) has indicated that intactness of the hippocampus may not be essential to mnemonic organisation of semantically related words.

Another study examining word-list recall among paranoid schizophrenic patients is that of Sengel and Lovallo (1983). Like that of Broga and Neufeld (1981a), findings can be compared to those obtained from patients with known lesions or damage. In particular, comparisons are drawn to results from Jetter et al (1986), first, where their measures and performance conditions resemble those of Sengel and Lovallo (1983) and, second, where secondary analyses of the latters' results, addressing specifically paranoid patients' performance, are tractable from presented statistics. Note, however, that even with maximum matching, parallelisms are incomplete. Hence, the risk of drawing inferences about implicated brain loci, according to similarities in performance to patients with documented injury or lesions, is exacerbated by remaining differences in procedures and measures. For example, although declaring to subjects that presented words could be categorised, Jetter et al (1986) conveyed their items in scrambled order and did not declare the categories involved. Lists were presented twice, with a free-recall trial after each presentation. On the other hand, Sengel and Lovallo (1983) presented their lists once in blocks of category-related words and stated explicitly the categories involved.

This having been said, Sengel and Lovallo's paranoid (and non-paranoid) patients recalled significantly fewer words than depressives and normals, after a 10-minute delay, with an intervening cognitive task (Shipley Abstraction or Vocabulary Test). Frontal patients tested by Jetter et al (1986), tested fifteen minutes after list presentation, with no intervening task, showed no deficits relative to mixed non-frontal patients.

Turning to "categories recalled" (the number with at least one of their words reproduced), the closest conditions across studies under which group differences could be compared were as follows: Sengel and Lovallo's (1983) combination of "delayed and uncued" conditions, and Jetter et al's (1986) "free recall, same day, delayed" conditions. In this case, the paranoid (and non-paranoid) patients again were significantly lower than both depressives and non-patients. No group differences, on the other hand, were found by Jetter et al (1986).

Observe that the controls of Jetter et al (1986) were non-frontal lobe damaged patients, while those of Broga and Neufeld (1981a) were non-patients (and non-paranoids), and those of Sengel and Lovallo (1983) were depressive patients, normal subjects and, apropos the present context, non-paranoid patients. Quite possibly, if a non-patient group had been employed, differences between Jetter et al's (1986) frontal and non-frontal groups and the non-patient controls may have emerged, not unlike the present instances of paranoid–control differences. However, given the comparable performance between the frontal and non-frontal groups in the above instances, it still would not be possible to point to the frontal area as "the source" of the above instances of paranoid schizophrenic deviation from controls in recall performance. Frontal damage may be sufficient, but not necessary.

Finally, a distinction concerning stimulus encoding is in order. The deficit emphasised in the preceding section pertained to the translating of presenting stimuli into a task-facilitative format by implementing stimulus properties according to task demands mediated through working memory (Yates' "basic data assembly"; Yates, 1966). Encoding of this form denotes the investment of preliminary organising activity according to task requirements, as presented in pre-trial instructions. In the case of categorised word lists, especially those presented in an enriched, blocked sequence, stimulus features pertaining to task requirements more or less are self evident. Chunking of stimuli into categories of relatedness facilitates recall, and here the stimuli essentially operationally are "chunked" *ab initio* in their format of presentation. Mnemonic organisation, then, likely involves a lower level of "encoding" from that referred to earlier. The latter encoding may involve frontal and augmenting structures to a greater degree than does mnemonic organisation of enriched word presentations.

LATERALISATION ABNORMALITIES

A fairly prominent hypothesis has been put forth that paranoid schizophrenic subtypes suffer from overactivation of the left cerebral hemisphere (Gruzelier, 1981; Gruzelier & Hammond, 1980; see also Gruzelier, chapter 8). Supporting evidence, for example, has taken the form of possibly increased right hand grip strength (reviewed in Levin et al, 1989, p. 347), as well as apparently greater sensitivity to right ear stimulation in dichotic listening tasks (e.g. Lerner et al, 1977; Nachson, 1980).

Results bearing on this hypothesis, however, have been relatively inconsistent. They appear to be affected by experimental procedures, not the least of which comprise task format and modality of stimulus presentation. Such variations include the administration of psychometric tests whose scores are related to efficiency of certain left versus right hemisphere functions, dichotic listening, and visual field of stimulus presentation. George & Neufeld (1987) varied systematically the task demands embedding the recognition of items presented tachistoscopically in the alternate visual fields. Results concerning differential right-field speed of detection among the paranoid patients were negative (error rates were non-contributory). A very simple task, but one known to be relatively sensitive to differential hemispheric functioning, that of bisection of a line by traversing it to midpoint with the finger, produced similar findings (Mather et al, 1990). Using psychometric measures, Shallice et al (1991) found no evidence that performance neatly fell into a pattern signifying asymmetrical hemispheric activation. Finally, once again at some variance with the above hypothesis, there are observations from magnetic resonance imaging of selected brain regions reported by Williamson et al (1991). These authors reported that values of T2-weighted images, quite likely reflecting tissue pathology, were higher for the left frontal relative to left temporal regions among patients with comparatively higher scores on the SANS. Results for differing SAPS scores were negative. T2 relaxation values were also predominantly higher on the left side in the schizophrenic patient group compared to matched normals (Williamson et al, 1992).

Some of the early impetus for the left hemisphere overactivation hypothesis arose from dichotic listening experiments (e.g. Lerner et al, 1977; Nachson, 1980). For paranoid subgroups, "right ear superiority" in tracking presented stimuli appeared to be more pronounced than for others. A lesser cited study, but one highly relevant to this issue is that of Korboot & Damiani (1976). This study is noteworthy for its attention to detail in subject selection, stimulus presentation and response recording and quantification. Like that of Lerner et al (1977), the work stemmed from hypotheses set initially in terms of information processing (Yates, 1966; Yates & Korboot, 1970); the results, however, are potentially instructive regarding the issue of hemispheric activation. The following observations arise from secondary analyses of presented data as directed to the questions at hand.

First, during dichotic listening, both acute and chronic paranoid patients were significantly *slower* in shadowing specifically right ear stimuli (digits). Second, consider results from these investigators' signal detection task. We highlight conditions where the "signal" to be detected comprised a pair of successive identical digits to the right ear. Signal detection "false alarms" consisted of "signal present" responses to left ear presentations of the identical pair. The index of sensitivity to signal versus non-signal presentations, d', increases in this case as influence of right ear presentations dominates that of left ear presentations. For acute subjects (1–7 days since first admission), the value of d' for non-paranoid patients was significantly and substantially larger than that of paranoid patients ($F(1/14) = 222.66$, $p < 0.0001$). The percentage of variance accounted for by the source, diagnostic-group membership, in this comparison was 0.81, a value corresponding to a point biserial correlation between d' and group membership of 0.90 (e.g. Gardner & Neufeld, 1987). Associated values for more chronic patients (0.3–7 years since first admission), were in the opposite direction, paranoid patients' d' values exceeding those of non-paranoid patients ($F(1/14) = 8.46$, $p < 0.05$). Percentage of total variance in this comparison accounted for by group membership was 0.4826, corresponding to a point biserial value of 0.69. Obviously, the picture of paranoid–non-paranoid differences from dichotic listening tasks is quite mixed, with chronicity possibly playing a part in this mixture.

Let us return, for some final considerations, to the visual stimulus modality. In the study by George & Neufeld (1987), above, a highly significant interaction for response latencies was obtained between visual field of stimulus presentation and the type of target stimulus to be recognised. As might be expected, words were detected more quickly in the left hemifield, and pictures of faces, more quickly in the right hemifield. This effect statistically was invariant across groups, overall task load, and their combination. However, a main effect for groups indicated that, generally, the schizophrenic subgroups were slower at encoding the target stimulation. Once again, a 2×2 factorial data layout may be extracted from this configuration, by considering one stimulus type, words or pictures, at a time. The first factor is that of group membership: control versus paranoid schizophrenic. The second is one of hemispheric specialisation: more versus less specialisation, in the case of words implying the left versus right hemisphere. Stochastic modelling of response latency means and variances led to the conclusion described in the earlier section, Structure of Stimulus Encoding Deficit. Subprocesses of encoding the target stimulus were transacted at the same rate for both groups, indicating intact attentional capacity. The paranoid (and, separately, non-paranoid) schizophrenic subgroups applied this capacity less efficiently, however, in that additional subprocesses were required (Appendix A).

Note that a recent report by Elkins et al (1992) indicated a schizophrenic right hemisphere deficit in recognising briefly presented visual stimuli. In a modified Estes–Taylor (Estes & Taylor, 1964) span-of-apprehension task, the (mixed) schizophrenic group had a lower percentage of correct indications of whether one of two alphabetic letters was present amidst distractors, when items were in the left visual field. A close comparison between Elkins et al's (1992) paradigm (see also Breitmeyer, 1984) and that of George & Neufeld (1987), however, suggests differences that may reconcile the apparent divergence in findings. Elkins et al's results may be interpreted more or less as depicting performance under given time intervals *vis-à-vis* those of George & Neufeld, where subjects simply were asked to respond as quickly and accurately as possible. In the former study, an illuminated blank screen ended trials at specified times from display onset; this stimulus may have tended to interrupt processing (Dilollo, 1977; Miller et al, 1979; Elkins et al, 1992). Reduced accuracy attendant to a given interval of processing can be shown potentially to be compatible with the above interpretation of group differences in response latencies. A technical basis for this statement is presented in Appendix B. On balance, then, the findings for differential hemispheric processing of brief visual displays are in keeping with a (bilateral) reduced efficiency in the implementation of intact attentional capacity.

IMPAIRMENT OF INTERHEMISPHERIC COMMUNICATION

The suggestion of impairment in interhemispheric transfer of information (Green, 1978; Walker et al, 1981; see also Gruzelier, chapter 8) has been one rallying an appreciable amount of empirical attention. It has been suspected that deficient integration of processing for which the respective hemispheres are specialised may foster, for example, misinterpretations underlying thought content disorder and the disorganisation involved in thought form disorder, among other symptoms. Evidence surrounding this initially intriguing idea, unfortunately, of late has tended to be more negative than positive. Raine et al (1989) corrected methodological frailties of earlier studies in administering two batteries of tests differentially compelling cross-hemisphere transfer of information. Lack of support for the central hypothesis was fairly consistent in this study. Ditchfield & Hemsley (1990) as well improved upon the rigour of earlier work and found no evidence of interhemispheric communication impediments either among paranoid or non-paranoid subgroups. There was some indication of left hemisphere dysfunction on their manual performance tasks among the non-paranoid subgroup.

George & Neufeld (1984) presented stimuli consisting of pairs either of schematic figures, or names of items, to paranoid, non-paranoid and control groups. Subjects were required to indicate which item was the largest in its real-life size ("overall volume") or, in a second condition, which had the more pronounceable name (Paivio, 1975). It is conceivable that the verbal stimulus format was more conducive to left hemisphere processing and the non-verbal format to right hemisphere processing. To the degree that phonemic property and spatial property comparisons in a similar vein are differentially compatible with processing specialisations of the alternate hemispheres, the combinations of stimulus modality and property comparison in this experiment would be expected to instigate differing degrees of interhemispheric communication. Results from analyses potentially revealing impairment in this respect again were negative for both schizophrenic subgroups.

SUMMARY AND IMPLICATIONS

While neuropsychological deficits have been associated more frequently with non-paranoid patients (Crow, 1980), it is clear that patients with predominant delusions and hallucinations demonstrate neuropsychological deficits as well. These are evident in tests of frontal lobe functions such as the Wisconsin Card Sorting Test but are also seen in a variety of paradigms which depend on stimulus encoding. It is likely that a number of brain regions, including the mesial temporal region, participate in this process. However, evidence for a selective lateralised involvement is equivocal.

It has been suggested that patients with predominant hallucinations and delusions suffer from a different disease process possibly related to the dopamine system (Crow, 1980). However, more recent studies have failed to provide evidence of dopamine hyperactivity *in vivo* or in postmortem brain tissue (Crow,

1987; Carlsson, 1988; Reynolds, 1989). The absence of a linkage between the D2 dopamine receptor gene region and the presence of schizophrenia has been even more disappointing (Moises et al, 1991). These findings suggest that the primary neuronal abnormality may involve neuronal circuits utilising other transmitters and connecting prefrontal, temporal, and subcortical regions. It is tempting to speculate that these neuronal circuits mediate stimulus encoding and that deficits in stimulus encoding could promote selected positive symptoms of schizophrenia.

On a more general note, research activity on the neuropsychology of delusions, hallucinations and other symptoms has escalated in tandem with technological advances. The latter notably have involved PET and MRI measures. Such technology has enabled increased precision of measurement of brain activation patterns accompanying the performance of cognitive tasks. Prospects of more exact mapping of abnormalities in activation patterns accompanying impaired cognitive functions have risen substantially. We believe that, among other innovations, the implementation of quantitative models of cognitive-task performance will accelerate progress in mapping function–activation associations.

Such models foster a rigorous specification of cognitive functions involved in the negotiation of tasks, during which activation patterns are monitored. Examples of these "functions" include parallel versus serial handling of stimulus elements; number of constituent operations making up component cognitive transactions, such as stimulus encoding, memory search, visual scanning, and so on; speed of carrying out the constituent operations; deployment of attentional capacity across stimulus features, or stages of processing; and resistance to task-irrelevant stimulus features. Use of such models provides a means of specifying quantitatively alterations in functions at the root of observed deviations in performance speed and/or accuracy. The identified alterations, in turn, may be aligned with activation abnormalities.

With the use of formal methods, then, functional changes associated with psychopathology are described according to specific shifts in model structure and/ or parameters accommodating observed changes in performance measures. The implicated functions, in turn, may have symptomatological significance (e.g., Neufeld et al, 1993). If so, the functions presumably educe, as well, potential symptomatological significance of corresponding activation abnormalities along with candidate neuronal circuits on which they bear. Innovations in quantitative cognitive psychology relevant to this arena of investigation continue to take place (see, for example, Townsend & Nozawa, 1995). It is possible to adapt these methodologies to the exigencies of applied settings (cf. Neufeld & McCarty, 1994; Neufeld, 1995; McFall et al, 1995). We suggest that doing so will enhance precision of function measurement, facilitating advances toward the ideal of a "one-to-one mapping" of functional deficits and activation anomalies. Note that formal models also potentially accommodate the dynamic character of cognitive activities and activation patterns, in as much as the unfolding of events over time often is a main focus.

Perhaps one of the more important assets of formalising statements regarding hypothesised cognitive functions involves the salience of continuing ambiguities. Constraints of rigour in specifying cognitive operations imposed by formal procedures can help to throw into relief questions that remain unanswered (e.g., which of two or more cognitive functions may be responsible for observed deviance in task-performance). Pinpointing unresolved issues can help to restrain unwarranted claims and to identify areas where further developments in "function diagnostics" are needed.

ACKNOWLEDGEMENTS

Preparation of this paper was supported in part by an Operating Grant from the Medical Research Council of Canada, an Ontario Mental Health Foundation Senior Research Fellowship, and a Joey and Toby Tannenbaum Schizophrenia Research Distinguished Scientist Award to R.W.J. Neufeld, and by an Ontario Mental Health Foundation, Medical Research Council of Canada, and National Institute of Mental Health Operating Grants to P.C. Williamson. Material appearing in the appendices was prepared during a Visiting Professorship by R.W.J. Neufeld to the Irvine Research Institute for Mathematical Behavioural Sciences, University of California, Irvine. Thanks are extended to Ross Norman for comments on the original draft of this manuscript.

REFERENCES

American Psychiatric Association (1994) *Diagnostic and Statistical Manual of Mental Disorders*, 4th edn, American Psychiatric Association, Washington, DC.

Andreasen, N.C. (1982) Negative symptoms in schizophrenia. *Archives of General Psychiatry*, **39**, 784–788.

Andreasen, N.C., Olson, S. (1982) Negative vs positive schizophrenia. *Archives of General Psychiatry*, **39**, 789–794.

Arndt, S., Alliger, R.J., Andreasen, N.C. (1991) The distinction of positive and negative symptoms: The failure of a two dimensional model. *British Journal of Psychiatry*, **158**, 317–322.

Asberg, M., Perris, C., Schalling, O., Sedvall, G. (1978) CPRS—The Comprehensive Psychopathological Rating Scale. *Acta Psychiatrica Scandinavica*, **58** (Suppl. 271), 69.

Avery, T.L. (1971) Seven cases of frontal tumour with psychiatric presentation. *British Journal of Psychiatry*, **119**, 19–23.

Bartfai, A., Lavender, S.E., Nyback, H., Berggren, B., Schalling, D. (1985) Smooth pursuit eye tracking, neuropsychological test performance and computed tomography in schizophrenia. *Psychiatry Research*, **15**, 49–62.

Bleuler, E. (1911) *Dementia Praecox or the Group of Schizophrenias* (translated by J. Zinkin, 1950), International Universities Press, New York.

Bornstein, R., Leason, M. (1985) Effects of localized lesions on the Verbal Concept Attainment Test. *Journal of Clinical and Experimental Neuropsychology*, **7**, 421–429.

Bornstein, R.A., Nasrallah, H.A., Olson, S.C., Coffman, J.A., Torello, M., Schwarzkopf, S.B. (1990) Neuropsychological deficit in schizophrenic subtypes: Paranoid, nonparanoid, and schizoaffective groups. *Psychiatry Research*, **31**, 15–24.

Bourne, L.E. (1970) Knowing and using concepts. *Psychological Review*, **77**, 546–556.

Braithwaite, R.B. (1968) *Scientific Explanation*, Cambridge University Press, London.

Breitmeyer, B.G. (1984) *Visual Masking: An Integrative Approach*, Oxford University Press, New York.

Broga, M.I., Neufeld, R.W.J. (1981a) Multivariate cognitive performance levels and response styles among paranoid and nonparanoid schizophrenics. *Journal of Abnormal Psychology*, **90**, 495–509.

Broga, M.I., Neufeld, R.W.J. (1981b) Evaluation of information-sequential aspects of schizophrenic performance, I: Framework and current findings. *Journal of Nervous and Mental Disease*, **169**, 559–568.

Buchsbaum, M.S., Neuchterlein, K.H., Haier, K.J., Wu, J., Sicotte, N., Hazlett, E., Asarnow, R., Potkin, S., Guich, S. (1990) Glucose metabolic rate in normals and schizophrenics during the continuous performance test assessed by positron emission tomography. *British Journal of Psychiatry*, **156**, 216–227.

Burack, J.A., Zigler, E. (1989) Age at first hospitalization and premorbid social competence in schizophrenia and affective disorder. *American Journal of Orthopsychiatry*, **59**, 188–196.

Carlsson, A. (1988) The current status of the dopamine hypothesis of schizophrenia. *Neuropsychopharmacology*, **1**, 179–186.

Carter, J.R. (1994) Encoding for similarity judgements among paranoid and nonparanoid schizophrenics. Unpublished Master's thesis, University of Western Ontario, Department of Psychology, London, Ontario.

Carter, J., Neufeld, R.W.J. (submitted) A process model of salience deficits in multidimensional judgments.

Chechile, R.A. (1987) Trace susceptibility theory. *Journal of Experimental Psychology*, **116**, 203–222.

Cochran, W.G. (1957) Analysis of covariance: Its nature and uses. *Biometrics*, **13**, 261–281.

Cromwell, R.L., Dokecki, P. (1968) Schizophrenic language: A disattention interpretation. In: *Developments in Applied Psychology Research* (Eds S. Rosenberg, J.H. Koplin), Macmillan, New York.

Crow, T.J. (1980) Molecular pathology of schizophrenia: more than one disease process?. *British Medical Journal*, **280**, 66–68.

Crow, T.J. (1987) The dopamine hypothesis survives, but there must be a way ahead. *British Journal of Psychiatry*, **151**, 460–465.

Dilollo, V. (1977) Temporal characteristics of iconic memory. *Nature*, **267**, 241–243.

Ditchfield, H., Hemsley, D.R. (1990) Interhemispheric transfer of information and schizophrenia. *European Archives of Psychiatry and Neurological Sciences*, **239**, 309–313.

Dobson, D., Neufeld, R.W.J. (1982) Paranoid–nonparanoid schizophrenic distinctions in the implementation of external conceptual constraints. *Journal of Nervous and Mental Disease*, **170**, 614–621.

Elkins, I.J., Cromwell, R.L., Asarnow, R.F. (1992) Span of apprehension in schizophrenic patients as a function of distractor masking and laterality. *Journal of Abnormal Psychology*, **101**, 53–60.

Estes, W.K., Taylor, H.A. (1964) A detection method and probabilistic models for assessing information processing from brief visual displays. *Proceedings of the National Academy of Science* **52**, 446–454.

Farmer, A.E. McGuffin, P., Spitznagel, E.L (1983) Heterogeneity in schizophrenia: A cluster-analytic approach. *Psychiatry Research*, **8**, 1–12.

Fenton, W.S., McGlashan, T.H. (1991) Natural history of schizophrenia subtypes II. Positive and negative symptoms and long-term course. *Archives of General Psychiatry*, **48**, 978–986.

Fisher, D.L., Goldstein, W.M. (1983) Stochastic PERT networks as models of cognition: Derivation of the mean, variance and distribution of reaction time using order-of-processing (OP) diagrams. *Journal of Mathematical Psychology*, **27**, 121–151.

Frith, C.R., Done, D.J. (1988) Towards a neuropsychology of schizophrenia. *British Journal of Psychiatry*, **153**, 437–443.

Gardner, R.C., Neufeld, R.W.J. (1987) The simple difference score in correlational analyses. *Educational and Psychological Measurement*, **47**, 849–864.

George, L. (1985) *Structures and Strategies of Attention Deployment in Schizophrenia*. Unpublished doctoral dissertation, University of Western Ontario.

George, L., Neufeld, R.W.J. (1984) Imagery and verbal aspects of schizophrenic informational-performance. *British Journal of Clinical Psychology*, **23**, 9–18.

George, L., Neufeld, R.W.J. (1987) Attentional resources and hemispheric functional asymmetry in schizophrenia. *British Journal of Clinical Psychology*, **26**, 35–45.

Goldman-Rakic, P.S. (1987) Circuitry of primate prefrontal cortex and regulation of behaviour by representation memory. In: *Handbook of Physiology*, Vol. 5 (Ed. S.R. Geiger), pp. 373–417, American Physiology Society, Bethesda, MD.

Goldstein, G., Zubin, J., Pogue-Geile, M.F. (1991) Hospitalization and the cognitive deficits of schizophrenia: The influences of age and education. *Journal of Nervous and Mental Disease*, **179**, 202–206.

Gordon, A.V., Gregson, R. (1970) The Symptom Sign Inventory as a diagnostic differentia for paranoid and nonparanoid schizophrenics. *British Journal of Social and Clinical Psychology*, **9**, 347-356.

Green, P. (1978) Defective interhemispheric transfer in schizophrenia. *Journal of Abnormal Psychology*, **87**, 472–480.

Gruzelier, J.H. (1981) Hemispheric imbalances masquerading as paranoid and nonparanoid syndromes? *Schizophrenia Bulletin*, **7**, 662-673.

Gruzelier, J.H., Hammond, N.V. (1980) Lateralized deficits and drug influences on the dichotic listening of schizophrenic patients. *Biological Psychiatry*, **15**, 759–779.

Heaton, R. (1981) *Wisconsin Card Sorting Manual*, Psychological Assessment Resources, Odessa, FL.

Hiatt, G.J. (1978) Impairment of cognitive organization in patients with temporal-lobe lesions. *Dissertation Abstracts International*, **39(B)**, 1996–1997.

Highgate-Maynard, S. (1984) *Information Processing among Schizophrenics: Extraction and Manipulation of Nonverbal Stimulation*, unpublished Master's thesis, University of Western Ontario, London, Ontario.

Highgate-Maynard, S., Neufeld, R.W.J. (1986) Schizophrenic memory-search performance involving nonverbal stimulus properties. *Journal of Abnormal Psychology*, **95**, 67–73.

Humphreys, L.G. (1978) Differences between correlations in a single sample: A correction and amplification. *Psychological Reports*, **43**, 657–658.

Jetter, W., Poser, U., Freeman, R.B.Jr., Markowitsch, H.J. (1986) A verbal long term memory deficit in frontal lobe damaged patients. *Cortex*, **22**, 229–242.

Just, M.A., Carpenter, P.A. (1976) Eye fixations and cognitive processes. *Cognitive Psychology*, **8**, 441–480.

Just, M.A., Carpenter, R.A. (1987) *The Psychology of Reading and Language Comprehension*, Allyn & Bacon, Newton, MA.

Katsanis, J., Iacono, W.G. (1991) Clinical, neuropsychological, and brain structural correlates of smooth-pursuit eye tracking performance in chronic schizophrenia. *Journal of Abnormal Psychology*, **100**, 526–534.

Kay, S.R. (1990) Significance of the positive–negative distinction in schizophrenia. *Schizophrenia Bulletin*, **16**, 635–652.

Kay, S.R. (1991) *Positive and Negative Syndromes in Schizophrenia: Assessment and Research*. Brunner/Mazel, New York.

Kay, S.R., Opler, L.A. (1987) The positive–negative dimension in schizophrenia: Its validity and significance. *Psychiatric Developments*, **2**, 79–103.

Kenny, J.F., Keeping, E.S. (1965) *Mathematics of Statistics*, Vol. 2, Van Nostrand, New York.

Khurana, B., Kowler, E. (1987) Shared attentional control of smooth eye movement and perception. *Vision Research*, **27**, 1603–1618.

Kolb, B., Whishaw, I.Q. (1980) *Fundamentals of Human Neuropsychology* (2nd edn), Freeman, New York.

Korboot, P.J., Damiani, N. (1976) Auditory processing speed and signal detection in schizophrenia. *Journal of Abnormal Psychology*, **85**, 287–295.

Kowler, E., van der Steen, J., Tamminga, E.P., Collewijn, H. (1984) Voluntary selection of the target for smooth eye movement in the presence of superimposed, full-field stationary and moving stimuli. *Vision Research*, **24**, 1789–1798.

Lees, M.C., Neufeld, R.W.J. (1994) Matching the limits of clinical inference to the limits of quantitative methods: A formal appeal to practice what we consistently preach. *Canadian Psychology*, **35**, 268–282.

Lenzenweger, M.F., Dworkin, R.H., Wethington, E. (1989) Models of positive and negative symptoms in schizophrenia: An empirical evaluation of latent structures. *Journal of Abnormal Psychology*, **98**, 62–70.

Lenzenweger, M.F. Dworkin, R.H. and Wethington, E. (1991) Examining the underlying structure of schizophrenic phenomenology: Evidence for a three-process model. *Schizophrenia Bulletin*, **17**, 515–524.

Lerner, J., Nachson, I., Carmon, A. (1977) Responses of paranoid and nonparanoid schizophrenics in a dichotic listening task. *Journal of Nervous and Mental Disease*, **164**, 247–252.

Levin, S. (1984) Frontal lobe dysfunctions in schizophrenia. I. Eye movement impairments. *Journal of Psychiatric Research*, **18**, 27–55.

Levin, S., Yurgelun-Todd, D., Craft, S. (1989) Contributions of clinical neuropsychology to the study of schizophrenia. *Journal of Abnormal Psychology*, **98**, 341–356.

Liddle, P.F. (1987) Schizophrenic syndromes, cognitive performance and neurological dysfunction. *Psychological Medicine*, **16**, 49–57.

Liddle, P.F., Morris, D. (1991) Schizophrenic syndromes and frontal lobe performance. *British Journal of Psychiatry*, **158**, 340–345.

Liddle, P.F., Barnes, T.R.E., Morris, D., Haque, S. (1989) Three syndromes in chronic schizophrenia. *British Journal of Psychiatry*, **155** (Suppl. 7), 119–122.

Liddle, P.F., Friston, K.J., Frith, C.D., Hirsch, S.R., Jones, T, Frackowiak, R.S.J. (1992) Patterns of cerebral blood flow in schizophrenia. *British Journal of Psychiatry*, **160**, 179–186.

Magaro, P., Abrams, L., Cantrell, P. (1981) The Maine scale of paranoid and nonparanoid schizophrenia: Reliability and validity. *Journal of Consulting and Clinical Psychology*, **49**, 438–447.

Marks, R.C., Luchins, D.J. (1990) Relationship between brain imaging findings in schizophrenia and psychopathology: A review of the literature relating to positive and negative symptoms. In: *Schizophrenia: Positive and Negative Symptoms and Syndromes* (Ed. N.C. Andreasen), pp. 89–123, Karger, Basel.

Mather, J.A., Neufeld, R.W.J., Merskey, H., Russell, N.C. (1990) Schizophrenic performance on line bisection: No simple defects. *Journal of Psychiatric Research*, **24**, 185–190.

Mather, J.A., Neufeld, R.W.J., Merskey, H., Russell, N.C. (1992) Disruption of saccade production during oculomotor tracking in schizophrenia and the use of its changes across target velocity as a discriminator of the disorder. *Psychiatry Research*, **43**, 93–109.

Mattes, R., Cohen, R., Berg, P, Canavan, A.G., Ilopmann, G. (1991) Slow cortical potentials (SCPs) in schizophrenic patients during performance of the Wisconsin card-sorting test (WCST). *Neuropsychology*, **29**, 195–205.

McClelland, J.L., Rummelhart, D.E. (Eds) (1986) *Parallel Distributed Processing: Explorations in the Microstructure Of Cognition, Vol. 2: Psychological and Biological Models*, pp. 170–215, MIT Press, Cambridge, MA.

McFall, R.M., Townsend, J.T., Viken, R.J. (1995) Diathesis stress model or "just so" story? *Behavioural and Brain Sciences*, **18**, 365–566.

McGlashan, T.H., Fenton, W.S. (1992) The positive–negative distinction in schizophrenia: Review of natural history validators. *Archives of General Psychiatry*, **49**, 63–72.

Miller, L. (1984) Hemispheric asymmetry of cognitive processing in schizophrenics. *Psychological Reports*, **55**, 932–934.

Miller, R. (1989) Schizophrenia is a progressive disorder: Relations to EEG, CT, neuropathological and other evidence. *Progress in Neurobiology*, **33**, 17–44.

Miller, S., Saccuzzo, D., Braff, D. (1979) Information processing deficits in remitted schizophrenics. *Journal of Abnormal Psychology*, **88**, 446–449.

Moises, H.W., Gelernter, J., Giuffra, L.A., Zarcone, V., Wetterberg, L., Civelli, O., Kidd, K.K., Cavalli-Sforza, L.A. (1991) No linkage between D2 dopamine receptor gene region and schizophrenia. *Archives of General Psychiatry*, **48**, 643–647.

Morrison, D.G. (1979) An individual differences pure extination process. *Journal of Mathematical Psychology*, **19**, 307–315.

Morrison-Stewart, S.L., Williamson, P.C., Corning, W.C., Kutcher, S.P., Snow, W.G., Merskey, H. (1992) Frontal and non-frontal lobe neuropsychological test performance and clinical symptomatology in schizophrenia. *Psychological Medicine*, **22**, 353–359.

Nachson, I. (1980) Hemispheric dysfunctioning in schizophrenia. *Journal of Nervous and Mental Disease*, **168**, 241–242.

Neufeld, R.W.J. (1975) A multidimensional scaling analysis of schizophrenics' and normals' perceptions of verbal similarity. *Journal of Abnormal Psychology*, **84**, 498–507.

Neufeld, R.W.J. (1976) Simultaneous processing of multiple stimulus dimensions among paranoid and nonparanoid schizophrenics. *Multivariate Behavioral Research*, **4**, 425–442.

Neufeld, R.W.J. (1977) Components of processing deficit among paranoid and nonparanoid schizophrenics. *Journal of Abnormal Psychology*, **86**, 60–64.

Neufeld, R.W.J. (1978) Paranoid and nonparanoid schizophrenics' deficit in the interpretation of sentences: An information-processing approach. *Journal of Clinical Psychology*, **34**, 333–339.

Neufeld, R.W.J. (1990a) *Stimulus encoding in schizophrenia, and the capacity deficit hypothesis*, paper presented at the Meetings of the Society for Mathematical Psychology, Toronto.

Neufeld, R.W.J. (1990b) *Abnormalities in the lateralisation of functions in schizophrenia: The perspective of mathematical neuropsychology*, paper presented at Schizophrenia 1990: Poised for Discovery. An International Conference. Vancouver.

Neufeld, R.W.J. (1991) Memory deficit in paranoid schizophrenia. In: *The Cognitive Bases of Mental Disorders: Annual Review of Psychopathology* (Ed. P.A. Magaro), pp. 31–61, Sage, New York.

Neufeld, R.W.J. (1994) Theoretical stress and stress-proneness effects on information processing in light of mathematical models of stochastic processes. *Department of Psychology Research Bulletin No. 720*, University of Western Ontario.

Neufeld, R.W.J. (1995) Formal touchstones of abnormal personality theory. *Behavioural and Brain Sciences*, **18**, 567–568.

Neufeld, R.W.J., Gardner, R.C. (1990) Data aggregation in evaluating psychological constructs: Multivariate and logical deductive considerations. *Journal of Mathematical Psychology*, **24**, 276–296.

Neufeld, R.W.J., McCarty, T. (1994) A formal analysis of stressor and stress-proneness effects on basic information processing. *British Journal of Mathematical and Statistical Psychology*, **47**, 193–226.

Neufeld, R.W.J., Mothersill, K. (1980) Stress as an irritant of psychopathology. In: *Stress and Anxiety*, Vol. 7 (Eds I.G. Saraon, C.D. Spielberger), pp. 31–56, Hemisphere, New York.

Neufeld, R.W.J., Vollick, D., Highgate, S. (1993) Stochastic modelling of stimulus encoding and memory search in paranoid schizophrenia: Clinical and theoretical implications. In: *Schizophrenia: Origins, Processes, Treatment and Outcome* (Eds R.L. Cromwell, R. Snyder), pp. 176–196, Oxford University Press, New York.

Neufeld, R.W.J., Mather, J.A., Merskey, H., Russell, N.A. (1995) Multivariate structure of eye-movement dysfunction distinguishing schizophrenia. *Multivariate Experimental Clinical Research*, **11**, 1–21.

Nicholson, I.R., Neufeld, R.W.J. (1993) The classification of the schizophrenias according to symptomatology: A two-factor model. *Journal of Abnormal Psychology*, **102**, 259–270.

Nicholson, I.R., Neufeld, R.W.J. (submitted) The latent structure of paranoid and nonparanoid symptom distributions: A taxometric analysis.

Nicholson, I.R., Chapman, J.E., Neufeld, R.W.J. (1995) Cautions in the use of the BPRS in schizophrenia research. *Schizophrenia Research*, **17**, 177–185.

Paivio, A. (1975) Perceptual comparisons through the mind's eye, *Memory and Cognition*, **3**, 635–647.

Paulman, R.G., Devous, M.D., Gregory, R.R., Herman, J.H., Jennings, L., Bonte, F.J., Nasrallah, H.A., Raese, J.D. (1990) Hypofrontality and cognitive impairment in schizophrenia: Dynamic single-photon tomography and neuropsychological assessment of schizophrenic brain function. *Biological Psychiatry*, **27**, 377–399.

Pickar, D., Litman, R.E., Konicki, P.E., Wolkowitz, O.M., Breier, A. (1990) Neurochemical and neural mechanisms of positive and negative symptoms in schizophrenia. In: *Schizophrenia: Positive and Negative Symptoms and Syndromes* (Ed. N.C. Andreasen), pp. 124–151, Karger, Basel.

Raine, A., Andrews, H., Sheard, C., Walder, C., Manders, D. (1989) Interhemispheric transfer in schizophrenics, depressives, and normals with schizoid tendencies. *Journal of Abnormal Psychology*, **98**, 35–41.

Reynolds, G.P. (1989) Beyond the dopamine hypothesis: The neurochemical pathology of schizophrenia. *British Journal of Psychiatry*, **155**, 305–316.

Ross, S.M. (1983) *Stochastic Processes*, Wiley, New York.

Rosse, R.B., Schwartz, B.L., Mastropaolo, J., Goldberg, R.L., Deutsch, S.I. (1991) Subtype diagnosis in schizophrenia and its relation to neuropsychological and computerised tomography measures. *Biological Psychiatry*, **30**, 63–72.

Russell, P.N., Knight, R.G. (1977) Performance of process schizophrenics on tasks involving visual search. *Journal of Abnormal Psychology*, **86**, 16–26.

Schulderg, D., Quinlan, D.M. Morgenstern, H., Glazer, W (1990). Positive and negative symptoms in chronic psychiatric outpatients: Reliability, Stability, and factor structure. *Psychological Assessment*, **2**, 262–268.

Schweikert, R. (1989) Separable effects of factors on activation functions in discrete and continuous models: d' and evoked potentials. *Psychological Bulletin*, **106**, 318–328.

Sengel, R.A., Lovallo, W.R. (1983) Effects of cueing on immediate and recent memory in schizophrenics, *Journal of Nervous and Mental Disease*, **171**, 426–430.

Sengel, R.A., Lovallo, W.R., Pishkin, V. (1985) Verbal recall in schizophrenia: Differential effect of retroactive interference in nonparanoid patients, *Comprehensive Psychiatry*, **26**, 164–174.

Shallice, T., Burgess, D.W., Frith, C.O. (1991) Can the neuropsychological case-study approach be applied to schizophrenia? *Psychological Medicine*, **21**, 661–673.

Silbersweig, D.A., Stern, E., Frith, C., Cahill, C., Holmes, A., Grootoonk, S., McKenna, P., Chua, S.E., Schnorr, L., Jones, T., Frackowiak, R.S.T. (1995) A functional neuroanatomy of hallucinations in schizophrenia. *Nature*, **378**, 176–179.

Smith, M.L., Milner, B. (1981) The role of the right hippocampus in the recall of spatial location. *Neuropsychologia*, **19**, 781–793.

Snodgrass, J.G., Townsend, J.T. (1980) Comparing parallel and serial models: Theory and implementation. *Journal of Experimental Psychology: Human Perception and Performance*, **6**, 330–354.

Spohn, H.E., Strauss, M.E. (1989) Relation of neuroleptic and anticholinergic medication to cognitive functions in schizophrenia. *Journal of Abnormal Psychology*, **98**, 367–380.

Staddon, J.E.R. (1984) Social learning theory and the dynamics of interaction. *Psychological Review*, **91**, 502–507.

Steinman, R.M. (1986) The need for an eclectic rather than systems approach to the study of primate oculomotor system. *Vision Research*, **26**, 101–112.

Strauss, M.E., Sirotkin, R.A., Griswell, J. (1974) Length of hospitalization and rate of readmission in paranoid and nonparanoid schizophrenics. *Journal of Consulting and Clinical Psychology*, **42**, 105–110.

Suddath, R.L., Cassanova, M.F., Goldberg, T.E., Daniel, D.G., Kelsoe, J.R., Weinberger, D.R. (1989) Temporal lobe pathology in schizophrenia: A quantitative magnetic resonance imaging study. *American Journal of Psychiatry*, **146**, 464–492.

Taylor, J. (Ed.) (1932) *Selected Writings of John Hughlings Jackson*, Vol. 2, Hodder & Stoughton, London.

Townsend, J.T. (1984) Uncovering mental processes with factorial experiments. *Journal of Mathematical Psychology*, **28**, 363–400.

Townsend, J.T. (1990) Truth and consequences of ordinal differences in statistical distributions: Toward a theory of hierarchical inference. *Psychological Bulletin*, **108**, 551–567.

Townsend, J.T. (1994) Review of G. Karen, C. Lewis. A handbook for data analysis in the behavioural Sciences. *Psychological Science*, **5**, 321–325.

Townsend, J.T., Ashby, F.G. (1978) Methods of modelling capacity in simple processing systems. In: *Cognitive Theory*, Vol. 3 (Eds J. Castellan, F. Restle), Erlbaum, Hillsdale, NJ.

Townsend, J.T., Ashby, F.G. (1983) *Stochastic Modelling of Elementary Psychological Processes*, Cambridge University Press, London.

Townsend, J.T., Nozawa, G. (1995) Spatio-temporal properties of elementary perception: An investigation of parallel, serial, and coactive theories. *Journal of Mathematical Psychology*, **39**, 321–359.

Townsend, J.T, Thomas, R.D. (1994) Stochastic dependencies in parallel and serial models: Effects on systems factorial interactions. *Journal of Mathematical Psychology*, **38**, 1–34.

Vanderwolf, C.H., Robinson, T.E. (1981) Reticulo-cortical activity and behavior: A critique of theoretical theory and new synthesis. *Behavioral and Brain Science*, **4**, 454–514.

Vollick, D. (1994) *Stochastic Modelling of Stimulus Encoding and Memorial Comparison in Paranoid and Nonparanoid Schizophrenia*, PhD Dissertation, Department of Psychology, University of Western Ontario, London, Canada.

Walker, E., Lewine, R.J. (1988) The positive/negative symptom distinction in schizophrenia: Validity and etiological relevance. *Schizophrenia Research*, **1**, 315–328.

Walker, E., Hoppes, E., Emory, E. (1981) A reinterpretation of findings on hemispheric dysfunction in schizophrenia. *Journal of Nervous and Mental Disease*, **169**, 378–380.

Weinberger, D.R., Berman, K.F. (1988) Speculation on the meaning of cerebral metabolic hypofrontality in schizophrenia. *Schizophrenia Bulletin*, **14**, 157–168.

Weinberger, D.R., Berman, K.F., Daniel, D.G. (1991) Prefrontal cortex dysfunction in schizophrenia. In: *Frontal Lobe function and Dysfunction* (Eds H.S. Levin., H.M. Eisenberg, A.L. Benton), pp. 275–287, Oxford University Press, New York.

Williamson, P.C., Pelz, D., Merskey, H., Morrison, S., Conlon, P. (1991) Frontal MRI correlates of negative symptoms in schizophrenia. *British Journal of Psychiatry*, **159**, 130–134.

Williamson, P.C., Pelz, D., Merskey, H., Morrison, S., Karlik, S., Drost, D., Carr, T., Conlon, P. (1992) Frontal, temporal, and striatal proton relaxation times in schizophrenic patients and normal comparison subjects. *American Journal of Psychiatry*, **149**, 549–551.

Winne, P.H. (1983) Distortions of construct validity in multiple regression analysis. *Canadian Journal of Behavioural Sciences*, **15**, 187–202.

Wishner, J., Stein, M.K., Paestrel, A.L. (1978) Stages of information processing in schizophrenia: Sternberg's paradigm. In: *The Nature of Schizophrenia: New Approaches to Research and Treatment* (Eds L. Wynne, R.L. Cromwell, S. Matthysse), pp. 233–243, Wiley, New York.

World Health Organization (1994) *The International Statistical Classification of Diseases, Injuries, and Causes of Death (ICD-X)*. WHO, Geneva.

Yates, A. (1966) Psychological deficit. *Annual Review of Psychology*, **17**, 111–114.

Yates, A., Korboot, P. (1970) Speed of perceptual functioning in chronic nonparanoid schizophrenics. *Journal of Abnormal Psychology*, **76**, 453–461.

Zec, R.F., Weinberger, D.R. (1986) The brain areas implicated in schizophrenia: A selective overview. In: *The Neurology of Schizophrenia*, Vol. 1 (Eds H.A. Nasrallah, D.R. Weinberger), Elsevier, New York.

Zemlan, F.P., Hirschowitz, J., Sautter, F.J., Garver, D.L. (1986) Relationship of psychotic symptom clusters in schizophrenia to neuroleptic treatment and growth hormone response to apomorphine. *Psychiatry Research*, **18**, 239–255.

APPENDIX A

MODELS ACCOMMODATING ADDITIVITY OF $E(T)$, COMBINED WITH SUBADDITIVITY OF $Var(T)$, AND WITH ADDITIVITY OF $Var(T)$

First, note that additivity of $E(T)$ implies that the mixed second order difference in the expected total completion times is equal to 0 (Townsend, 1984):

$$E(T; x_{a(1)}, x_{b(2)}) - E(T; x_{a(1)}, x_{b(1)}) - [E(T; x_{a(2)}, x_{b(2)}) - E(T; x_{a(2)}, x_{b(1)})] = 0$$

Here, $x_{a(1)}$ and $x_{a(2)}$ denote the absence and presence of the focal symptomatology, and $x_{b(1)}$ and $x_{b(2)}$ denote the lower and higher values of the encoding load factor. Subadditivity of $Var(T)$ implies the following inequality:

$$Var(T; x_{a(1)}, x_{b(2)}) - Var(T; x_{a(1)}, x_{b(1)}) - [Var(T; x_{a(2)}, x_{b(2)}) - Var(T; x_{a(2)}, x_{b(1)})] < 0$$

Throughout, an increase in encoding load is implemented by an increase in the subprocess-number parameter, or where this parameter is stochastic, a change in its distribution toward increased probabilities of higher values. It is stated, without proof, here, that a change in the processing-rate parameter, or where this parameter is stochastic, in its distribution toward greater densities of lower values, would prevent the necessary configuration of $E(T)$ and $Var(T)$, regardless of the model, below.

In the first model, the rate parameter, v, is stochastic, conveying its random variation over trials. Its distribution is ordinary gamma (e.g. Kenny & Keeping, 1965) with parameters r and k. The base distribution, representing that of the given instances of encoding latencies, T, also is ordinary gamma, with parameters, v and k', the number of encoding subprocesses. Thus, we have a mixture on mixing variable, v. (This compound gamma distribution has some interesting properties, including conditions of moment tractability.) The mixture on v introduces a positive covariance across the k' stages of the base distribution, under certain conditions making for subadditivity of encoding latency variance, below.

In terms of this model, then, increased encoding demands imply an increase in k'. Impairment associated with paranoid schizophrenia may be represented by (i) a further increase in k', or (ii) higher densities of lower values of v, effected, here, through an increase in r. Case (i) represents added subprocesses and case (ii), the erosion of attentional capacity.

Convenient indexes of additive effects on $E(T)$ include the following: for case (i), the second order difference equation with respect to k' for the model-generated $E(T) = 0$. The first-order difference equation is

$$E(T)_{k'+1} - E(T)_{k'} = \Delta E(T)_{k'}/\Delta_{k'} = \Delta E(T)_{k'}$$

The second-order difference equation is

$$\Delta^2 E(T)_{k'} = \Delta E(T)_{k'+1} - \Delta E(T)_{k'} = E(T)_{k'+2} - E(T)_{k'+1} - (E(T)_{k'+1} - E(T)_{k'})$$

For case (ii),

$$\partial \Delta E(T)_{k'}/\partial r = 0$$

Proposition A.1

Given the representation of encoding latencies by a compound gamma distribution, with mixing parameter, v, the rate parameter of the base distribution, v being gamma distributed (see, for example, Morrison, 1979) with parameters r and k, and k' being the shape parameter of the base distribution, and given that increased task load implies increased k', additivity of $E(T)$, and subadditivity of $Var(T)$, will occur, (i) if impairment implies further increase in k', and (ii) will not occur if impairment implies increased r.

Proof

$$\text{Compute } E(T^n) = \int_0^\infty \int_0^\infty f(t \mid v) f(v) dv t^n dt$$

$$= \int_0^\infty \int_0^\infty (r^k t^{(k'-1)} v^{(k'+k-1)} e^{-(r+t)v}) / [(k'-1)! \Gamma(k)] dv t^n dt$$

$$= \int_0^\infty (r^k (k'+n-1)! \Gamma(k-n+1)) / [\Gamma(k)(k'-1)!(r+t)^{(k-n+1)}] dt$$

by a Laplace transform on $v^{k'+k-1}$, $\mathscr{L}\{v^{k'+k-1}\}$, $(r+t)$ being the parameter of transform, followed by integration by parts (elaborated in Neufeld, 1994). The solution to the foregoing integral then readily is available as

$$(r^k (k'+n-1)! \log(r+t)) / (\Gamma(k)(k'-1)!)]_{t=0}^{t=\infty}|_{k=n} = \infty|_{k=n}$$

$$= [r^k (k'-n-1)! (\Gamma(k-n) / (\Gamma(k)(k'-1)!(r+t)^{k-n}]_{t=0}^{t=\infty}|_{k>n}$$

$$= [r^n (k'+n-1)! \Gamma(k-n) / [(k'-1)! \Gamma(k)]]|_{k>n}$$

$$\text{Letting } k > 2, \quad E(T) = k'r/(k-1), \quad \text{and} \quad \Delta^2 E(T)_{k'} = 0;$$

$$Var(T) = E(T^2) - (E(T))^2 = [r^2 k'((k-1) + (k'))] / [(k-1)^2 (k-2)],$$

$$\text{and} \quad \Delta^2 Var(T)_{k'} > 0, \quad \text{as required}$$

Finally,

$$\partial \Delta E(T)_{k'} / \partial r = 1/(k-1) \neq 0$$

In the following model, both the rate of the base distribution, v, and its subprocesses, k', are distributed randomly over trials.

Proposition A.2

Given a second-order mixture, where the base distribution of encoding latencies, T, is gamma distributed, its rate parameter, v, also being gamma distributed with parameters r and k, and its shape parameter, k' being Poisson distributed, with parameter m, and given that increased task load implies increased m, additivity of $E(T)$, and subadditivity of $Var(T)$, will occur, (i) if impairment implies further increase in m, and (ii) will not occur if impairment implies increased r.

Proof

$$\text{Compute } E(T^n) = \int_0^\infty f(v) \sum_{k'=0}^\infty Pr(k') E(T^n | k' \cap v) dv$$

$$= \int_0^\infty f(v) E(T^n | v) dv$$

$$= \int_0^\infty [(rv)^{k-1}] / [\Gamma(k)] r e^{-rv} E(T^n | v) dv$$

$$= \int_0^\infty [(rv)^{k-1}] / [\Gamma(k)] r e^{-rv} m E(T_i | v) dv|_{n=1}$$

$$= \int_0^\infty [(rv)^{k-1}] / [\Gamma(k)] r e^{-rv} m E(T_i^2 | v) + m^2 (E(T_i | v))^2 dv|_{n=2},$$

since, based on Ross (1983),

$$E(T|m \cap v) = mE(T_i|v) \text{ and } Var(T|m \cap v) = mE(T_i^2|v)$$

where $E(T_i)$ is the expected latency for each of the k' subprocesses.

As the base distribution is gamma, with rate parameter v, $E(T_i|v) = 1/v$, and $E(T_i^2|v) = 2/v^2$. Consequently, allowing $k > 2$, upon solving the above integral for $n = 1$, $E(T)$ is found to be equal to $mr/(k-1)$, and $\partial^2 E(T)/\partial m^2 = 0$. Solving the above integral for $n = 2$, and then computing $E(T)^2 - (E(T))^2$, $Var(T)$ is found to be equal to $r^2m(2(k-1) + m)/((k-1)^2(k-2))$, and $\partial^2 Var(T)/\partial m^2$ becomes $2r^2/((k-1)^2(k-2)) > 0$, as required. Finally,

$$\partial^2 E(T)/(\partial m \ \partial r) = \partial(r/(k-1))/\partial r = 1/(k-1) > 0$$

Proposition A.3

Given a moderately limited capacity, independent parallel model, and given that an increased task load implies an increase in subprocesses, additivity of $E(T)$, and subadditivity of $Var(T)$, will occur (i) if impairment implies further increase in subprocesses, and, (ii) will not occur if impairment implies reduced processing rate.

This proposition will not be proven here. The model has been formulated by Townsend & Ashby (1983), and developments pertaining to the above proposition appear in Neufeld et al (1993).

We turn, now, to models generating additivity both of $E(T)$, and $Var(T)$.

The following model once again represents a mixture, but this time on k' only.

Proposition A.4

Given a compound Poisson distribution, whereby the number of subprocesses of the base distribution, k', is Poisson distributed with parameter m, and where the base distribution is ordinary-gamma with rate parameter v, and assuming that an increase in task load implies an increase in encoding subprocesses, additivity of $E(T)$ and of $Var(T)$ will occur (i) if impairment implies further increase in subprocesses, and (ii) will not occur if impairment implies reduced processing rate.

Proof

$E(T)$ for this model $= m(E(T_i))$, and $Var(T) = mE(T_i^2)$ (Ross, 1983), whereby $\partial^2 E(T)/\partial m^2 = \partial^2 Var(T)/\partial m^2 = 0$. As the base distribution is gamma, the subprocess (intercompletion) time, $E(T_i) = 1/v$. Consequently,

$$\partial[\partial E(T)/\partial m]/\partial v = -v^{-2} \neq 0$$

Proposition A.5

Given an ordinary gamma distribution, with parameters k' and v, and given that an increase in task load implies an increase in encoding subprocesses, additivity of $E(T)$ and of $Var(T)$ will occur (i) if impairment implies further increase in subprocesses, and (ii) will not occur if impairment implies reduced processing rate.

Proof

$E(T)$ for this model $= k'/v$, and $Var(T) = k'/v^2$. The necessary results follow obviously.

APPENDIX B

Proposition B.1

Additivity of completion-time latency, $E(T)$, does not imply additivity of percentage of correct responses, given a processing interval, t.

Proof

Let processing times be described by a compound gamma distribution. Then $E(T)$ will be additive under the conditions stated in Proposition A.1. Define the probability of a correct response as $F(t) + (1 - F(t))g$, where $F(t)$ is the probability of completing the processing necessary to an informed response, and g is the probability of a correct response strictly through guessing (e.g. 0.50, for a two-item recognition task). Note that $F(t) + (1 - F(t))g = F(t)(1 - g) + g$. As g is a constant, we focus simply on $\Delta^2 F(t)_{k'}$. First, compute, for the present model, $F(t)$:

$$\int_0^t \int_0^\infty f(t'|v)f(v)dv\ dt'$$

$$\int_0^t \int_0^\infty [r^k t'^{k'-1} v^{k+k'-1} e^{-(r+t')v}]/[(k'-1)!\Gamma(k)]dv\ dt'$$

$$= 1 - \sum_{j=0}^{k'-1} r^k \left(\frac{\Gamma(k+j)}{j!\Gamma(k)} \right) t^j/(r+t)^{k+j}$$

(Each term of the summation is a mixture on the rate parameter, v, of the Poisson probability of exactly j subprocesses occurring, given t, and is equal to the negative binomial for the probability of j failures before k "successes", given the special case of $t = 1 - r$, $r < 1$, and, as before, $r > 0$.)

$$\text{Compute} \quad \Delta^2 F(t)_{k'} \neq 0 \qquad \square$$

Inspection of response surfaces for $F(t)$ indicates that the subadditive or superadditive status of $\Delta^2 F(t)$ for a given t, varies with k, k', and r (Neufeld, 1994).

Addendum to Proposition B.1

$F(t)$, for an ordinary gamma distribution, with parameters k' and v, is

$$= \sum_{j=k'}^\infty (vt)^j/j!e^{-vt} = 1 - \sum_{j=0}^{k'-1} (vt)^j e^{-vt}/j! \ ;\Delta^2 F(t)_{k'} \neq 0$$

Comment

Emphasis in the above developments has been on processing structures and rates, with response selection and registration latencies being put aside for the present. Response processes are considered not to contribute to latency deviations of the schizophrenic patients discussed in this paper. Reasons for this position are enumerated in Neufeld et al (1993).

12

Abnormal Involuntary Movements in Schizophrenia and their Association with Cognitive Impairment

SIMON L. COLLINSON, CHRISTOS PANTELIS and
THOMAS R.E. BARNES

INTRODUCTION

In recent years, an increasing number of neuropsychological studies of schizophrenia have centred on the subcortex and allocortex as important sites of pathogenesis. While some authors have focused principally on limbic structures and
their cortical connections (Weinberger, 1991), others consider that the evidence
implicates the basal ganglia and diencephalon (Buchsbaum, 1990; Pantelis et al,
1992). Recent explanations have also suggested that schizophrenia may be a
"frontostriatal" disorder involving the selective dysfunction of circuitry subserving
the frontal cortex and basal ganglia (Robbins, 1990; Pantelis & Brewer, 1995 and
chapter 16). Increasingly, it has been suggested that localised dysfunction in the
subcortex may be responsible for some of the major cognitive abnormalities
underlying schizophrenia.

To date, much of the supporting evidence for a specific subcortical pathology in
schizophrenia has been derived from similarities with disorders affecting the basal
ganglia, such as Parkinson's and Huntington's diseases. Patients with subcortical
disorders often exhibit disturbances of behaviour, emotion and cognition similar
to those observed in schizophrenia and studies have reported a high incidence of
psychiatric morbidity, particularly in Huntington's disease (Jeste et al, 1984;
Shoulson, 1990). Furthermore, similarities have been reported in the neuropsychological profiles of patients with schizophrenia and those with basal ganglia

Schizophrenia: A Neuropsychological Perspective. Edited by C. Pantelis, H.E. Nelson and T.R.E. Barnes
© 1996 John Wiley & Sons Ltd

disorders (Reading, 1991; Pantelis et al, 1992; Joyce et al, 1996; Hanes et al, 1995, 1996). While these are important parallels, the defining clinical feature of basal ganglia disorders is the presence of abnormal movements. The presence of involuntary movements in a significant proportion of patients with schizophrenia has therefore been cited as supporting evidence for subcortical compromise in this disorder.

Although the presence of abnormal movements in idiopathic disorders is considered indicative of subcortical compromise (Cummings, 1986), it is only recently that they have been examined in the same way with respect to schizophrenia. Due to the widespread use of neuroleptic medication since the 1950s and the putative belief that abnormal movements emerged some time after their introduction, such abnormalities have traditionally been classified as iatrogenic. However, abnormal movements were considered an integral feature of the schizophrenic illness long before the advent of antipsychotic medication (Kahlbaum, 1874; Kraepelin, 1913; see also Rogers, 1992). Indeed, disorders of movement have also been observed in some but not all contemporary studies of patients with schizophrenia who have never been exposed to neuroleptics (Owens et al, 1982; Rogers, 1985; Waddington, 1989; McCreadie et al, 1996; Chorfi & Moussaoui, 1989; Moussaoui et al, 1992) and, more recently, there are reports of possible motor precursors of the illness in children who later developed schizophrenia (Walker, 1994; Walker et al, 1994).

Schizophrenia has been associated with a range of abnormal movements, usually referred to as catatonic symptoms, but also in these patients there are a range of medication-induced movements. The latter include akathisia, parkinsonian type symptoms and late-onset dystonia (for review: Barnes, 1988, 1990). However, the movement disorder which occurs frequently in schizophrenia and is perhaps the most suggestive of an insidious subcortical pathology, is tardive dyskinesia. Tardive dyskinesia is broadly similar in form and severity to disorders affecting the basal ganglia, such as Huntington's disease, and has in common with these disorders a late onset and chronic course. Importantly, basal ganglia disorders are also accompanied, particularly in their declining stages, by cognitive changes of varying severity. Given recent interest in basal ganglia pathology in schizophrenia it is relevant that there have been reports of similarities in neuropsychological profile between schizophrenia and the disorders affecting the basal ganglia (Hanes et al, 1995, 1996; Pantelis et al, in submission). Taken together with recent evidence suggesting that the basal ganglia are important in normal cognition, it is possible that the neuropsychological aspects of tardive dyskinesia may reveal much about the neural substrates of abnormal cognition in schizophrenia.

In this chapter we review the evidence linking cognitive deficits and tardive dyskinesia. We suggest a possible frontostriatal explanation for this association and present possible hypotheses. The importance of theory-driven research is emphasised including directions for future research. Finally, on the basis of the evidence outlined below, an approach is proposed which considers the reported association of tardive dyskinesia and neuropsychological deficits within the framework of a theory of brain reserve capacity.

OVERVIEW OF TARDIVE DYSKINESIA

Abnormalities of movement were described in schizophrenia prior to the introduction of neuroleptic medication. However, more recently the syndrome of tardive dyskinesia has been related to the use of neuroleptic drugs in patients with this condition. Although chiefly associated with schizophrenia, tardive dyskinesia has also been reported in patients with affective disorders (Kane et al, 1985), Alzheimer's disease (Molsa et al, 1987) and mental retardation (Gaultieri et al, 1986; Richardson et al 1986; for review: Waddington, 1989). With regard to schizophrenia, conservative estimates suggest that tardive dyskinesia occurs in approximately 15–20% of patients (Yassa & Jeste, 1992) but may range from 30% to 50% in older patients (Harris et al, 1992).

While dyskinetic movements may potentially be sited in any body region, they typically take the form of choreic movements of the perioral area, including tongue thrusting, chewing, pouting, lip smacking and sucking movements, grimacing or frowning (orofacial dyskinesia). A second group of abnormal movements is also common and consists of choreiform and athetoid movements of the trunk, limbs and distal extremities. These include spreading/flexion of the toes or fingers, choreoathetoid movements of the upper or lower limbs, or writhing twisting movements of the trunk (trunk and limb dyskinesia) (for review: Lohr et al, 1986; Barnes, 1990).

The neurochemical basis of tardive dyskinesia is thought to be dopaminergic. The putative explanation of the disorder is that long term blockade by antipsychotic drugs causes a compensatory proliferation of dopamine receptors in the striatum. This in turn leads to postsynaptic receptor supersensitivity and greater dopamine uptake. Greater uptake or increased sensitivity then results in an imbalance of dopamine–acetylcholine transmission in the striatum which manifests in hyperkinesis (Klawans et al, 1980). This has come to be known as the supersensitivity theory and has gained general acceptance. More recent explanations have incorporated the inhibitory GABAergic neurotransmitter system which is also known to modulate nigrostriatal dopamine transmission (Thaker et al, 1987, 1989).

Although the supersensitivity hypothesis provides a plausible explanation, there are specific criticisms of the theory (see Waddington 1992). For example, if neuroleptic exposure results in progressive chemical denervation of the striatum it would be expected that longer exposure or more concentrated exposure (i.e. greater quantities of neuroleptics) would result in higher incidence and possibly severity of dyskinetic movements. To date, this has not been established. Another major criticism is the fact that not all patients who receive antipsychotic medication later develop abnormal movements. This suggests that other factors operate in determining risk, which may be intrinsic to the individual or their illness, a consequence of some aspect of an individual's treatment, or a combination of these variables (Kane & Smith, 1982; Barnes et al, 1983).

Given the likelihood of individual or treatment risk factors, studies to date have sought to determine additional sources of influence which may predispose individuals to the development of abnormal movements. A number of variables have been suspected, including lifetime exposure to medication, electroconvulsive therapy (ECT), insulin coma therapy and duration of hospitalisation (for reviews: Barnes 1988; Kane et al, 1992). Presently, none of these have proven to be reliable predictors. However, specific signs suggestive of organicity have appeared which add to the suspicion of a predisposing neurological deficit. Among these are increasing age, negative symptoms, neurological soft signs and neuropsychological impairment.

THE INFLUENCE OF AGE IN TARDIVE DYSKINESIA

Although tardive dyskinesia can occur in young patients as little as 3 months after the introduction of medication, the disorder is more likely to occur in the later decades of life. A consistent finding in the literature is the correlation between the prevalence of tardive dyskinesia and increasing age (Kane & Smith 1982; for review: Waddington, 1989). In addition the expression of tardive dyskinesia varies according to age in terms of prognosis. For example, in a follow-up study over 3 years, Barnes et al (1983) found spontaneous remission in half of those patients who were under 50 years of age, whereas remission occurred in only one-third of those over 50. While some authors have reported that a linear relationship exists between tardive dyskinesia prevalence and age (Smith & Baldessarini, 1980), more recent studies using regression methodologies have reported age to be the only consistent predictor of tardive dyskinesia when other cumulative variables have been accounted for, such as lifetime hospitalisation, neuroleptic exposure and ECT treatment (Brown et al, 1992; Waddington et al, 1993). This contradicts the commonly held belief that age is merely a proxy for these cumulative treatment variables and suggests that the ageing process itself has an important role in the development of tardive dyskinesia.

The significance of age in the development of dyskinesias is further demonstrated when it is considered that such disorders occur in a sizeable proportion of the normal elderly without psychiatric diagnosis nor prior exposure to neuroleptics (Kane et al, 1982; Blowers et al, 1982; Blowers & Borinson, 1983). In a study examining the occurrence of orofacial tardive dyskinesia, Kidger et al (1980) compared a group of drug treated patients with schizophrenia with a group of normal drug-naive individuals across a large age range. These authors reported that neuroleptic-treated patients were most likely to exhibit orofacial dyskinesia in the sixth decade of life, whereas such movements did not appear in normal individuals until about 15 years later. This was interpreted as evidence that the administration of neuroleptic medication might hasten the development of orofacial tardive dyskinesia. More interestingly, the study provides evidence that the same pathophysiological process may underlie the development of dyskinesia in both the normal elderly and in patients with schizophrenia. While the exact nature of this process is unknown one possibility is that dyskinesias occur as a result of a failure to inhibit an inherent motor pattern, akin to a primitive reflex. The observation of primitive reflexes in newborns and in the elderly suggests that acquisition and retention of motoric control are dependent upon developmental processes which gain control with maturation (neuronal development) and lose control with ageing (neuronal attrition). This loss of control over inhibitory systems, especially in the cerebral cortex, may also occur in disorders such as schizophrenia resulting in involuntary movements (Rafal & Henik, 1994). The administration of neuroleptic medication may serve to accelerate this process of disinhibition, thereby bringing forward in time the emergence of tardive dyskinesia.

An important factor to emphasise in the above explanation is that the notion of a hypothesised cortical compromise leading to tardive dyskinesia may occur as a function of normal ageing or as a result of the schizophrenic disease process. That is, in the study by Kidger et al (1980) the patients differed from controls not only in their exposure to medication but also the pathophysiological processes that generate the symptoms of schizophrenia. Thus, a further possibility raised by this finding is that the pathological processes integral to schizophrenia might act synergistically with age (Liddle et al, 1993). If this were the case, then it might be predicted that, first, dysfunction of this system might lead to abnormal involuntary movements even in patients with schizophrenia who have never been exposed to neuroleptics. There is evidence to support this prediction, as suggested earlier. Second, it might be expected that tardive dyskinesia would be associated with particular symptoms of schizophrenia. In support of this prediction, as described below, both negative symptoms and cognitive dysfunction have consistently been associated with tardive dyskinesia, with the relationship being generally more robust for orofacial rather than trunk and limb dyskinesia.

RELATIONSHIP OF NEGATIVE SYMPTOMS TO TARDIVE DYSKINESIA

The presence of negative symptoms has been shown to be related to both normal ageing and tardive dyskinesia. Waddington and Youssef (1986a) found that negative symptoms occurred more frequently in patients with tardive dyskinesia when compared to age-matched controls. Davis et al (1992) reported significantly greater subscale scores of the SANS in dyskinetic patients when compared to non-dyskinetic age matched controls. In this study, higher scores were reported on avolition/apathy and anhedonia/asociality subscales. Similar findings have been reported by others (Owens & Johnstone, 1980; Itil et al, 1981; Waddington, et al, 1987; Karson et al, 1990; Manschreck et al, 1990).

In a recent study by Liddle and colleagues (1993) the presence of negative symptoms was proposed as a risk factor for the earlier development of tardive dyskinesia. In this cross-sectional study, the relationship between negative symptoms, age and tardive dyskinesia was examined. The prevalence of tardive dyskinesia was significantly greater in patients with negative symptoms compared to those patients without such symptoms. There was an interaction between the effects of negative symptoms and age in patients with orofacial tardive dyskinesia, such that the group with prominent negative symptoms developed orofacial tardive dyskinesia at an earlier age than those without negative symptoms. At the extremes of the age spectrum, the curves came together, so that any association with negative symptoms was lost. In addition there was no such association between trunk and limb dyskinesia and age. These results may explain the contradictory findings in this area.

Liddle and colleagues proposed that several different pathological factors act synergistically to bring forward the appearance of orofacial tardive dyskinesia in individuals with schizophrenia. With regard to the previously presented hypotheses, it would appear that there is a complex interaction between the ageing process, exposure to dopamine antagonists and the pathological changes underlying the schizophrenic illness, particularly those implicated in negative symptoms. This synergistic effect may act to accelerate the pathophysiological disturbance implicated in the development of tardive dyskinesia, especially orofacial tardive dyskinesia. What is unclear at this stage is which of these factors are directly implicated in the underlying pathophysiology of the disorder as opposed to those which act as catalysts in accelerating this process.

The common denominator characterising the factors which influence the development of tardive dyskinesia is that each involves compromise of brain systems. Other factors have also been implicated in this way, providing further support to the notion of organicity and tardive dyskinesia. In a study by Edwards (1970), organic signs were more common in a sample of elderly female patients without psychiatric diagnoses but who had developed tardive dyskinesia. More recently, Yassa et al (1984) investigated over 300 psychiatric patients and reported that significantly greater numbers displayed tardive dyskinesia when associated with an organic diagnosis. Associations have also been reported between the development of dyskinesia and head injury, epilepsy and mental retardation (Hunter et al, 1964; Crane & Paulson, 1967; Yassa et al, 1984; Barnes & Liddle, 1985). Further, in a recent study of alcohol use in patients with schizophrenia, the highest levels of alcohol use were associated with more severe orofacial dyskinesia (Duke et al, 1994). Thus, there appears to be a strong association between the presence of tardive dyskinesia and organic compromise. However, the exact nature of the involved neuronal systems requires elaboration. In order further to support this argument markers of organicity may be examined, such as the presence of structural brain changes, neurological soft signs and cognitive impairment.

THE NATURE OF BRAIN CHANGES IN TARDIVE DYSKINESIA

Clinical markers suggestive of structural pathology are reported in studies, such as that by Altshuler and colleagues (1988) who found significant asymmetry of facial dyskinesia in their sample of 27 patients. In this case there was a predilection for more severe movements on the left side of the face, although a previous study found a predilection for the right side (Myslobodsky et al, 1984). While these studies appear contradictory, such lateralised deficits implicate organic changes involving specific neuronal systems in tardive dyskinesia. In addition to these reports, a number of studies have found that dyskinetic patients display "neurological soft signs" more frequently than non-dyskinetic patients (Wegner et al, 1985; Youssef & Waddington, 1988; King et al, 1991). However, a recent study by Barnes et al (1995) found no relationship between primitive reflexes and tardive dyskinesia. From these studies, no specific sign has emerged to indicate a common site of dysfunction. Instead dyskinetic patients would appear to display more neurological signs overall than their matched counterparts.

Postmortem studies of tardive dyskinesia have revealed a non-specific pattern of atrophy in both cortical and subcortical sites including a number of reports of basal ganglia pathology, particularly in the striatum and substantia nigra (for review: Lohr et al, 1986). Neuroradiological investigations have also reported both cortical and subcortical changes. For example, Gellenberg (1976) reported diffuse cerebral atrophy on examination of computerised tomographic (CT) scans of eight patients with tardive dyskinesia, whereas other CT studies have reported increased lateral ventricle size and reduced caudate size (Famuyiwa et al, 1979; Bartels & Themelis, 1983). These results should be viewed cautiously, however, as recent magnetic resonance imaging (MRI) studies have failed to report any significant structural differences between patients with and without tardive dyskinesia (Elkashef et al, 1994; Waddington et al, 1995). Presently the small literature pertaining to structural changes is inconclusive.

TARDIVE DYSKINESIA AND COGNITIVE IMPAIRMENT

GLOBAL INTELLECT

Examinations of patients with schizophrenia and dyskinesia have generally sought to assess the presence of cognitive impairment by using short form measures of global cognition. A series of controlled studies by Waddington and colleagues (1985, 1987; Waddington & Youssef, 1986a, 1986b) have reported that dyskinetic patients with schizophrenia perform significantly worse than non-dyskinetic patients on such measures. Though some have failed to demonstrate any significant difference between tardive dyskinesia and non-tardive dyskinesia groups (Famuyiwa et al, 1979; Richardson et al, 1989; Karson et al, 1990) the findings of Waddington and colleagues have generally been supported by others using similar measures (Gureje, 1988; Davis et al, 1992; King et al, 1991; Manschreck et al, 1990).

While these studies constitute a great percentage of the neuropsychological investigations of tardive dyskinesia, interpretation of the findings should take account of the limitations of the short-form measures of cognition used. Although diagnostically useful, short-form measures such as the Mini Mental State Examination (MMSE) (e.g. Richardson et al, 1985; Davis et al, 1992), Ten Question Test and the Roth–Hopkins test (Waddington et al, 1986) assess only a small array of functions such as attention, orientation and immediate memory, and do not generally test conceptual abilities or abstraction. Furthermore, not all of these tests have been standardised against a normative or non-normative population. Without collaborative evidence drawn from standardised intelligence tests, it is difficult to determine whether tardive dyskinesia is associated with a specific type of cognitive abnormality.

Studies which have examined intelligence using standardised batteries have found contradictory results. Two studies (Wolf et al, 1983; Gold et al, 1991) failed to find any significant decrement in performance on full versions of the WAIS and WAIS-R. However, there were limitations to both of these studies, namely, the former sample consisted of less than 10 subjects, whereas in the latter only young patients with tardive dyskinesia were examined. In contrast, DeWolfe and colleagues (1988) examined an older, age-matched sample and found a significant negative relationship between severity of tardive dyskinesia and WAIS IQ. In this study, the magnitude of the association was influenced by the location of symptoms in that severity of orofacial dyskinesia was significantly correlated with nine of the WAIS subtests whereas trunk and limb dyskinesia was only significantly correlated with two.

In accordance with Dewolfe et al, Barnes and colleagues (1994) examined a cohort of 61 patients with schizophrenia and found that both orofacial and trunk and limb tardive dyskinesia showed significant negative correlations with current WAIS-R IQ. Further, the two subsyndromes of tardive dyskinesia were associated with a differential pattern of impaired performance on subscale scores from the WAIS-R. In another recent and well controlled study, Paulsen et al (1994) reported significant global impairment in patients with tardive dyskinesia when compared to a non-dyskinetic matched comparison group. In this study a large battery of tasks were administered and converted into a "global deficit score" as well as seven subscores (verbal ability, psychomotor skills, abstraction and cognitive flexibility, attention, learning and incidental memory, memory and motor skills). The severity of impairments in global functioning were found to be significantly related to both topography and severity of tardive dyskinesia.

The dissociation of topography of movement disorder on cognitive testing was also apparent when compared directly within groups. While these more recent studies have identified differential patterns of performance between orofacial and trunk and limb dyskinesias, earlier studies tended to find associations between cognitive measures and orofacial tardive dyskinesia but not trunk and limb dyskinesia. Indeed, Waddington et al (1993) reviewed the cognitive literature with reference to topography and suggested that the association of abnormal movements with cognitive dysfunction was more robust for orofacial dyskinesia. This is in accord with the findings of Liddle et al (1993) regarding an interaction between age, negative symptoms and orofacial dyskinesia specifically, as discussed above. Taken together these studies lend support to the notion of separate subsyndromes of tardive dyskinesia, with differing characteristics and neuropsychological profiles.

There may be a number of possible explanations for the differing characteristics of the two types of dyskinesia. First, it is possible that orofacial tardive dyskinesia is pathophysiologically distinct from trunk and limb dyskinesia and therefore represent separate "core" syndromes of the disorder (Waddington 1989). Another explanation, which would support the tendency for studies to find associations between neurocognitive measures and orofacial rather trunk and limb dyskinesia, might be that areas which are most susceptible to tardive dyskinesia, such as the extremities and buccolingual musculature, are affected as a consequence of their greater somatotopic representation on the cortex when compared to those of the limbs and trunk (e.g. as represented by the homunculus in the primary motor cortex). Such areas may be more vulnerable because the brain regions required to control fine movement are disrupted more easily than those which require less cortical control. Finally, it is possible that the distinction between orofacial dyskinesia and trunk and limb dyskinesia simply reflects the difficulty in detecting and rating distal abnormal movements (Barnes, 1990). The differing associations between these subsyndromes of tardive dyskinesia may have aetiological significance and future studies should investigate the two separately.

A factor which may explain the association between low scores on global measures of intelligence and tardive dyskinesia is the presence of bradyphrenia. Bradyphrenia, or slowness of thought, has been recognised as a core symptom of schizophrenia (for review: Pantelis et al, 1992) and is considered a characteristic feature of basal ganglia disorders (Cummings, 1986). Babcock (1933) hypothesised that abnormal slowness among patients with psychosis could account almost entirely for the general intellectual deterioration observed. Robbins (1990) notes that patients with this feature are often capable of completing cognitive tasks accurately if given adequate time. In the study by DeWolfe et al (1988), subtests of the WAIS which had the highest correlations with tardive dyskinesia had timed responses or penalties, suggesting that the greater cognitive impairment found in those patients with tardive dyskinesia could be accounted for by the presence of more profound bradyphrenia. The established findings of associations between negative symptoms and orofacial dyskinesia on the one hand and of orofacial dyskinesia and slowed cognition on the other provide some support for the notion of subcortical involvement in schizophrenia (Pantelis et al, 1992).

MEMORY AND LEARNING

In addition to impairments in global intellect, it has been suggested that patients with tardive dyskinesia are more vulnerable to disruption of learning and memory than non-dyskinetic patients. Studies which have examined global memory functioning have reported contradictory findings. DeWolfe et al (1988) found that severity of orofacial tardive dyskinesia was associated with impairment on a number of the summary indices of the Wechsler Memory Scale (WMS; Wechsler, 1974). In contrast, Wolf et al (1983) examined a small sample of matched dyskinetic patients with tardive dyskinesia on the WMS and reported no significant difference on summary scores. Similarly, Kolakowska et al (1986) used a series of verbal and non-verbal memory tests and failed to find any significant association between tardive dyskinesia and performance. However, the latter study only examined younger patients with the disorder. The methodological differences between these studies may help to explain these disparate findings. In particular, few studies have examined orofacial and trunk and limb dyskinesia separately while other studies have not examined patients across the age range. Another possibility is that global measures of memory are inadequate in delineating the nature of the memory impairment.

Many studies of memory have attempted to differentiate between deficits in recognition and recall as a means of distinguishing a failure to access stored memories and degeneration of the memory store, respectively. There have been relatively few studies relating specifically to tardive dyskinesia. However, Myslobodsky et al (1985) reported a significant difference between tardive dyskinesia and non-tardive dyskinesia groups on a picture recall task but not on a picture recognition task, suggesting difficulties in accessing stored memories. Furthermore, this pattern was evident even when those with low MMSE scores were excluded, thereby arguing against the possibility that such impairment was a part of a wider process of cognitive decline. In support of this study, Manschreck et al (1990) reported poorer recall memory but not recognition memory in tardive dyskinesia patients compared with controls. However, Sorokin et al (1988) found significant differences between tardive dyskinesia and non-tardive dyskinesia groups on both recall and recognition tests in the visual modality.

In addition to specific impairments of memory, impairments of learning have been reported in patients with tardive dyskinesia, although few studies have systematically addressed this issue. Famuyiwa et al (1979) examined a group of schizophrenic patients with and without tardive dyskinesia. They reported significantly impaired performance in the patients with tardive dyskinesia on a test of paired associate learning. This effect could not be explained by age. Further, Wolf et al (1983) reported significantly impaired performance of dyskinetic patients on a test of serial word learning, the Rey Auditory Verbal Test (RAVLT). In a recent study, Paulsen et al (1994) found significantly impaired learning in a large sample of patients with tardive dyskinesia when compared to a matched non-tardive dyskinesia control group. In this study, as already mentioned, a large battery of tasks were administered which provided a "global deficit score". In addition, seven subscores were derived relating to verbal ability, psychomotor skills, abstraction and cognitive flexibility, attention, learning and incidental memory, memory and motor skills. The groups differed only on the global deficit score and the learning subscore. These scores were also related to severity and topography of the movement disorder, specifically being associated with orofacial tardive dyskinesia.

While the above reported studies have identified deficits on declarative tasks, there has also been particular interest in non-declarative forms of skill acquisition. The latter, termed procedural learning, refers to the ability to acquire a motor skill through repeated exposure to a task. On these tasks, patients with schizophrenia demonstrate markedly reduced learning in comparison to normal controls (Schwartz et al, 1992). To date, few studies have specifically examined procedural learning in patients with tardive dyskinesia. Manschreck et al (1990) failed to find any significant differences between tardive dyskinesia and non-tardive dyskinesia groups on a maze learning test. However, in a study by Granholm et al (1993), increased severity of tardive dyskinesia was associated with poorer procedural learning. Using MRI, the authors also identified shortened T2 relaxation times in the caudate nuclei of these patients, suggesting pathology in the basal ganglia.

Before conclusions can be made regarding the status of memory and learning impairment in tardive dyskinesia, a number of potential artifacts should be considered. First, it is not entirely clear if impairments are part of a global intellectual decline or whether they are functionally and perhaps pathologically distinct from other changes occurring. However, in the few studies which have controlled for global intellectual deficits, memory impairments have been identified. Second, the influence of anticholinergic treatment on test performance has not been adequately established. These agents, which are used to treat extrapyramidal conditions and are known to affect normal memory function (Tune et al 1992), have not been accounted for in the majority of studies. Third, there are reports that patients with tardive dyskinesia demonstrate ocular motor and perceptual dysfunctions including impaired volitional/smooth pursuit eye tracking (Thaker et al, 1989; Henderson et al, chapter 13) and visuoperceptual function (Donnelly et al, 1981). This might account for learning and memory impairments tested via the visual modality in that poor performance is secondary to abnormalities in perception.

Differences between tardive dyskinesia and non-tardive dyskinesia patients on tests of memory and learning may provide important clues to the neural substrates implicated in the genesis of tardive dyskinesia. The finding that there are dissociations between recall and recognition memory between these tardive dyskinesia groups suggests involvement of subcortical systems, particularly those involving the basal ganglia. There is a growing understanding of the importance for the involvement of the basal ganglia in specific cognitive processes (Saint-Cyr & Taylor, 1992) which has mainly derived from neuropsychological investigations of disorders with known basal ganglia pathology, such as Huntington's and Parkinson's diseases, which have been described as frontal–subcortical dementias (Cummings, 1986). A cardinal feature of memory impairment in basal ganglia disorders is the finding of a specific pattern of impaired recall but intact recognition memory. This is reported in both Parkinson's disease (Tweedy et al, 1982) and Huntington's disease (Butters et al, 1976; Martone et al, 1984) but not Alzheimer's dementia (Zec, 1994). The interpretation of this pattern of impairment is that in disorders affecting the basal ganglia there is a failure to access memory, whereas in cortical dementia there is a degeneration of stored memories (Butters et al, 1985; Randolph et al, 1993). Further, impairments in skill-based (procedural) learning have been reported in Huntington's disease (Martone et al, 1984) but not in cortical dementias, such as Alzheimer's disease (Eslinger & Damasio, 1986). Given the striking similarities between patterns of neuropsychological impairment in these disorders of the basal ganglia and those found in patients with tardive dyskinesia, there is evidence to suggest the involvement of similar neuronal systems.

In summary, the evidence to date indicates marked impairment of memory and learning in patients with tardive dyskinesia. While such impairments could suggest limbic system involvement, the observed pattern of impairment in patients with tardive dyskinesia would appear to be more consistent with a frontal–subcortical dementia, as opposed to a classical amnesia. The impairment of recall but not recognition memory, the failure to learn new material, including the failure of procedural learning, and poor performance on tasks sensitive to executive dysfunction, such as the RAVLT (Lezak, 1995), suggests that impairments represent a failure adequately to commit and retrieve memories. Such impairments are characteristic of frontal lobe involvement but are also common in basal ganglia disorders. Given the neuroanatomical links between prefrontal areas, the basal ganglia and thalami (Alexander et al, 1986), it is hypothesised that disturbances in frontal–striatal–thalamic circuits are specifically involved in the development of tardive dyskinesia in patients with schizophrenia. Such a hypothesis would suggest that there is disturbance of prefrontal cortical function in patients with tardive dyskinesia.

FRONTAL-EXECUTIVE FUNCTION IN TARDIVE DYSKINESIA

Reports of poor performance on frontal-executive tasks have been repeatedly observed in the literature. Wegner et al (1985) reported significant impairment on a traditional test of frontal function, the Trail Making Test, in patients with tardive dyskinesia in comparison to controls. Furthermore, these differences were observed after the influence of movement errors and medication exposure were accounted for. This was later replicated by O'Callaghan et al (1990) who examined a number of likely sources of organicity and found the primary variable associated with tardive dyskinesia was performance on the trails B section of the Trail Making Test.

In a recent study using regression analysis, Waddington et al (1993) found performance on the Trail Making Test to be the only significant independent predictor of tardive dyskinesia when examined with other putative markers of organicity. More recently, Waddington and co-workers (1995) found evidence of executive dysfunction using the Wisconsin Card Sorting Test (WCST) in that patients with orofacial tardive dyskinesia achieved fewer categories than non-dyskinetic patients. Interestingly, this study was performed on groups of young patients in their mid thirties who could not be distinguished by age. This may suggest that frontal lobe deficits precede the development of chronic dyskinesia by decades.

The relationship between tardive dyskinesia, negative symptoms and executive function was examined by Brown and colleagues (Brown & White, 1991; Brown et al, 1992). In their first study, the authors reported that patients with negative symptoms had more severe dyskinesia and poorer performance on three separate tests sensitive to frontal lobe function. The authors also reported a significant association between negative symptoms and cognition, although, with the exception of WCST perseveration score, this relationship did not withstand correction for the presence of tardive dyskinesia. In a follow-up study, Brown and colleagues (1992) established a significant linear relationship between frontal lobe test performance and tardive dyskinesia which remained after global impairment (MMSE) and negative symptoms had been accounted for.

The discovery of frontal-executive impairments in patients with tardive dyskinesia is interesting in relation to the commonly reported association of frontal impairments and negative symptoms in schizophrenia. As previously reported, Liddle and colleagues (1993) found that negative symptoms were a risk factor in the precocious development of tardive dyskinesia and it has been suggested that the pathological processes underlying the development of negative symptoms may also be implicated in tardive dyskinesia. The discovery of a neuropsychological impairment common to both phenomena emphasises the possibility of a shared pathophysiological basis for tardive dyskinesia and negative symptoms, specifically implicating frontal–subcortical systems. Such an association may be relevant to our understanding of the underlying disturbance inherent to schizophrenia (for review: Pantelis & Brewer, 1995 and chapter 16).

While there is evidence to suggest that tardive dyskinesia is associated with impairments in executive functioning, the specific pattern of frontal deficits in patients with tardive dyskinesia has yet to be fully described. In recent work comparing patients with frontal lesions and those with abnormalities of movement secondary to basal ganglia pathology, separable patterns of deficits have been identified. In a series of studies of patients with frontal lobe lesions, Parkinson's disease, multiple system atrophy, and progressive supranuclear palsy syndrome, subjects were examined using a battery of tasks deemed sensitive to frontal–striatal dysfunction (Owen et al, 1990, 1991, 1992; Robbins et al, 1994). While patients displayed some similarities in the overall pattern of performance on these tasks, some characteristic differences emerged in patients with striatal pathology as compared to the frontal lesioned group. Such investigations, using tasks which identify specific patterns of neuropsychological deficits in patients with known pathology, may help to inform investigations regarding the pathophysiological basis of tardive dyskinesia, with specific regard to the nature of frontal–striatal compromise.

In terms of the cognitive processes subserved by the frontal lobes, it has been proposed that a fundamental component of tasks of executive function is the requirement to inhibit inappropriate or overlearned responses to meet challenging circumstances. For example, the failure to shift set on tasks such as the Wisconsin Card Sorting Test or section B of the Trail Making task may be interpreted as a failure to inhibit a previously acquired schema. Therefore, the above findings would be consistent with the notion that patients with tardive dyskinesia have significant difficulty in the inhibition of a previously learned response such that they perform poorly on tasks involving shifts between different modes of responding. With regard to the previously presented hypothesis pertaining to the relationship between ageing and tardive dyskinesia it is interesting that schizophrenic patients with the disorder display more significant impairments than their non-dyskinetic counterparts. It has been proposed that the presence of abnormal movements in itself is suggestive of disinhibition in that they occur as a consequence of a loss of control over previously inhibited motoric reflexes. Thus, it is possible to conceptualise tardive dyskinesia as a disorder of disinhibition such that both the involuntary movements and the neuropsychological deficits inherent to the phenomena represent an inability to inhibit instinctive, environmentally driven responses.

Further evidence of inhibitory failure in patients with tardive dyskinesia has been reported in studies of ocular motor function (Spohn et al, 1985; Spohn & Coyne, 1993). In these studies, patients with tardive dyskinesia were shown to have impaired eye tracking and an increased rate of scanning. The implication of these findings is that the pathophysiological processes underlying tardive dyskinesia are also involved in the disinhibition of eye movements. In a study by

Thaker et al (1989) patients were required to perform a task which involved the inhibition of saccades to a peripheral stimulus. They found a two-fold increase in oculomotor distractibility in schizophrenic patients with tardive dyskinesia when compared to matched non-dyskinetic patients and normal controls. The authors explained their findings in terms of disruption of inhibitory pathways in the basal ganglia which are involved in eye movements. Such pathways have intimate connections with prefrontal cortical areas, particularly involving the frontal eye fields. Future studies which examine inhibitory processes in patients with tardive dyskinesia may serve to clarify the neural mechanisms of disinhibition.

TARDIVE DYSKINESIA AS A FRONTAL–STRIATAL DISORDER

The evidence cited implicates disruption to both prefrontal and striatal areas in patients with tardive dyskinesia. A framework to interpret these findings is provided by the recent characterisation of five parallel segregated circuits subserving the prefrontal cortex via reciprocal connections through the basal ganglia and thalamus (Alexander et al, 1986; Delong et al 1990). The anatomical proximity of these frontal–striatal–thalamic circuits may help to explain the co-occurrence of both frontal and subcortical patterns of neuropsychological impairment in tardive dyskinesia. These pathways are organised such that they originate in separate areas of the prefrontal cortex, remaining parallel and segregated as they converge within the basal ganglia. Thus, disturbances in the subcortex may result in a more diverse range of symptoms and neuropsychological impairments than more circumscribed lesions of the prefrontal cortex (Pantelis & Nelson, 1994). The observation that there are similar impairments of movement, affect and cognition in neurological disorders involving the basal ganglia supports this hypothesis.

It is possible to conceptualise the association of negative symptoms, abnormal movements and impaired cognition in terms of deafferentation of prefrontal areas at the level of the subcortex (Pantelis et al, 1992; Pantelis & Nelson, 1994). Of particular relevance to the neuropsychology of schizophrenia are the three circuits which subserve cognitive function, that is, those involving the dorsolateral and orbitofrontal cortices and the anterior cingulate (Robbins, 1990; Pantelis & Brewer, 1995 and chapter 16). The motor loop which terminates in the supplementary motor area may be of specific relevance to tardive dyskinesia (Gold et al, 1992). Further, evidence from ocular motor studies, cited earlier, implicates a second motor circuit involving frontal eye fields. These frontal–striatal–thalamic circuits may be relevant to understanding the hypothesised disinhibitory processes underlying tardive dyskinesia.

The implication of these separable loops is that they each subserve separable cognitive operations. However, these "circuit-specific" impairments are difficult to isolate primarily because the loops are unlikely to work in isolation and, if lesioned at the level of the basal ganglia, more than one circuit is likely to be affected by the insult (Pantelis & Nelson, 1994). Given the evidence that the neuropsychological impairments in schizophrenic patients with dyskinesia are more severe than those of non-dyskinetic patients, it is likely that the involvement of the loops is in some way different between the two groups. Investigations which explore the functions of individual loops may help to clarify this hypothesis. The notion of "circuit-specific" (or "network-specific") impairments is discussed further by Pantelis and Brewer (chapter 16).

TARDIVE DYSKINESIA AND BRAIN RESERVE CAPACITY

While the association of abnormal movements with cognitive and other symptomological factors would seem robust, as yet there is still no explanation as to why some patients develop abnormal movements while others do not. One explanation which may account for the available evidence is provided by Satz (1993) who proposes the theoretical notion of "brain reserve" to explain individual differences which determine the onset of clinical symptoms.

It is well known that individuals with degenerative disorders, such as Parkinson's disease, Huntington's disease and Alzheimer's dementia differ markedly in the age at which symptoms occur (Roth, 1994). Furthermore, such patients show qualitative differences in cognitive functioning from the normal age related cognitive changes. It is conceivable, therefore, that these differences are mediated by an individual's ability to withstand cerebral pathological changes. Such explanations imply that individuals differ in the degree of cerebral insult sustainable before overt symptoms become manifest. In essence, Satz's (1993) model seeks to explain threshold differences in degenerative disease in the light of possible predisposing and protective factors. Within this formulation brain insult can be degenerative or traumatic, however, it is central that thresholds of neuronal attrition exist and must be exceeded before the clinical features of a disorder are overt. The model proposes that the level of this threshold is mediated by each individual's "brain reserve capacity" (BRC). Brain reserve is operationally defined by anatomical parameters such as overall brain weight or psychosocial measures, such as level of general intelligence or education. Thus, increased brain weight or higher intelligence acts as protection against degeneration or injury, whereas low IQ or low brain weight confers vulnerability. Included in the theory are a number of sub-postulates which suggest that, under sufficient challenge, subthreshold injury will become overt as a result of multiple factors which have aggregate effects, such as secondary lesions or neuronal attrition with ageing.

As also suggested by Satz, this notion can be directly applied to tardive dyskinesia. In this disorder, the combined effects of ageing and exposure to neuroleptics are considered compounding factors in lowering the threshold at which abnormal movements become overt. In this respect, prolonged chemical denervation of dopamine containing cells in the striatum, in conjunction with normal neuronal attrition, results in supersensitivity and the presence of abnormal movements. When the additional effects of a possible disease or developmental process are also considered, such as schizophrenia, it is likely that the threshold of brain reserve in these patients may be dramatically lower than in the normal brain. This would explain why abnormal movements develop in schizophrenia decades before they appear in the normal elderly population.

Satz's theory provides an explanation for individual vulnerability to the development of tardive dyskinesia. A paradox of tardive dyskinesia is that while all patients with schizophrenia are subject to the effects of neuroleptic exposure, increasing age and the disease itself, not all develop the disorder. Within the theory, it is possible to account for this discrepancy as a function of the individuals' brain reserve. Hence, factors which confer greater brain reserve, such as greater neuronal density, are protective against the prolonged denervation caused by pathogenic factors. As such, indices of BRC, such as high intelligence, would be expected to be associated with lower risk of developing abnormal movements. This prediction was supported by a cross-sectional study of patients with chronic schizophrenia (Collinson et al, 1994) which found an interaction between age and current WAIS-R IQ, such that patients with low IQ were found to have tardive dyskinesia at a younger age than non-dyskinetic patients. While cross-sectional studies provide evidence to support the notion of BRC in tardive dyskinesia, the application of longitudinal research designs are required to examine this question more conclusively.

SUMMARY AND CONCLUSIONS

The purpose of this chapter has been to explore the nature of the underlying pathophysiological basis of tardive dyskinesia and its implications for our understanding of schizophrenia. Research has shown that there are a number of factors implicated in the genesis of the disorder and it has been proposed that increasing age, neuroleptic medication and negative symptoms act synergistically to bring forward in time the onset of tardive dyskinesia in patients with schizophrenia (Liddle et al, 1993). That there is some organic pathology underlying the onset of abnormal movements is suggested by the fact that each of these risk factors is associated with cerebral compromise. In addition, studies have shown that patients with known organic pathology also display dyskinetic movements.

Recent neuropsychological research has also provided evidence for an organic basis to tardive dyskinesia. Studies have shown that patients with tardive dyskinesia have greater cognitive impairments than their non-dyskinetic counterparts on tests of global intellect. When more specific functions are examined, patients with orofacial dyskinesia have been shown to display deficits on tasks of executive functioning and in learning and memory. The pattern of neuropsychological impairment found in patients with tardive dyskinesia has been likened to that of patients with basal ganglia pathology and it has been hypothesised that the existing findings suggest a pattern of neuropsychological impairment consistent with disturbances of frontal–striatal–thalamic circuitry.

An interesting corollary to the neuropsychological studies is the suggestion that tardive dyskinesia is reflective of a more general failure of inhibitory processes. It is possible to conceptualise tardive dyskinesia as a disorder of disinhibition such that both the motor disturbances and the cognitive impairment reflect an inability to inhibit instinctive, environmentally driven responses. This notion of disinhibition has been linked to the process of neuronal attrition which is thought to occur as a consequence of ageing and is perhaps exacerbated by the schizophrenic disease process itself. Within this context the propensity to the development of tardive dyskinesia may be understood by the concept of a "brain reserve capacity" which corresponds to the level of neuronal redundancy within the brain.

REFERENCES

Alexander, G.E., DeLong, M., Strick, P.E. (1986) Parallel organization of functionally segregated circuits linking basal ganglia and cortex. *Annual Review of Neuroscience*, **9**, 357–381.

Altshuler, L.L., Cummings, J.L., Bartzokis, G., Hill, M.A., May, P.R.A.(1988) Lateral asymmetries of tardive dyskinesia in schizophrenia. *Biological Psychiatry*, **24**, 83–86.

Babcock, H. (1933) *Dementia Praecox, a Psychological Study*, The Science Press, Lancaster, Philadelphia.

Barnes, T.R.E. (1988) Tardive dyskinesia: Risk factors, pathophysiology and treatment. *Recent Advances in Clinical Psychiatry*, **6**, 185–207.

Barnes T.R.E (1990) Movement disorders associated with antipsychotic drugs: The tardive syndromes. *International Review of Psychiatry*, **2**, 355–366.

Barnes, T.R.E., Crichton, P., Nelson., H.E., Halstead, S. (1995) Primitive (developmental) reflexes, tardive dyskinesia and intellectual impairment in schizophrenia. *Schizophrenia Research*, **16**, 47–52.

Barnes, T.R.E., Kidger, T., Gore, S.M. (1983) Tardive dyskinesia: A 3-year follow-up study. *Psychological Medicine*, **13**, 71–81.

Barnes, T.R.E., Liddle, P.F. (1985) Tardive dyskinesia: implications for schizophrenia. In: *Schizophrenia: New Pharmacological and Clinical Developments* (Eds M.A. Schiff, M. Roth, H.L. Freeman), pp. 81–88, Royal Society of Medicine Services International Conference and Symposium, Series 94, UK.

Barnes, T.R.E., Pantelis, C., Collinson, S., Nelson, H.E., Carruthers, K., Halstead, S.M. (1994) Relationship between tardive dyskinesia, intellectual impairment and bradyphrenia in a chronic schizophrenic inpatient population. *Schizophrenia Research*, **11**, 192.

Bartels, M., Themelis, J. (1983) Computerised tomography in TD: Evidence of structural abnormalities in the basal ganglia system. *Archives of Psychiatry and Neurological Sciences*, **233**, 371–329.

Blowers, A.J., Borinson, R.L. (1983) Dyskinesias in the geriatric population. *Brain Research Bulletin*, **11**, 175–178.

Blowers, A.J., Borinson, R.L., Blowers, C.M. et al (1982) Abnormal involuntary movements in the elderly. *British Journal of Psychiatry*, **139**, 363–364.

Brown, K.W., White, T. (1991) The association among negative symptoms, movement disorders, and frontal lobe psychological deficits in schizophrenic patients. *Biological Psychiatry*, **30**, 1182–1190.

Brown, K.W., White, T., Palmer, D. (1992) Movement disorders and psychological tests of frontal lobe function in schizophrenic patients. *Psychological Medicine*, **22**, 69–77.

Buchsbaum, M.S. (1990) The frontal lobes, basal ganglia, temporal lobes as sites for schizophrenia. *Schizophrenia Bulletin*, **16**, 379–390.

Butters, N., Tarlow, S., Cermak, L.S., Sax, D. (1976) A comparison of the information processing deficits of patients with Huntington's chorea and Korsakoff's syndrome. *Cortex*, **12**, 134–144.

Butters, N., Wolfe, J., Martone, M., Granholm, E., Cermak, L.S. (1985) Memory disorders associated with Huntington's disease: verbal recall, verbal recognition and procedural memory. *Neuropsychologia*, **23**, 729–743.

Chorfi, M., Moussaoui, D. (1989) Lack of dyskinesias in unmedicated schizophrenics. *Psychopharmacology*, **97**, 423.

Collinson, S.L., Barnes, T.R.E., Pantelis, C., Nelson, H.E., Carruthers, K., Halstead, S. (1994) Level and Speed of Cognitive Functioning in Schizophrenia with Tardive Dyskinesia. *Proceedings of the Australian Society for Psychiatric Research (Perth)*, (Abstract).

Crane, G.E., Paulson, G. (1967) Involuntary movements in a sample of chronic mental patients and their relation to treatment with neuroleptics. *International Journal of Neuropsychiatry*, **3**, 286–291.

Cummings, J.L. (1986) Subcortical dementia: Neuropsychology, neuropsychiatry, and pathophysiology. *British Journal of Psychiatry*, **149**, 682–697.

Davis, E.J.B., Borde, M., Sharma, L.N. (1992) TD and type II schizophrenia. *British Journal of Psychiatry*, **160**, 253–256.

DeLong, M.R., Alexander, G.E., Miller, W.C., Crutcher, M.D. (1990) Anatomical and functional aspects of basal ganglia–thalamocortical circuits. In: *Function and Dysfunction in the Basal Ganglia* (Eds A.J. Franks, J.W. Ironside, H.S. Mindham, R.J. Smith, E.G.S. Spokes, W. Winlow), pp. 3–32, Manchester University Press, Manchester.

DeWolfe, A.S., Ryan, J.J., Wolf, M.E. (1988) Cognitive sequelae of tardive dyskinesia. *Journal of Nervous and Mental Disorders*, **176**, 270–274.

Donnelly, E.F., Jeste, D.V., Wyatt, R.J. (1981) Tardive dyskinesia and perceptual dysfunction. *Perceptual and Motor Skills*, **55**, 689–690.

Duke, P.J., Pantelis, C., Barnes, T.R.E. (1994) South Westminster Schizophrenia Survey. Alcohol use and its relationship to symptoms, tardive dyskinesia and illness onset. *British Journal of Psychiatry*, **164**, 630–636.

Edwards, H. (1970) The significance of brain damage in persistent oral dyskinesia. *British Journal of Psychiatry*, **116**, 271–275.

Elkashef, A.M., Buchanan, R.W., Gellad, F., Munson, R.C., Breier, A. (1994) Basal ganglia pathology in schizophrenia and TD: An MRI quantitative study. *American Journal of Psychiatry*, **151**, 752–755

Eslinger, P.J., Damasio, A.R. (1986) Preserved motor learning in Alzheimer's disease: Implications for anatomy and behaviour. *Journal of Neuroscience*, **6**, 3006–3009.

Famuyiwa, O.O., Eccleston, D., Donaldson, A.A., Garside, R.F. (1979) Tardive dyskinesia and dementia. *British Journal of Psychiatry*, **135**, 500–504.

Gaultieri, C.T., Schroeder, S.R., Hicks, R.E., Quade, H. (1986) TD in young mentally retarded individuals. *Archives of General Psychiatry*, **43**, 335–340.

Gellenberg, A.J. (1976) Computerised tomography in patients with TD. *American Journal of Psychiatry*, **133**, 578–579.

Gold, J.M., Egan, M.F., Kirch, D.G., Goldberg, T.E., Daniel, D.G., Bigelow, L.B., Wyatt, R.J. (1991) Tardive dyskinesia: Neuropsychological, computerized tomographic, and psychiatric symptom findings. *Biological Psychiatry*, **30**, 587–599.

Granholm, E., Bartzokis, G., Asarnow, R.F., Marder, S.R. (1993) Preliminary associations between motor procedural learning, basal ganglia T2 relaxation times, and tardive dyskinesia in schizophrenia. *Psychiatry Research*, **50**, 33–44.

Gureje, O. (1988) Topographic subtypes of tardive dyskinesia in schizophrenic patients aged less than 60 years: Relationship to demographic, clinical, treatment, and neuropsychological variables. *Journal of Neurology, Neurosurgery and Psychiatry*, **51**, 1525–1530.

Hanes, K.R., Andrewes, D.G., Pantelis, C. (1995) Cognitive flexibility and complex integration in Parkinson's disease, Huntington's disease and schizophrenia. *Journal of the International Neuropsychological Society*, **1**, 545–553.

Hanes, K.R., Andrewes, D.G., Pantelis, C., Chiu, E. (1996) Subcortical dysfunction in schizophrenia: A comparison with Parkinson's and Huntington's disease. *Schizophrenia Research*, **19**, 121–128.

Harris, M.J., Panton, D., Caligiuri, M.P., Krull, A.J., Tran-Johnson, T.K., Jeste, D.V. (1992) High incidence of tardive dyskinesia in older outpatients on low doses of neuroleptics. *Pharmacology Bulletin*, **28**, 87–92.

Hunter, R., Earl, C.J., Thornicroft, S. (1964) An apparently irreversible syndrome of chronic movements following phenothiazine medication. *Proceedings of The Royal Society of Medicine*, **57**, 758–762.

Itil, T.M., Reisberg, B., Augue, M., Mehta, D. (1981) Clinical profiles of TD. *Comprehensive Psychiatry*, **22**, 282–290.

Jeste, D.V., Karson, C.N., Wyatt, R.J. (1984) Movement disorders and psychopathology. In: *Neuropsychiatric Movement Disorders* (Eds D.V. Jeste, R.J. Wyatt), pp. 119–150, American Psychiatric Press, Washington, DC.

Joyce, E.M., Collinson, S.L., Crichton, P. (1996) Verbal fluency in schizophrenia: Relationship with executive function, semantic memory and clinical alogia. *Psychological Medicine*, **26**, 39–49.

Kahlbaum, K.L. (1874) *Catatonia* (translated by Y. Levij, T. Priden, 1973), John Hopkins University Press, Baltimore, MD.

Kane, J.M., Smith, J.M. (1982) Tardive dyskinesia: Prevalence and risk factors 1959–1979. *Archives of General Psychiatry*, **39**, 473–481.

Kane, J.M., Jeste, D.V., Barnes, T.R.E., Casey, D.E., Cole, J.O., Davis, J.M., Gaultieri, C.T., Schooler, N.R., Sprague, R.L., Wettstien, R.M. (1992) *Tardive dyskinesia: A Task Force Report of the American Psychiatric Association*, American Psychiatric Association, Washington, DC.

Kane, J.M., Wienhold, P., Kinon, B., Wegner, J., Leader, M. (1982) Prevalence of abnormal involuntary movements ("spontaneous dyskinesia") in the normal elderly. *Psychopharmacology*, **77**, 105–108.

Kane, J.M., Woerner, M., Lieberman, J. (1985) Tardive dyskinesia: Prevalence, incidence and risk factors. In: *Dyskinesia: Research and Treatment* (Eds D.E. Casey, T.N. Chase, A.V. Christensen, J. Gerlach), pp. 72–78, Springer-Verlag, Berlin.

Karson, C.N., Bracha, S., Powell, A., Adams, L. (1990) Dyskinetic movements, cognitive impairment and negative symptoms in elderly neuropsychiatric patients. *American Journal of Psychiatry*, **147**, 1646–1649.

Kidger, T., Barnes, T.R.E., Trauer, T., Taylor, P.J. (1980) Subsyndromes of tardive dyskinesia. *Psychological Medicine*, **10**, 513–520.

King, D.J., Wilson, A., Cooper, S.J., Waddington, J.L. (1991) The clinical correlates of neurological soft signs in chronic schizophrenia. *British Journal of Psychiatry*, **158**, 770–775.

Klawans, H.L., Goetz, C.G., Perlick, S. (1980) TD: Review and update. *American Journal of Psychiatry*, **137**, 900–908.

Kolakowska, T., Williams, A.O., Arden, M., Revely, M. (1986) Tardive dyskinesia in schizophrenics under 60 years of age. *Biological Psychiatry*, **21**, 161–169.

Kraepelin, E. (1913) *Dementia Praecox and Paraphrenia* (translated by R.M. Barclay, 1919), Livingstone, UK.

Lezak, M.D. (1995) *Neuropsychological Assessment* (3rd edn), Oxford University Press, NY.

Liddle, P.F., Barnes, T.R.E., Speller, J., Kibel, D. (1993) Negative symptoms as a risk factor for tardive dyskinesia in schizophrenia. *British Journal of Psychiatry*, **163**, 776–780.

Lohr, J.B., Wisniewski, A., Jeste, D.V. (1986) Neurological aspects of TD. In: *Handbook of Schizophrenia, Vol. 1: The Neurology of Schizophrenia* (Eds H.A. Nasrallah, D.R. Weinberger), Elsevier, Amsterdam.

Manschreck, T.C., Keuthen, N.J., Schneyer, M.L., Celada, M.T., Laughery, J., Collins, P. (1990) Abnormal involuntary movements and chronic schizophrenic disorders. *Biological Psychiatry*, **27**, 150–158.

Martone, M., Butters, N., Payne, M., Becker, J., Sax, D.S. (1984) Dissociations between skill learning and verbal recognition in amnesia and dementia. *Archives of Neurology*, **41**, 965–970.

McCreadie, R.G., Kamath, S., Padmavathy, R., Latha, S., Mathrublotham, N., Menon, M.S. (1996) Abnormal movements in never-medicated Indian patients with schizophrenia. *British Journal of Psychiatry*, **168**, 221–226.

Molsa, P.K., Sako, E., Paljarvi, L., Rinne, J.O., Rinne, U.K. (1987) Alzheimer's disease: Neuropathological correlates of cognitive and motor disorders. *Acta Neurologica Scandinavica*, **75**, 376–384.

Moussaoui, D., Fenn, D., Kadri, N., Bentounsi, B., Khomais, M., Tilane, A., Hoffman, W. (1992) Never treated schizophrenics do present tardive dyskinesia-like abnormal movements. *European Neuropsychopharmacology*, 339.

Myslobodsky, M.S., Tomer, R., Holden, T., Kempler, S., Sigal, M. (1985) Cognitive impairment in patients with tardive dyskinesia. *Journal of Nervous and Mental Disorders*, **173**, 156–160.

Myslobodsky, M.S., Holden, T,., Saundler, R. (1984) Asymmetry of abnormal involuntary movements: A prevalence study. *Biological Psychiatry*, **9**, 623–628.

O'Callaghan, E., Larkin, C., Kinsella, A., Waddington, J.L. (1990) Obstetric complications, the putative familial–sporadic distinction and TD in schizophrenia. *British Journal of Psychiatry*, **157**, 578–584.

Owen, A.M., Downes, J.J., Sahakian, B.J., Polkey, C.E., Robbins, T.W. (1990) Planning and spatial working memory following frontal lobe lesions in man. *Neuropsychologia*, **28**, 1021–1034.

Owen, A.M., James, M., Leigh, P.N., Summers, B.A., Marsden, C.D., Quinn, N.P., Lange, K.W., Robbins, T.W. (1992) Fronto-striatal cognitive deficits at different stages of Parkinson's disease. *Brain*, **115**, 1727–1751.

Owen, A.M., Roberts, A.C., Polkey, C.E., Sahakian, B.J., Robbins, T.W. (1991) Extra-dimensional versus intra-dimensional set shifting performance following frontal lobe excisions, temporal lobe excisions or amygdalo-hippocampectomy in man. *Neuropsychologia*, **29**, 993–1006.

Owens, D.G.C., Johnstone, E.C. (1980) The disabilities of chronic schizophrenia: Their nature and factors contributing to their development. *British Journal of Psychiatry*, **136**, 384–395.

Owens, D.G.C., Johnstone, E.C., Frith, C.D. (1982) Spontaneous involuntary disorders of movement, their prevalence, severity, and distribution in chronic schizophrenics with and without treatment with neuroleptics. *Archives of General Psychiatry*, **39**, 452–481.

Pantelis, C., Barnes, T.R.E., Nelson, H.E. (1992) Is the concept of frontal–subcortical dementia relevant to schizophrenia? *British Journal of Psychiatry*, **160**, 442–460.

Pantelis, C., Barnes, T.R.E., Nelson, H.E., Tanner, S., Weatherley, L., Owen, A.M., Robbins, T.W. Frontal–striatal cognitive deficits in patients with chronic schizophrenia. (MS in submission).

Pantelis, C., Brewer, W.J. (1995) Neuropsychological and olfactory dysfunction in schizophrenia: relationship of frontal syndromes to syndromes of schizophrenia. *Schizophrenia Research*, **17**, 35–45.

Pantelis, C., Nelson, H.E. (1994) Cognitive functioning and symptomatology in schizophrenia. In: *The Neuropsychology of Schizophrenia* (Eds A.S David, J.C. Cutting), pp. 215–230, Erlbaum, Hove, UK.

Paulsen, J.S., Heaton, R.K., Jeste, D.V. (1994) Neuropsychological impairment in tardive dyskinesia. *Neuropsychologia*, **8**, 227–256.

Rafal, R., Henik, A. (1994) The neurology of inhibition: integrating controlled and automatic processes. In: *Inhibitory Processes In Attention, Memory and Language* (Eds D. Dagenbach, T.H. Carr), pp. 1–50, Academic Press, NY.

Randolph, C., Braun, A., Goldberg, T., Chase, T. (1993) Semantic fluency in Alzheimer's, Parkinson's and Huntington's disease: Dissociation of storage and retrieval failures. *Neuropsychology*, **7**, 82–88.

Reading, P.J. (1991) Frontal lobe dysfunction in schizophrenia and Parkinson's disease: A meeting point for neurology, psychology and psychiatry: discussion paper. *Journal of the Royal Society of Medicine*, **84**, 349–353.

Richardson, M.A., Pass, R., Bregman, Z., Craig, T.J. (1985) TD and depressive symptoms in schizophrenics. *Psychopharmacology Bulletin*, **21**, 130–135.

Richardson, M.A., Haugland, G., Pass, R., Craig, T.J. (1986) The prevalence of tardive dyskinesia in a mentally retarded population. *Psychopharmacology Bulletin*, **22**, 243–249.

Robbins, T.W. (1990) The case for fronto-striatal dysfunction in schizophrenia. *Schizophrenia Bulletin*, **16**, 391–402.

Robbins, T.W., James, M., Owen, A.M., Lange, K.W., Lees, A.J., Leigh, P.N., Marsden, C.D., Quinn, N.P., Summers, B.A. (1994) Cognitive deficits in progressive supranuclear palsy, Parkinson's disease, and multiple system atrophy in tests sensitive to frontal lobe dysfunction. *Journal of Neurology, Neurosurgery and Psychiatry*, **57**, 79–88.

Rogers, D. (1985) The motor disorders of severe psychiatric illness: A conflict of paradigms. *British Journal of Psychiatry*, **147**, 221–232.

Rogers (1992) *Motor Disorders in Psychiatry: Towards a Neurological Psychiatry*, Wiley, Chichester.

Roth, M. (1994) The relationship between dementia and normal ageing of the brain. In: *Dementia and Normal Ageing* (Eds F.A. Huppert, C. Brayne, D.W. O'Connor), Cambridge University Press, Cambridge.

Saint-Cyr, J.A., Taylor, A.E. (1992) The mobilisation of procedural learning: The key signature of the basal ganglia. In: *The Neuropsychology of Memory*, 2nd edn (Eds C.R. Squire, N. Butters), pp. 188–202, Guilford Press, New York.

Satz, P. (1993) Brain reserve capacity on symptom onset after brain injury: A formulation and review of evidence for threshold theory. *Neuropsychology*, 7, 273–295.

Schwartz, B.L., Rosse, R.B., Deutsch, S.I. (1992) Toward a neuropsychology of memory in schizophrenia. *Psychopharmacology Bulletin*, 28, 341–344.

Shoulson, I. (1990) Huntington's disease: cognitive and psychiatric features. *Neuropsychiatry, Neuropsychology, and Behavioural Neurology*, 3, 15–22.

Smith, J.M., Baldessarini, R.J. (1980) Changes in prevalence, severity and recovery in tardive dyskinesia with age. *Archives of General Psychiatry*, 37, 1368–1373.

Sorokin, J.E., Giordani, B., Mohs, R.C., Losonczy, M.F., Davidson, M., Siever, L.J., Ryan, T.A., Davis, K.L. (1988) Memory impairment in schizophrenic patients with tardive dyskinesia. *Biological Psychiatry*, 23, 129–135.

Spohn, H.E., Coyne, L. (1993) The effect of attention/information processing impairment of TD and neuroleptics in chronic schizophrenics. *Brain and Cognition*, 23, 28–39.

Spohn, H.E., Coyne, L., Lacoursiere, R., Mazur, D., Hayes, K. (1985) Relation of neuroleptic dose and TD to attention, information processing and psychophysiology on medicated schizophrenics. *Archives of General Psychiatry*, 42, 849–859.

Thaker, G., Nguyen, J., Tamminga, C. (1989) Increased saccadic distractibility in tardive dyskinesia: Functional evidence for subcortical GABA dysfunction. *Biological Psychiatry*, 25, 49–59.

Thaker, G.K., Tamminga, C.A., Alphs, L.D., Lafferman, J., Ferraro, T.N., Hare, T.A. (1987) Brain gamma-aminobutyric acid abnormality in tardive dyskinesia: Reduction in cerebrospinal fluid GABA levels and therapeutic response to GABA agonist treatment. *Archives of General Psychiatry*, 44, 522–529.

Tune, L., Strauss, M.E., Lew, M.F., Breitlinger, E., Coyle, J.T. (1992) Serum levels of anticholinergic drugs and impaired recent memory in chronic schizophrenic patients. *American Journal of Psychiatry*, 139, 1460–1462.

Tweedy, J.R., Langer, K.G., McDowell, F.H. (1982) The effect of semantic relations on the memory deficit associated with Parkinson's disease. *Journal of Clinical Neuropsychology*, 4, 235–247.

Waddington, J.L. (1987) Tardive dyskinesia in schizophrenia and other disorders: Associations with ageing, cognitive dysfunction and structural brain pathology in relation to neuroleptic exposure. *Human Psychopharmacology*, 2, 11–22.

Waddington, J.L. (1989) Schizophrenia, affective psychosis and other disorders treated with neuroleptic drugs: The enigma of TD, its neurobiological determinants and the conflict of paradigms. *International Review of Neurobiology*, 31, 297–351.

Waddington, J.L. (1992) Mechanisms of neuroleptic-induced extrapyramidal side-effects. In: *Adverse Effects of Psychotropic Drugs* (Eds J.M. Kane, J.A. Lieberman), pp. 246–265, Guilford Press, New York.

Waddington, J.L., O'Callaghan, E., Larkin, C., Kinsella, A. (1993) Cognitive dysfunction in schizophrenia: Organic vulnerability factor or state marker for TD? *Brain and Cognition*, 23, 56–70.

Waddington, J.L., O'Callaghan, E., Buckley, P., Madigan, C., Redmond, O., Stack, J.P., Kinsella, A., Larkin, C., Ennis, J.T. (1995) Tardive dyskinesia in schizophrenia: Relationship to minor physical anomalies, frontal lobe dysfunction and cerebral structure on magnetic resonance imaging. *British Journal of Psychiatry*, 167, 41–44.

Waddington, J.L., Youssef, H.A. (1986a) Late onset involuntary movements in chronic schizophrenia: relationship of "tardive" dyskinesia to intellectual impairment and negative symptoms. *British Journal of Psychiatry*, 149, 616–620.

Waddington, J.L., Youssef, H.A. (1986b) An unusual cluster of tardive dyskinesia in schizophrenia: association with cognitive dysfunction and negative symptoms. *American Journal of Psychiatry*, **143**, 1162–1165.

Waddington, J.L., Youssef, H.A., Dolphin, C., Kinsella, A. (1987) Cognitive dysfunction, negative symptoms, and tardive dyskinesia in schizophrenia: Their association in relation to topography of involuntary movements and criterion of their abnormality. *Archives of General Psychiatry*, **44**, 907–912.

Waddington, J.L., Youssef, H.A., O'Boyle, K.M., Molloy, A.G. (1986) A reappraisal of abnormal, involuntary movements (tardive dyskinesia) in schizophrenia and other disorders: animal models and alternative hypotheses. In: *The Neurobiology of Dopamine Systems* (Eds W. Winlow, R. Harkstein), pp. 266–286, Manchester University Press, Manchester.

Walker, E.F., Savoie, T., Davis, D. (1994) Neuromotor precursors of schizophrenia. *Schizophrenia Bulletin*, **20**, 441–451.

Walker, E.F. (1994) Developmentally moderated expressions of the neuropathology underlying schizophrenia. *Schizophrenia Bulletin*, **20**, 453–480.

Wechsler, D. (1974) *Wechsler Memory Scale Manual*. The Psychological Corporation, San Antonio, TX.

Wegner, J.T., Catalano, F., Gibralter, J., Kane, J.M. (1985) Schizophrenics with tardive dyskinesia: Neuropsychological deficit and family psychopathology. *Archives of General Psychiatry*, **42**, 860–865.

Weinberger, D.R. (1991) Anteromedial temporo-prefrontal connectivity: A functional neuroanatomical system implicated in schizophrenia. In: *Psychopathology and the Brain* (Eds B.J. Carroll, J.E. Barrett), pp. 25–43, Raven Press, New York.

Wolf, M.E., Ryan, J.J., Mosnaim, A.D. (1983) Cognitive functions in TD. *Psychological Medicine*, **13**, 671–674.

Yassa, R., Jeste, D.V. (1992) Gender differences in TD: A critical review of the recent literature. *Schizophrenia Bulletin*, **18**, 701–715.

Yassa, R., Nair, V., Schwartz, G. (1984) Tardive dyskinesia and the primary psychiatric diagnosis. *Psychosomatics*, **25**, 135–138.

Youssef, H.A., Waddington, J.L. (1988) Primitive (developmental) reflexes and diffuse cerebral dysfunction in schizophrenia and bipolar affective disorder: Overrepresentation in patients with tardive dyskinesia. *Biological Psychiatry*, **23**, 791–796.

Zec, R.F. (1994) Neuropsychological functioning in Alzheimer's disease. In: *Neuropsychology of Alzheimers and other dementias* (Eds R.W. Parks, R.F. Zec, R.S. Wilson), pp. 3–80, Oxford University Press, New York.

13

Neuropsychology of Eye Movement Abnormalities in Schizophrenia

LESLIE HENDERSON, TREVOR J. CRAWFORD and
CHRISTOPHER KENNARD

DISORDERS OF SACCADIC EYE MOVEMENTS IN PATIENTS WITH SCHIZOPHRENIA

The great attractiveness of the saccadic system as an object of enquiry and as a means of investigating the integrity of brain function stems from the following considerations: (i) the movements of the eye afford the opportunity for precise but unobtrusive measures of the performance of a complete sub-system of action control; (ii) various biomechanical properties of the saccade, notably its limited degrees of freedom, allow ready access to the kinematics of the system; (iii) impairments of the mechanical plant are sufficiently rare for the kinematics to yield a fairly transparent window onto the neural control processes; (iv) our considerable ability to manipulate the attributes of saccadic tasks permits us to engage selectively a variety of attentional, perceptual, cognitive and motor processes; (v) we can also vary the attentional demands of saccadic tasks over a broad span from automaticity to effortful strategic control; (vi) at several levels of control, the neural pathways serving saccades and their functional roles are unusually well charted.

It is curious, therefore, and disappointing, to find that the great bulk of saccadic studies of psychiatric patients have made minimal use of these advantages. Until very recently, such investigations typically employed the eyeball merely as a device for generating reaction times, confining the field of view to REFLEX saccades and adhering to insensitive and artefact-prone measurement techniques.

We can distinguish four levels of measurement that reveal inadequacies in psychiatric investigations of saccades. At the transducer level, the persistence of electro-oculographic (EOG) methods has imposed fundamental restrictions on

Schizophrenia: A Neuropsychological Perspective. Edited by C. Pantelis, H.E. Nelson and T.R.E. Barnes
© 1996 John Wiley & Sons Ltd

what can be measured and how finely. Analogue to digital conversion has commonly been accomplished by hand from the recording trace, yielding poor resolution and the possibility of human error. The range of performance variables considered has often been restricted to a single parameter, usually the latency of the primary saccade. Finally, employment of saccadic tasks that require a level of sustained attention likely to reveal disturbances of the strategic control of action had to await the 1990s. In view of these deficiencies, the common failure to detect robust differences between patients with schizophrenia and controls seems neither surprising nor illuminating. To conclude, as did most reviewers in the 1980s, that "there is no gross dysfunction of oculomotion associated with this disorder" (Iacono's, 1988, verdict) now appears to have been somewhat premature.

There is an ever present danger in literatures such as this that a great mass of narrow or defective studies, few of which are, on their own, capable of sustaining any general conclusion will, nevertheless, somehow impel us, by their sheer weight into drawing conclusions which a single, well-constructed investigation might overthrow. The null hypothesis is never more adhesive than when caught in the feeble embrace of studies that lack the resolving power to see beyond it.

Lipton and colleagues (1983) provided a wide-ranging review of methods and findings in oculomotor studies of patients with schizophrenia. As with Iacono (1988), their major concern lay in abnormalities of smooth pursuit eye movements (SPEM) but they devoted a few paragraphs to disposal of the notion of any saccadic deficit. From this putative dissociation they somehow concluded that the schizophrenic's difficulties neither lay in the strategic control of attention nor in a "generalised motor dysfunction".

A narrower but altogether more penetrating review was provided by Levin (1984) with special regard to frontal lobe functioning. Amongst the important points made by Levin, was the fact that the saccadic and SPEM systems are designed to work in concert. The saccadic intrusions in SPEM which formed the central preoccupation of these reviewers could therefore be construed either as a defect in SPEM, such as inability to generate adequate tracking velocities, or a pathological disinhibition of the saccadic system, itself. A major theme of Levin's was the possibility that a more general distractibility factor, could be found both in frontal disorders and in the negative aspects of schizophrenia. Levin also argued that, since patients with schizophrenia apparently fail to exhibit the eye movement impairments found in Parkinson's disease, the functioning of their basal ganglia must be intact. As we shall see, the role of a frontal-type distractibility factor and a Parkinsonian pattern of impairment are the two major issues that have arisen from saccadic studies of patients with schizophrenia appearing subsequent to Levin's review.

A PARKINSONIAN PATTERN OF ABNORMALITY ASSOCIATED WITH NEUROLEPTIC TREATMENT

Diefendorf & Dodge's (1908) remarkable investigation of eye movements in schizophrenia had at least three methodological virtues which have somehow eluded most subsequent researchers. Their patients were perforce free from neuro-leptic medication. By including other psychotic patients, they were in a position to assess the specificity of any abnormalities in schizophrenia. Moreover, by studying more than one type of eye movement they were able to search for selective deficits. Their analysis of saccades, however, suffered from one major technical limitation, latency being the only measure available to them. Another study from the pre-chlorpromazine era succeeded in filling that lacuna. Couch & Fox (1934) were able to add a measure of spatial accuracy. This, taken in conjunction with adoption of a task requiring *voluntary* initiation of the saccade, allowed them to detect abnormalities in the spatial metrics of their schizophrenics' fast eye movements.

One indulgence of modern technology was to perform a minimalist analysis (primarily saccadic reaction times) on patients without regard for the fact that almost all of them were receiving neuroleptic treatment. With hindsight, there is some solace in the thought that this was unlikely to lead to confusion of treatment and disease effects, since the methods adopted were very unlikely to succeed in detecting any treatment effects. Nevertheless, given the propensity of neuroleptics to induce extrapyramidal side effects, this indifference seems puzzling. These motor side-effects stem from the neuroleptic blockade of the nigrostriatal dopamine pathway, the degeneration of which causes Parkinson's disease. The significance of this for the student of saccades is that other circuits within the basal ganglia intimately related to the dopaminergic pathway are known to play an important role in saccadic control. These facts acquire greater significance through recent demonstrations that, in the relatively circumscribed neuro-pathology of mild–moderate Parkinson's disease, the patients show a character-istic abnormality in the kinematics of their saccades. They tend to exhibit *multistepping hypometria*, with fixation arriving at the correct final eye position by means of a train of miniature saccadic steps. In particular, the primary saccade, which would normally cover about 90% of the distance, is markedly hypometric (e.g. Crawford et al, 1989a).

As the top panel of Table 13.1 shows, patients with Parkinson's disease cannot usually be distinguished from controls on other performance parameters, though a few studies have found slight prolongation of saccade latency. Moreover, the hypometria is limited to saccades generated towards the locus where a target is expected (PRED saccades: e.g. Crawford et al, 1989b), or where a target has recently been extinguished (REM saccades: e.g. Lueck et al, 1990). In contrast, there is little detectable deficit in saccades directed to an imaginary location in the opposite hemi-field to that of the target (ANTI saccades). In a synoptic discus-sion, Lueck et al (1992) have concluded that *target visibility* during the period leading up to generation of the movement is a necessary condition for saccades to be executed normally by patients with Parkinson's disease.[1]

---

[1]These experiments are performed in the dark; at the time of generating REM and PRED saccades nothing is visible at the target locus. Note that saccades executed as part of a planned sequence also exhibit MSH but since this requirement has not been investigated in schizophrenia, we do not discuss it further here. Since ANTI saccades are normal in Parkinson's disease the presence of an ANTI target must be sufficient to satisfy the *target visibility* condition.

Table 13.1. The principal types of saccadic eye movement investigated in Parkinson's disease, schizophrenia and bipolar affective disorder and the parameters of saccadic performance in which abnormalities have been detected.

Saccade-eliciting paradigm:	Reflex	Remembered	Predicted	Antisaccade	Previewed	Multiple[a]
Target characteristics:	Novel			Mirror image	Not novel	Novel
Target visibility:	Visible	Internal	Internal	Visible	Visible	Visible
Nature of the imperative signal:	Target onset	Buzzer onset	Internal model	Visual stimulus onset	Buzzer onset	Target onset

The Parkinsonian abnormality (PDs versus age-matched normals)[1]

Saccade-eliciting paradigm:	Reflex	Remembered	Predicted	Antisaccade	Previewed	Multiple[a]
Latency:	Normal?	Normal	Normal	Normal	Normal	Prolonged
Primary gain:	Normal	Abnormal?	V. abnormal	Normal	Normal	V. abnormal
FEP gain:	Normal	Normal				
Peak velocity:	Normal	Normal		Normal	Normal	Normal
Distractibility:	Normal	Normal		Normal	Normal	

The neuroleptic effect (NL-treated versus NL-free SZ/BPs)[3]

Saccade-eliciting paradigm:	Reflex	Remembered	Predicted	Antisaccade	Previewed	Multiple[a]
Latency:	Normal	Normal	Normal	Normal	N/S[b]	N/A[b]
Primary gain:	Normal	Normal?	V. abnormal	Normal	N/A[b]	N/A[b]
FEP gain:	Normal	Normal?	V. abnormal	Normal	N/A[b]	N/A[b]
Distractibility:		Normal?		Normal?	N/A[b]	N/A[b]

The schizophrenic abnormality (NL-free SZ versus normal or other controls)[2]

Saccade-eliciting paradigm:	Reflex	Remembered	Predicted	Antisaccade	Previewed	Multiple[a]
Latency:	Normal	Normal	Normal	Normal?	N/A[b]	N/A[b]
Primary gain:	Normal	Normal	Normal	Abnormal?	N/A[b]	N/A[b]
FEP gain:	Normal	Normal	Normal	Abnormal?	N/A[b]	N/A[b]
Distractibility		SZ abnormal		SZ abnormal	N/A[b]	N/A[b]

Abbreviations: SZ, schizophrenic; BP, bipolar affective; PD, mild–moderate idiopathic Parkinson's disease; FEP, final eye position; NL, (typical) neuroleptics; ?, robustness questionable (marginal statistically or with lack of consensus across studies).

[a] The table entry for the MULTIPLE saccade paradigm is based on the first saccade of a reciprocating, four-saccade sequence. Save for the sequencing requirement, this saccade is executed under REFLEX conditions, in the sense that the *when?* and *where?* information is supplied by the arrival of a novel visual target.

[b] Neither of these paradigms appears yet to have been employed on psychotic patients.

[1] The Parkinsonian pattern of abnormality is defined by comparison of mild–moderate Parkinson's disease patients with age-matched (thus usually elderly) normal control subjects (top panel). The Parkinsonian abnormality is a kinematic one, in which the primary saccade falls short of the target. While the patient often attains a normal final eye position, this tends to require multiple saccadic steps, often varying in amplitude.

[2] The schizophrenic abnormality emerges from a comparison of neuroleptic-free SZs with age-matched controls (bottom panel). Whilst normal controls are usually employed, comparison with other psychotic patients (e.g. BPs) presents a more rigorous test of a specifically schizophrenic abnormality. Distractibility errors, in which the subject has failed to suppress a REFLEX saccade where the task requires it, can be used to distinguish SZs from BPs as well as normal controls. Other converging measures have been proposed for what may turn out to be a general disinhibitory syndrome.

[3] The neuroleptic treatment effect is defined by comparison of neuroleptic-treated psychotic patients with neuroleptic-free psychotic patients, matched as closely as possible (middle panel). Such effects should be indifferent to nosological category.

[4] Peak velocity not available for studies of psychosis.

Crawford et al (1995a, 1995b) investigated several types of eye movement in 90 psychotic patients in order to determine whether the Parkinsonian pattern was detectible when closely matched groups of neuroleptic-treated and neuroleptic-free schizophrenic patients were compared. A detailed clinical description of the patients was provided. This included a formal assessment of positive and negative symptoms, neurological examination and neuropsychological testing. The middle panel of Table 13.1 shows that neuroleptic treatment was, indeed, associated with the Parkinsonian abnormality. The primary saccades of neuroleptic-treated patients with schizophrenia showed much more hypometria than the saccades of neuroleptic-free patients with schizophrenia and, as predicted, this difference was only found in the PRED and REM tasks. Moreover, we can reject any idea that this reflects a highly specific neuroleptic/schizophrenia interaction since the same neuroleptic treatment effect was found amongst patients with bipolar affective disorder.[2] For the psychotic patients, taken as a whole, the characteristics which best predicted neuroleptic treatment were (in descending order): hypometric predictive saccades, tardive dyskinesia and rated Parkinsonism score.

In sum, the hypothesis that protracted neuroleptic treatment can induce specific abnormalities of saccade execution received strong support. The neuroleptic-treated, especially those showing other Parkinsonian signs, exhibited greater hypometria. This only occurred when saccades had to be generated in the absence of a visible target, precisely the condition where hypometria distinguishes Parkinson's disease patients from controls.[3]

It has proved surprisingly difficult to detect effects of chronic neuroleptic treatment in other cognitive and motor tasks (see Cassens et al, 1990; see also King and Green, chapter 20). So these findings have important methodological as well as substantive implications. Moreover, the robustness of the saccadic effects stand in sharp contrast to a controversy regarding the claimed resistance of neuroleptic effects to detection in SPEM (Litman et al, 1989; Friedman et al, 1992; Sweeney et al, 1994; Crawford et al, 1995c).

FAILURE OF PSYCHOTIC PATIENTS TO CORRECT RETINAL ERROR

In the studies by Crawford et al (1995a, 1995b, 1996) an effect which obtained for all the psychotic groups, compared to neurotic and normal control groups, was a tendency not to eliminate with corrective saccades the residual retinal error resulting from shortfall of the primary saccade. Thus, the hypometria found in the REM and PRED saccades of the neuroleptic-treated psychotic patients obtained not only for the primary saccade (as in Parkinson's disease patients) but

---

[2]Though these groups were less well matched and we suspect that amongst bipolar disorder patients those who attract neuroleptic treatment may have some inherently different attributes.

[3]The fact that the Parkinson's disease pattern has been obtained in patients taking dopamine replacement therapies must be reckoned with. Also, the great capacity of the dopamine system to compensate for even major cell loss.

also, though in lesser degree, for the final eye position. This effect was not restricted to neuroleptic-treated patients since it obtained for all the psychotic groups in the ANTI saccade task. So it appears that, whatever the particular cause of hypometria in their primary saccades, psychotic patients show a tendency not to eliminate the distance off target in subsequent corrective saccades. Evidence that this is truly a distinctive feature of psychotic patients was available in the ANTI saccade paradigm because here the neurotic group also had hypometric primary saccades but they alone brought the eye onto the target locus with their corrective saccades.

We are disinclined to take seriously the idea that in all these conditions psychotic patients suffer a shrinkage of spatial memory such that they believe their eyes to have come to rest on the remembered target location (but cf. Hommer et al, 1991; note also that in the PRED task the target arrives short after execution of the primary saccade). However, further studies are necessary before we can determine the role of spatial memory in these saccadic tasks.

An interesting possibility is that psychotic patients have a specific problem with error correction in the absence of the direct feedback provided by a visible target. This account might seem to fit comfortably with a suggestion first advanced by Feinberg (1978) and developed more fully by Frith (1992; see also Cahill and Frith, chapter 18). This posits a key schizophrenic deficit in Central Monitoring of Efference (CME). While this general thesis can be made to supply an ingenious explanation of vocal hallucinations and delusions, as an account of uncorrected retinal error in these saccadic studies it is unsatisfactory. Note, first, the alarmingly abrupt shift in level of discourse between postulating defective monitoring of intentionality in order to explain delusional and hallucinatory positive symptoms and, in the present instance, postulation of defective monitoring of the amplitude of a saccade that is being generated! Furthermore, defective monitoring of the efference copy associated with execution of a saccade would result in disastrous instability of the visual image, for which there is no evidence. Finally, Crawford et al (1995a, 1995b) found that almost all the patients with schizophrenia they studied spontaneously corrected their antisaccade errors. That is, they followed any saccade that had been incorrectly directed *towards* the target with a reverse saccade towards the (originally appropriate) mirror-image location. Moreover, this spontaneous correction was usually executed before the visual feedback stimulus was delivered at the ANTI target location. This implies capacity to monitor efference that is at least sufficient to detect gross errors in direction.

It is of interest that a recent study in the monkey has identified a region of the dorsolateral prefrontal cortex (DLPFC), area 46, which appears to contain spatially organised memory fields active during retention (Funahashi et al, 1993) and which involve dopamine D1 receptors (Sawaguchi & Goldman-Rakic, 1991; Williams & Goldman-Rakic, 1995). Interestingly, when the saccade has to be directed to the location of a remembered target, local blockade of these receptors results in reduced amplitude saccades, both of the primary saccade and the final eye position. This is reminiscent of the abnormalities found in our study of psychotic patients.

All that would seem to remain is our unglamorous, but testable, working hypothesis. This asserts that, in the absence of a motive for achieving precise foveation of our targets, psychotic patients lack any compelling incentive to correct the retinal error resulting from the shortfall of their primary saccade. Since the targets are merely light-emitting diodes, which scarcely merit close scrutiny, who can blame them?

SACCADIC DISTRACTIBILITY: A PROTOTYPICAL FRONTAL SIGN?

As a result of extensive anatomical and physiological studies in the non-human primate and clinical studies in patients with focal lesions, a fairly comprehensive outline of the major centres involved in saccade generation is now available (Wurtz & Goldberg, 1989). Equally, the known disturbances in the metrics of saccades, such as reduced amplitude or peak velocity, and prolonged latency are attributable to functional deficits in specific neural centres (Kennard & Lueck, 1989). This knowledge, although incomplete, at least allows the saccadic deficits in schizophrenia to be considered in terms of possible specific neural pathophysiology.

Attempts to define the neural basis for saccade generation started with the observations of Ferrier, who electrically stimulated the prefrontal cortex in monkeys and elicited contralateral eye movements (Ferrier, 1874). This area is called the frontal eye field (FEF), which, in recent years as a result of stimulation studies in monkeys (Bruce et al, 1985) and humans (Penfield & Baldrey, 1937) as well as lesion studies (Holmes, 1938) and electrophysiological recordings (Bruce & Goldberg, 1985; Segraves & Goldberg, 1987), has been shown to be involved in the generation of volitional saccades, even in the absence of a visual stimulus. Similar experimental techniques have defined two other frontal lobe areas involved in the generation of saccades – the supplementary eye field (SEF) which lies medially in the rostral part of the supplementary motor area (Schlag & Schlag-Rey, 1987; Schall, 1991a, 1991b) and the arcuate sulcus (area 46) in the dorsolateral prefrontal cortex (DLPFC) (Funahashi et al, 1989). There is a convergence of inputs on the FEF, which represents sensory, motor and cognitive responses, and may serve as an important outflow from the cortex to the brainstem saccade generators. The saccadic generator for horizontal saccades lies in the paramedian reticular formation while that for vertical saccades is located in the rostral interstitial nucleus of the medial longitudinal fasciculus (Henn, 1992).

The "automatic" attraction of saccades by novel extrafoveal events takes place for each of us many thousand times a day without demanding our attention. Turning to the converse situation, we find that suppression of reflexive saccades is relatively easy when we have been instructed simply to maintain fixation. It becomes more difficult when the saccade has to be executed, but not until a symbolic cue is supplied (the REM and PREVIEW paradigms), and yet more difficult when an immediate but spatially transformed (ANTI) saccade is required. Failures of saccadic suppression in these tasks have become known as *distractibility errors*.

Studies of humans with frontal lesions in the region of the FEF, using the ANTI saccade paradigm, have found abnormal distractibility (Guitton et al, 1985). A few cases with exceptionally focal lesions led Pierrot-Deseilligny et al (1991) to propose that the critical frontal region is the DLPFC, although a similar increased distractibility was recently found in a steady fixation task with ventrolateral lesions (Paus et al, 1991).

The frontal cortex connects with the striatum, which projects with inhibitory (GABA) fibres to the substantia nigra pars reticulata, which in turn projects to the superior colliculus (Hikosaka & Wurtz 1989). This system could well act as an inhibitory gate on the activation of the superior colliculus by inputs from other saccade related centres. Bilateral lesions of either the FEF or the superior colliculus result in only minor saccadic deficits, whereas lesions of both produce a marked impairment of saccade generation. This suggests two parallel saccadic pathways to the midbrain and pontine premotor saccadic generators, one from the FEF and the other from the superior colliculus (Schiller et al, 1980).

Abnormal saccadic distractibility has been found in pathological disorders of this basal ganglia-mediated saccade pathway, as observed in Huntington's disease (Lasker et al, 1987) and progressive supranuclear palsy (Pierrot-Deseilligny et al, 1989), whereas in the substantia nigra pars compacta degeneration of Parkinson's disease it appears to be absent (Crawford et al, 1989a; Lueck et al, 1990, 1992a, 1992b).

Several reports of elevated rates of distractibility in schizophrenia have recently appeared (e.g. Fukushima et al, 1990; Thaker et al, 1989; Sereno & Holzman, 1995; Crawford et al, 1995a, 1995b, 1996). The abnormality has appeared especially marked in patients exhibiting tardive dyskinesia (Thaker et al, 1989), frontal atrophy (Fukushima et al, 1990) and either perseverative errors in card sorting or an abundance of negative signs (Crawford et al, 1995a). Crawford et al (1995b) showed that distractibility sets neuroleptic-free patients with schizophrenia apart from patients with either bipolar disorder or anxiety neurosis, as well as from Parkinson's disease (see Table 13.1).

These findings pose the question whether ANTI and REM errors are but two manifestations of a broader syndrome of saccadic disinhibition. Arguably this syndrome might embrace spontaneous saccades that occur in schizophrenia despite instructions to maintain fixation (Paus, 1991), a disposition towards antici-patory saccades when the target locus is known (Hommer et al, 1991), saccadic intrusions in smooth pursuit and a proneness of distractible patients to generate express saccades (Pierrot-Deseilligny et al, 1989; Matsue et al, 1994) although Currie et al (1993) reported a paucity of express saccades at selective gap durations. It is tempting also to consider the possibility that certain schizophrenic abnormalities reported in recent studies of patterns of exploratory eye movements (Kojima et al, 1992; Kurachi et al, 1990) might find a place in this schema. Indeed, the breadth of this putative disinhibition syndrome raises the question (pursued in the next section) whether saccadic disinhibition might serve as a sensitive experimental model of a more general, frontal-type dysfunction of strategic control processes in schizophrenia.

Robbins (1990) has used differences in the performance profile exhibited by patients with Parkinson's disease and schizophrenia on neuropsychological tests purportedly sensitive to frontal dysfunction to argue that these two classes of disorder are associated with different types of frontal syndrome. Our saccadic data indicate an even sharper double dissociation between a "nigrostriatal dopamine effect", consisting of an abnormal dependence of saccadic gain on target visibility, and a "prefrontal disinhibition effect" that is associated (inter alia) with negative type schizophrenia and consists of high saccadic distractibility. These seem to be the most powerful discriminators currently available for distinguishing schizophrenic from Parkinson's disease hypofrontality.

ATTENTION, INTENTION, STRATEGIC PLANNING AND THE SACCADIC MODEL OF DISTRACTIBILITY

The postulation of attentional deficits dominated early clinical descriptions of the schizophrenic syndrome (Kraepelin, 1919; Bleuler, 1911) and returned to favour with the importation of concepts like that of selective filtering of sensory input from a renascent cognitive psychology (e.g. McGhie & Chapman, 1961). The eclipse of these attentional accounts seems to have been due to at least two factors. First, they were focused almost entirely on the positive symptoms. As negative/deficit signs came to be regarded as equally primary this restricted focus became a liability. Second, the type of channel selection invoked was an essentially passive data driven one, whereas, increasingly it seemed that the key deficits lay in strategic planning (e.g. Callaway & Naghdi, 1982) or more generally in processes involving intentionality (Frith, 1992). This contrast echoes a distinction drawn by Denny-Brown (1966) between automatic, parietally mediated attention and frontally mediated deliberative process control.

The saccadic system offers a convenient model for examining this distinction (see also Maruff and Currie, chapter 6). On the one hand, we find the REFLEX saccade and various associated phenomena, such as spatial cuing and express saccades, which seem to share posterior parietal involvement and have to do with the automatic capture and release of spatial attention (see e.g. Posner & Peterson, 1990). On the other hand, we find voluntary types of saccade that require a planned series of cognitive operations. For instance, in the REMEMBERED target paradigm, the subject must suppress the disposition to look reflexively towards the arriving target, commit its location to memory, program the appropriate saccade and activate that program when the command signal is decoded. Even that account is over-simplified. Consider the matter of encoding and retrieving target location information. This might be conducted within the coordinates of retinal space. It might require a complex mapping of the retinal address of the target into an egocentric representation of environmental space. It might even involve a motor code, with the subject storing the saccadic vector required to foveate the target.

Several issues can readily be discerned, here. Even something as simple as a REM saccade necessitates the construction of an action plan consisting of a number of do's and don'ts, involving a mix of automatic parallel computations and contingent sequential steps, often accompanied by timing parameters and conditional loops. These are likely to involve processes widely dispersed throughout the brain and failure may be due to a defective component in the plan or a global defect in the organisation of planning, itself.

Distractibility, as we recognise it in everyday conduct, involves an inability to adhere to a plan so as to produce coherent and sustained purposive action. It has often been regarded as the hallmark of frontal disorders (e.g. Fuster, 1980; Stuss & Benson, 1986). It is also recognisable amongst the signs and symptoms of schizophrenia, where it seems to straddle the traditional positive/negative boundary, being evident in positive thought disorder (e.g. derailment or distractible speech) as well as in such negative features as complaints of difficulty in sustaining attention (Andreasen, 1985; see also Liddle & Morris, 1991). In normal but inattentive individuals, it can be witnessed in those bizarre slips of action sometimes called "capture errors" (e.g. Reason, 1990).

What might make for distractibility? One way to make this question tractable is to consider appropriate paradigms for investigating distraction. The vigilance task reminds us that in some situations the deficit may consist of an inability to sustain alertness. This can, in turn, be decomposed either into inadequate nonspecific arousal or insufficient intentness. Slips of action may occur because we are fatigued or because, having ascended to the bedroom and undressed without refreshing our internal representation of the goal (changing for dinner), the prepotent (i.e. default) option in this stimulus context takes priority and we climb into bed! Even in this rudimentary example we can identify three possible contributions to distractibility: inadequate arousal, inadequate intentness (colloquially referred to as "being on autopilot") and inability to modulate prepotency.

If prepotency itself is of the essence, then the saccadic model commends itself. One way forward on this issue is to examine the nature of those neuropsychological tasks that are widely held to be valid indicators of negative frontal-type signs. Many tests appear to share the salient feature of the saccadic distractibility tasks: the requirement to suppress a prepotent response. In these terms, the saccadic tasks seem ideal since only in them is prepotency biologically established. In contrast, the Wisconsin Card Sort Test (WCST) relies only on the relatively weak and transient interference exercised by a prepotent response that is acquired and replaced many times in the course of the experiment. Consequently, in order even to generate interference the tester must arbitrarily change the rules. So different are these situations that we would no more speak of "distractibility" in the WCST than we would speak of "perseveration" in the antisaccade task. Stroop interference is intermediate, the prepotency of word naming becoming fixed with the acquisition of literacy and the "lesser meaning task" (Cohen & Servan-Schreiber, 1992) reflects a weaker form of linguistic habit strength.[4] However, this evaluation assumes that the property of the WCST that makes it a

---

[4]Note too that, whereas an abundance of evidence based upon functional brain imaging points to DLPFC as the crucial structure in WCST performance and some evidence by Pierrot-Deseilligny et al (1991) implicates DLPFC in saccadic distractibility, the PET study by Pardo et al (1990) implicates anterior cingulate but not DLPFC.

valid instrument is prepotency. Consider, to the contrary, that an attribute of the WCST measure that is not shared by the saccadic tasks is the attention shift requirement which stems precisely from the transient nature of its response prepotency.

Two aspects of this emphasis on prepotency are worrying. One is that it supplies no explanation of why the WCST is by far the most widely validated predictor of metabolically imaged hypofrontality, frontal lesion and schizophrenic negative state (or even why it predicts saccadic distractibility). The other aspect of the WCST's status worth noting is that it was constructed to mimic the predominant frontal test used on primates, the delayed spatial response task which is in turn mimicked by the 'A not-B' task developed for use on infants (see Goldman-Rakic, 1987; Diamond, 1990; see also Pantelis and Brewer, chapter 16).

Thus, we are led to the idea that perhaps the biologically hard-wired prepotency of the reflexive saccade is not of the essence. The significance of an inappropriate but prepotent response may merely be to allow us to detect a primary deficit in strategic planning. This line of thinking bears some resemblance to Cohen & Servan-Schreiber's (1992) thesis that the primary schizophrenic deficit consists of a disability of internal representation of what they call (rather opaquely) "context", but which we prefer to call an action plan. Such a plan is necessary for the Tower of Hanoi test because the inherent structure of the test is that of a set of discrete goal-directed steps. In contrast, the Continuous Performance Task (CPT) is sensitive to strategic planning because of the vigilance-like property of requiring sustained attention, arguably also a feature of WCST.

SACCADIC AND SPEM ABNORMALITY: A COMMON MECHANISM?

The primary function of smooth pursuit eye movements in the service of vision is to maintain a relatively stable image of a moving target on the retina. In order to achieve efficient and accurate pursuit, this remarkable oculomotor system must solve a number of neuro-computational problems stretching from selective attention to transduction of target velocity (see Thurston et al, 1988) and the programming of an appropriate motor output for the ocular muscles. It is not surprising, therefore, that SPEM impairments have been observed following a wide range of brain lesions (see Leigh & Zee, 1991). In normal subjects efficient smooth pursuit can also break down when, for example, the target velocity exceeds that permissible for smooth pursuit. When SPEM is overstretched the visuomotor system may switch to saccadic eye movements in order to monitor the target, but there will usually be a high cost in target visibility. The saccadic and SPEM systems, therefore, interact to achieve the final objective of maintaining a stable target image at the fovea and together they provide a prime example of an integrated visuomotor network involving many levels of brain function.

Diefendorf & Dodge (1908) were the first to recognise that patients with schizophrenia were unable to generate accurate SPEM. This finding has since been extensively confirmed in many laboratories (see Levy, 1994). Interest in the possible genetic basis of the abnormality was heightened by the demonstration that a SPEM abnormality is present in approximately 50% of first-degree relatives of patients with schizophrenia (Holzman et al, 1974). However, until recently, there has been relatively little advance in the understanding of the under-lying neuropsychological mechanisms of the SPEM abnormality.

Although a detailed analysis of the SPEM deficit has been more forthcoming in recent years (Friedman et al, 1991; Yee et al, 1987; Hommer et al, 1991) the source of the abnormality is still unclear as few studies have attempted to distin-guish between the different levels at which the SPEM abnormality might arise. Many of the early studies on SPEM were conducted under photopic conditions in normal room lighting conditions with many potentially distracting visual targets. Under these conditions a complex pattern of optical flow will occur on the retina, providing a powerful stimulus for attentional capture (i.e. distract-ibility). This provides a mechanism by which the distractibility effect could have direct implications for both saccadic and SPEM abnormalities. The possibility of a direct relationship of the saccadic distractibility and SPEM deficits is an issue of some importance since a SPEM abnormality has been claimed to be a promising candidate for the elusive biological marker of schizophrenia (e.g. see Clementz & Sweeney, 1990; Bell et al, 1994). Kaufman & Abel (1986) demon-strated that normal subjects show a smooth pursuit gain deficit (i.e. reduced velocity pursuit) when pursuit was elicited across a distracting background. In our laboratory (Lawden et al, 1995) we have found that a wide range of cortical lesions impair SPEM at target velocities above 10 degrees/s, which is then signifi-cantly worsened when smooth pursuit is generated across a patterned background.

However, one form of a distractibility hypothesis suffers from a major diffi-culty. SPEM across a contoured surround generates a motion percept in which the contoured visual field appears to move at the angular velocity of the eye but in the opposite direction. The optokinetic nystagmus (i.e. OKN) that would otherwise occur in response to the movement of the visual field must, therefore, be suppressed at some level. If patients with schizophrenia are unable to inhibit the influence of the visual field motion on SPEM, as appears to be the case following cortical lesions (Lawden et al, 1995), the fast phases would be in the opposite direction to the field of motion. In addition, SPEM in the direction of the field of motion, and thus, paradoxically, in the direction opposite to foveal target, should also be evident. To our knowledge such records have not yet been widely reported as a characteristic of SPEM in schizophrenia.

Much of the early work in this field relied on purely qualitative judgements of SPEM (e.g. Holzman et al, 1973) or used measures such as the natural log ratio of pursuit frequencies at the target waveform frequency (derived from Fourier analysis) to frequencies outside the target bandwidth (usually denoted by "ln S/N"). Such measures are unable to distinguish between the various forms of smooth pursuit dysfunction (Friedman et al, 1995a). More recently, detailed quantitative measures of saccadic–pursuit interactions during SPEM have been applied in schizophrenia research. Abel et al (1991) have distinguished between several different forms of saccadic intrusions that are observed in smooth pursuit tracking. The saccadic system can compensate to some extent when SPEM velocity gain is compromised with a catch-up saccade (CUS) of the appropriate amplitude to bring the eye back on target (see Gellman & Carl, 1991). Square wave jerks (SWJ) are pairs of saccades (usually between 0.5 and 3 degrees) separated by an inter-saccadic interval (150–450 ms) during which pursuit continues (e.g. Dell'Osso et al, 1975). Anticipatory saccades (AS) are large saccades that take the eye ahead of the target after which pursuit ceases until the target is re-foveated either by a return saccade or by simply waiting for the target image to arrive at the fovea (Abel & Ziegler, 1988). Most studies of eye movements in schizophrenia have reported an increase in saccadic activity during pursuit but have not distinguished between intrusive and corrective saccades.

Low pursuit gain (i.e. the ratio of eye velocity to target velocity) itself does not distinguish between a disorder that is primarily saccadic and one that is primarily pursuit based, since if saccades become disinhibited, thus taking the eye ahead of the target, pursuit may be disrupted. Similarly, CUS per se are not informative on this distinction since they can arise from either a SPEM dysfunction in which CUS compensate for low SPEM velocity gain (as is normally assumed) or be part of a defective circuit whereby intrusive saccades are followed by low velocity pursuit as the oculomotor system waits for the target before issuing the next intrusive saccade.

A more profitable search for clues to the cause of the SPEM impairment would combine quantitative analysis of the various forms of saccadic intrusions and assessment of their relation to other measures of visuomotor programming. For example, evidence in favour of a distractibility hypothesis of pursuit comes from recent studies showing an association between SPEM dysfunction and excessive express saccades in schizophrenia (Kamijo et al, 1991; Sereno & Holzman, 1993; Matsue et al, 1994). This hypothesis would, however, be strengthened by further evidence in schizophrenia showing significant correlations between intrusive saccades during SPEM and other neuropsychological measures of distractibility. However, a recent study (Friedman et al, 1995b) found SPEM and performance on the Wisconsin Card Sort Test in schizophrenia to be uncorrelated. Abel and co-workers (1991) have recently distinguished between anticipatory saccades and other types of saccadic intrusions in SPEM abnormalities. Of the several types of saccadic intrusions this appears to be the most likely candidate relating to saccadic distractibility.

Currently there is no direct evidence linking the saccadic distractibility and SPEM dysfunction to a common mechanism. Research directly addressing this question is still awaited, but the current evidence suggests that although the incidence of saccadic intrusions is negatively correlated with saccadic gain (showing unsurprisingly that catch-up saccades are used to compensate for low velocity SPEM gain) this relationship is weak or non-existent in schizophrenia (Abel et al, 1991). This suggests that, not only are both SPEM and saccadic inhibition mechanisms impaired, but the functional relationship between the two systems is also disturbed.

CONCLUSIONS

In this chapter our primary concerns have been two-fold. We have attempted to evaluate the utility of saccadic eye movement paradigms and measures in the search for a biological basis for schizophrenia. We have also attempted to integrate certain saccadic findings into a coherent neuropsychology of schizophrenia.

Detailed research in schizophrenia with an emphasis on saccadic abnormalities is still in its infancy, as most of these studies are flawed by a failure to control for the use of neuroleptic medication. As we have indicated, many of the purported abnormalities in the smooth pursuit system, reported in the 1970s and 1980s, may relate more to the general problem of increased saccadic distractibility than to any primary deficit in the modulation of eye velocity.

In light of the fact that a biological marker for the disease has eluded us thus far we believe this is a timely point at which to re-open the question of whether the search for a marker is not wholly compromised from the start by the heterogeneity of, what Bleuler called, "the schizophrenias". Rather than proceeding from the assumption of a unitary disease entity, we prefer to view "schizophrenia" as heterogeneous in its neuropathological and cognitive processing substrates and to be guided by the procedural heuristic that the power, range and sensitivity of oculomotor measures is more likely to result in direct mappings onto neural and functionally defined cognitive networks than have so far been demonstrated.

REFERENCES

Abel, L.A., Ziegler, A.S. (1988) Smooth pursuit eye movements in schizophrenics: What constitutes quantitative assessment? *Biological Psychiatry*, **24**, 747–761.

Abel, L.A., Friedman, J., Jesberger, J., Malki, A., Meltzer, H.Y. (1991) Quantitative assessment of smooth pursuit gain and catch-up-saccades in schizophrenia and affective disorders. *Biological Psychiatry*, **29**, 1063–1072.

Anderson, R.A. (1989) Visual and eye movement functions of the posterior parietal cortex. *Annual Review of Neuroscience*, **12**, 377–403.

Anderson, T.J., Jenkins, I.H., Brooks, D.J., Hawken, J.B., Frackowiak, R.S., Kennard, C. (1994) Cortical control of saccades and fixation in man: A PET study. *Brain*, **117**, 1073–1084.

Andreasen, N.C. (1985) *The Comprehensive Assessment of Symptoms and History*, University of Iowa Press, Iowa City.

Bell, B.B., Able, A.A., Li, W., Yee, R.D. (1994) Concordance of smooth pursuit and saccadic measures in normal monozygotic twin pairs. *Biological Psychiatry*, **36**, 522–526.

Bleuler, E. (1911) *Dementia Praecox or the Group of Schizophrenias* (translated by H. Zinkin, 1950), International Universities Press, New York.

Bruce, C.J., Goldberg, M.E. (1985) Primate frontal eye fields. I. Single neurones discharging before saccades. *Journal of Neurophysiology*, **53**, 603–635.

Bruce, C.J., Goldberg, M.E., Bushnell, M.C., Stanton, G.B. (1985) Primate frontal eye fields. II. Physiological and anatomical correlates of electrically evoked eye movements. *Journal of Neurophysiology*, **54**, 714–734.

Callaway, E., Naghdi, S. (1982) An information processing model for schizophrenia. *Archives of General Psychiatry*, **39**, 339–347.

Cassens, G., Inglis, A., Appelbaum, P.S., Gutheil, G. (1990) Neuroleptics: Effects on neuro-psychological function in chronic schizophrenic patients. *Schizophrenia Bulletin*, **16**, 477–492.

Clementz, B.A., Sweeney, J.A. (1990) Is eye movement dysfunction a biological marker for schizophrenia? A methodological review. *Psychological Bulletin*, **108**, 1,77–92.

Cohen, J.D., Servan-Schreiber, D. (1992) Context and dopamine: A connectionist approach to behaviour in schizophrenia. *Psychological Review*, **99**, 45–77.

Couch, F.H., Fox, J.C. (1934) Photographic study of ocular movements in mental disease. *Archives of Neurology and Psychiatry*, **34**, 556–578.

Crawford, T.J., Henderson, L., Kennard, C. (1989a) Abnormalities of nonvisually-guided eye movements in Parkinson's disease. *Brain*, **112**, 1573–1586.

Crawford, T.J., Goodrich, S., Henderson, L., Kennard, C. (1989b) Anticipatory responses to predictable visual signals in Parkinson's disease: Manual key presses and saccadic eye-movements. *Journal of Neurology, Neurosurgery and Psychiatry*, **52**, 1033–1042.

Crawford, T.J., Haegar, B., Kennard, C., Reveley, M.A., Henderson, L. (1995a) Saccadic abnormalities in psychotic patients. I. Neuroleptic-free psychotic patients. *Psychological Medicine*, **25**, 461–471.

Crawford, T.J., Haegar, B., Kennard, C., Reveley, M.A., Henderson, L. (1995b) Saccadic abnormalities in psychotic patients. II. The role of neuroleptic treatment. *Psychological Medicine*, **25**, 473–483.

Crawford, T.J., Lawden, M.C., Haegar, B., Henderson, L., Kennard, C. (1995c) Smooth pursuit eye movement abnormalities in patients with schizophrenia and focal cortical lesions. In: *Eye Movement Research: Mechanisms, Processes and Applications* (Eds R.W. Findlay, J. Walker, R. Kentridge), Elsevier, Amsterdam.

Crawford, T.J., Puri, B.K., Nijran, K.S., Jones, B., Kennard, C., Lewis, S.W. (1996) Abnormal saccadic distractibility in patients with schizophrenia: A 99mTc-HMPAO SPET study. *Psychological Medicine*, **26**, 265–277.

Currie, J., Joyce, S., Maruff, P., Ramsden, B., McArthur Jackson, C., Malone, V. (1993) Selective impairment of express saccade generation in patients with schizophrenia. *Experimental Brain Research*, **97**, 343–348.

Dell'Osso, L.F., Troost, B.T., Daroff, R.B. (1975) Macro square wave jerks. *Neurology*, **25**, 975–979.

Denny-Brown, D. (1966) *The Cerebral Control of Movement*, Liverpool University Press, Liverpool.

Diamond, A. (1990) Developmental time course in human infants and infant monkeys and the neural basis of inhibitory control in reaching. *Annals of New York Academic Sciences*, **608**, 637–669.

Diefendorf, A.R., Dodge, R. (1908) An experimental study of the ocular reactions of the insane from photographic records. *Brain*, **31**, 451–489.

Feinberg, I. (1978) Efference copy and corollary discharge: Implications for thinking and its disorders. *Schizophrenia Bulletin*, **4**, 636–640.

Ferrier, D. (1874) Experiments on the brains of monkeys. *Philosophical Transactions, London*, **165**, 433–488.

Friedman, L., Jesberger, J.A., Meltzer, H.Y. (1991) A model of smooth pursuit performance illus-trates the relationship between gain, catch-up saccade rate and catch-up saccade amplitude in normal controls and patients with schizophrenia. *Biological Psychiatry*, **30**, 537–556.

Friedman, L., Jesberger, J.A., Meltzer, H.Y. (1992) Effect of typical antipsychotic medications and clozapine on smooth pursuit performance in patients with schizophrenia. *Psychiatry Research*, **41**, 25–36.

Friedman, L., Jesberger, J.A., Siever, L.J., Thompson, P., Mohs, R., Meltzer, H.Y. (1995a) Smooth-pursuit performance in patients with affective disorders or schizophrenia and normal controls: Analysis with specific oculomotor measures, RMS error and qualitative ratings. *Psychological Medicine*, **25**, 387–403.

Friedman, L., Kenny, J.T., Jesberger, J.A., Choy, M.M., Meltzer, H.Y. (1995b) Relationship between smooth-pursuit eye-tracking and cognitive performance in schizophrenia. *Biological Psychiatry*, **37**, 265–272.

Frith, C. (1992) *The Cognitive Neuropsychology of Schizophrenia*, Erlbaum, London.

Fukushima, J., Fukushima, K., Chiba, T., Tanaka, S., Yamashita, I., Kata, M. (1988) Disturbances of voluntary control of saccadic eye movements in schizophrenic patients. *Biological Psychiatry*, **23** (7), 670–677.

Fukushima, J., Fukushima, K., Nobuyuki, M., Yamashita, I. (1990) Further analysis of the control of voluntary saccadic eye movements in schizophrenic patients. *Biological Psychiatry*, **28**, 943–958.

Funahashi, S., Bruce, C.J., Goldman-Rakic, P.S. (1989) Mnemonic coding of visual space in the monkey's dorsolateral prefrontal cortex. *Journal of Neurophysiology*, **61**, 331–349.

Funahashi, S., Chafee, M., Goldman-Rakic, P.S. (1993) Prefrontal neuronal activity in rhesus monkeys performing a delayed anti-saccade task. *Nature*, **365**, 753–756.

Fuster, J.M. (1980) *The Prefrontal Cortex*, Raven Press, New York.

Gellman, R.S., Carl, J.R. (1991) Motion processing for saccadic eye movements in humans. *Experimental Brain Research*, **84**, 660–667.

Goldman-Rakic, P.S. (1987) Circuit basis of a cognitive function in non-human primates. In: *Cognitive Neurochemistry* (Eds S.M. Stahl, S.D. Iversen, E.C. Goodman), pp. 91–109, Oxford University Press, Oxford.

Guitton, D., Buchtal, H.A., Douglas, R.M. (1985) Frontal lobe lesions in man cause difficulties in suppressing reflexive glances and in generating goal directed saccades. *Experimental Brain Research*, **58**, 455–474.

Henn, V. (1992) Pathophysiology of rapid eye movements in the horizontal, vertical and torsional directions. In: *Ocular Motor Disorders of the Brain Stem* (Eds V. Buttner, T.H. Brandt), Baillière Tindall, London.

Hikosaka, O., Wurtz, R.H. (1989) The basal ganglia. In: *the Neurobiology of Saccadic Eye Movements* (Eds R.H. Wurtz, M.E. Goldberg), pp. 257–282, Elsevier, Amsterdam.

Holmes, G. (1938) The cerebral integration of the ocular movements. *British Medical Journal*, **2**, 107–112.

Holzman, P.S., Proctor, L.R., Hughes, D.W. (1973) Eye-tracking patterns in schizophrenia. *Science*, **181**, 179–180.

Holzman, P.S., Proctor, L.R., Levy, D.L., Yasillo, N.J., Meltzer, H.Y., Hurt, S.W. (1974) Eye-tracking dysfunctions in schizophrenic patients and their relatives. *Archives of General Psychiatry*, **31**, 143–151.

Hommer, D.W., Clem, T., Litman, R., Pickar, D. (1991) Maladaptive anticipatory saccades in schizophrenia. *Biological Psychiatry*, **30**, 779–794.

Iacono, W.G. (1988) Eye movement abnormalities in schizophrenic and affective disorders. In: *Neuropsychology of Eye Movements* (Eds C.W. Johnston, F.J. Pirozzolo), pp. 115–145, Erlbaum, Hillsdale, NJ.

Kamijo, Y., Nakajima, K., Matsushima, E., Morya, H., Ando, H., Ando, K., Kojima, T., Swa, H., Miyasaka, M. (1991) Saccadic eye movements in schizophrenics: Concerning tardive dyskinesia. *Biological Psychiatry*, **29** (Suppl. 11S), 654S.

Kaufman, S.R., Abel, L.A. (1986) The effects of distraction on smooth pursuit in normal subjects. *Acta Otolaryngologica*, **102**, 57–64.

Kennard, C., Lueck, C.J. (1989) Oculomotor abnormalities in diseases of the basal ganglia. *Revue Neurologique (Paris)*, **145**, 587–595.

Kojima, T., Matsushima, E., Ando, K., Ando, H., Sakurada, M., Ohta, K., Moriya, H., Shimazono, Y. (1992) Exploratory eye-movements and neuropsychological tests in schizophrenic patients. *Schizophrenia Bulletin*, **18**, 85–94.

Kraepelin, E. (1919) Dementia Praecox and Paraphrenia (translated by R.M. Barclay, 1986), Chicago Medical Book, Chicago.

Kurachi, M., Yuasi, S., Tsunoda, M., Kadono, Y. (1991) Neural mechanisms underlying negative symptoms in schizophrenia. *Biological Psychiatry*, **29**, 655S.

Lasker, A.G., Zee, D.S., Hain, T.C., Folstein, S.E., Singer, H.S. (1987) Saccades in Huntington's disease: Initiation defects and distractibility. *Neurology*, **37**, 364–370.

Lawden, M.C., Bagelmann, H., Crawford, T.J., Matthews, T.D., Kennard, C. (1995) An effect of structured backgrounds on smooth pursuit eye movements in patients with cerebral lesions. *Brain*, **118**, 37–48.

Leigh, R.J., Zee, D.S. (1991) *The Neurology of Eye Movements* (2nd edn), Davis, Philadelphia.

Levin, S. (1984) Frontal lobe dysfunction in schizophrenia. I. Eye movement impairments. *Journal of Psychiatric Research*, **18**, 27–55.

Levy, D.L., Holzman, P.S., Matthysse, S., Mendell, N.R. (1994) Eye tracking and schizophrenia: A selective review. *Schizophrenia Bulletin*, **20**, 47–62.

Liddle, P.F., Morris, D.L. (1991) Schizophrenic syndromes and frontal lobe performance. *British Journal of Psychiatry*, **158**, 340–345.

Lipton, R.B., Levy, D.L., Holzman, P.S., Levin, S. (1983) Eye movement dysfunctions in psychiatric patients: A review. *Schizophrenia Bulletin*, **9**, 13–32.

Litman, R.E., Hommer, D.W., Clem, T., Rapaport, M.H., Pato, C.N., Pickar, D. (1989) Smooth pursuit eye movements in schizophrenia: Effects of neuroleptic treatment and caffeine. *Psychopharmacology Bulletin*, **25**, 473–478.

Lueck, C.J., Tanyeri, S., Crawford, T.J., Henderson, L., Kennard, C. (1990) Antisaccades and remembered saccades in Parkinson's disease. *Journal of Neurology, Neurosurgery and Psychiatry*, **53**, 284–288.

Lueck, C.J., Crawford, T.J., Henderson, L., Kennard, C. (1992b) Saccadic eye movements in Parkinson's diseases: II. Remembered saccades: Towards a unified hypothesis. *Quarterly Journal of Experimental Psychology*, **45A**(2), 211.

Lueck, C., Tanyerim, S., Crawford, T.J., Henderson, L., Kennard, C. (1992a) Saccadic eye movements in Parkinson's diseases: I. Delayed saccades. *Quarterly Journal of Experimental Psychology*, **45A**(2), 193–210.

Matsue, Y., Goto, H., Saito, T., Ueno, H., Matsuoka, Y., Fuse, H., Chiba, H., Sato, M. (1991) Pursuit eye movement dysfunction and disinhibition of saccades in schizophrenia. *Biological Psychiatry*, **29** (Suppl. 11S), 387S.

Matsue, Y., Osakabe, K., Saito, H., Goto, Y., Ueno, T., Matsuoka, H., Chiba, H., Fuse, Y., Sato, M. (1994) Smooth-pursuit eye-movements and express saccades in schizophrenic patients. *Schizophrenia Research*, **12**, 121–130.

McGhie, A., Chapman, J. (1961) Disorders of attention and perception in early schizophrenia. *British Journal of Psychiatry*, **34**, 103–116.

Pardo, J.V., Pardo, P.J., Janer, K.W., Raichle, M.E. (1990) The anterior cingulate cortex mediates processing in the Stroop attentional conflict paradigm. *Proceedings of the National Academy of Sciences USA*, **87**, 256–259.

Paus, P. (1991) Modes of central gaze fixation maintenance and oculomotor distractibility in schizophrenics. *Schizophrenia Research*, **5**, 145–152.

Paus, T., Kalina, M., Patockova, L., Angerova, Y., Cerny, R., Mecir, P., Bauer, J., Krabec, P. (1991) Medial vs lateral frontal lobe lesions and differential impairment of central-gaze fixation maintenance in man. *Brain*, **114**, 2051–2067.

Penfield, W., Baldrey, E. (1937) Somatic motor and sensory representation in the cerebral cortex of man as studied by electrical stimulation. *Brain*, **60**, 389–433.

Pierrot-Deseilligny, C.H., Rivaud, S., Pillon, B., Fournier, E., Agid, Y. (1989) Lateral visually-guided saccades in progressive supranuclear palsy. *Brain*, **112**, 471–487.

Pierrot-Deseilligny, C.H., Rivaud, S., Gaymaud, B., Agid, Y. (1991) Cortical control of reflexive visually-guided saccades. *Brain*, **114**, 1473–1485.

Posner, M.I., Peterson, S.E. (1990) The attention system of the human brain. *Annual Review of Neuroscience*, **13**, 25–42.

Reason, J. (1990) *Human Error*, Cambridge University Press, Cambridge.

Robbins, T. (1990) The case for frontostriatal dysfunction in schizophrenia. *Schizophrenia Bulletin*, **16**, 391–402.

Sawaguchi, T., Goldman-Rakic, P.S. (1991) *Science*, **251**, 947–950.

Schall, J.D. (1991a) Neuronal activity related to visually guided saccadic eye movements in the supplementary motor area of Rhesus monkeys. *Journal of Neurophysiology*, **66**, 530–558.

Schall, J.D. (1991b) Neuronal activity related to visually guided saccades in the frontal eye fields of Rhesus monkeys: Comparison with supplementary eye fields. *Journal of Neurophysiology*, **66**, 559–579.

Schiller, P.H., True, S.D., Conway, J.L. (1980) Deficits in eye movements following frontal eye field and superior colliculus ablations. *Journal of Neurophysiology*, **44**, 1175–1189.

Schlag, J., Schlag-Rey, M. (1987) Evidence for a supplementary eye field. *Journal of Neurophysiology*, **57**, 179–200.

Segraves, M.A., Goldberg, M.E. (1987) Functional properties of corticotectal neurons in the monkey's frontal eye field. *Journal of Neurophysiology*, **58**,1387–1419.

Sereno, A.B., Holzman, P.S. (1993) Express saccades and smooth-pursuit eye-movement function in schizophrenic, affective-disorder, and normal subjects. *Journal of Cognitive Neuroscience*, **5**, 303–316.

Sereno, A.B., Holzman, P.S. (1995) Antisaccades and smooth-pursuit eye-movements in schizophrenia. *Biological Psychiatry*, **37**, 394–401.

Stuss, D.T., Benson, D.F. (1986) *The Frontal Lobes*, Raven Press, New York.

Sweeney, J.A., Haas, G.L., Li, S.H., Weiden, P.J. (1994) Selective effects of antipsychotic medications on eye-tracking performance in schizophrenia. *Psychiatry Research*, **54**, 185–198.

Thaker, G.K., Nguyen, J.A., Tamminga, C.A. (1989) Increased saccadic distractibility in tardive dyskinesia: Functional evidence for subcortical GABA dysfunction. *Biological Psychiatry*, **25**, 45–59.

Thurston, S., Leigh, J., Crawford, T.J., Thompson, A., Kennard, C. (1988) Two distinct deficits of visual tracking caused by unilateral lesions of cerebral cortex in man. *Annals of Neurology*, **23**, 266–273.

Williams, G.V., Goldman-Rakic, P.S. (1994) Modulation of memory fields by dopamine D1 receptors in prefrontal cortex. *Nature*, **376**, 572–575.

Wurtz, R.H., Goldberg, M.E. (1989) *The Neurobiology of Saccadic Eye Movements*, Elsevier, Amsterdam.

Yee, R.D., Baloh, R.W., Marder, S.R., Levy, D.L., Sakala, S.M., Honrubia, V. (1987) Eye movements in schizophrenia. *Investigative Ophthalmological Visual Sciences*, **28**, 366–374.

14

Structural Neuroimaging and Neuropsychological Impairments

ROBERT M. BILDER and PHILIP R. SZESZKO

INTRODUCTION

Since the landmark demonstration of ventricular enlargement in patients with schizophrenia by Johnstone and colleagues (1976), *in vivo* neuroimaging studies have led to the identification of additional structural anomalies in these patients. Unfortunately, both the causes and functional significance of these abnormalities remain largely unknown. In this context, neuropsychological methods may be employed to understand the nature and development of brain dysfunction. Using information gained in the study of disorders with known aetiology and pathophysiology, neuropsychological techniques may help to identify both the precursors and functional correlates of structural abnormalities. These techniques may help distinguish whether an observed pattern of brain dysfunction reflects an early developmental compromise or later deteriorative processes.

In addition, delineation of patterns of neuropsychological impairment may be a useful approach to aid the identification of the dysfunctional systems that accompany any given structural abnormality. Such an approach is similar to that used in the differential diagnosis and localisation of neurological insults. A combination of these neuropsychological approaches (i.e. those which examine the course and nature of impairment and those which identify the affected neuroanatomical systems) may be especially valuable in understanding the significance of structural abnormalities in syndromes with unknown pathophysiology, such as schizophrenia.

A review of existing evidence supports the identification of at least three independent pathological processes, each of which may be marked by a set of gross anatomical features and accompanying functional deficits. First, general

Schizophrenia: A Neuropsychological Perspective. Edited by C. Pantelis, H.E. Nelson and T.R.E. Barnes
© 1996 John Wiley & Sons Ltd

deficits in lateralised cerebral specialisation may interfere with the acquisition of basic cognitive competencies but also decrease vulnerability to deteriorative processes. Second, periventricular damage may interfere with learning and memory functions. Each of these processes may be relatively non-specific but contribute to the diathesis for schizophrenia. Third, a medial frontolimbic abnormality, involving disturbed development of the dorsal cytoarchitectonic trend and marked by structural abnormalities in hippocampus, cingulate and medial/dorsal premotor and prefrontal regions, may be more specific to the schizophrenia syndrome. Damage to this system may lead to deficits in the executive control of behaviour and underlie a range of the attentional, organisational and neuromotor disturbances that are characteristic of patients with schizophrenia.

ANATOMICAL ABNORMALITIES AND THEIR FUNCTIONAL CORRELATES: OVERVIEW

Although a variety of anatomical abnormalities have been identified in schizophrenia, most work has failed to indicate a focal or specific pathological process. Structural brain imaging using computerised tomography (CT) has yielded reports of the most widely documented abnormalities: ventricular enlargement (VE) and cortical sulcal enlargement (SE). These comprise the least specific abnormalities detectable on neuroradiological examination. Some other findings such as "atrophy" of the cerebellar vermis, densitometric anomalies, abnormalities in the normal pattern of hemispheric asymmetry and abnormalities in the shape and/or size of the corpus callosum have been less widely replicated and are also of uncertain significance. There have been several reviews of this CT literature to which the reader is referred (e.g. Goetz & Van Kammen, 1986; Raz, 1989), including two meta-analyses of the major findings (Raz & Raz, 1990; van Horn & McManus, 1992).

The more recent application of magnetic resonance imaging (MRI) has corroborated earlier findings based on CT scanning. Additionally, MRI has a number of advantages over CT which provide greater scope for studies investigating the nature of structural brain abnormalities in schizophrenia. First, MRI provides high-resolution imaging of structures without artefact of nearby bony surfaces. Thus, there is greater potential for examining and measuring structures that are juxtaposed to the inner surfaces of the skull, such as the basal forebrain and anterior temporal lobe. Second, the absence of ionising radiation with MRI is more appropriate for longitudinal, repeated-measures designs and, therefore, allows the evaluation of parallel deterioration of brain structure and function. Third, three-dimensional MRI acquisition, along with advanced image reconstruction methods applied to MRI data, offers greater promise for simultaneous examination of multiple morphologic features in the same patients. This also allows imaging of different structures that are best visualised in different planes. The simultaneous assessment of multiple anatomical features in the same subjects offers hope that their patterns of co-variation will become better understood, which would foster a better understanding of the degree to which specific structural abnormalities reflect one or more different pathological processes.

RELATIONSHIP OF STRUCTURAL AND OTHER MEASURES

Clues to the significance of structural abnormalities have been sought in studies attempting to relate structure to a number of other phenomena associated with the disease, such as symptoms, biological correlates and neuropsychological findings. These comparisons have met with limited success. Most attention has been directed to the study of the relationship between structural abnormalities and symptoms. Generally, these studies have been disappointing and little evidence has been found to support widely held hypotheses that structural abnormalities, such as VE and/or SE, are related to either the presence of "negative" symptoms or the absence of "positive" symptoms. For example, Raz (1989) reviewed 16 studies, among which only two reported significant associations of structural abnormality with negative symptoms. Studies attempting to link structural abnormalities with movement disorders, premorbid social adjustment and response to neuroleptic treatment have generally found no association (for review: Bilder, 1992).

However, these equivocal findings may reflect failure to identify structural abnormalities that are germane to key clinical features of the syndrome and/or a failure to identify clinical constructs that are relevant to the structural abnormalities. For example, two recent studies using MRI, which focused on the superior temporal gyrus, demonstrated a relationship to certain positive symptoms and thought disorder (Barta et al, 1990; Shenton et al, 1992). Other MRI studies have shown that detailed morphometry of the ventricular system (Degreef et al, 1992) and of the hippocampo-amygdaloid complex (Bogerts et al, 1993) may yield measures of brain structure that relate more clearly to symptoms than the kinds of measures that were available in older CT scan studies.

One area demonstrating a consistent relationship to structural abnormalities is that of neurochemistry. Specifically, more severe VE and SE have been related to low concentrations of homovanillic acid (HVA) and 5-hydroxyindoleacetic acid (5-HIAA) (chief metabolites of dopamine and serotonin, respectively) in the cerebrospinal fluid (CSF) of patients with schizophrenia. Unfortunately, it remains unclear whether this finding reflects decreased levels in patients with structural abnormality or is a result of increased levels among patients with no structural abnormality (see Raz, 1989 for a discussion of this and other methodological problems with this work).

Another consistently robust finding has been the relationship between structural abnormalities and neuropsychological dysfunction. Although some reviews have suggested that findings are mixed (e.g. Goetz & Van Kammen, 1986; Zec & Weinberger, 1986), the majority of studies have indicated significant associations between structural abnormality and neuropsychological deficit. Moreover, compared to the findings of other correlative studies these associations have been relatively robust. This literature has been reviewed in detail elsewhere (Bilder,

1992). The chapter briefly summarises these findings and aims to highlight some additional directions for future research.

METHODOLOGICAL ISSUES

A range of methodological problems affect the interpretation of studies of structure–function relations in schizophrenia. First, it should be recognised that only ventricular enlargement has been studied in any detail. Results from these studies are difficult to compare because of the variability in methods used to assess ventricular size. These methods have included the use of qualitative ratings, linear indices and planimetric measures such as the ventricular brain ratio (VBR). Indeed, Raz et al (1987) obtained different values for measures of the cerebral ventricles using volumetric, linear and planimetric indices. Another methodological problem is that even among studies reporting the VBR, there are machine related differences and different criteria for slice selection which make comparisons across studies difficult.

To complicate matters further there is much variability in neuropsychological assessment (see Goldstein, chapter 3). Some studies used only brief mental status examinations while others employed more comprehensive test batteries. When brief tests are used, positive results do little to discern the specific pathological systems that may mediate functional deficits, whereas negative results are uninformative because of the insensitivity of the measurement instruments. There are also problems with studies that have used more extensive batteries. In general, these problems include: (1) the use of cut-off scores, to differentiate normal from abnormal groups, or summary measures of neuropsychological performance, neither of which utilise the full discriminating power of the measuring instrument; (2) the failure to assure comprehensive assessment of relevant functional brain systems; (3) the failure to determine that certain morphological abnormalities are accompanied by a specific, rather than a generalised neuropsychological deficit; and (4) the failure to consider possible effects of neuroleptic and ancillary medications on neuropsychological performance.

Sampling is one of the most difficult issues to contend with in schizophrenia research since there are so many variables that could confound results when interpreting relationships between neuropsychological test results and morphological data. These include age, sex, education, handedness, obstetric complications, cultural and socioeconomic factors, family history of psychiatric disorder, history of medical illness, substance abuse, head trauma, age at which symptoms first appeared, duration of illness and treatment, type of treatment, treatment response, side effects (e.g. tardive dyskinesia or extra-pyramidal symptoms), overall level of neuropsychological functioning and the extent of morphological abnormality. Since it is unlikely that any investigation could control for all these potentially confounding variables, a more prudent course of action might be standardisation of assessment methods and data analysis that would enable comparisons across research centres.

NEUROPSYCHOLOGICAL DEFICITS ASSOCIATED WITH STRUCTURAL ABNORMALITIES

CSF SPACE ENLARGEMENTS AND DETERIORATION-SENSITIVE FUNCTIONS

In a detailed review of the literature on structure–function relations in schizophrenia, Bilder (1992) suggested that the most widely studied morphological abnormalities, primarily VE and to some extent SE, are associated with deficits on measures of memory, attention, speed of performance and "fluid" cognitive abilities. However, no associations are found with impairments on tests of basic language competencies and general knowledge. This pattern may explain why studies relating VE or SE to performance on neuropsychological test batteries have most often yielded associations of deficit with structural abnormality, while studies using intelligence tests have more often found no association.

Even among studies using intelligence tests, structural abnormalities have more often been related to deficits on deterioration-sensitive subtests ("don't hold" subtests; e.g. Digit Symbol or Digit Span) than to performance on subtests that are relatively resistant to deterioration ("hold" subtests; e.g. Information or Vocabulary). This distinction between "hold" and "don't hold" tests is used clinically to estimate premorbid intellectual ability and deterioration from premorbid levels (Wechsler, 1958; Lezak, 1983). A clinical neuropsychologist, seeing the average test profile of patients with VE or SE, might conclude that these profiles reflected deterioration. Several independent groups of investigators contrasted performance on "hold" and "don't hold" tests to form composite indices and found that VE and/or SE were more strongly related to these more general indices than to deficits on individual tests (Bilder, 1985; Bilder et al, 1988; DeQuardo et al, 1994; Nyman et al, 1986).

Interpreting these findings at face value would suggest that VE and SE reflect degeneration. This simple interpretation would be supported if it could be demonstrated that either VE or SE were typical, atrophic, degenerative processes. When VE and SE were first observed in schizophrenia, investigators speculated that they were due to atrophic changes since they resembled the findings in degenerative diseases such as dementia (Weinberger, 1984). However, subsequent research showed that: (1) structural changes may be found in young, untreated, first episode patients; (2) VE may be associated with poor premorbid social adjustment; (3) VE may be associated with obstetric complications or other perinatal traumata (for review: Bilder, 1992). These findings indicated that these structural abnormalities were not the results of long-term illness or treatment. Moreover, the possible links to early developmental antecedents suggested that the pathological process(es) responsible for these structural abnormalities might operate before or near the time of birth and certainly well before overt manifestations of the schizophrenia syndrome.

Still more compelling evidence that VE and SE might reflect developmental dysplasia rather than degenerative encephalopathy can be found in post-mortem studies. Although some studies have yielded histological evidence compatible with cellular death and tissue degeneration there have been a number of failures to replicate these findings. This has led to suggestions that the changes resulting in VE and/or SE must occur in the immature brain before it is capable of reactive gliosis (see Bogerts, 1990). While none of these findings have enabled unequivocal specification of the pathological processes leading to VE and SE, they have fostered controversy about the relative abilities of "neurodevelopmental" (dysplastic) and "neurodegenerative" hypotheses to account for both these structural abnormalities and their correlates (see Lieberman & DeLisi, 1991).

Longitudinal follow-up studies could determine whether deterioration of structure occurs in schizophrenia. Existing studies of structural change are not definitive due to methodological problems. However, positive findings are compatible with the impression that a subset of patients with schizophrenia (from 17% to 30%) show progression of structural abnormality after the onset of symptoms and that this structural change is paralleled by clinical deterioration (for review: Bilder, 1992). These figures are compatible with the estimated proportions of patients likely to show moderate to severe functional decline, based on detailed clinical observations of large samples (Bleuler, 1972; Ciompi, 1980, 1989; Huber et al, 1975). Unfortunately, recent studies, including those of first episode patients, may have failed to detect progression of structural abnormality within a subgroup of patients due to small sample sizes and a corresponding difficulty distinguishing subsets of patients in whom clinical deterioration occurred (DeLisi et al, 1991; Degreef et al, 1991). It is likely that definitive answers will await the results of large scale, prospective follow-up studies of patients starting when symptoms first emerge.

More attention should be focused on the possibility that significant deterioration may occur prior to the onset of overt symptoms. According to family informants, patients first hospitalised for psychosis may have had psychotic symptoms for over a year as well as signs of behavioural change for several years (Lieberman et al, 1992). Thus, even studies of first episode patients may fail to recognise a progressive pathological process appearing concomitantly with the emergence of overt symptoms. It remains unclear whether there may be significant decline even earlier. Ratings of premorbid social and academic adjustment may show patterns of decline in childhood and early adolescence, well before the emergence of behavioural changes that family members associate with incipient psychosis (Mukherjee et al, 1989). Studying "premorbid deterioration" obviously involves difficulties in ascertainment. High risk samples might offer logical targets for the study of premorbid deterioration, although the cost of these efforts is daunting.

Until such studies can be conducted, neuropsychological findings may offer clues to the pathological processes underlying VE and/or SE. As noted above, the pattern of neuropsychological deficits associated with enlargement of CSF spaces suggests deterioration of function. This pattern appears to be sufficiently robust in that some investigators have reported paradoxical findings of better performance on certain tests among patients with more severe VE and/or SE (Bilder et al, 1988; Carr & Wedding, 1984; DeQuardo et al, 1994; Nyman et al, 1986; Obiols et al, 1987). When paradoxical results have been found, they have been most selective to those tests considered good indices of premorbid ability. Sampling differences that might lead to this pattern of results are considered in detail elsewhere (Bilder, 1992). The observations that VE and SE are associated with impairment of deterioration-sensitive functions, but not with impairment of premorbid ability, has suggested two non-exclusive possibilities:

1. VE/SE have their cognitive effects after the successful acquisition of basic cognitive competencies and, thus, they may be considered markers of a deteriorative process; or,
2. some independent process, unrelated to (or negatively correlated with) VE/SE, has a more pronounced effect on the customary indices of "premorbid" ability, which are thought to reflect the acquisition of language and general knowledge.

The latter interpretation could help explain the apparently paradoxical findings of Johnstone et al (1989), who reported that neuropsychological function was poorest among patients with the smallest and the largest ventricles, while patients with intermediate ventricular size had better neuropsychological function. This "inverted-U" relation might be expected if there are independent pathological processes, one related to VE and the other predominating specifically in patients without VE. Some independent pathological process is further suggested by findings that neuropsychological morbidity is more prevalent than structural abnormality as manifest in VE or SE. This finding cannot be explained by differences in the criteria for defining abnormality of structure and function (Bilder, 1992). Furthermore, the findings are consistent with the view that some threshold of brain dysfunction may be sufficient to produce vulnerability to schizophrenia. Bilder and colleagues (Bilder & Degreef, 1991; Bilder, 1992) hypothesised that for some patients this vulnerability is expressed in poor performance on tests of "fluid" neuropsychological functions and may be marked by VE or SE. For others, the vulnerability is seen in a pattern of failed development of basic cognitive competencies and is unrelated to VE or SE.

CEREBRAL SPECIALISATION TRENDS AND COGNITIVE DEVELOPMENT

If poor early cognitive development is not associated with VE or SE, it is possible that there may be some other structural abnormalities that could explain these deficits. Bilder and colleagues have argued previously that failures of "cerebral specialisation", including reductions of brain size and asymmetry, might be involved (Bilder, 1992; Bilder & Degreef, 1991). To the extent that both sets of morphological features have been studied simultaneously, these cerebral specialisation abnormalities have been statistically independent from both VE and SE. In fact, findings of reversed occipital asymmetry were found selectively among patients who did not have either VE or SE (Luchins et al, 1982). Overall brain volume has also been found to be unrelated to either VE or SE (Andreasen et al,

1986; Johnstone et al, 1989; Pearlson et al, 1989). These findings are compatible with the suggestion that general neurodevelopmental processes governing overall brain size and cerebral asymmetries are unrelated to the processes underlying VE and SE. While there is so far little information about the relation between brain size and asymmetry, we found no clear relations between overall cortical volume and asymmetry in a sample of first episode patients and healthy controls; further, in this sample, patients did not have smaller brain volumes but did lack the normal cortical asymmetries (Bilder et al, 1994).

Are abnormalities in these general brain growth trends related to clinical features of early developmental failure? Examining the symptom correlates of occipital asymmetry, Luchins & Meltzer (1983) found that "poor quality of interview" from the Present State Examination (PSE; Wing et al, 1974) distinguished the patients who had reversals of the normal asymmetry. This PSE item is most critically affected by failures in verbal communication abilities. Patients with reversed asymmetry were also distinguished by a highly atypical psychometric pattern; specifically, Verbal IQ was lower than Performance IQ (Luchins et al, 1982). Although there is evidence supporting "left hemisphere" hypotheses of the neuropsychological deficits in schizophrenia almost all studies of intellectual functioning in samples of patients with schizophrenia reveal the opposite pattern with higher Verbal IQ (for reviews: Goldberg & Seidman, 1991; Barber et al, chapter 4). In a sample of first episode patients, we recently reported that absence of the normal cortical asymmetries was more common in patients who received diagnoses of the "undifferentiated" compared to the "paranoid" subtype of schizophrenia and that men who lacked the normal asymmetries had more severe negative symptoms (Bilder et al, 1994). These findings, together with those of Luchins and his colleagues, suggest that patients who lack the normal asymmetries may be less likely to develop systematised psychotic symptoms. Failure to develop typical patterns of manual preference have also been associated with a particularly poor developmental profile (Green et al, 1989). These findings suggest that abnormalities in the development of normal cerebral asymmetries may be associated with prominent disturbances of language and other cognitive competencies that develop early in the lifespan (see also Wolf and Cornblatt, chapter 9).

While deviations from the normal pattern of cerebral asymmetry may have adverse consequences with respect to the development of language and other specialised cognitive coding schemata, there may also be advantages associated with lesser degrees of cerebral specialisation (Geschwind & Galaburda, 1985). It has been hypothesised that the less lateralised (less specialised) brain may be less vulnerable to the effects of insults. This hypothesis was invoked to explain the association of reversed occipital asymmetry and lower degrees of manual dominance with a *decreased* risk for the development of persistent tardive dyskinesia (TD). Barr et al (1989) found that non-dextral patients with schizophrenia without normal occipital asymmetry had less persistent TD movements than those with normal dominance and asymmetry patterns. Similarly, Kern et al (1991) found that, in comparison to non-dextral patients, dextral patients with schizophrenia exhibited more TD movements on clinical measures. In another study, Waddington et al (1990) suggested that cognitive deterioration was associated with the emergence of TD. Together, these studies support the notion that cerebral specialisation may be associated with the emergence of TD movements and deterioration in cognitive functioning (for review: Collinson et al, chapter 12).

Absence or reversal of the normal asymmetry of the Sylvian fissure, which has been identified in both MRI (Hoff et al, 1992) and post-mortem (Falkai et al, 1992) studies of schizophrenia, may also be related to better neuropsychological functioning (Hoff et al, 1992). Analysing differences between first episode and chronic patients with schizophrenia, the authors concluded that dextral patients appeared to be at greater risk of intellectual deterioration following the onset of illness (Bilder et al, 1992). Taken together, these findings suggest that patients with atypical patterns of cerebral specialisation may have a lower capacity for establishing certain developmental cognitive competencies but are less vulnerable to other pathological insults.

DO LOCALISED PATHOLOGICAL PROCESSES UNDERLIE SPECIFIC DEFICITS IN CEREBRAL AUTOREGULATION?

Not only do atypical patterns of cerebral specialisation appear to be independent of enlargement of the CSF spaces but VE and SE themselves may comprise markers of independent pathological processes. Meta-analysis of studies in which both abnormalities were examined together showed that VE was not associated with SE (Raz & Raz, 1990). Moreover, in an analysis of the familial and environmental antecedents of VE and SE in schizophrenia (Cannon et al, 1989), VE was associated with both obstetric complications and familial risk, while SE was associated with family history alone. This possible dissociation of the pathological processes underlying VE and SE has been replicated (Cannon et al, 1993), suggesting that VE might mark a process of environmental insult superimposed on a congenital vulnerability, while SE might mark a more exclusively genetic predisposition.

Unfortunately, there have been few attempts to determine whether other clinical features may distinguish VE from SE. It was noted above that clinical symptoms have been essentially unrelated to either VE or SE. Retrospective analysis of early social and academic functioning suggested that VE was associated more with persistent deficits of social functioning, while SE was linked more to a pattern of decline in academic functioning during late childhood (Mukherjee et al, 1989). In the same sample, other analyses suggested that VE was associated more with both social maladjustment and deterioration of memory functions, while SE was linked more strongly to deficits in "anterior" (motor and executive) cortical functions (Bilder, 1985; Bilder et al, 1988). Some other findings suggest that disturbances of learning and memory may be prominent correlates of VE (Johnstone et al, 1989; Keilp et al, 1988; Lawson et al, 1988). There is intuitive appeal to the notion that SE may be associated with predominantly anterior cortical dysfunction, with impairments of executive, motor and attentional abilities; while VE may be associated with predominantly subcortico-limbic dysfunction, manifest as learning and memory deficits. However, the existing evidence is not consistent enough to reject the null hypothesis that both types of structural abnormality are associated with a pattern of diffuse brain dysfunction.

The failure so far to identify consistent neuropsychological deficits associated with VE or SE may reflect a lack of refinement in both sets of measures, rather than the absence of genuine associations. Thus, few studies have attempted to determine whether enlargement of different components of the ventricular system, or regionally focal patterns of sulcal prominence, may have unique neuropsychological correlates. There are suggestions that different components of the ventricular system may be differentially affected (Degreef et al, 1992; Bornstein et al, 1992) and that SE in different loci may have different functional correlates (McCarley et al, 1989). It would therefore appear worthwhile to focus more closely on regional variations of structural abnormalities in attempts to identify localised patterns of cerebral dysfunction.

Moreover, few neuropsychological studies have used a comprehensive approach to assessment that enables reliable and valid assessment of multiple, distinct functional domains. Of 42 published reports, eight used the Halstead Reitan Battery (HRB) or Luria–Nebraska Neuropsychological Battery (LNNB) with only one of these studies using both, seven studies used other non-standard composite batteries, while the remainder used either brief mental status examinations, single neuropsychological tests or an IQ test (or selected subtests) alone. Use of the HRB without supplemental tests may be criticised specifically for the lack of learning and memory measures; use of the LNNB alone may be criticised for a range of issues involving its validation and scale construction (see Lezak, 1983). If one takes these criticisms seriously, only six of these 42 reports included adequate methods to assess functionally specific impairment.

There is a further problem that prompts questions about the adequacy of standard neuropsychological methods to investigate the functional correlates of abnormal cerebral morphology in schizophrenia or in other disorders with suspected neurodevelopmental bases. Even using a comprehensive battery of neuropsychological tests there is no assurance that we are assessing relevant functions. The validation of almost all neuropsychological constructs derives from studies of patients with focal cortical pathology following relatively healthy development. There are good reasons to wonder whether these methods are useful in the study of syndromes such as schizophrenia. In schizophrenia focal cortical damage is either not present or very rare. Indeed, cases with focal cortical damage, even if presenting with symptoms characteristic of schizophrenia, would satisfy exclusion criteria according to most diagnostic systems. Moreover, there is ample evidence that at least some of the pathological processes underlying brain dysfunction in schizophrenia are neurodevelopmental.

When comprehensive batteries of neuropsychological tests are administered to patients with schizophrenia the resulting profiles are most often interpreted as evidence of frontotemporal, frontolimbic or subcortical dysfunction (Flor-Henry, 1983; Goldberg & Seidman, 1991; Kolb & Whishaw, 1983; Seidman, 1983; Gruzelier et al, 1988; Pantelis et al, 1992). These inferences are drawn from findings that patients with schizophrenia are most impaired on measures of attentional, executive and memory functions. Such neuropsychological disturbances may indeed be associated with focal disruptions of limbic, diencephalic or striatal nuclei. Unfortunately, there is sparse data about the effects of highly focal lesions to these regions and comparable deficit profiles may be seen in "diffuse" disorders, including toxic-metabolic encephalopathies and closed head injury. What is needed, to enable a better understanding of schizophrenia generally and to gain insights into structure–function relations in this syndrome, is an improved neuropsychology of the mechanisms underlying cerebral arousal, activation and effort (used here in the sense advocated by Pribram & McGuinness, 1975). These mechanisms clearly involve the key frontal, striatal, limbic, diencephalic and mesencephalic centres that have become suspect in schizophrenia. However, their specific roles remain difficult if not impossible to disentangle using traditional neuropsychological methods. Moreover, while dysfunction in these "primary drivers" of cortical activation states may be sufficient to explain the neuropsychological impairments of schizophrenia, it is plausible that similar deficits may reflect aberrant patterns of cortico-cortical connectivity. A failure in the organisation of parallel re-entrant neural networks at the cortical level alone could explain the same disorders of activational tone and would also be parsimonious with the evidence (Edelman, 1987).

Bilder & Degreef (1991) previously suggested that a "medial frontolimbic" defect might prove sufficient as an essential vulnerability to schizophrenia and that this disturbance might be marked by specific cerebral morphological features, including volume reductions in the anterior hippocampus and certain multi-site cortical abnormalities. Periventricular damage and cerebral specialisation deficits were seen as potentially contributing to the diathesis but neither necessary nor sufficient to produce psychosis. In specifying the *medial* (or dorsal) frontolimbic system as central to the schizophrenia syndrome these authors wished to distinguish this from the *lateral* (or ventral) system. This distinction follows the duality in cytoarchitectonic patterns that was proposed by Sanides (1969) in his evolutionary model and which has been supported by further detailed anatomical studies of both long-range connectivity patterns and shorter-range patterns of laminar organisation (Pandya & Barnes, 1987; Yeterian & Pandya, 1988). The medial frontolimbic trend is seen by these investigators as originating from a primordial archicortical moiety (hippocampus); the next phase in development of this trend is proisocortical (cingulate); the highest phase of development in this trend is represented by true, six-layered isocortex, comprising the medial aspects of the dorsal neocortices and the most dorsal aspects of the lateral neocortices. This system can be distinguished from the lateral (paleocortical) cytoarchitectonic trend which originates in the olfactory cortex and has higher phases of development in peri-insular and ventral neocortices.

The functional significance of this distinction between medial and lateral cytoarchitectonic trends has been elaborated by Goldberg (1985, 1987) in elegant studies of the premotor cortex. He drew the distinction between the medial system's involvement in the "projectional" control of behaviour and its sensitivity to internal contexts; while the lateral system is more involved in responsive control of behaviour and is sensitive to external contexts. A clinical example, that is particularly germane to schizophrenia, involves effects of lesions to the supplementary motor area, which is the medial-trend component of the premotor cortex. These lesions may lead to the "alien hand syndrome" in which patients may lack volitional control over the hand contralateral to the lesion but, still more dramatically, frequently attribute spontaneous actions of the "alien" hand to external agents (see also Cahill and Frith, chapter 18). There is a clear parallel of these phenomena to certain symptoms seen in schizophrenia, including thought insertion and withdrawal and ideas of reference. This general defect in appreciating the intentional source of actions has further been used to explain such phenomena as hallucinations (Frith, 1987; Frith & Done, 1989; Gray et al, 1991).

Evidence supporting the specificity of defects in schizophrenia to the medial trend includes:

1. Cytoarchitectonic or gross anatomical abnormalities have been found in the hippocampal formation (Scheibel & Kovelman, 1981; Kovelman & Scheibel, 1984; Bogerts et al, 1985, 1990, 1993; Conrad & Scheibel, 1987; Becker et al, 1990; Rossi et al, 1991; Breier et al, 1992; Conrad et al, 1992; Buchanan et al, 1993). Moreover, when structural defects have been found in the hippocampal formation, the anterior hippocampus has been implicated most frequently (Suddath et al, 1989, 1990; DeLisi et al, 1988; Shenton et al, 1992). The anterior hippocampus is more dedicated to efferent projections to the medial frontolimbic system while posterior hippocampus is more involved in receiving afferents from posterior neocortices.

2. Cytoarchitectonic defects have been found in cingulate and medial frontal cortices (Benes et al, 1986; Benes, 1987; Akbarian et al, 1993). These comprise the intermediate proisocortical and true, six-layered isocortical divisions of the medial "archicortical" cytoarchitectonic trend.

3. Studies of cerebral metabolism showing impairments in activation of dorsolateral prefrontal cortex show these deficits specifically in the most dorsal and medial regions, as well as in the cingulate gyrus (Weinberger et al, 1986; Berman, 1987; Early et al, 1987).

4. The dorsal cytoarchitectonic trend has unique and relatively specific relations with the striatopallidal system (Pandya & Barnes, 1987) which has been implicated in the mediation of antipsychotic drug effects. It may have a role in the pathophysiology of key symptoms of the schizophrenia syndrome (see Early et al, 1989a, 1989b; Gray et al, 1991) and has shown abnormal patterns of activation in functional brain imaging studies (for review: Buchsbaum, 1990).

5. Many of the findings of attentional and executive dyscontrol that have been observed in schizophrenia may be classified as reflecting deficits in the "projectional" control of behaviour which has been seen as the key functional role played by the medial trend (Goldberg, 1985, 1987). Similar deficits are the predicted result of failures in frontostriatal "activation" which was hypothesised to be one of three major systems regulating cerebral activity (Pribram & McGuinness, 1975; McGuinness & Pribram, 1980; Tucker & Williamson, 1984) and which maps onto the medial frontolimbic system, as described above. The principal functional role of these systems involves the maintenance

of stable response sets, particularly in the face of environmental irrelevancies. Examples of cognitive or neuropsychological deficits in schizophrenia that may be understood as reflecting dysfunctions within the medial frontolimbic trend include: (a) continuous performance test deficits (Neuchterlein & Dawson, 1984; Cornblatt et al, 1988, 1990); (b) the reaction time "crossover" phenomenon (Steffy & Galbraith, 1980; Galbraith et al, 1983; DeAmicis et al, 1986); (c) Wisconsin Card Sorting Test errors (Goldberg et al, 1987; Goldberg & Weinberger, 1988); (d) deficits in motor synchrony (Manschreck et al, 1981, 1982); (e) deficits on tests of "covert orienting" (Posner et al, 1988); (f) increased redundancy in two-choice guessing behaviour (Frith & Done, 1983; Lyon et al, 1986); (g) deficits in perceptual organisation (Place & Gilmore, 1980; Wells & Leventhal, 1984); (h) deficits in semantic priming (Manschreck et al, 1988; Kwapil et al, 1990); (i) deficits in sensory gating (Freedman et al, 1983; Braff & Geyer, 1990; Waldo et al, 1991); and (j) deficits on tests of "working memory" (Sawaguchi & Goldman-Rakic, 1991; Park & Holzman, 1992).

The hypothesis that there is a deficit in this aspect of attentional control accords well with prior hypotheses of the "core" neurocognitive deficits in schizophrenia, as advanced by: Shakow (1962), in his specification of "response set" abnormalities as possibly underlying RT deficits; Kahnemann (1973), who identified "pigeon-holing" of responses as more important than "filtering" of stimuli; Neuchterlein & Dawson (1984), who specified the "effortful" attentional processes as those comprising the most promising markers of vulnerability; Frith (1987) and Frith & Done (1988), who hypothesised that failures in the monitoring of willed intentions might underlie positive symptoms; and Cohen & Servan-Schreiber (1992), who saw deficits in "memory for context" as the central defect in neural network models of schizophrenic patients' performance of cognitive tests (see Maruff and Currie, chapter 6).

There is some recent direct evidence suggesting that structural abnormalities in the medial frontolimbic system may underlie some of the deficits in projectional control as described above. One recent report showed that prefrontal cortex volume predicted performance selectively on a context-rich list-learning task; further, when the frontal lobe was subdivided, performance on this task was correlated significantly only with the most dorsal part (Maher et al, 1995). In another report, of relations between mesiotemporal lobe tissue volumes and neuropsychological functions, decreased volume selectively in the anterior hippocampal formation was associated with lower scores on measures of executive and motor functions that are usually considered sensitive to the integrity of frontal lobe systems (Bilder et al, 1995). These results corroborate the report that anterior hippocampal volume predicted metabolic activation of the prefrontal cortex during performance of the Wisconsin Card Sorting Test, in contrasts of monozygotic twins discordant for schizophrenia (Weinberger et al, 1992). These latter studies converge in suggesting that abnormalities of anterior hippocampal structure may predict "frontal lobe" dysfunction in schizophrenia, and support the likelihood that deficits within this frontolimbic network may be sufficient to explain the high level executive deficits in schizophrenia.

These findings in patients can be integrated well with attempts to develop "animal models" of schizophrenia. Recent studies in both primates (Bachevalier, 1993; Bachevalier, 1994; Beauregard et al, 1992) and rodents (Lipska et al, 1993) suggest that early developmental lesions to the hippocampal formation may yield both behavioural and psychopharmacologic abnormalities that are more similar to those seen after frontal lobe lesions in adult animals. Particularly important is the observation that these developmentally lesioned animals show evidence of "frontal dysfunction" only when they mature into adolescence or adulthood. A recent study of patients with seizure disorders showed that lesions affecting the left mesiotemporal region may yield dysfunction of the "frontal" type selectively among patients with damage occurring before the first year of age (Strauss et al, 1993). These studies may thus provide a model for, and help to resolve, a major problem faced by current pathophysiologic hypotheses of schizophrenia: that a primary neurodevelopmental lesion has its clinical manifestations only in adolescence or adulthood. These results are most compatible with the hypotheses that a developmental abnormality affecting the volume of the hippocampus disrupts integrated frontohippocampal function in adulthood.

There is thus converging evidence that altered development of the medial frontolimbic system, whether this is observed in hippocampal, cingulate or dorsal frontal cortical divisions, may comprise a core pathologic process underlying vulnerability to schizophrenia. Further investigations aimed at identifying the structural covariation of the components of this system and the functional implications of damage to its different elements at varying times during ontogeny, may prove useful to understanding both the normal development of executive control functions in humans and the disturbances of these functions in schizophrenia.

SUMMARY

This review of structure–function relations in schizophrenia and presentation of a hypothesis about multiple pathological processes is presented to assist researchers in reducing the complexity of the daunting tasks that face them. The richness of comprehensive neuropsychological databases and the magnitude of data generated in modern brain imaging studies together make it essential that research focuses on simple testable hypotheses about the nature of structure–function correlations. The model specified above may offer a starting point for the integration of some apparently discrepant and seemingly paradoxical findings already in the literature. Also, it is expected that as new experimental data come to bear on this model its tenets shall be either modified or abandoned. It is hoped that, in the process, a more effective synthesis and a better understanding of the structural bases of the schizophrenia syndrome will be forthcoming.

REFERENCES

Akbarian, S., Vinuela, A., Kim, J.J., Potkin, S.G., Bunney, W.E. (1993) Distorted distribution of nicotinamide-adenine dinucleotide phosphate-diaphorase neurons in temporal lobe of schizophrenics implies anomalous cortical development. *Archives of General Psychiatry*, **50**, 178–187.

Andreasen, N.C., Nasrallah, H.A., Dunn, V., Olson, S.C., Grove, W.M., Ehrhardt, J.C., Coffman, J.A., Crossett, J.H.W. (1986) Structural abnormalities in the frontal system in schizophrenia. *Archives of General Psychiatry*, **43**, 136–144.

Bachevalier, J. (1993) Cognition, localization, and schizophrenia. Paper presented at the International Congress for Schizophrenia Research, Colorado Springs, CO.

Bachevalier, J. (1994) Medial temporal lobe structures and autism: A review of clinical and experimental findings. *Neuropsychologia*, **32**, 627–648.

Barr, W.B., Mukherjee, S., Degreef, G., Caracci, G. (1989) Anomalous dominance and persistent tardive dyskinesia. *Biological Psychiatry*, **25**, 826–834.

Barta, P.E., Pearlson, G.D., Powers, R.E., Richards, S.S., Tune, L.E. (1990) Auditory hallucinations and smaller superior temporal gyral volume in schizophrenia. *American Journal of Psychiatry*, **147**, 1457–1462.

Beauregard, L., Malkova, L., Bachevalier, J. (1992) Is schizophrenia a result of early damage to the hippocampal formation? A behavioral study in primates. Paper presented at the Society for Neuroscience Annual Meeting, Anaheim, CA. *Society for Neuroscience Abstracts*.

Becker, T., Elmer, K., Mechela, B., Schneider, F., Taubert, S., Schroth, G., Grodd, W., Bartels, M., Beckmann, H. (1990) MRI findings in medial temporal lobe structures in schizophrenia. *European Neuropsychopharmacology*, **1**, 83–86.

Benes, F.M. (1987) An analysis of the arrangement of neurons in the cingulate cortex of schizophrenic patients. *Archives of General Psychiatry*, **44**, 608–616.

Benes, F.M., Davidson, B., Bird, E.D. (1986) Quantitative cytoarchitectural studies of the cerebral cortex of schizophrenics. *Archives of General Psychiatry*, **43**, 31–35.

Berman, K.F. (1987) Cortical "stress tests" in schizophrenia: Regional cerebral blood flow studies. *Biological Psychiatry*, **22**, 1304–1326.

Bilder, R.M. (1985) *Subtyping in Chronic Schizophrenia: Clinical, Neuropsychological and Structural Indices of Deterioration*, University Microfilms, Ann Arbor, MI.

Bilder, R.M. (1992) Structure–function relations in schizophrenia: Brain morphology and neuropsychology. In: *Progress in Experimental Personality and Psychopathology Research*, Vol. 15 (Eds E.F. Walker, R.H. Dworkin, B.A. Cornblatt), pp. 183–251, Springer, New York.

Bilder, R.M., Degreef, G. (1991) Morphologic markers of neurodevelopmental paths to schizophrenia. In: *Developmental Neuropathology of Schizophrenia* (Eds S.A. Mednick, T.D. Cannon, C.E. Barr, J.M. LaFosse), pp. 167–190, Plenum Press, New York.

Bilder, R.M., Degreef, G., Pandurangi, A.K., Rieder, R.O., Sackeim, H.A., Mukherjee, S. (1988) Neuropsychological deterioration and CT-scan findings in chronic schizophrenia. *Schizophrenia Research*, **1**, 37–47.

Bilder, R.M., Lipschutz-Broch, L., Reiter, G., Geisler, S.H., Mayerhoff, D.I., Lieberman, J.A. (1992) Intellectual deficits in first-episode schizophrenia: Evidence for progressive deterioration. *Schizophrenia Bulletin*, **18**, 437–448.

Bilder, R.M., Wu, H., Bogerts, B., Degreef, G., Ashtari, M., Alvir, J.Ma.J., Snyder, P.J., Lieberman, J.A. (1994) Regional hemispheric volume asymmetries are absent in first episode schizophrenia. *American Journal of Psychiatry*, **151**, 1437–1447.

Bilder, R.M., Bogerts, B., Ashtari, M., Wu, H., Alvir, J.Ma.J., Jody, D., Reiter, G., Bell, L., Lieberman, J.A. (1995) Anterior hippocampal volume reductions predict frontal lobe dysfunction in first episode schizophrenia. *Schizophrenia Research*, **17**, 47–58.

Bleuler, M. (1972) *The Schizophrenic Disorders: Long-Term Patient and Family Studies*, Yale University Press, New Haven.

Bogerts, B. (1990) The neuropathology of schizophrenia: Pathophysiological and neurodevelopmental implications. In: *Fetal Neurodevelopmental and Adult Schizophrenia* (Eds S.A. Mednick, T.D. Cannon, C.E. Barr, M. Lyon), Cambridge University Press, Cambridge.

Bogerts, B., Meertz, E., Schonfeld-Bausch, R. (1985) Basal ganglia and limbic system pathology in schizophrenia. *Archives of General Psychiatry*, **42**, 784–791.

Bogerts, B., Ashtari, M., Degreef, G., Alvir, J.Ma.J., Bilder, R.M., Lieberman, J.A. (1990) Reduced temporal limbic structure volumes on magnetic resonance images in first episode schizophrenia. *Psychiatry Research: Neuroimaging*, **35**, 1–13.

Bogerts, B., Lieberman, J.A., Ashtari, M., Bilder, R.M., Degreef, G., Lerner, G., Johns, C., Masiar, S. (1993) Hippocampus–amygdala volumes and psychopathology in chronic schizophrenia. *Biological Psychiatry*, **33**, 236–246.

Bornstein, R.A., Schwarzkopf, S.B., Olson, S.C., Nasrallah, H.A. (1992) Third ventricle enlargement and neuropsychological deficit in schizophrenia. *Biological Psychiatry*, **31**, 954–961.

Braff, D.L., Geyer, M.A. (1990) Sensorimotor gating and schizophrenia: Human and animal studies. *Archives of General Psychiatry*, **47**, 181–188.

Breier, A., Buchanan, R.W., Elkashef, A., Munson, R.C., Kirkpatrick, B., Gellad, F. (1992) Brain morphology and schizophrenia: A magnetic resonance imaging study of limbic, prefrontal cortex and caudate structures. *Archives of General Psychiatry*, **49**, 921–926.

Buchanan, R.W., Breier, A., Kirkpatrick, B., Elkashef, A., Munson, R.C., Gellad, F., Carpenter, W.T., Jr (1993) Structural abnormalities in deficit and nondeficit schizophrenia. *American Journal of Psychiatry*, **150**, 59–65.

Buchsbaum, M.S. (1990) The frontal lobes, basal ganglia and temporal lobes as sites for schizophrenia. *Schizophrenia Bulletin*, **16**, 379–389.

Cannon, T.D., Mednick, S.A., Parnas, J. (1989) Genetic and perinatal determinants of structural brain deficits in schizophrenia. *Archives of General Psychiatry*, **46**, 883–889.

Cannon, T.D., Mednick, S.A., Parnas, J., Schulsinger, F., Praestholm, J., Vestergaard, A. (1993) Developmental brain abnormalities in the offspring of schizophrenic mothers, I: contributions of genetic and perinatal factors. *Archives of General Psychiatry*, **50**, 551–564.

Carr, E.G., Wedding, D. (1984) Neuropsychological assessment of cerebral ventricular size in chronic schizophrenics. *International Journal of Clinical Neuropsychology*, **21**, 106–111.

Ciompi, L.C. (1980) The natural history of schizophrenia. *British Journal of Psychiatry*, **136**, 413–420.

Ciompi, L. (1989) The dynamics of complex biological–psychosocial systems. Four fundamental psycho-biological mediators in the long-term evolution of schizophrenia. *British Journal of Psychiatry*, **155**, 15–21.

Cohen, J.D., Servan-Schreiber, D. (1992) Context, cortex and dopamine: A connectionist approach to behaviour and biology in schizophrenia. *Psychological Review*, **99**, 45–77.

Conrad, A.J., Scheibel, A.B. (1987) Schizophrenia and the hippocampus: The embryological hypothesis extended. *Schizophrenia Bulletin*, **13**, 577–587.

Conrad, A.J., Abebe, T., Austin, R., Forsythe, S., Scheibel, A.B. (1992) Hippocampal pyramidal cell disarray in schizophrenia as a bilateral phenomenon. *Archives of General Psychiatry*, **48**, 413–417.

Cornblatt, B.A., Risch, N.J., Faris, G., Friedman, D., Erlenmeyer-Kimling, L. (1988) The continuous performance test, identical pairs version (CPT-IP): 1. New findings about sustained attention in normal families. *Psychiatry Research*, **26**, 223–238.

Cornblatt, B.A., Lenzenweger, M.F., Erlenmeyer-Kimling, L. (1990) *The Continuous Performance Test, Identical Pairs Version (CPT-IP): Ii. Contrasting Attentional Profiles in Schizophrenic and Depressed Patients* (unpublished).

DeAmicis, L.A., Wagstaff, D.A., Cromwell, R.L. (1986) Reaction time crossover as a marker of schizophrenia and of higher functioning. *Journal of Nervous and Mental Disease*, **174**, 177–179.

Degreef, G., Ashtari, M., Wu, H., Borenstein, M., Geisler, S., Lieberman, J. (1991) Follow up MRI study in first episode schizophrenia. *Schizophrenia Bulletin*, **5**, 204–206.

Degreef, G., Ashtari, M., Bogerts, B., Bilder, R.M., Jody, D.N., Alvir, J.Ma.J., Lieberman, J.A. (1992) Volumes of ventricular system subdivisions measured from magnetic resonance images in first-episode schizophrenic patients. *Archives of General Psychiatry*, **49**, 531–537.

DeLisi, L.E., Dauphinias, I.D., Gershon, E.S. (1988) Perinatal complications and reduced size of brain limbic structures in familial schizophrenia. *Schizophrenia Bulletin*, **14**, 185–191.

DeLisi, L.E., Stritzke, P.H., Holan, V., Anand, A., Boccio, A., Kuschner, M., Riordan, H.,

McClelland, J., VanEyle, O. (1991) Brain morphological changes in 1st episode cases of schizophrenia: Are they progressive? *Schizophrenia Bulletin*, **5**, 206–208.

DeQuardo, J.R., Tandon, R., Goldman, R., Meador-Woodruff, J.H., McGrath-Giroux, M., Brunberg, J.A., Kim, L. (1994) Ventricular enlargement, neuropsychological status, and premorbid function in schizophrenia. *Biological Psychiatry*, **35**, 517–524.

Early, T.S., Reiman, E.R., Raichle, M.E., Spitznagel, E.C. (1987) Left globus pallidus abnormality in never medicated patients with schizophrenia. *Proceedings of the National Academy of Sciences USA*, **84**, 561–563.

Early, T.S., Posner, M.I., Reiman, E.M., Raichle, M.E. (1989a) Hyperactivity of the left striato-pallidal projection. Part 1: Lower level theory. *Psychiatric Developments*, **2**, 85–108.

Early, T.S., Posner, M.I., Reiman, E., Raichle, M.E. (1989b) Left striato-pallidal hyperactivity in schizophrenia. Part II: Phenomenology and thought disorder. *Psychiatric Developments*, **2**, 109–121.

Edelman, G.M. (1987) *Neural Darwinism*, Basic Books, New York.

Falkai, P., Bogerts, B., Greve, B., Pfeiffer, E., Machus, B., Fölsch-Reetz, B., Majtenyi, C., Ovary, I. (1992) Loss of Sylvian fissure asymmetry in schizophrenia: A quantitative post-mortem study. *Schizophrenia Research*, **7**, 23–32.

Flor-Henry, P. (1983) *Cerebral Basis of Psychopathology*, John Wright, Boston.

Freedman, R., Adler, L.E., Waldo, M.C., Pachtman, E., Franks, R.D. (1983) Neurophysiological evidence for a defect in inhibitory pathways in schizophrenia: Comparison of medicated and drug-free patients. *Biological Psychiatry*, **18**, 537–551.

Frith, C.D. (1987) The positive and negative symptoms of schizophrenia reflect impairments in the perception and initiation of action. *Psychological Medicine*, **17**, 631–648.

Frith, C.D., Done, D.J. (1983) Stereotyped responding by schizophrenic patients on a two-choice guessing task. *Psychological Medicine*, **13**, 779–786.

Frith, C.D., Done, D.J. (1988) Towards a neuropsychology of schizophrenia. *British Journal of Psychiatry*, **153**, 437–443.

Frith, C.D., Done, D.J. (1989) Experiences of alien control in schizophrenia reflect a disorder in the central monitoring of action. *Psychological Medicine*, **19**, 359–363.

Galbraith, K.J., MacCrimmon, D.J., Steffy, R.A. (1983) Preparatory interval effects of redundancy deficit reaction time patterns in schizophrenic and normal subjects using the embedded-set procedure. *Journal of Nervous and Mental Disease*, **171**, 670–675.

Geschwind, N., Galaburda, A.M. (1985) Cerebral lateralization. Biological mechanisms, associations and pathology: I. A hypothesis and a program for research. *Archives of Neurology*, **42**, 428–459.

Goetz, K.L., Van Kammen, D.P. (1986) Computerized axial tomography scans and subtypes of schizophrenia. *Journal of Nervous and Mental Disease*, **174**, 31–41.

Goldberg, E., Seidman, L.J. (1991) Higher cortical functions in normals and in schizophrenia: A selective review. In: *Handbook of Schizophrenia, Vol. 5: Neuropsychology, Psychophysiology and Information Processing* (Eds S.R. Steinhauer, J.H. Gruzelier, J. Zubin), pp. 553–597, Elsevier, Amsterdam.

Goldberg, G. (1985) Supplementary motor area: Review and hypotheses. *Behavioral and Brain Sciences*, **8**, 567–588.

Goldberg, G. (1987) From intent to action: Evolution and function of the premotor systems of the frontal lobe. In: *The Frontal Lobes Revisited* (Ed. E. Perecman), pp. 273–306, IRBN Press, New York.

Goldberg, T.E., Weinberger, D.R. (1988) Probing prefrontal function in schizophrenia with neuropsychological paradigms. *Schizophrenia Bulletin*, **14**, 179–183.

Goldberg, T.E., Weinberger, D.R., Berman, K.F., Pliskin, N.H., Podd, M.H. (1987) Further evidence for dementia of the prefrontal type in schizophrenia. *Archives of General Psychiatry*, **44**, 1008–1014.

Gray, J.A., Feldon, J., Rawlins, J.N.P., Hemsley, D.R., Smith, A.D. (1991) The neuropsychology of schizophrenia. *Behavioural and Brain Sciences*, **14**, 1–84.

Green, M.F., Satz, P., Smith, C., Nelson, L. (1989) Is there atypical handedness in schizophrenia. *Journal of Abnormal Psychology*, **98**, 57–61.

Gruzelier, J., Seymour, K., Wilson, L., Jolley, A., Hirsch, S. (1988) Impairments on neuropsychologic tests of temporohippocampal and frontohippocampal functions and word fluency in remitting schizophrenia and affective disorders. *Archives of General Psychiatry*, **45**, 623–629.

Hoff, A.L., Rioordan, H., O'Donnell, D., Stritzke, P., Neale, C., Boccio, A., Anand, A.K., DeLisi, L.E. (1992) Anomalous lateral sulcus asymmetry and cognitive function in first-episode schizophrenia. *Schizophrenia Bulletin*, **18**, 257–270.

Huber, G., Gross, G., Schutter, R. (1975) A long-term follow-up study of schizophrenia: Clinical course and prognosis. *Acta Psychiatrica Scandinavica*, **52**, 49–57.

Johnstone, E.C., Crow, T.J., Frith, C.D., Husband, J., Kreel, L. (1976) Cerebral ventricular size and cognitive impairment in chronic schizophrenia. *Lancet*, **ii**, 924–926.

Johnstone, E.C., Owens, D.G.C., Bydder, G.M., Colter, N., Crow, T.J., Frith, C.D. (1989) The spectrum of structural brain changes in schizophrenia: Age of onset as a predictor of cognitive and clinical impairments and their cerebral correlates. *Psychological Medicine*, **19**, 91–103.

Kahnemann, D. (1973) *Attention and Effort*, Prentice Hall, Englewood Cliffs, NJ.

Keilp, J.G., Sweeney, J.A., Jacobsen, P., Solomon, C., St Louis, L., Deck, M., Frances, A., Mann, J.J. (1988) Cognitive impairment in schizophrenia: Specific relations to ventricular size and negative symptomatology. *Biological Psychiatry*, **24**, 47–55.

Kern, R.S., Green, M.F., Satz, P., Wirshing, W.C. (1991) Patterns of manual dominance in patients with neuroleptic-induced movement disorders. *Biological Psychiatry*, **30**, 483–492.

Kolb, B., Whishaw, I.Q. (1983) Performance of schizophrenic patients on tests sensitive to left or right frontal, temporal, or parietal function in neurological patients. *Journal of Nervous and Mental Disorders*, **171**, 435–443.

Kovelman, J.A., Scheibel, A.B. (1984) A neurohistological correlate of schizophrenia. *Biological Psychiatry*, **19**, 1601–1621.

Kwapil, T.R., Hegley, D.C., Chapman, L.J., Chapman, J.P. (1990) Facilitation of word recognition by semantic priming in schizophrenia. *Journal of Abnormal Psychology*, **99**, 215–221.

Lawson, W.B., Waldman, I.N., Weinberger, D.R. (1988) Schizophrenic dementia. Clinical and computed axial tomography correlates. *Journal of Nervous and Mental Disease*, **176**, 207–212.

Lezak, M.D. (1983) *Neuropsychological Assessment*, Oxford University Press, New York.

Lieberman, J.A., DeLisi, L. (1991) American College of Neuropsychopharmacology Satellite Meeting, Longitudinal Perspectives on the pathophysiology of schizophrenia: Examining the neurodevelopmental versus neurodegenerative hypotheses. *Schizophrenia Research*, **5**, 183–210.

Lieberman, J.A., Alvir, J.Ma.J., Woerner, M., Degreef, G., Bilder, R.M., Ashtari, M., Bogerts, B., Mayerhoff, D.I., Geisler, S.H., Loebel, A., Levy, D.L., Hinrichsen, G., Szymanski, S., Chakos, M., Koreen, A., Borenstein, M., Kane, J.M. (1992) Prospective study of psychobiology in schizophrenia at Hillside Hospital. *Schizophrenia Bulletin*, **18**, 351–371.

Lipska, B.K., Jaskiw, G.E., Weinberger, D.R. (1993) Postpubertal emergence of hyperresponsiveness to stress and to amphetamine after neonatal excitotoxic hippocampal damage: A potential animal model of schizophrenia. *Neuropsychopharmacology*, **9**, 67–75.

Luchins, D.J., Meltzer, H.Y. (1983) A blind, controlled study of occipital asymmetry in schizophrenia. *Psychiatry Research*, **10**, 87–95.

Luchins, D.J., Weinberger, D.R., Wyatt, R.J. (1982) Schizophrenia and cerebral asymmetry detected by computed tomography. *American Journal of Psychiatry*, **139**, 753–757.

Lyon, N., Mejsholm, B., Lyon, M. (1986) Stereotyped responding by schizophrenic outpatients: Cross-cultural confirmation in perseverative switching on a two-choice task. *Journal of Psychiatric Research*, **20**, 137–150.

Maher, B.A., Manschreck, T.C., Woods, B.T., Yurgelun-Todd, D.A., Tsuang, M.T. (1995) Frontal brain volume and context effects in short-term recall in schizophrenia. *Biological Psychiatry*, **37**, 144–150.

Manschreck, T.C., Maher, B.A., Rucklos, M.E., Vereen, D.R., Ader, D.N. (1981) Deficient motor synchrony in schizophrenia. *Journal of Abnormal Psychology*, **90**, 321–328.

Manschreck, R.C., Maher, B.A., Rucklos, M.E., Vereen, D.R. (1982) Disturbed voluntary motor activity in schizophrenic disorder. *Psychological Medicine*, **12**, 73–84.

Manschreck, T.C., Maher, B.A., Milavetz, J.J., Ames, D. (1988) Semantic priming in thought disordered schizophrenic patients. *Schizophrenia Research*, **1**, 61–66.

McCarley, R.W., Faux, S.F., Shenton, M., LeMay, M., Cane, M., Ballinder, R., Duffy, F.H. (1989) CT abnormalities in schizophrenia. A preliminary study of their correlations with P300/P200 electrophysiological features and positive/negative symptoms. *Archives of General Psychiatry*, **46**, 698–708.

McGuinness, D., Pribram, K.H. (1980) The neuropsychology of attention: Emotional and motivational controls. In: *The Brain and Psychology* (Ed. M.C. Wittrock), pp. 95–139, Academic Press, New York.

Mukherjee, S., Reddy, R., Schnur, D.B. (1989) A developmental model of negative syndromes in schizophrenia. In: *Negative Schizophrenic Symptoms: Pathophysiology and Clinical Aspects* (Eds J. Greden, R. Tandon), American Psychiatric Press, Washington, DC.

Neuchterlein, K.H., Dawson, M.E. (1984) Information processing and attentional functioning in the developmental course of schizophrenic disorders. *Schizophrenia Bulletin*, **19**, 160–202.

Nyman, H., Nybäck, H., Wiesel, F.A., Oxenstierna, G., Schalling, D. (1986) Neuropsychological test performance, brain morphological measures and CSF monoamine metabolites in schizophrenic patients. *Acta Psychiatrica Scandinavica*, **74**, 292–301.

Obiols, J.E., Marcos, T., Salamero, M. (1987) Ventricular enlargement and neuropsychological testing in schizophrenia. *Acta Psychiatrica Scandinavica*, **76**, 199–202.

Pandya, D.N., Barnes, C.L. (1987) Architecture and connections of the frontal Lobe. In: *The Frontal lobes Revisited* (Ed. E. Perecman), pp. 41–72, IRBN Press, New York.

Pantelis, C., Barnes, T.R.E., Nelson, H.E. (1992) Is the concept of frontal–subcortical dementia relevant to schizophrenia? *British Journal of Psychiatry*, **160**, 442–460.

Park, S., Holzman, P.S. (1992) Schizophrenics show spatial working memory deficits. *Archives of General Psychiatry*, **49**, 975–982.

Pearlson, G.D., Kim, W.S., Kubos, K.L., Moberg, P.J., Jayaram, G., Bascom, M.J., Chase, G.A., Goldfinger, A.D., Tune, L.E. (1989) Ventricle–brain ratio, computed tomographic density and brain area in 50 schizophrenics. *Archives of General Psychiatry*, **46**, 690–697.

Place, E.J.S., Gilmore, G.C. (1980) Perceptual organization in schizophrenia. *Journal of Abnormal Psychology*, **89**, 409–418.

Posner, M.I., Early, T.S., Reiman, E.M., Pardo, P.J., Dhawan, M. (1988) Asymmetries in hemispheric control of attention in schizophrenia. *Archives of General Psychiatry*, **45,** 814–821.

Pribram, K.H., McGuinness, D. (1975) Arousal, activation and effort in the control of attention. *Psychological Review*, **82**, 116–149.

Raz, S. (1989) Structural brain abnormalities in the major psychoses. In: *Neuropsychological Function and Brain Imaging* (Eds E.D. Bigler, R.A. Yeo, E. Turkheimer), pp. 245–268, Plenum Press, New York.

Raz, S., Raz, N. (1990) Structural brain abnormalities in the major psychoses: A quantitative review of the evidence from computerized imaging. *Psychological Bulletin*, **108**, 93–108.

Raz, S., Raz, N., Neinberger, D.R., Boronow, J., Pickar, D., Bigler, E.D., Turkheimer, E. (1987) Morphological brain abnormalities in schizophrenia determined by computed tomography: A problem of measurement? *Psychiatry Research*, **22**, 910–998.

Rossi, A., Stratta, P., DiMichele, V., Gallucci, M., Splendiani, A., Casacchia, M. (1991) Temporal lobe structure by magnetic resonance imaging in bipolar affective disorders and schizophrenia. *Journal of Affective Disorders*, **21**, 19–22.

Sanides, F. (1969) Comparative architectonics of the neocortex of mammals and their evolutionary interpretation. *Annals of the New York Academy of Sciences*, **167**, 404–423.

Sawaguchi, T., Goldman-Rakic, P.S. (1991) D1 dopamine receptors in prefrontal cortex: Involvement in working memory. *Science*, **251**, 947–950.

Scheibel, A.B., Kovelman, J.A. (1981) Correspondence: Disorientation of the hippocampal pyramidal cell and its processes in the schizophrenic patient. *Biological Psychiatry*, **16**, 101–102.

Seidman, L.J. (1983) Schizophrenia and brain dysfunction: An integration of recent neurodiagnostic findings. *Psychological Bulletin*, **94**, 195–238.

Shakow, D. (1962) Segmental set. *Archives of General Psychiatry*, **6**, 1–17.

Shenton, M.E., Kikinis, R., Jolesz, F.A., Pollak, S.D., LeMay, M., Wible, C.G., Kokama, H., Martin, J., Metcalf, D., Coleman, M., McCarley, R.W. (1992) Abnormalities of the left temporal lobe and thought disorder in schizophrenia: A quantitative magnetic resonance imaging study. *New England Journal of Medicine*, **327**, 604–612.

Steffy, R.A., Galbraith, K.J. (1980) Relation between latency and redundancy-associated deficit in schizophrenic reaction time performance. *Journal of Abnormal Psychology*, **89**, 419–427.

Strauss, E., Hunter, M., Wada, J. (1993) Wisconsin card sorting performance: Effects of age of onset of damage and laterality of dysfunction. *Journal of Clinical and Experimental Neuropsychology*, **15**, 896–902.

Suddath, R.L., Casanova, M.F., Goldberg, T.E., Daniel, D.G., Kelsoe, J.R.Jr., Weinberger, D.R. (1989) Temporal lobe pathology in schizophrenia: A quantitative magnetic resonance imaging study. *American Journal of Psychiatry*, **146**, 464–472.

Suddath, R.L., Christison, G.W., Torrey, E.F., Casanova, M.F., Weinberger, D.R. (1990) Anatomical abnormalities in the brains of monozygotic twins discordant for schizophrenia. *New England Journal of Medicine*, **322**, 789–794.

Tucker, D.M., Williamson, P.A. (1984) Asymmetric neural control systems in human self-regulation. *Psychological Review*, **91**, 185–215.

van Horn, J.D., McManus, I.C. (1992) Ventricular enlargement in schizophrenia. A meta-analysis of studies of the ventricle:brain ratio (VBR). *British Journal of Psychiatry*, **160**, 687–697.

Waddington, J.L., Youssef, H.A., Kinsella, A. (1990) Cognitive dysfunction in schizophrenia followed up over 5 years and its longitudinal relationship to the emergence of tardive dyskinesia. *Psychological Medicine*, **20**, 835–842.

Waldo, M.C., Carey, G., Myles-Worsley, M., Cawthra, E., Adler, L.E., Nagamoto, H.T., Wender, P., Byerly, W., Plaetlke, R., Freedman, R. (1991) Co-distribution of a sensory gating deficit and schizophrenia in multi-affected families. *Psychiatry Research*, **39**, 257–268.

Wechsler, D. (1958) *The Measurement and Appraisal of Adult Intelligence*, Williams & Wilkins, Baltimore.

Weinberger, D.R. (1984) Computed tomography (CT) findings in schizophrenia: Speculation on the meaning of it all. *Journal of Psychiatric Research*, **18**, 477–490.

Weinberger, D.R., Berman, K.F., Zec, R.F. (1986) Physiological dysfunction of dorsolateral prefrontal cortex in schizophrenia: I. Regional cerebral blood (rCBF) flow evidence. *Archives of General Psychiatry*, **43**, 114–124.

Weinberger, D.R., Berman, K.F., Suddath, R., Torrey, E.F. (1992) Evidence of dysfunction of a prefrontal–limbic network in schizophrenia: A magnetic resonance imaging and regional cerebral blood flow study of discordant monozygotic twins. *American Journal of Psychiatry*, **149**, 890–897.

Wells, D.S., Leventhal, D. (1984) Perceptual grouping in schizophrenia: Replication of Place and Gilmore. *Journal of Abnormal Psychology*, **93**, 231–234.

Wing, J.K., Cooper, J.E., Sartorius, N. (1974) *The Measurement and Classification of Psychiatric Symptoms*, Cambridge University Press, London.

Yeterian, E.H., Pandya, D.N. (1988) Architectonic features of the primate brain: Implications for information processing and behavior. In: *Information Processing by the Brain* (Ed. H.J. Markowitsch), pp. 7–37, Hans Huber, Switzerland.

Zec, R.F., Weinberger, D.R. (1986) Brain areas implicated in schizophrenia: A selective overview. In: *Handbook of Schizophrenia, Vol. 1: The Neurology of Schizophrenia* (Eds H.A. Nasrallah, D.R. Weinberger), pp. 175–206, Elsevier, New York.

15

Syndromes in Schizophrenia and their Neuropsychological and Neuroanatomical Correlates

PETER F. LIDDLE

INTRODUCTION

Schizophrenia is a disorder of the higher mental functions that enable a human being to function as an autonomous person. It presents an enigma, not only because these higher mental functions are subtle and complex, but also because the expression of the illness is diverse. The clinical features include: the experience of thought, action and affect being imposed by an alien influence; the fragmentation of thinking and behaviour that leads to incoherent speech, bizarre behaviour and incongruous affect; and the impoverishment of mental activity that is reflected in poverty of speech, decreased movement and blunted affect. The disease can produce disorder spanning the entire gamut of mental activity from perception to thought, affect, volition and motor activity.

As well as being diverse, the manifestations of schizophrenia are also changeable in response to circumstances. Eugen Bleuler (1911) remarked that "even the most demented patient with schizophrenia can under proper conditions suddenly demonstrate productions of a rather highly integrated type". It is a commonplace observation that, in both neuropsychological tests and in daily life, the performance of patients with schizophrenia can be highly variable. Poor neuropsychological performance is often associated with increased inconsistency.

The task of understanding schizophrenia is the task of understanding how a subtle derangement of the neural tissue that supports the highest human capacities modifies the interactions between the patient and his surroundings to produce a diverse and potentially devastating disruption of his life. This chapter is an

Schizophrenia: A Neuropsychological Perspective. Edited by C. Pantelis, H.E. Nelson and T.R.E. Barnes
© 1996 John Wiley & Sons Ltd

account of a series of studies designed to relate the protean clinical manifestations of the disorder to the neuronal systems involved in the higher mental
functions. The underlying strategy guiding these studies is based on the assumption that exploration of the relationships between the diverse clinical features,
and between clinical features and indices of neuronal function, will reveal a
pattern that can be understood in terms of the structure and function of the
normal human brain.

CROW'S CONCEPTS OF TYPE 1 AND TYPE 2 SCHIZOPHRENIA

The stimulus to this series of studies was Crow's (1980) proposal that there are
two distinct pathological processes in schizophrenia. The proposed *type 1* process
entails potentially reversible dopaminergic imbalance and is manifest as positive
symptoms such as delusions, hallucinations and formal thought disorder. In
contrast, the proposed *type 2* process involves irreversible structural damage to
the brain and is manifest as negative symptoms, such as poverty of speech and
flat affect. Some of the available evidence supports Crow's hypothesis. In particular, 5 of the 18 computed tomography (CT) studies that have examined the
issue have found an association between ventricular enlargement and negative
symptoms (Lewis, 1990). Furthermore, there is evidence that negative symptoms
are associated with more extensive neuropsychological impairment. For example,
Johnstone et al (1978) found that negative symptoms were associated with poor
performance on the Withers and Hinton test battery which assesses a broad
range of aspects of mental function such as attention, memory and abstract
reasoning.

However, other studies which attempted to identify more specific relationships
between symptom type and deficits in neuropsychological performance have
revealed a more complex picture, in which positive and negative symptoms are
associated with differing patterns of impairment in the processing of information. For example, Cornblatt et al (1985) employed an information overload
task to demonstrate that negative symptoms were associated with lowered
processing capacity while positive symptoms were associated with increased
distractibility.

In general, studies that have examined the relationships between positive
symptoms and neuropsychological performance in detail find that formal thought
disorder is the positive symptom that is associated with the most extensive impairment. In particular, formal thought disorder is associated with a variety of
impairments of attention and of language processing (McGrath, 1992). Insofar as
formal thought disorder is associated with relatively extensive cognitive impairment, it has something of the character of a deficit or negative symptom. Thus,
the positive symptoms of schizophrenia do not form a homogeneous syndrome.
Delusions and hallucinations might be considered as core positive symptoms
while formal thought disorder has some of the characteristics of a negative
symptom.

Crow's proposal that there are two groups of schizophrenia symptoms reflecting two distinct pathological processes (one entailing a biochemical imbalance and the other consisting of structural damage) accounts for the observation that positive symptoms tend to be transient, while negative symptoms tend to be chronic. However, in some cases positive symptoms are persistent, while in others negative symptoms are transient. Thus, it is unclear whether the distinction between type 1 and type 2 schizophrenia is essentially a matter of symptom type or of symptom chronicity. This speculation raises the question of whether or not symptoms of uniform chronicity segregate into two groups exhibiting differing relationships with indices of brain structure and function.

THREE SYNDROMES OF SCHIZOPHRENIC SYMPTOMS

To examine the segregation of symptoms of relatively homogeneous chronicity, a sample of patients with persistent, stable symptoms were recruited and the pattern of correlations between their symptoms was examined (Liddle, 1984, 1987a). The symptoms segregated into three distinguishable syndromes: *psychomotor poverty* (poverty of speech, blunted affect and decreased spontaneous movement); *disorganisation* (formal thought disorder, poverty of content of speech and inappropriate affect); and *reality distortion* (various delusions and hallucinations).

The three syndromes do not reflect three types of illness but, rather, three distinct dimensions of psychopathology within a single illness. An individual patient might exhibit evidence of more than one syndrome. Many other studies (e.g. Bilder et al, 1985; Kulhara et al, 1986; Liddle & Barnes, 1990; Mortimer et al, 1990; Arndt et al, 1991; Pantelis et al 1991; Schroder et al, 1992; Liddle et al, 1992a, 1992b; Brown & White, 1992; Peralta et al, 1992; Frith, 1992), using different cohorts of patients and differing symptom rating scales, have identified three similar syndromes. Several of the subsequent studies (e.g. Arndt et al, 1991; Peralta et al, 1992) have included acute patients, suggesting that the three syndromes are discernible in both acute and chronic phases of the illness.

The range of symptoms embraced by the three syndromes includes neither depression nor elation. These symptoms are often relatively transient and were not entered into the factor analysis in the original study of persistent symptoms (Liddle, 1987a). Studies that have embraced a broader range of symptoms (e.g. Kay, 1991) have identified separate depression and excitement factors in addition to three factors resembling those identified in Liddle's original study.

Insofar as the psychomotor poverty syndrome comprises the core negative symptoms, while reality distortion comprises the core positive symptoms, the three-syndrome model has substantial overlap with the positive/negative dichotomy. The distinctive feature of the three-syndrome model is the identification of the disorganisation syndrome, comprising symptoms such as formal thought disorder and inappropriate affect. These symptoms appear to reflect the fragmentation of mental activity that is implied by the semantic origin of the word schizophrenia.

NEUROPSYCHOLOGICAL CORRELATES OF THE THREE SYNDROMES

If the three syndromes reflect three distinguishable neuropathological processes, it might be expected that each syndrome would be associated with a distinct pattern of neuropsychological impairment. This was examined in a study of the correlations between severity of each syndrome and performance in a battery of neuropsychological tests embracing aspects of cognitive function such as attention, perception, memory and abstract reasoning (Liddle, 1987b). The findings of this study revealed that psychomotor poverty is associated with impairment of abstract reasoning and of long term episodic memory, including memory for events pre-dating onset of illness, while disorganisation is associated with impairments of attention and of the ability to learn new material. In contrast, reality distortion showed only a weak association with impaired figure ground perception but no significant association with other neuropsychological deficits, confirming that delusions and hallucinations reflect a tightly circumscribed deficit in cognitive processing.

The Initiation and Selection of Mental Activity

Consideration of the nature of the individual items of each syndrome suggests that the common feature underlying the symptoms of the psychomotor poverty syndrome is a difficulty in the initiation of activity, while the common feature underlying symptoms of the disorganisation syndrome is an impaired ability to select appropriate mental activity in the face of conflicting impulses to act. Initiation and selection of mental activity are characteristic functions of multimodal association cortex, especially prefrontal cortex (see also Pantelis and Brewer, chapter 16).

Blumer & Benson (1975) have described two syndromes that arise from frontal lobe injury. The first of these syndromes, which they called "pseudodepression", is virtually identical in composition with the psychomotor poverty syndrome and is characterised by impoverished speech and blunted affect. They attributed this syndrome to damage to the dorsolateral prefrontal cortex, though others (Kolb & Whishaw, 1980) have attributed it to predominantly left-sided prefrontal damage. The second frontal syndrome, which Blumer and Benson designated the "pseudopsychopathic" syndrome, consists of garrulousness and an inability to maintain specific meanings. These clinical features resemble the symptoms of the disorganisation syndrome. Blumer and Benson attributed the pseudopsychopathic syndrome to ventral prefrontal damage, while Kolb & Whishaw (1980) considered it reflects predominantly right-sided frontal damage.

To test the hypothesis that psychomotor poverty and disorganisation reflect impairment of different aspects of the function of the prefrontal cortex, Liddle & Morris (1991) examined the relationship between syndrome severity and performance in a battery of frontal lobe tests in a group of chronic, stable, medicated patients with schizophrenia. They found that both psychomotor poverty and disorganisation syndrome scores were correlated with impairment in frontal lobe tests but the pattern of association suggested impairment of different aspects of frontal lobe function. In contrast to the psychomotor poverty and disorganisation syndromes, reality distortion was not associated with impaired performance in any of the frontal lobe tests.

The psychomotor poverty syndrome was associated with reduced number of words produced in the FAS verbal fluency task, in which the subject has to generate words beginning with a specified letter. Psychomotor poverty was also associated with slow performance in other tasks requiring the articulation of words. After allowing for variation in speed of articulation, the magnitude of the correlation between psychomotor poverty and impaired verbal fluency was reduced, but nonetheless remained significant, indicating that psychomotor poverty is associated not only with slowing of articulation but also with impairment of higher mental processing.

The disorganisation syndrome was associated with impaired performance in tasks that entail the suppression of an inappropriate response, such as the Stroop task, Trails B from the Halstead–Reitan battery and with increased proportion of perseverative errors in the Modified Wisconsin Card Sorting Test (MWCST). In the Stroop test the subject is presented with colour names printed in ink that is not congruent with the colour name and asked to state the colour of the ink. In Trails B the subject traces a path connecting points labelled with letters or numbers in a sequence that demands alternation between letters and numbers. In the MWCST, the subject is required to sort cards according to a changing rule. Perseverative errors reflect a tendency to persist with a particular response even when feedback indicates the need to change strategy. The common feature of all of these tasks is the need to select between competing responses and suppress the tendency to respond to the inappropriate response.

Liddle & Morris (1991) also found that disorganisation was associated with impaired verbal fluency performance and that this correlation was not diminished by allowing for variation in speed of articulation of words. Performance on a self-directed task such as verbal fluency would be expected to be sensitive to the effects of distractibility. In light of the evidence from tasks such as the Stroop test and Trails B, that disorganisation is associated with impaired ability to suppress inappropriate activity, it is possible that the association with poor verbal fluency and disorganisation reflects distractibility.

In a comprehensive study of 283 patients, representative of a wide range of levels of severity of illness, Frith et al (1992a) found a very similar pattern of correlation between symptoms and neuropsychological performance to that found by Liddle & Morris (1991). In particular, psychomotor poverty symptoms such as poverty of speech and motor retardation were associated with impaired verbal fluency, while disorganisation symptoms such as incoherence of speech and incongruity of affect were associated with poor suppression of inappropriate responses in the Continuous Performance Test (CPT) and with the production of odd words in the verbal fluency task. Frith et al (1992a) also found an association between disorganisation symptoms and reduced number of words produced in the verbal fluency task.

Allen et al (1993) carried out a more detailed study of the association between symptoms and verbal fluency performance. Poverty of speech was associated with production of a reduced number of words in a verbal fluency task in which the subject was asked to generate words belonging to a given semantic category. By repeating the task on multiple occasions they demonstrated that even the patients with poverty of speech produced a substantial number of different words on repetition of the test. This suggested that the problem lay in the ability to access stored words, rather than in the number of words stored. By extrapolation to the expected number of different words that would be produced in a very large number of repetitions of the test, they estimated the total pool of words in each category. Even patients with poverty of speech did not have a significant reduction in the word pool, thus confirming that the difficulty appears to be in accessing stored words. On the other hand, formal thought disorder was associated with a significant tendency to produce words that were inappropriate to the nominated category.

McGrath (1992) examined the relationships between neuropsychological performance and three categories of thought disorder: poverty of speech; positive formal thought disorder, including derailment and loss of goal; and perseveration. He found that poverty of speech was associated with impaired verbal fluency performance, while positive thought disorders were associated with impaired Stroop performance, in agreement with the findings of Liddle & Morris (1991). Clinically observed perseveration was associated with perseverative errors in the Wisconsin Card Sorting Test (WCST) and impaired Trails B performance.

Despite relatively minor differences in detail, there is a substantial degree of consensus between the various studies that have examined the correlation of putative frontal lobe functions with psychomotor poverty and disorganisation symptoms. These studies support the conclusion that psychomotor poverty is associated with impairment in the initiation and planning of mental activity and in speed of processing, whereas disorganisation is associated with impaired selection of mental activity, especially with impaired ability to suppress inappropriate responses.

The Evaluation and Monitoring of Mental Activity

In the studies by Liddle & Morris (1991), Frith et al (1992a) and Allen et al (1993) there was no evidence for an association of delusions and hallucinations with the types of executive function assessed by tests such as FAS verbal fluency, Stroop, Trails B or WCST. This is consistent with the previously noted lack of evidence for an association between reality distortion and extensive cognitive impairment. What then might be the nature of the disorder that generates the reality distortion syndrome? Consideration of the nature of the delusions and hallucinations suggests that such symptoms might arise from a disorder of the executive functions responsible for evaluation of mental activity. Delusions reflect an impaired ability to evaluate the evidence in support of a particular belief. Hallucinations reflect an impaired ability to recognise the source of an internally generated mental process.

However, reality distortion entails more than a simple impairment of ability to evaluate evidence. Jaspers (1963) emphasised that schizophrenic symptoms such as alien control of thought and action are experiences rather than beliefs and imply a disturbance of the sense of self. Frith & Done (1989) demonstrated that patients with these symptoms had an impaired ability to correct errors when aiming at a target under circumstances in which the ability to make the correction was dependent on internal monitoring of the selection of action. This study supports the proposal that at least one factor contributing to reality distortion in schizophrenia is defective monitoring of self-generated activity (see also: Cahill and Frith, chapter 18; Nayani and David, chapter 17; Neufeld and Williamson, chapter 11).

Synthesis and Hypothesis

In the introduction we noted both the diversity and the variability of the manifestations of the illness. Despite the protean nature of the illness, examination of the relationships between symptoms and between symptoms and neuropsychological performance has revealed a consistent pattern of relationships between symptoms and neuropsychological deficits. Although the evidence is incomplete, that which is available suggests that the diverse symptoms typical of schizophrenia arise from three distinguishable pathophysiological processes reflecting disorder of three aspects of the supervision of mental activity. There is substantial evidence supporting the proposal that psychomotor poverty reflects an impaired ability to initiate mental activity, while disorganisation arises from defective selection of mental activity. In the case of the reality distortion syndrome, the evidence is less extensive but supports the proposal that this syndrome entails a defect in the internal monitoring of self-generated mental activity.

The hypothesis that the essential deficit is in the domain of the supervisory mental processes, rather than in the constituent elements of routine mental processing, is consistent with both the diversity and variability of the manifestations of schizophrenia. Furthermore, it accounts for the clinical observation that the disorder is most apparent in circumstances where there is ambiguity in deciding what behaviour is most appropriate, since it is under such circumstances that the greatest demands are placed upon the supervisory mental functions.

What is known of the neuroanatomical structures that underlie the supervisory mental processes? It might be expected that the association cortex, which integrates information from various internal and external sources, would be implicated. In particular, we have already referred to the evidence that left and/or dorsolateral prefrontal damage can produce a syndrome that closely resembles psychomotor poverty while right and/or ventral prefrontal damage can produce a syndrome resembling disorganisation (Blumer & Benson, 1975; Kolb & Whishaw, 1980). The clinical observation that temporal lobe epilepsy can be associated with psychosis characterised by delusions and hallucinations, but with relative paucity of symptoms typical of the psychomotor poverty and disorganisation syndromes (Slater et al, 1963), suggests that the reality distortion syndrome arises from disorder of the medial temporal lobe.

Thus, comparison of the three syndromes of schizophrenia with recognised syndromes arising from focal brain lesions, together with the pattern of associa-tion between the schizophrenic syndromes and neuropsychological performance, leads to the prediction that each of the three syndromes is associated with a specific deficit in supervisory mental processes and with altered brain activity in specified frontal or temporal sites. These predictions can be tested by employing functional brain imaging techniques, such as positron emission tomography (PET).

PATTERNS OF CEREBRAL BLOOD FLOW IN SCHIZOPHRENIA

Regional cerebral blood flow (rCBF) is a sensitive index of local neuronal activity and can be measured using PET, by determining the distribution in the brain of carbon dioxide or water labelled with the positron-emitting isotope ^{15}O. In a study of 30 medicated schizophrenic patients with persistent symptoms during a stable phase of the illness, Liddle and colleagues (1992a) carried out a PET study in which the correlations between rCBF and severity of each of the three syndromes were examined. We found that each of the three syndromes was associated with a different pattern of rCBF in multimodal association cortex and related subcortical nuclei.

In particular, psychomotor poverty was negatively correlated with rCBF in left prefrontal cortex and parietal cortex and positively correlated with rCBF in the head of the caudate nucleus. There was a similar though less extensive pattern of correlation with rCBF in the right hemisphere, consisting of negative correlations with right prefrontal rCBF and a positive correlation with rCBF in the head of the right caudate nucleus. Disorganisation was associated with decreased rCBF in right ventral prefrontal cortex, contiguous right insula and bilateral parietal cortex, and with increased rCBF in the right medial prefrontal cortex, anterior cingulate and thalamus. Reality distortion was associated with increased rCBF in left medial temporal lobe, left temporal pole, left lateral prefrontal cortex and left ventral striatum.

The selection criteria for this study were designed to ensure that all patients were in a stable state with persistent symptoms, in order to minimise confounding influences arising from variation in clinical state around the time of scanning and from variation in the pattern of brain activity with phase of illness. Therefore, it is necessary to be cautious in extending these findings to other groups of patients such as acutely disturbed, drug-naive cases.

To what extent might the findings have been influenced by medication? All patients were receiving regular antipsychotic treatment, though none were taking atypical antipsychotic drugs such as clozapine. Since all patients were receiving similar medication, the observed patterns of correlation between syndromes and rCBF cannot be attributed to effects of medication independent of the symptom profile. Furthermore, for each syndrome, the partial correlations between syndrome score and rCBF allowing for variation in antipsychotic drug dose were virtually identical to the first order correlations. However, it is possible that pharmacological treatment interacts with symptom profile such that the pattern of cerebral activity associated with symptoms in the presence of medication differs from that which might be seen in the absence of medication.

Nonetheless, evidence from studies of unmedicated patients indicates that the major features of the pattern of cerebral activity associated with the psychomotor poverty and disorganisation syndromes are similar in medicated and unmedicated patients. Studies that have examined the correlation between severity of psycho-motor poverty symptoms and either rCBF or regional cerebral metabolic rate for glucose (rCMRglu) in unmedicated patients have found an association with hypofrontality. Ebmeier et al (1993), using single-photon emission tomography (SPET), found a negative correlation between resting left prefrontal rCBF and psychomotor poverty score in a group of 20 unmedicated patients, 10 of whom were first episode, treatment-naive cases. In a study of 20 chronic patients with schizophrenia, scanned while free of medication, Wolkin et al (1992) found a negative correlation between right frontal rCMRglu and negative symptoms, especially affective flattening. The difference in laterality between the findings of Ebmeier et al and Wolkin et al raises the possibility that poverty of speech reflects left frontal underactivity while affective flattening reflects right frontal underactivity.

Andreasen et al (1992) using SPET found that unmedicated patients with negative symptoms (alogia, affective flattening, avolition, anhedonia) failed to activate left medial prefrontal cortex during the Tower of London task, which entails planning a sequence of actions. Patients without negative symptoms did produce significant activation in left medial prefrontal cortex during this task. Furthermore, there were no significant differences between medication-naive patients and those who had been withdrawn from long-term antipsychotic medication. There was actually a weak trend for the drug naive patients to have more marked hypofrontality. Thus, it does not appear that hypofrontality is a product of prolonged prior antispychotic treatment. It appears unlikely that the frontal underactivity that occurs in association with psychomotor poverty symptoms can be ascribed either to acute effects of concurrent medication or to the sustained effects of prior medication.

Ebmeier et al (1993), in a study of acute unmedicated patients, found that disorganisation syndrome score was negatively correlated with left parietal rCBF and there was a trend for a positive correlation with right anterior cingulate rCBF. These findings were in agreement with those reported by Liddle et al (1992a) in stable medicated patients. However, in the case of the reality distortion syndrome, Ebmeier et al reported a negative correlation with left lateral temporal rCBF, whereas Liddle et al (1992a) had found a positive correlation with left medial temporal rCBF. Thus, the question of whether or not the pattern of association between syndrome severity and rCBF varies with treatment or with phase of illness has yet to be fully resolved. Notwithstanding the inconsistencies regarding the reality distortion syndrome, the available evidence does provide consistent support for the hypothesis that psychomotor poverty is associated with frontal underactivity, while disorganisation is associated with right medial frontal overactivity and with parietal underactivity.

CEREBRAL ACTIVATION ASSOCIATED WITH THE SUPERVISORY MENTAL FUNCTIONS

The sites involved in the type of supervisory mental process implicated in each syndrome can be located by using PET to measure changes in rCBF associated with the cerebral activation in normal individuals engaged in the relevant supervisory mental activity.

Internal Generation of Activity

Frith et al (1991) carried out two experiments in which they compared rCBF during the performance of a task in which the subject was required to plan the activity, compared with rCBF while the subject carried out a similar task according to a plan generated by the experimenter. In the first experiment, rCBF during articulation of a list of words generated by the subject was compared with rCBF during the articulation of a list of words generated by the experimenter. In the second experiment, the subject performed a random series of movements of middle or index finger of the right hand. In the internal generation condition, the subject generated the sequence of movements, while in the external generation condition, the sequence was determined by the experimenter. In both types of task, there was activation of the lateral and medial prefrontal cortex in the internal generation condition relative to the control external generation condition. In the case of the word generation task the activation was mainly confined to the left side but in the finger movement task the activation was bilateral.

This study demonstrates that, for two quite different types of activity, internal generation of action is associated with increased activity of the lateral and medial prefrontal cortex in normal individuals. Furthermore, the site of maximal activation during the internal generation of words coincided with the locus of negative correlation between rCBF and psychomotor poverty in schizophrenia (see Figure 15.1).

Suppression of Inappropriate Activity: The Stroop Task

Pardo et al (1990) measured cerebral activation in normal individuals performing the Stroop task, in which the subject names the colour of the ink in a list of colour names where ink colour is not congruent with the colour name. They compared rCBF in the condition where ink and colour name were incongruent with rCBF when the ink and colour name were congruent. The site of maximum difference in rCBF between the two conditions was located in the right anterior cingulate cortex at a site lying within the area in which Liddle et al (1992a) had found a positive correlation between rCBF and disorganisation in schizophrenia (see Figure 15.2).

In contrast to the psychomotor poverty syndrome (for which there was a negative correlation between syndrome severity and rCBF at the site maximally activated in normal individuals engaged in the initiation of mental activity), in the case of the disorganisation syndrome there was a positive correlation between

PSYCHOMOTOR POVERTY

Decreases in rCBF ≡≡≡

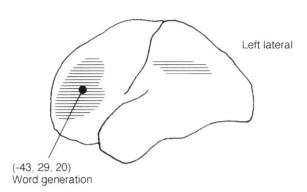

Left lateral

(-43, 29, 20)
Word generation

Figure 15.1. Locus of maximal activation of the prefrontal cortex during the internal generation of words in normal subjects superimposed on the areas of decreased cortical blood flow associated with psychomotor poverty in schizophrenia. Coordinates specify distance in millimetres from an origin at the midpoint of the anterior commissure with reference to a coordinate frame whose x axis is directed from left to right, y axis is directed from posterior to anterior and z axis is perpendicular to the horizontal plane containing the anterior and posterior commissures (Reprinted from Liddle et al, 1992b, with permission)

DISORGANISATION

Increases in rCBF ||||||||

Right medial

(10, 18, 30)
Stroop test

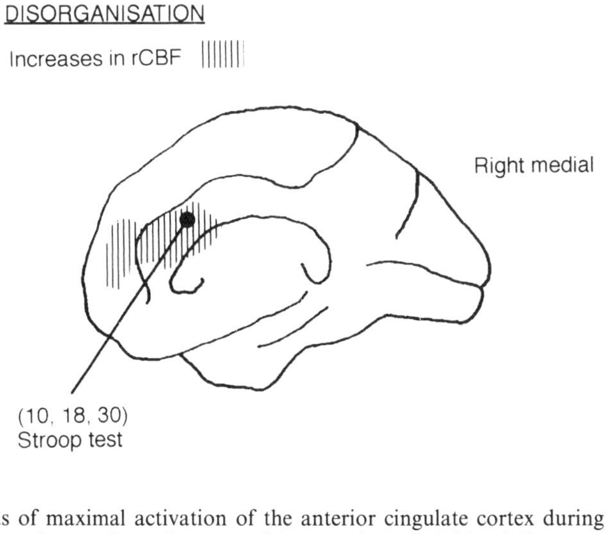

Figure 15.2. Locus of maximal activation of the anterior cingulate cortex during performance of the Stroop test superimposed on the area of increased cortical blood flow associated with disorganisation in schizophrenia (Reprinted from Liddle et al, 1992b, with permission)

syndrome severity and rCBF at the site of maximal activation in normal individuals engaged in the suppression of inappropriate activity. It is possible that the explanation of this apparently paradoxical finding lies in the observation that disorganisation was negatively correlated with rCBF in right ventral prefrontal cortex. In monkeys, lesions of ventral prefrontal cortex result in impaired ability to suppress previously learned responses that are inappropriate to current circumstances (Fuster, 1980). This suggests that, in patients with schizophrenia with the disorganisation syndrome, underactivity of ventral prefrontal cortex creates a tendency for inappropriate activity to intrude in the stream of concurrent mental processing, giving rise to a pathological increase in activity in the anterior cingulate and medial prefrontal cortex.

Internal Monitoring

Normally, a person is not consciously aware of ocular muscle movements. Nonetheless, one can distinguish the situation in which a visual image of an object moves across the retina as a result of movement of the object, from the situation in which the motion of the image across the retina arises from movement of the eyes. The ability to make this distinction implies internal monitoring of the intention to move the eyes. Frith et al (1992b) carried out an experiment in which they measured rCBF during the learning of a novel task involving eye movement with the object of identifying brain regions involved in internal monitoring. An electrode attached to the skin overlying the lateral rectus muscle detected the electrical signal generated by contraction of the muscle. This electrical signal was employed to drive a diamond-shaped object across the screen of a visual display unit in such a manner that, when the subject moved his eyes horizontally, the diamond moved horizontally but in a direction contrary to the anticipated direction. The subject was asked to attempt to make the diamond move regularly to and fro across the screen of the visual display unit. It would be expected that this task would place heavy demands upon the internal monitoring of internally generated activity during initial attempts, but that this demand would decrease as the task became more automatic. If so, the cerebral sites involved in internal monitoring might be identified by comparing rCBF during initial attempts at the task with rCBF after the task had been well learned. Frith and colleagues found that the maximal changes between initial and subsequent performance of the task were in the visual area for motion and in the left parahippocampal gyrus at a site within the area of positive correlation between rCBF and reality distortion (see Figure 15.3).

CONCLUSION

Each of the three syndromes is associated with a specific pattern of neuropsychological impairment and with a specific pattern of rCBF in multimodal association cortex of the frontal, parietal and temporal lobes and in related

REALITY DISTORTION

Increases in rCBF ‖‖‖‖‖

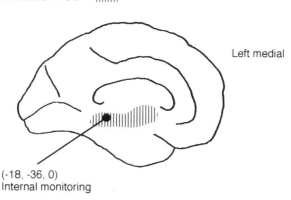

Left medial

(-18, -36, 0)
Internal monitoring

Figure 15.3. Locus of maximal activation of the parahippocampal gyrus during the internal monitoring of eye movements superimposed on the area of increased medial temporal blood flow associated with reality distortion in schizophrenia (Reprinted from Liddle et al, 1992b, with permission)

subcortical nuclei. Furthermore, for each syndrome the rCBF pattern involves the sites that are maximally activated in normal individuals during the performance of the type of supervisory mental process that is implicated in that syndrome.

The psychomotor poverty syndrome, which appears to reflect impaired ability to initiate self-generated mental activity, is associated with underactivity in the prefrontal sites that are activated in normal individuals during the internal generation of a word list and also during the internal generation of a sequence of simple finger movements. The disorganisation syndrome, which is associated with impaired ability to suppress inappropriate mental activity, is associated with decreased rCBF in the right ventral prefrontal cortex and with increased rCBF at the right anterior cingulate and medial prefrontal sites maximally activated during the Stroop task in normal individuals. The evidence with regard to the reality distortion syndrome is less consistent but indicates an association with increased rCBF in medial temporal lobe, at a site that is activated in normal individuals during a task that places heavy demands on the internal monitoring of self-generated mental activity. This is consistent with the proposal that reality distortion entails a pathologically increased level of internal monitoring of self-generated mental activity.

In view of the complexity and variability of schizophrenia it is necessary to be cautious in the interpretation of these findings. Nonetheless, they indicate an emerging understanding of schizophrenia in which symptom profiles can be described in terms of impairment of specific aspects of the supervisory mental processes and related to patterns of activity in the distributed neural networks that subserve each relevant supervisory mental process.

REFERENCES

Allen, H.A., Frith, C.D., Liddle, P.F. (1993) Negative features, retrieval processes and verbal fluency in schizophrenia. *British Journal of Psychiatry*, **163**, 769–775

Andreasen, N.C., Rezai, K., Alliger, R., Swayze, V.W., Flaum, M., Kirchner, P., Cohen, G., O'Leary D.S. (1992) Hypofrontality in neuroleptic-naive patients and in patients with chronic schizophrenia: Assessment with xenon 133 single-photon emission computed tomography and the Tower of London. *Archives of General Psychiatry*, **49**, 943–958.

Arndt, S., Alliger, R.J., Andreasen, N.C. (1991) The distinction of positive and negative symptoms: The failure of a two dimensional model. *British Journal of Psychiatry*, **158**, 317–322.

Bilder, R.M., Mukherjee, S., Reider, R.O., Pandurangi, A.K. (1985) Symptomatic and neuropsychological components of defect states. *Schizophrenia Bulletin*, **11**, 409–419.

Bleuler, E. (1911) *Dementia Praecox or the Group of Schizophrenias* (translated by J. Zinkin, 1950), International Universities Press, New York.

Blumer, D., Benson, D.F. (1975) Personality changes with frontal lobe lesions. In: *Psychiatric Aspects of Neurological Disease* (Eds D. Blumer, D.F. Benson), pp. 151–170, Grune & Stratton, New York.

Brown, K.W., White, T.W. (1992) Syndromes of chronic schizophrenia and some clinical correlates. *British Journal of Psychiatry*, **161**, 317–322.

Cornblatt, B.A., Lenzenweger, M.F., Dworkin, R.H., Erlenmeyer-Kimling, L. (1985) Positive and negative schizophrenic symptoms: Attention and information processing. *Schizophrenia Bulletin*, **11**, 397–405.

Crow, T.J. (1980) The molecular pathology of schizophrenia: More than one disease process. *British Medical Journal*, **280**, 66–68.

Ebmeier, K.P., Blackwood, D.H.R., Murray, C., Souza, V., Walker, M., Dougall, N., Moffoot, A.P.R., O'Carroll, R.E., Goodwin, G.M. (1993) Single photon emission tomography with 99mTc-exametazime in unmedicated schizophrenic patients. *Biological Psychiatry*, **33**, 487–495.

Frith, C.D. (1992) *The Cognitive Neuropsychology of Schizophrenia*, Erlbaum, Hove, UK.

Frith, C.D., Done, D.J. (1989) Experiences of alien control in schizophrenia reflect a disorder in the central monitoring of action. *Psychological Medicine*, **19**, 359–363.

Frith, C.D., Friston, K.J., Liddle, P.F., Frackowiak, R.S.J. (1991) Willed action and the prefrontal cortex in man: A study with PET. *Proceedings of the Royal Society (London) B*, **244**, 241–246.

Frith, C.D., Leary, J., Cahill, C., Johnstone, E.C. (1992a) Disabilities and circumstances of schizophrenic patients: A follow-up study. IV. Performance on psychological tests. *British Journal of Psychiatry*, **159** (Suppl. 13), 26–29.

Frith, C.D., Friston, K.J., Liddle, P.F., Frackowiak, R.S.J. (1992b) PET imaging and cognition in schizophrenia. *Journal of the Royal Society of Medicine*, **85**, 222–224.

Fuster, J.M. (1980) *The Prefrontal Cortex*, Raven Press, New York.

Jaspers, K. (1963) *General Psychopathology* (translated by J. Hoenig, M.W. Hamilton). Manchester University Press, Manchester.

Johnstone, E.C., Crow, T.J., Frith, C.D., Stevens, M., Kreel, L., Husband, J. (1978) The dementia of dementia praecox. *Acta Psychiatrica Scandinavica*, **57**, 305–324.

Kay, S.R. (1991) *Positive and Negative Syndromes in Schizophrenia*, Brunner Mazel, New York.

Kolb, B., Whishaw, I.Q. (1980) *Fundamentals of Human Neuropsychology*, Freeman, San Francisco.

Kulhara, P., Kota, S.K., Joseph, S. (1986) Positive and negative subtypes of schizophrenia: A study from India. *Acta Psychiatrica Scandinavica*, **74**, 353–379.

Lewis, S.W. (1990) Computerised tomography in schizophrenia 15 years on. *British Journal of Psychiatry*, **157** (Suppl. 9), 16–24.

Liddle, P.F. (1984) *Chronic Schizophrenic Symptoms, Cognitive Function and Neurological Impairment*, Membership Examination Thesis, Royal College of Psychiatrists, London.

Liddle, P.F. (1987a) The symptoms of chronic schizophrenia: A re-examination of the positive–negative dichotomy. *British Journal of Psychiatry*, **151**, 145–151.

Liddle, P.F. (1987b) Schizophrenic syndromes, cognitive performance and neurological dysfunction. *Psychological Medicine*, **17**, 49–58.

Liddle, P.F., Barnes, T.R.E. (1990) Syndromes of chronic schizophrenia. *British Journal of Psychiatry*, **157**, 558–561.

Liddle, P.F., Morris, D.L. (1991) Schizophrenic syndromes and frontal lobe performance. *British Journal of Psychiatry*, **158**, 340–345.

Liddle, P.F., Friston, K.J., Frith, C.D., Jones, T., Hirsch, S.R., Frackowiak, R.S.J. (1992a) Patterns of cerebral blood flow in schizophrenia. *British Journal of Psychiatry*, **160**, 179–186.

Liddle, P.F., Friston, K.J., Frith, C.D., Frackowiak, R.S.J. (1992b) Cerebral blood flow and mental processes in schizophrenia. *Journal of the Royal Society of Medicine*, **85**, 224–227.

McGrath, J.J. (1992) The neuropsychology of thought disorder. *Schizophrenia Research*, **6**, 157.

Mortimer, A.M., Lund, C.E., McKenna, P.J. (1990) The positive–negative dichotomy in schizophrenia. *British Journal of Psychiatry*, **157**, 41–49.

Pantelis. C., Harvey, C., Taylor, J., Campbell, P.G. (1991) The Camden schizophrenia surveys: Symptoms and syndromes in schizophrenia. *Biological Psychiatry*, **29** (Suppl.), 646S.

Pardo, J.V., Pardo, P.J., Janer, K.W., Raichle, M.E. (1990) The anterior cingulate mediates processing selection in the Stroop attentional conflict paradigm. *Proceedings of the National Academy of Sciences USA*, **87**, 256–259.

Peralta, V., deLeon, J., Cuesta, M.J. (1992) Are there more than two syndromes in schizophrenia? A critique of the positive–negative dichotomy. *British Journal of Psychiatry*, **161**, 335–343.

Schroder, J., Geider, F.J., Binkert, M., Reitz, C., Jauss, M., Sauer, H. (1992) Sub-syndromes in chronic schizophrenia: Do their psychopathological characteristics correspond to cerebral alterations? *Psychiatry Research*, **42**, 209–220.

Slater, E., Beard, A.W., Glitherow, E. (1963) The schizophrenia-like psychoses of epilepsy. *British Journal of Psychiatry*, **109**, 95–105.

Wolkin, A., Sanfilipo, M., Wolf, A.P., Angrist, B., Brodie, J.D., Rotrosen, J. (1992) Negative symptoms and hypofrontality in chronic schizophrenia. *Archives of General Psychiatry*, **49**, 959–965.

Part D

NEUROPSYCHOLOGICAL MODELS OF SCHIZOPHRENIA

16

Neurocognitive and Neurobehavioural Patterns and the Syndromes of Schizophrenia: Role of Frontal–Subcortical Networks

CHRISTOS PANTELIS and WARRICK BREWER

INTRODUCTION

There is a growing literature indicating that patients with schizophrenia have problems in generalised neurocognitive processing (Hemsley, 1982; Goldstein, 1986; see also this volume: Rogers, chapter 2; Barber et al, chapter 4). More recently, however, the use of increasingly refined neuropsychological tasks has revealed that there may be specific patterns of neurocognitive deficits in schizophrenia or subtypes of schizophrenia (Crow, 1980; Liddle, 1987b) as is suggested in a number of chapters of this volume. Perhaps the most common cognitive deficits found in schizophrenia are observed with neuropsychological tests of executive function. These tests typically assess the ability to plan, organise or generate novel problem solving strategies and have been considered sensitive to frontal lobe function. They include the Wisconsin Card Sorting Test (WCST), the Stroop task, the antisaccade task, the controlled oral word association task (COWAT) and the Tower of London task (Kolb & Whishaw, 1983; Weinberger et al, 1986; Liddle, 1987b; Morice, 1990; Shallice et al, 1991; Andreasen et al, 1992; Maruff et al, 1995; Pantelis et al, 1993, 1996b, 1996c). The literature has focused particularly on the WCST, which is thought to implicate the dorsolateral prefrontal cortex (DLPFC) (Kolb & Whishaw, 1983; Weinberger et al, 1986 & 1988, Berman et al, 1986 & 1988; Goldberg et al, 1987; Morice, 1990), although the specificity of this task has been questioned (David, 1992; Corcoran & Upton, 1993).

Schizophrenia: A Neuropsychological Perspective. Edited by C. Pantelis, H.E. Nelson and T.R.E. Barnes
© 1996 John Wiley & Sons Ltd

While the frontal lobes have received a great deal of attention in schizophrenia, careful examination has attributed performance deficits to dysfunction or pathology in other areas with which they connect, such as the temporal lobes, basal ganglia and thalami (Buchsbaum, 1990; Pantelis et al, 1992; Weinberger et al, 1992; Gold & Harvey, 1993). For example, in their review of neuropsychological studies in schizophrenia, Gold and Harvey (1993) identified impairments in attention, memory and problem solving and suggested that these findings implicated multi-system dysfunction involving frontal, temporal, thalamic and basal ganglia areas. Recently, researchers have sought to link the range of phenomena observed in schizophrenia to the neurocognitive deficits by utilising distributed neuronal network models (Mesulam, 1990; Goldman-Rakic, 1988). According to this approach the control of any cognitive function is distributed across a number of interconnected nuclei through the brain. Disruption to any of these nuclei or their interconnections result in changes in cognitive function. A recent and influential model used to explain deficits in executive function in schizophrenia has been proposed by Weinberger and colleagues (1992). These authors have drawn on the animal literature for working memory (Goldman-Rakic, 1987) to suggest that the consistent findings of deficits of frontal lobe functioning may result from disruption of the circuitry connecting with limbic structures. Specifically, they argue that the neuropsychological dysfunction in schizophrenia results from disruption of the circuitry connecting the DLPFC with the hippocampus. However, other authors (Robbins, 1990, 1991; Pantelis et al, 1992; Pantelis & Nelson, 1994; Pantelis & Brewer, 1995) have marshalled evidence, including the results from functional imaging studies of schizophrenia (for review: Velakoulis & Pantelis, 1996), which has implicated dysfunction of the fronto-striato-thalamic networks. The latter include the frontal eye fields (FEF), the supplementary motor area (SMA), the orbitofrontal cortex (OFC) and anterior cingulate (AC) as well as the DLPFC. As discussed below, the DLPFC, OFC and AC are involved in mediating cognitive processes found to be disturbed in schizophrenia, while the FEF has been implicated in the eye movement disturbances in schizophrenia (see Henderson et al, chapter 13) and the SMA may be important in mediating certain symptoms of schizophrenia (see Cahill and Frith, chapter 18).

Pantelis and colleagues (Pantelis et al, 1992; Pantelis & Nelson, 1994; Pantelis & Brewer, 1995) have drawn parallels between the features of schizophrenia and the frontal–subcortical dementias and have argued that the apparent frontal hypofunctioning observed in schizophrenia may result from deafferentation of the circuitry connecting the basal ganglia with these various prefrontal areas. These and other authors (e.g. Robbins, 1991) suggest that fronto-striato-thalamic pathways connecting cortex with subcortex are important in understanding the range of deficits observed. They have also suggested that the associations found in schizophrenia between cognitive deficits and the symptoms (Liddle, chapter 15), behavioural deficits (Pantelis & Brewer, 1995) and both motor (Collinson et al, chapter 12) and ocular motor (Henderson et al, chapter 13) disturbances seen in this disorder may be better understood by examining the topography of the neural circuitry connecting prefrontal areas with other sites, particularly the striatum and thalami (Pantelis et al, 1992), as well as medial temporal structures

(Weinberger, 1991). In this chapter we discuss the notion of separate prefrontal syndromes which are characterised by specific patterns of behavioural and neuro-cognitive impairment and which therefore suggest the presence of patterns of functional specialisation. We will argue that these specialised patterns of impairment are associated with the different clinical (both symptom-based and behavioural) syndromes of schizophrenia. Furthermore, we propose that some of the observed deficits of executive function in schizophrenia may be explained as secondary to disruptions of neurocognitive networks distributed through fronto-striato-thalamic regions, while others may be mediated through mesolimbic circuits. Because of the interconnectedness of these neuronal networks, disruptions at any point in the circuit will generally produce similar functional deficits. It is suggested that *"network-specific"* components of neurocognitive tasks can be identified and may be used as probes to examine the integrity of each cortical–subcortical (or indeed cortico-cortical) network. Other tasks which have been shown to be affected by disruption of specific elements of the circuit are more useful in identifying the circumscribed cortical relative to subcortical disruptions to components within the circuit, which we term *"component-specific"* functions. This strategy of using *"network-specific"* functions or *"component-specific"* functions may be useful in examining the contribution of separate neuronal networks, such as prefrontal–hippocampal versus prefrontal–striatal systems.

FRONTAL-STRIATO-THALAMIC PATHWAYS: STRUCTURAL AND FUNCTIONAL ORGANISATION

The prefrontal area is considered to subserve aspects of executive function which may be considered as integral to the functions embraced by Shallice's "supervisory attentional system" (Shallice, 1988). These functions have been considered to be mediated by prefrontal cortical areas. Alexander and colleagues, in their investigations of the structure and neuronal connections of the prefrontal cortex, have identified a highly organised system of circuits connecting the basal ganglia and the thalami with discrete areas within the prefrontal cortex. These frontal-striato-thalamic pathways are highly organised with parallel, segregated circuits which maintain their anatomical and functional segregation (Alexander et al, 1986; DeLong et al, 1990; Groenewegen et al, 1991; see Figure 16.1). As depicted in Figure 16.2, at least five distinct basal ganglia-thalamo-cortical circuits have been identified (Alexander et al, 1986), which funnel through the basal ganglia from the prefrontal cortex, returning to the prefrontal area of origin via the thalami. Therefore, these prefrontal–subcortical circuits implicate the basal ganglia and thalami, not only in motor and ocular motor function via their connections with the FEF and SMA, but also in cognitive function via their connections with prefrontal cortical areas (i.e. DLPFC, AC and OFC). Basal ganglia connections with the limbic lobe via the AC circuit also suggest that they play a role in emotion and behaviour. Lesions anywhere within this extended neuronal framework would be expected to produce a similar functional deficit. Further, despite their close proximity subcortically, it also appears that there is very little

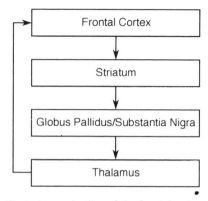

Figure 16.1. Central organisation of the frontal–subcortical circuits.

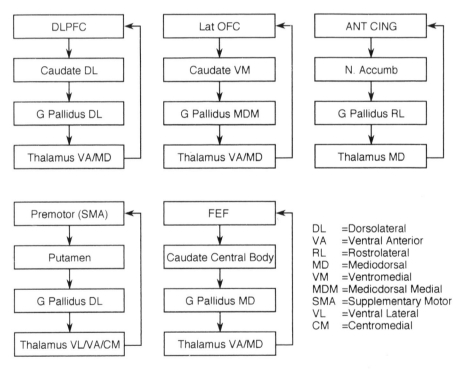

Figure 16.2. Organisation of the frontal-subcortical circuits (see also Cummings, 1993). (NB: indirect circuits of the substantia nigra and subthalamic nucleus are not shown.)

cross-communication among these circuits and these loops remain segregated (Duffy & Campbell, 1994) and consequently their functions may be described as "circuit-specific" (Cummings, 1993; Mega & Cummings, 1994) or "*network-specific*".

Another corollary of the organisation of the circuits and their close proximity in the basal ganglia is that a disturbance of their pathophysiology subcortically might generate a range of symptoms, including disorders of movement, affect and cognition. While outside of the basal ganglia these pathways are not so closely aligned and lesions would be expected to produce more limited and discrete impairments of cognitive, limbic or motor function, disruption occurring within subcortical nuclei would be more likely to produce symptoms involving all of these functions (Pantelis & Nelson, 1994). For example, small lesions of the head of the caudate are likely to produce marked deficits in executive function while, conversely, relatively large areas of frontal ablation may result in relatively minor behavioural deficits (Duffy & Campbell, 1994). Thus, the topographical arrangement of these pathways would seem to be consistent with evidence of cognitive, psychiatric and motor disturbance occurring together in disorders of the basal ganglia, such as Huntington's disease and Parkinson's disease (Cummings, 1993; Litvan et al, 1991). The implication of similar disturbances coexisting in schizophrenia is that basal ganglia and/or thalamic pathology may be relevant in this condition (Pantelis et al, 1992). While recent work with MRI has identified structural abnormalities in the hippocampi of patients with schizophrenia (e.g. Suddath et al, 1989, 1990; Velakoulis et al, 1996), post-mortem studies have reported reduced volumes of basal ganglia and thalamic structures (Bogerts et al, 1985; Pakkenberg & Gundersen, 1989). A recent MRI study has also identified significant differences in the thalami between patients and controls (Andreasen et al, 1994), while PET studies also suggest involvement of basal ganglia and their connections with prefrontal areas (Buchsbaum et al, 1992; Andreasen et al, 1992).

"*NETWORK-SPECIFIC*" VERSUS "*COMPONENT-SPECIFIC*" FUNCTIONS

Each of the prefrontal-striato-thalamic pathways described have been associated with a specific pattern of cognition and behaviour, which Cummings (1993) has described as "*signature behavioural syndromes*". He later referred to these as "signature" prefrontal syndromes (Mega & Cummings, 1994). Similarly, each of the schizophrenia syndromes (Liddle, 1987a; Harvey et al, 1996), elaborated below, has been associated with relatively independent patterns of cognition and behaviour. The degree of overlap between these prefrontal behavioural and schizophrenia syndromes suggests a useful framework could be formulated for reducing the heterogeneity of this disorder. Furthermore, elucidating the presence of relatively more discrete cognitive and clinical disturbances associated with each circuit is consistent with the notion that the sum behaviour generated through interaction of each circuit can be "fractionated" into component processes. Frith considers that defining the component cognitive processes and linking these to schizophrenic phenomena is a necessary prerequisite to elucidating the underlying brain dysfunction (Frith, 1992). The principle of "fractionation" of cognitive processes has been described by Shallice and colleagues (Shallice, 1988; Shallice & Burgess, 1991a). Research in schizophrenia which attempts to "fractionate" cognitive processes has been relatively limited, yet this approach can be particularly powerful (Frith, 1992; Neufeld and Williamson, chapter 11). For example, poor performance on the WCST may implicate a number of component cognitive processes involved in task performance, each of which may implicate different neuronal systems. The component processes in performing this task would include working memory, abstraction, maintenance of set and response to feedback. While patients with schizophrenia have demonstrated poor ability in completing the WCST, the component processes which might be implicated are unclear. The development of tasks which separate individual components is necessary in order to examine the cognitive processes underlying deficits in more complex tasks, such as the WCST, which may then provide clues to the underlying pathophysiological disturbance.

Some recent studies attempt to address these issues and provide the possibility to develop *"network-specific"* and *"component-specific"* cognitive tasks. Owen and colleagues (1991, 1993) have developed set-shifting tasks which decompose the WCST into component processes and distinguish the types of failure in set shifting as either a problem of perseveration (failure to shift attention from a previously relevant dimension) or learned irrelevance (failure to shift attention to a previously irrelevant dimension). While patients with frontal lesions demonstrate a marked deficit due to perseveration, the deficits of set shifting in medicated patients with Parkinson's disease are due to learned irrelevance. In this example, differences in component cognitive processes illustrate a differential pattern of impairment along the cortical/subcortical axis. These tasks have been utilised in recent studies of patients with schizophrenia (Elliott et al, 1995; Pantelis et al, 1996a). In the study by Elliott and colleagues (1995) patients with schizophrenia demonstrated set shifting abnormalities akin to frontal lesioned patients due to marked perseveration. In the study by Pantelis and colleagues, chronic hospitalised patients with schizophrenia demonstrated a failure of set shifting at a much earlier stage than patients with frontal lesions, suggesting a more severe deficit of set shifting ability than in patients with focal frontal damage.

Another similar example, developed by the same group, has identified dissociations between planning times and execution times using a computerised Tower of London task (Owen et al, 1990, 1992). Using this task to assess both motor and cognitive speed, dissociations were found between frontal lesioned patients and disorders of the basal ganglia. While the frontal patients showed significant prolongation of subsequent thinking time (time to complete the problem after planning) they showed no deficit of initial thinking (planning) time. In contrast, patients with pathology in the basal ganglia, such as those with Parkinson's disease, showed the opposite pattern with significantly prolonged planning times rather than subsequent thinking times. Recent studies in schizophrenia (Morris et al, 1995; Hanes et al, 1996; Pantelis et al, 1993, 1996) have demonstrated that patients with schizophrenia were prolonged in their subsequent thinking times rather than planning times, thereby demonstrating similarities to those patients with frontal lesions.

Eslinger & Grattan (1993) provide further evidence in support of the notion of a cortical–subcortical distinction in their study of cognitive flexibility. Patients with frontal ischaemic damage and patients with ischaemic damage of the basal ganglia were compared to a group of patients with posterior cortical lesions and normal controls, on tasks of "reactive" flexibility (shifting response set) and "spontaneous" flexibility (producing a diversity of ideas). Pathology in the frontal lobe or the basal ganglia both resulted in a similar degree of impairment in "reactive flexibility" in comparison to the other groups, suggesting that this function is "*network-*" rather than "*component-specific*". In contrast, only frontal damage resulted in impairment of "spontaneous flexibility", providing evidence for this function as "*component-specific*", at least within the frontal–subcortical circuit. Few studies have examined cognitive flexibility in schizophrenia in this way. In a recent study of reasoning behaviour, Hanes and colleagues (1995) examined cognitive flexibility and cognitive integration in patients with schizo-phrenia, Huntington's and Parkinson's diseases in comparison with normal control subjects. These investigators identified deficits in reactive flexibility in patients with schizophrenia and Huntington's disease but not medicated Parkin-son's disease patients, while aspects of spontaneous flexibility were impaired in all groups. Further, patients with schizophrenia and Huntington's disease patients were impaired in their ability to integrate information, which may have resulted either from a deficit of inductive reasoning or, alternatively, from a tendency to be impulsive suggesting a deficit in response inhibition. The authors suggest that these data are consistent with involvement of frontal–striatal circuits in schizo-phrenia.

Experimental designs which provide the possibility of double dissociations, as described above, provide clues to the nature of the pathophysiological disturbance in conditions such as schizophrenia. However, "*component-specific*" functions such as these tend to be the exception rather than the rule, as dysfunction at any locus of an integrated neuronal network generally produces similar functional deficit. This overlap was exemplified in the extensive review of the notion of subcortical dementia by Brown & Marsden (1988). As was evident in this review, the number of "*network-specific*" functions was far in excess of the functions deemed to be "*component-specific*". Brown & Marsden (1988) indicated that some cognitive functions may provide a distinction along a cortical–subcortical axis. While they may be relatively few, such "*component-specific*" functions may be particularly relevant in helping to identify the site of pathophysiological disturbance in schizo-phrenia (Table 16.1).

We propose that, in schizophrenia, an examination of the relationship between the cognitive or behavioural functions related to each of the parallel, segregated frontal-striato-thalamic circuits ("*network-specific*" functions) versus those which provide a cortical–subcortical distinction (which are better described as "*component-specific*" functions) may provide clues to the pathophysiological processes underlying this disorder. "*Component-specific*" cognitive functions, which may provide further evidence of a cortical–subcortical distinction, are shown in Table 16.1. As well as those discussed above, other neuropsychological functions which may provide a cortical–subcortical distinction include recall versus recognition memory deficits, and procedural versus declarative knowledge and learning; these are discussed more fully elsewhere (Pantelis et al, 1992;

Table 16.1 Neuropsychological evidence for a 'cortical' (frontal)/'subcortical' (striatal) distinction ('*component-specific*' functions)

	Frontal disorders/lesions	Basal ganglia disorders (e.g. Parkinson's and Huntington's disease)	Schizophrenia
Set shifting	Perseveration (Owen et al, 1993)	Perseveration and learned irrelevance: unmedicated Parkinson's disease (Owen et al, 1993) Learned irrelevance: medicated Parkinson's disease (Owen et al, 1993) Perseveration and learned irrelevance: Huntington's disease (Lawrence et al; cited in Elliott et al, 1995)	Perseveration (Elliott et al, 1995)
Cognitive speed	Subsequent thinking time prolonged (Owen et al, 1990) Initial thinking time not affected (Owen et al, 1990)	Subsequent thinking time not affected (Owen et al, 1992) Initial thinking time prolonged (Owen et al, 1992)	Subsequent thinking time prolonged (Pantelis et al, 1993; Morris et al, 1995) Initial thinking time not affected (Pantelis et al, 1993; Morris et al, 1995; Hanes et al, 1996)
Cognitive flexibility	Reactive flexibility impaired (Eslinger and Grattan, 1993) Spontaneous flexibility impaired (Eslinger and Grattan, 1993)	Reactive flexibility impaired (Eslinger and Grattan, 1993) Spontaneous flexibility *not* impaired (Eslinger and Grattan, 1993)	Reactive flexibility impaired (Hanes et al, 1995) Spontaneous flexibility impaired (Hanes et al, 1995)

Pantelis & Nelson, 1994; Collinson et al, chapter 12). The following discussion will focus largely on prefrontal–subcortical networks and their (*"network-specific"*) functions and relate prefrontal syndromes to the syndromes of schizophrenia.

PREFRONTAL BEHAVIOURAL SYNDROMES: FRACTIONATION OF THE PREFRONTAL CORTEX

Frith (1987) commented that "putting all patients with frontal lobe injury together is a rather unfortunate practice, since the frontal lobes represent a very large area accounting for about 33% of total cortical area" (p. 642). That different prefrontal areas subserve different functions is supported by the parallel segregated nature of the prefrontal-striato-thalamic circuitry described by Alexander and colleagues (1986) and discussed above (Figure 16.1). Attempts, therefore, to model deficits of schizophrenia to deficits consequent on compromise of frontal–subcortical systems should take into account the heterogeneity of function of these circuits. Shallice & Burgess (1991a, 1991b) conceptualise that the supervisory aspects of a problem-solving process involve a number of subprocesses, involving distinct subsystems. Such fractionation supports the notion of separable prefrontal syndromes with distinct behavioural features.

While Cummings (1993) has described the *signature* prefrontal syndromes as patterns of behaviour associated with the appropriate prefrontal cortical and subcortical areas, most relevant to the study of neuropsychological functioning in schizophrenia are the circuits connecting with the DLPFC, OFC, AC and SMA. Duffy & Campbell (1994) have described three prefrontal syndromes and their clinical characteristics. The *"DLPFC syndrome"* (dysexecutive type) has been characterised by deficits in executive function and motor programming abnormalities, which result in impairments in temporal and sensory integration, planning and maintenance of goal-directed behaviour and behavioural flexibility. The behavioural manifestations of this syndrome have been characterised as apathy, lack of drive, inability to plan ahead and total unconcern, features which have previously been termed as the "pseudo-depressed" personality (Blumer & Benson, 1975) (Table 16.2).

Unlike the *"DLPFC syndrome"*, descriptions of the *"OFC syndrome"* (disinhibited type) have emphasised the presence of marked changes in personality, including irritability, disinhibition, inappropriate self-indulgence and lack of concern for others, which have been described as the "pseudo-psychopathic" personality (Blumer & Benson, 1975). Cummings further states that this syndrome is characterised by an "enslavement to environmental cues with automatic imitation of the gestures and actions of others, or enforced utilisation of objects in the environment" (Cummings, 1993, p. 875). Such "utilisation" behaviour has been described by Lhermitte and colleagues (Lhermitte, 1986; Lhermitte et al, 1986) and has been termed the "environmental dependency syndrome" (Lhermitte, 1986). This has been associated with lesions of the OFC.

The *"Mesial Frontal syndrome"* (Apathetic type) involves disturbance of the

Table 16.2. Prefrontal syndromes and schizophrenia syndromes

Prefrontal Syndrome	Description	Associated Behaviours (Personality type)	Cognitive Functions of Relevant Circuit ('Network-specific')	Proposed Schizophrenia Syndromes
DLPFC (dorsolateral prefrontal)	Dysexecutive	Apathy, Lack of drive Inability to plan ahead Total unconcern ('Pseudodepressed')	Appropriate selection Novelty Goal-directed behaviour Developing new strategies/ problem solving Set shifting	Psychomotor Poverty (Liddle, 1987a) Social Withdrawal and Depressed Behaviour factors (Harvey et al, 1996)
OFC (orbitofrontal)	Disinhibited	Changes in personality: Irritability Disinhibition Inappropriate self-indulgence Lack of concern for others Stimulus driven behaviour 'Utilisation' Behaviour/ Automatic imitation ('Pseudo-psychopathic')	Inhibition (internal) Inhibition of inappropriate responses (together with AC) Olfactory identification ability Impairments on Go/No Go and Delayed Alternation (DAT) tasks	Disorganisation (Liddle, 1987a) Thought disturbance factor and Antisocial Behaviour factors (Harvey et al, 1996)
AC (anterior cingulate)	Apathetic	Attentional deficits Impaired drive/motivation Deficits in affect Reduced inhibition Akinesis/Apathy Akinetic mutism ('Amotivational')	Attention for Action Inhibition of inappropriate responses (together with OFC) Intentional selection/ inhibition of external stimuli (internal volition) Acts with SMA for environmental search and inhibition of exploratory behaviour	Overactivity of AC identified with Disorganisation syndrome (Liddle, 1987a) Social Withdrawal and Thought Disturbance factor (Harvey et al, 1996)
SMA (supplementary motor area)	Ideomotor	Failure of internal monitoring of motor acts 'Alien-hand' syndrome	Inhibition (external) Initiator (internal generation) of motor programs	Delusions of Control (Frith, 1992; Cahill and Frith, chapter 18)

balance between AC and SMA. Goldberg & Bloom (1990) have proposed that the SMA and cingulate form a reciprocal system responsible for environmental search and inhibition of exploratory behaviour. However, both these areas subserve different functions, the AC being important to motivational aspects of behaviour and attention while the SMA is important for inhibition. We would suggest that the *"anterior cingulate syndrome"* be separate from a *"supplementary motor area syndrome"*. Indeed, Mega & Cummings (1994) describe the *"anterior cingulate syndrome"* as a separate prefrontal syndrome but do not elaborate on the role of the SMA and its connections. The AC circuit is linked to the hippocampus and forms part of the paralimbic cortex. It also has close connections with other prefrontal cortical areas, such as the DLPFC (Benes et al, 1992) and OFC circuits (Mesulam, 1985, 1990). As might be expected there is an overlap of function (Devinsky & Luciano, 1993), with these areas functioning in concert when engaged in tasks requiring initiation, motivation, selection and inhibition. The AC circuit enables the intentional selection of external stimuli based upon the internal relevance these stimuli have for the organism. Input about the internal relevance is provided by the activity of the OFC circuit, while the DLPFC is involved in developing novel strategies and appropriate response selection. Lesions to the AC circuit result in akinesis, impaired ability to inhibit inappropriate responses, and apathy. Bilateral lesions of the anterior cingulate result in akinetic mutism and impairments in the ability to express and experience affect (Damasio & Van Hoesen, 1983), these phenomena being very similar to the negative symptoms of schizophrenia. Further, apathy is prominent in patients with subcortical disorders, including Parkinson's disease, Huntington's disease and thalamic lesions (Vogt & Gabriel, 1993), thereby implicating the AC-striatothalamic circuit in these disorders. More recently, Devinsky et al (1995) have detailed the functions of the AC cortex, which they divide up into "affect" and "cognition" components.

The functions of the SMA have been investigated and described by Passingham (1993) and include "self initiated" movements not determined by "external" cues, a role in repetitive movements and in the performance of a well rehearsed sequence from memory. Disturbance of these functions has also been observed in disorders of the basal ganglia, such as Parkinson's disease (Cunnington et al, in press), thus implicating the SMA and its connections with basal ganglia structures. These functions may have significance for the stereotypies and other motor abnormalities observed in schizophrenia. The potential importance of the SMA region to the positive symptoms of schizophrenia is discussed in the model proposed by Frith (Frith, 1992; see Cahill & Frith, chapter 18). Cahill and Frith discuss the alien-hand syndrome, consequent on lesions of the SMA and relate this to some of the positive symptoms of schizophrenia, such as delusions of control.

Thus, while the DLPFC region is particularly important for executive function, the SMA/anterior cingulate areas are important mediators of motivational and volitional aspects of behaviour, while the OFC region is more important for emotional behaviour (Mega & Cummings, 1994). The latter has also been implicated in inhibitory processes, as exemplified by "utilisation" behaviour, and is also implicated in olfactory identification ability (Seidman et al, 1992).

Though the advocates of these prefrontal syndromes have emphasised that they are characterised by separate behavioural profiles, there is a lack of empirical evidence to assess accurately the degree of their independence. For example, "utilisation" behaviour of the OFC syndrome could also be conceived of as a deficit in executive function and would affect planning and the maintenance of goal-directedness, functions ascribed to the DLPFC syndrome. Similarly, overlap of the DLPFC and AC circuits and of the AC and SMA circuits was suggested above. It is likely that there is an interrelationship between the functions of two or more areas in the execution of any particular task and hence an overlap of function might be expected. However, the parallel segregated nature of the circuits involved in these networks (Alexander et al, 1986) would also predict some degree of independence of function. Studies which provide evidence for dissociable functions support the validity of separate prefrontal syndromes, which we term *"network-specific"*. Few studies to date have addressed these issues, although recently there are some promising areas of research seeking such distinctions (e.g. Dias et al, 1995, 1996; Anderson et al, 1995; Tranel et al, 1995). As already mentioned such dissociations may prove useful in helping to understand the nature of the heterogeneity in conditions such as schizophrenia.

It has been suggested that there are separable symptom profiles in schizophrenia which differ in their pathophysiology and may implicate separate prefrontal areas (Liddle, 1987b; see Liddle, chapter 15). A recent study, discussed below, has also identified separate behavioural syndromes of schizophrenia which are related to these symptom-based syndromes (Harvey et al, 1996). Though previous authors have examined "symptom-based syndromes" of schizophrenia and their relationship to frontal function, few have examined the behavioural disturbances of schizophrenia in this context. This is surprising given that disturbances of behaviour are integral features of the frontal syndromes.

NEUROPSYCHOLOGY OF THE FRONTAL SYNDROMES

In the following discussion, which examines these prefrontal syndromes in relation to schizophrenia, we will focus on the DLPFC, OFC and AC and their subcortical connections (Table 16.2). Neuropsychologically, patients with the *"OFC syndrome"* are impaired on "Go–No Go" tasks, indicating an inability to suppress inappropriate responses (Malloy et al, 1993), while they have been found to perform normally on card sorting tasks (e.g. Laiacona et al, 1989), traditionally associated with DLPFC impairment. Like patients with the "OFC syndrome", patients with the *"AC syndrome"* also demonstrate a failure of response inhibition on "Go–No Go" tasks. The anterior cingulate is important in initiation, motivation and goal-directed behaviours (Devinsky et al, 1995). The AC has been associated with the process of "attention for action", which is described as the process of assigning motivational significance to an act or event in order to select an appropriate response or behaviour over other competing and/or inappropriate responses (Mesulam, 1990; Vogt et al, 1992). Of relevance are the positron emission tomographic activation studies of the Stroop task in normal subjects (Pardo et al, 1990; Bench et al 1993; George et al, 1994; Pantelis et al, 1996c), a task that requires "attention for action" and inhibition of inappropriate responses but not novel responses (such as in card sort tasks). In this task patients are asked to name the colour of the ink words are written in when the letters spell the name of a different colour (incongruent condition) versus when they spell the name of the same colour (congruent condition). These studies identified activation of the anterior cingulate circuit during performance of this task.

These findings suggest that some of the cognitive functions of the OFC, AC and DLPFC circuits are dissociable, which also supports the notion of separable behavioural syndromes related to these circuits. Other tasks which may discriminate particularly DLPFC and OFC functions have included the delayed-response (DR) and delayed-alternation (DA) tasks (Oscar-Berman, 1991; Oscar-Berman et al, 1991) as well as object alternation (Mishkin et al, 1969; Freedman, 1990). DR tasks index the ability to guide behaviour by stored information or representational memory (Fuster, 1989; Goldman-Rakic, 1987). Evidence has suggested that performance on these tasks is mediated by DLPFC regions (Goldman-Rakic & Friedman, 1991). Correct response on DA tasks depends upon remembering the preceding response, which provides the key to the correct direction of subsequent moves (Goldman-Rakic, 1987).

In her elegant series of studies, Goldman-Rakic (1987) has used DR/DA tasks to examine prefrontal cortical function in primates. She has suggested that the cognitive functions mediated by the principal sulcus (PS) (Brodmann's area 46, i.e. the DLPFC) are subserved by specific classes of neurones and specific pathways linking the principal sulcus to other brain areas (Goldman-Rakic, 1987; Goldman-Rakic & Friedman, 1991). The PS is considered to be essential for guiding voluntary behaviour which is dependent upon the "remembered" location of visual cues. She has adopted Baddeley's (1986) notion of working memory to suggest that the PS may be the focus for visuospatial working memory. The PS and the areas with which it connects, including the mediodorsal (MD) nucleus of the thalamus (Fuster & Alexander, 1971), hippocampus (Watanabe & Niki, 1985) and head of the caudate nucleus (Hikosaka et al, 1989), are all implicated as important for adequate performance on visuospatial DR tasks.

While DR performance depends upon the integrity of the DLPFC, Oscar-Berman (1991) argued that DA tasks are specific indexes of the orbitofrontal regions. However, the experimental work would suggest some degree of overlap between performance on DA tasks and lesions in these areas (Mishkin, 1964), which may result from an overlap of functions between components of the DA task with those of the DR task. The importance of the parallel segregated circuits described earlier is that it should be possible to identify "*network-specific*" patterns of neurocognition and behaviour for the OFC as has been found for the DLPFC. For example, Freedman (1990) has discussed the "object alternation" task which may be more specific to OFC function than traditional DA tasks, as suggested in studies of non-human primates (Mishkin et al, 1969; Pribram & Mishkin, 1956), though there have been no studies to date in schizophrenia.

THE STROOP TASK IN SCHIZOPHRENIA

The evidence in patients with schizophrenia suggests that they are impaired in their ability to inhibit inappropriate responses (Maruff et al, in press) and that they have difficulty in the ability to exert internal control over the processing of word stimuli (Rafal & Henik, 1994). The Stroop task is a classic task of inhibition involving word stimuli. Neuropsychological studies have shown that patients with schizophrenia perform poorly on this task (Liddle & Morris, 1991; Joyce et al, 1996). In agreement with the findings of Liddle and colleagues, Joyce and colleagues (1996) found that impaired Stroop performance was associated with increased severity of the "disorganisation syndrome" described by Liddle (chapter 15; and see below). Liddle suggested that this implicated a common involvement of the anterior cingulate cortex. This was suggested by the findings of PET studies using the Stroop in normal subjects described earlier and the findings of a resting PET study (Liddle et al, 1992) which found that scores for the disorganisation syndrome were correlated with increased activity in the anterior cingulate. However, to date there are no published studies investigating patients with schizophrenia using the Stroop task under PET activation conditions.

DR/DA TASKS IN SCHIZOPHRENIA

The consistent findings of impaired frontal lobe functioning in patients with schizophrenia, particularly data which have implicated the DLPFC (Weinberger et al, 1986, 1988; Berman et al, 1986, 1988; Liddle, 1987b; Liddle et al, 1992) and the OFC (Liddle, 1987b; Brewer et al, in press) would predict impairment on DR/DA tasks, or other tasks of working memory. Differential impairment on these tasks may provide clues as to which systems are disrupted. There have been relatively few studies examining DR/DA task performance in patients with schizophrenia (Gold et al, 1991; Raine et al, 1992; Partiot et al, 1992; Park & Holzman, 1992; Brewer et al, in press), although such tasks have been used in patients with frontal lobe dysfunction (Freedman & Oscar-Berman, 1986; Lewisohn et al, 1972) and other neurological patients, including those with Korsakoff's amnesia and amnestic syndrome (see Frith et al, 1992) and patients with Huntington's disease (Oscar-Berman et al, 1982). One of the problems in adapting tasks from the animal work is to develop tasks of an appropriate difficulty level for use with human subjects (Fleming et al, 1994). Another potential problem concerns the nature of the modality of these tasks in primates. Goldman-Rakic (1987) suggested that the PS in primates subserves working memory restricted to the visuospatial domain. Some studies have employed additional non-visual DR tasks to examine such specificity (e.g. Park and Holzman, 1992).

In the study by Gold and colleagues (Gold et al, 1991; Fleming et al, 1994), a computerised Delayed Response Alternation task (DRA) was developed which combined the requirements of both DR and DA function. The DRA task required the subject simultaneously to keep track of the location of a visual stimulus and of an alternating principle. Maintenance of information in working memory was thus required while the appropriate response was determined, this being dependent on the previous response. In a group of normal control subjects, metabolic activation of the DLPFC was observed when this task was used while patients were examined using positron emission tomography (PET). Unfortunately, in this experiment any likely specific requirements of DR versus DA tasks were not explored. Future investigations of this kind should take account of likely differences between these tasks.

Partiot et al (1992) demonstrated a dissociation between DR and DA tasks in patients with schizophrenia compared with DLPFC lesioned patients and normal controls. The performance of the schizophrenic patients was similar to that of the frontal lobe patients, with impaired performance on the DR rather than the DA tasks. This study would support the notion that DR tasks are more specific to DLPFC dysfunction, however, patients with lesions of the OFC should also have been examined to help clarify the role of these brain areas in performance of these tasks.

To investigate spatial working memory in schizophrenia, Park & Holzman (1992) used DR tasks to assess working memory function in patients with schizophrenia in comparison with bipolar patients and normal controls. They used a DR task derived directly from the primate work (oculomotor DR task) as well as a haptic DR task to examine specificity of sensory modality. Their findings indicated that patients with schizophrenia were impaired in their performance on both tasks compared with the comparison groups, suggesting that the spatial working memory deficits were diagnosis specific. The findings of deficits in the two types of spatial working memory tasks suggested that such function was not specific to one sensory modality.

The results from these studies indicate that patients with schizophrenia are impaired in their performance on DR tasks, suggesting impaired "spatial working memory" performance, which implicates dysfunction of the DLPFC. However, such dysfunction may not necessarily be a consequence of damage at this site. In their study, Raine and colleagues (1992) compared patients with schizophrenia with psychiatric and normal controls using magnetic resonance imaging (MRI) and a number of neuropsychological measures, including a Spatial Delayed Response task. In comparison with the control groups, patients with schizophrenia had smaller prefrontal areas on MRI and demonstrated impairment in measures of prefrontal function, specifically the WCST, block design and the DR task. However, no association was found between the structural and functional deficits of this area. The authors speculated that the prefrontal cognitive deficits may have been secondary to structural damage at subcortical sites rather than being related to the structural findings in the frontal area. Such a hypothesis would be in keeping with the nature of the fronto-striato-thalamic circuits described above and would support the suggestion of frontal deafferentation as a result of subcortical damage (Pantelis et al, 1992) which would be in keeping with the functional interrelatedness of this circuitry. However, these results could also be explained by disruption of circuits connecting DLPFC and hippocampus as suggested by Weinberger and colleagues (Weinberger, 1991; Weinberger et al, 1992). In order to examine these possibilities it is necessary to select tasks which discriminate between the circuits connecting prefrontal cortex with hippocampus versus those connecting with the basal ganglia. Though there are few tasks providing such discriminative ability, some possibilities are discussed below.

The studies above have consistently demonstrated impaired performance on DR tasks in schizophrenia, thereby implicating dysfunction of the DLPFC or its connecting pathways. However, the findings related to OFC function have been less consistent. This has partly resulted from the difficulties in identifying tasks which adequately discriminate the functions of the DLPFC and the OFC. As well as DR and DA tasks and object alternation, it has been suggested that olfactory identification tasks may also provide such a useful discrimination (Seidman et al, 1992). The latter ability is of particular interest as it is suggested that olfactory identification ability and olfactory acuity may discriminate between OFC and hippocampal areas respectively. We discuss these in more detail in the following section.

OLFACTORY DEFICITS IN SCHIZOPHRENIA

Olfactory function may be divided conveniently into "olfactory acuity" (the ability to detect an odour) and olfactory "identification" (the ability to name a common odour). Inability to identify common odours has been termed olfactory agnosia (Kopala & Clark, 1990). These two different types of olfactory deficits have been found to be relatively independent and may implicate different neuronal systems. Thus, patients with lesions of the OFC are impaired in their ability to distinguish odour qualities reliably, whereas they demonstrate no impairment in odour detection (Potter & Butters, 1980). This dissociation of acuity and identification was also demonstrated in Korsakoff's amnestic syndrome, in which lesions of the mediodorsal thalamic nuclei have been consistently found (Adams & Victor, 1985). Jones-Gotman & Zatorre (1988) also showed that identification ability was impaired after unilateral excision (either side) of the OFC whilst acuity was unaffected. On the other hand, in the study by Rausch & Serafetinides (1975), temporal lobe excision resulted in threshold increases while odour recognition was intact. Potter & Butters (1980) have suggested that there is a hierarchical organisation of olfactory processing passing from the mediodorsal thalamic nucleus to the temporal (entorrhinal) lobe, and then to the OFC. Projections to the mediodorsal thalamus and the prefrontal cortex have been considered as the major neocortical representations involved in odour discrimination (Kopala & Clark, 1990). Thus, while olfactory acuity deficits have implicated the temporal lobes, impaired olfactory identification has implicated the OFC and thalamus. This pattern of deficits is consistent with the OFC loop identified by Alexander and colleagues (1986).

Recent studies in schizophrenia have also identified consistent deficits in olfactory ability. The results of those studies investigating olfactory identification have found that males with schizophrenia have significant impairment in their ability to identify common odours (Hurwitz et al, 1988; Kopala et al, 1989; Warner et al, 1990; Hurwitz & Clark, 1990; Serby et al, 1990; Seidman et al,

1992; Brewer et al, in press). Seidman and colleagues (1992) also used the WCST as a measure of DLPFC function, whilst they used tests of olfactory identification to examine the orbitofrontal system. They found no association between performance with the WCST and the olfactory deficits and suggested that the deficits in schizophrenia could be subdivided into subtypes of DLPFC, OFC and generalised prefrontal impairment. This would be consistent with the proposed segregated yet parallel nature of the fronto-striato-thalamic circuitry described above.

The relatively few studies investigating olfactory acuity have not all been consistent (Bradley, 1984; Isseroff et al, 1987), however, both males and females appear to have elevated thresholds (Isseroff et al, 1987; Kopala et al, 1989; Serby et al, 1990; Geddes et al, 1991). Also, Geddes and colleagues (1991) examined the relationship with symptomatology and found that the negative symptom patients had significantly higher olfactory thresholds than the positive symptom group.

Though some investigators have used tests of olfactory identification ability as a measure of the integrity of the orbitofrontal system in schizophrenia (Seidman et al, 1992), no studies have investigated the relationship of olfactory deficits to other tasks which have been deemed specific to this brain region. Also, no studies in schizophrenia have examined the relationship of such olfactory deficits to function deemed specific to medial temporal structures. We have recently examined the relationship between olfactory identification deficits and tests of both prefrontal function and tasks considered sensitive to medial temporal regions (Brewer et al, in press). In this study, 27 male patients with DSM-III-R schizophrenia were compared with a group of 19 sex, age and IQ matched controls. The patients were characterised by high scores for negative symptoms as assessed by the PANSS (Positive and Negative Syndromes in Schizophrenia) (Kay et al, 1987). In comparison to controls, the patients with schizophrenia demonstrated impaired performance on prefrontal tasks, including a version of the DR task and the modified WCST (Nelson, 1976). They were also significantly impaired on tests of memory (Wechsler Memory Scale subtests; Wechsler, 1987), considered to reflect function of medial temporal structures. The patients were significantly impaired in their ability to identify smells on the UPSIT (University of Pennsylvania Smell Identification Test [UPSIT]; Doty et al, 1984). In the patients rather than controls, poor performance on the UPSIT was associated with impairment on neuropsychological measures of executive function rather than poor memory ability. While in control subjects UPSIT scores were significantly associated with an index of verbal memory, no such association was found in the patients with schizophrenia. This suggested that in this group, putative function of the prefrontal cortex was not related to measures of left medial temporal lobe function. In support of these findings, the relationship between measures of frontal lobe function and UPSIT score remained significant after partialling out the performance on measures of memory. Thus, though identification ability in normal subjects was related to indices of medial temporal lobe function, the deficits of identification found in schizophrenia was not related to medial temporal lobe function. However, a significant association was found between identification ability and measures of frontal lobe function. This strategy of using tasks deemed specific to particular circuits (*"network-specific"* functions) or to components within the circuits (*"component-specific"* functions) may be useful in examining the relative contribution of separate neuronal networks, such as prefrontal–hippocampal versus prefrontal–striatal systems.

PREFRONTAL CORTICAL SYNDROMES AND SCHIZOPHRENIA SYNDROMES

The above discussion has highlighted the heterogeneity of function of the prefrontal cortex, and its multiple functional–anatomic subdivisions (for discussion: Goldman-Rakic, 1987). As already discussed, Cummings (1993) attempted to clarify this heterogeneity by adopting a syndromal classification. Such an approach is appealing and provides a framework for understanding the heterogeneity of function observed in disorders such as schizophrenia. In a recent, detailed neuropsychological evaluation of five patients with schizophrenia with different symptom profiles, Shallice and his colleagues (1991) used an extensive battery of tests, including a number of tests of executive function. They identified specific deficits in performance on the tests of executive function in addition to a more widespread decline in cognitive functioning. All five patients performed poorly on some but not all tests of executive function and there was no uniformity in the pattern of results suggesting that different frontal impairments might be implicated in these patients. The authors did not attempt to relate this heterogeneity to other characteristics of the patients, particularly their symptoms. The approach of Liddle (1987b; Liddle, chapter 15) may be relevant here. Liddle (1987a) used factor analysis of symptom measures to describe three syndromes in schizophrenia. These he described as the "reality-distortion" syndrome, characterised by positive symptoms such as delusions and hallucinations; the "psychomotor poverty" syndrome, characterised by negative symptoms including flatness of affect, poverty of speech and apathy; and the "disorganisation" syndrome, manifest as thought disorder and incongruous affect. He examined the relationship of each of these syndromes to neuropsychological impairments and identified different patterns of test performance associated with each syndrome (Liddle, 1987b). He has corroborated these findings in subsequent studies (Liddle & Morris, 1991; Liddle et al, 1992). On the basis of the pattern of performance on the various tests and the associations found with each of the three syndromes, Liddle postulated the existence of three distinguishable, but related neuropathological processes in schizophrenia. Specifically, he proposed that the "psychomotor poverty syndrome" results from dysfunction of the left DLPFC; that the "disorganisation syndrome" involves reduced activity of right ventral prefrontal cortex and associated increased activity of anterior cingulate cortex; and that the "reality distortion syndrome" involves abnormality of the medial temporal lobe (Liddle, 1987b; Liddle et al, 1992). It is relevant to the present discussion that the prefrontal areas related to two of these schizophrenic syndromes are the DLPFC, the OFC and the AC. These prefrontal areas are those regions outlined in the above fronto-striato-thalamic circuits, which also form the frontal syndromes described by Cummings (1993).

We propose that behaviours as well as symptoms should be examined in this context, particularly as the frontal lobe syndromes are characterised clinically by disturbances of behaviour and patients with schizophrenia also manifest such disturbances. In a study of 404 patients who met Feighner diagnostic criteria for probable or definite schizophrenia (Feighner et al, 1972), Harvey and colleagues (1996) examined the behavioural syndromes of schizophrenia. This study has been replicated in a further independent sample of patients with schizophrenia (Curson et al, in submission). These epidemiologically based studies assessed behaviour using the Social Behaviour Schedule (SBS; Wykes & Sturt, 1986) developed for use with psychotic patients (Pantelis & Curson, 1994). Factor analysis of the SBS in these studies, revealed four factors: (i) thought disturbance factor (incoherence of speech, odd/inappropriate conversation, poor attention span) (ii) social withdrawal factor (little spontaneous communication, poor self care, slowness, underactivity) (iii) depressed behaviour factor (depression, suicidal ideas or behaviour), and (iv) antisocial behaviour factor (hostility, socially unacceptable behaviour, destructive behaviour). These behavioural factors are correlated with the corresponding syndromes of clinical symptoms identified by Liddle and further support these symptom-based factors. Moreover, they also provide evidence for syndromes not fully identified by a symptom-based approach. For example, antisocial behaviour and depressed behaviour were not identified by Liddle. The potential relevance of these syndromes to frontal syndromes is indicated by the overlap in description between the depressed and social withdrawal behaviour factors of schizophrenia with the "pseudodepressed" syndrome described by Blumer & Benson (1975), on the one hand, and the antisocial behaviour factor of schizophrenia with the "pseudopsychopathic" personality of frontal lobe lesioned patients, on the other. The former frontal syndrome was related to pathology of either the anterior convexity and/or medial aspects of the frontal lobes, while the latter type was associated with lesions of the OFC. Thus, as well as identifying symptom-based syndromes, behavioural descriptions provide further support for a relationship between frontal and schizophrenia syndromes. The implication of the overlap of these clinical descriptions is that specific patterns of association would be expected between the syndromes of schizophrenia and the hypothesised neuropsychological profiles related to each of the frontal syndromes.

WHAT ARE THE IMPLICATIONS OF DISTURBANCE OF THESE FRONTAL–SUBCORTICAL CIRCUITS?

In a previous review Pantelis et al (1992) consider a subcortical disturbance of frontal–subcortical systems as important in explaining the range of disturbances observed in schizophrenia and postulate a subcortical pathogenesis of schizophrenia, specifically implicating the basal ganglia and thalami (see also Collinson et al, chapter 12). Other researchers have suggested that the observed deficit of function of the DLPFC is explained by dysfunction of the circuitry connecting the DLPFC with the hippocampus (Weinberger et al, 1992; Goldman-Rakic, 1994) and that the hippocampus may be the anatomical substrate of schizophrenia (Weinberger, 1991). The evidence reviewed above indicates that it is necessary to examine other prefrontal areas and their connections with subcortical structures in attempting to understand the range of deficits observed in schizophrenia. Of particular importance are the parallel-segregated frontal-striato-thalamic circuits described by Alexander and colleagues (1986) which appear to be affected to various degrees in different patients with schizophrenia (see Robbins, 1990; Pantelis & Nelson, 1994; Pantelis & Brewer, 1995).

In this chapter two approaches have been proposed to examine the nature of the prefrontal dysfunction in schizophrenia. First, an evaluation of "*component-specific*" versus "*network-specific*" functions may provide evidence for a cortical/subcortical distinction on the one hand, versus involvement of segregated frontal–subcortical circuits on the other. One useful method to assess the latter distinction is to relate the frontal syndromes described by recent authors (e.g. Cummings, 1993; Mega & Cummings, 1994) to the syndromes of schizophrenia. It is proposed that each frontal–subcortical network is characterised by differing behavioural profiles and subserves specific cognitive functions. Adopting such an approach in schizophrenia may help to account for the heterogeneity of the disorder. Although schizophrenia researchers to date have focused on symptom-based syndromes (e.g. Liddle, 1987a) the findings from factor analysis of behaviours would suggest that behavioural syndromes provide another dimension to the features apparent in this disorder (Harvey et al, 1996; Curson et al, in submission), which may provide closer parallels to the behavioural descriptions of the frontal syndromes. We recommend that, as well as symptoms and cognitive function, disturbances of behaviour in schizophrenia should also be related to the observed deficits of prefrontal functioning, with particular reference to the circuits implicating the DLPFC, OFC and AC.

The degree of overlap between the syndromes so described may prove useful in delineating the pathophysiological processes underlying various aspects of schizophrenia. Two approaches which would be useful here are first, to examine functions deemed specific to these frontal–subcortical circuits or their components (Pantelis & Brewer, 1995), and second to examine the degree of overlap between the various neurocognitive–symptom–behavioural syndromes. Such approaches would provide evidence for localisation and may help to differentiate subcortical from prefrontal pathophysiology and would delineate which neuronal networks are specifically implicated in subtypes or syndromes of schizophrenia.

ACKNOWLEDGEMENTS

We wish to thank Dr Paul Maruff for his helpful comments during the preparation of this manuscript. This work was supported by the NH&MRC Schizophrenia Research Unit and the Mental Health Research Institute of Victoria.

REFERENCES

Adams, R., Victor, M. (1985) *Principles of Neurology*, McGraw Hill, New York.

Alexander, G.E., DeLong, M., Strick, P.E. (1986) Parallel organization of functionally segregated circuits linking basal ganglia and cortex. *Annual Review of Neurosciences*, **9**, 357–381.

Anderson, S.W., Tranel, D., Damasio, H., Damasio, A.R. (1995). Consistency and specificity of acquired social and emotional defects following ventromedial frontal lobe damage. *Society for Neuroscience Abstracts*, **21**, 476.9.

Andreasen, N., Rezai, K., Alliger, R., Swayze, V., Flaum, M., Kirchner, P., Cohen, G., and O'Leary, D. (1992) Hypofrontality in neuroleptic naive patients and in patients with chronic schizophrenia: Assessment with xenon 133 single photon emission computed tomography and the Tower of London. *Archives of General Psychiatry*, **49**, 943–958.

Andreasen, N.C., Arndt, S., Swayze, V., Cizadlo, T., Flaum, M., O'Leary, D., Ehrhardt, J.C., Yuh, W.T.C. (1994). Thalamic abnormalities in schizophrenia visualized through magnetic resonance image averaging. *Science*, **266**, 294–298.

Baddeley, A. (1986) *Working Memory*, Clarendon Press, Oxford.

Bench, C.J., Frith, C.D., Grabsky, P.M., Friston, K.J., Paulesu, E., Frackowiak, R.S.J., Dolan, R.J. (1993) Investigations of the functional anatomy of attention using the Stroop test. *Neuropsychologia*, **31**, 907–922.

Benes, F.M., Sorensen, I., Vincent, S.L., Bird, E.D., Sathi, M. (1992). Increased density of glutamate-immunoreactive vertical processes in superficial laminae in cingulate cortex of schizophrenic brain. *Cerebral Cortex*, **2**, 503–512.

Berman, K.F., Zec, R.F., Weinberger, D.R. (1986) Physiologic dysfunction of dorsolateral prefrontal cortex in schizophrenia. II. Role of neuroleptic treatment, attention, and mental effort. *Archives of General Psychiatry*, **43**, 126–135.

Berman, K.F., Illowsky, B.P., Weinberger, D.R. (1988) Physiologic dysfunction of dorsolateral prefrontal cortex in schizophrenia. IV. Further evidence for regional and behavioural specificity. *Archives of General Psychiatry*, **45**, 616–622.

Blumer, D., Benson, D.F. (1975) Personality changes with frontal and temporal lobe lesions. In: *Psychiatric Aspects of Neurologic Disease* (Eds D.F. Benson, D. Blume), Grune & Stratton, New York.

Bogerts, B., Meertz, E., Schonfeldt-Bausch, R. (1985) Basal ganglia and limbic system pathology in schizophrenia. A morphometric study of brain volume and shrinkage. *Archives of General Psychiatry*, **42**, 784–791.

Bradley, E.A. (1984) Olfactory acuity to a pheromonal substance and psychotic illness. *Biological Psychiatry*, **19**, 899–905.

Brewer, W.J., Edwards, J., Anderson, V., Robinson, T., Pantelis, C. (in press) Neuropsychological, olfactory, and hygiene deficits in men with negative symptom schizophrenia. *Biological Psychiatry*.

Brown, R.G., Marsden, C.D. (1988) "Subcortical dementia": The neuropsychological evidence. *Neuroscience*, **25**, 363–387.

Buchsbaum, M.S. (1990) The frontal lobes, basal ganglia and temporal lobes as sites for schizophrenia. *Schizophrenia Bulletin*, **16**, 277–389.

Buchsbaum, M.S., Haier, R.J., Potkin, S.G., Nuechterlein, K., Bracha, H.S., Katz, M., Lohr, J., Wu, J., Lottenberg, S., Jerabek, P.A., et al (1992). Frontostriatal disorder of cerebral metabolism in never-medicated schizophrenics. *Archives of General Psychiatry*, **49**, 935–942.

Burgess, P.W., Shallice, T. (1993) Fractionation of the frontal lobe syndrome. Paper presented at the meeting "Neuropsychologie du lobe frontal" held by the Societe de Neuropsychologie de Langue Francaise, Angers.

Corcoran, R., Upton, D. (1993) A role for the hippocampus in card sorting? *Cortex*, **29**, 293–304.

Crow, T.J. (1980) Molecular pathology of schizophrenia: More than one disease process? *British Medical Journal*, **280**, 66–68.

Cummings, J.L. (1993) Frontal–subcortical circuits and human behaviour. *Archives of Neurology*, **50**, 873–880.

Cunnington, R., Iansek, R., Bradshaw, J.L., Phillips, J.G. (in press) Movement-related potentials in Parkinson's disease: Presence and predictability of temporal and spatial cues. *Brain*.

Curson, D.A., Duke, P.J., Harvey, C.A., Pantelis, C., Barnes, T.R.E. (MS in submission) Four behavioural syndromes of schizophrenia: A replication in a second inner London epidemiological sample.

Damasio, A.R., Van Hoesen, G.W. (1983) Focal lesions of the limbic frontal lobe. In: *Neuropsychology of Human Emotion* (Eds K.M. Heilman, P. Satz), pp. 85–110, Guilford Press, New York.

David, A.S. (1992) Frontal Lobology: Psychiatry's new pseudoscience. *British Journal of Psychiatry*, **61**, 244–248.

DeLong, M.R., Alexander, G.E., Miller, W.C., Crutcher, M.D. (1990) Anatomical and functional aspects of basal ganglia–thalamocortical circuits. In: *Function and Dysfunction in the Basal Ganglia* (Eds A.J. Franks, J.W. Ironside, H.S. Mindham, R.J. Smith, E.G.S. Spokes, W. Winlow), pp. 3–32, Manchester University Press, Manchester.

Devinsky, O., Luciano, D. (1993) The contributions of the cingulate cortex to human behaviour. In: *Neurobiology of Cingulate Cortex and Limbic Thalamus* (Eds B.A. Vogt, M. Gabriel), pp. 528–556, Birkhäuser, Boston.

Devinsky, O., Morrell, M.J., Vogt, B.A. (1995) Contributions of the anterior cingulate cortex to behaviour. *Brain*, **118**, 279–306.

Dias, R., Robbins, T.W., Roberts, A.C. (1995). Affective and attentional shifting: A functional dissociation between the dorsolateral and orbital prefrontal cortices of the monkey. *Society for Neuroscience Abstracts*, **21**, 566.22.

Dias, R., Robbins, T.W., Roberts, A.C. (1996) Dissociation in prefrontal cortex of affective and attentional shifts. *Nature*, **380**, 69–72.

Doty, R., Shaman, P., Dann, W. (1984) Development of the University of Pennsylvania Smell Test: Standardised micro-encapsulated test of olfactory function. *Physiological Behavior*, **32**, 489–502.

Duffy, J.D., Campbell, J.J. (1994) The regional prefrontal syndromes: A theoretical and clinical overview. *Journal of Neuropsychiatry and Clinical Neurosciences*, **6**, 379–387.

Elliott, R., McKenna, P.J., Robbins, T.W., Sahakian, B. (1995) Neuropsychological evidence for frontostriatal dysfunction in schizophrenia. *Psychological Medicine*, **25**, 619–630.

Eslinger, P.J., Grattan, L.M. (1993) Frontal lobe and fronto-striatal substrates for different forms of human cognitive flexibility. *Neuropsychologia*, **31**, 17–28.

Feighner, J.P., Rubins, E., Guze, S., et al (1972) Diagnostic criteria for use in psychiatric research. *Archives of General Psychiatry*, **26**, 57–62.

Fleming, K., Goldberg, T.E., Gold, J.M. (1994) Applying working memory constructs to schizophrenic cognitive impairment. In: *The Neuropsychology of Schizophrenia* (Eds A.S. David, J.C. Cutting), pp. 197–214, Erlbaum, Hove, UK.

Freedman, M. (1990) Object alternation and orbitofrontal system dysfunction in Alzheimer's and Parkinson's disease. *Brain and Cognition*, **14**, 134–143.

Freedman, M., Oscar-Berman, M. (1986) Bilateral frontal lobe disease and selective delayed-response deficits in humans. *Behavioral Neurosciences*, **100**, 337–342.

Frith, C.D. (1987) The positive and negative symptoms of schizophrenia reflect impairments in the perception and initiation of action. *Psychological Medicine*, **7**, 631–638.

Frith, C.D. (1992) *The Cognitive Neuropsychology of Schizophrenia*, Erlbaum, Hove, UK.

Frith, C.D., Cahill, C., Ridley, R.M., Baker, H.F. (1992) Memory for what it is and memory for what it means: A single case of Korsakoff's amnesia. *Cortex*, **28**, 53–67.

Fuster, J.M. (1989) *The Prefrontal Cortex*, Raven Press, New York.

Fuster, J.M., Alexander, G.E. (1971) Neuron activity related to short-term memory. *Science Wash.*, **173**, 652–654.

Geddes, J., Huws, R., Pratt, P. (1991) Olfactory acuity in the positive and negative symptoms of schizophrenia. *Biological Psychiatry*, **29**, 774–778.

George, M.S., Ketter, T.A., Parekh, P.I., Rosinsky, N., Ring, H., Casey, B.J., Trimble, M.R., Horwitz, B., Herscovitch, P., Post, R.M. (1994) Regional brain activity when selecting a response despite interference: An H_2O^{15} PET study of the Stroop and emotional Stroop. *Human Brain Mapping*, **9**, 194–209.

Gold J.M., Harvey P.D. (1993) Cognitive deficits in schizophrenia. *Psychiatric Clinics of North America*, **16**, 295–312.

Gold, J., Berman, K.F., Randolph, C., Goldberg, T.E., Weinberger, D.R. (1991) PET validation and clinical application of a novel prefrontal task. *Journal of Clinical and Experimental Neuropsychology*, **13**, 81.

Goldberg, G., Bloom, K.K. (1990) The alien hand sign: Localisation, lateralisation and recovery. *American Journal of Physiological Medical Rehabilitation*, **69**, 228–238.

Goldberg, T.E., Weinberger, D.R., Berman, K.F., Pliskin, N.H., Podd, M.H. (1987) Further evidence for dementia of the prefrontal type in schizophrenia? A controlled study of teaching the Wisconsin Card Sorting Test. *Archives of General Psychiatry*, **44**(11), 1008–1014.

Goldman-Rakic, P.S. (1987). Circuitry of primate prefrontal cortex and regulation of behaviour by representational memory. In: *Handbook of Physiology: The Nervous System*, Vol. 5 (Ed. F. Plum), pp. 373–417, American Physiological Society, Bethesda, USA.

Goldman-Rakic, P.S. (1988) Changing concepts of cortical connectivity: Parallel distributed cortical networks. In: *Neurobiology of Neocortex* (Eds P. Rakic, W. Singer), pp. 177–202, Wiley, New York.

Goldman-Rakic, P.S. (1994) Working memory dysfunction in schizophrenia. *Journal of Neuropsychiatry and Clinical Neurosciences*, **6**, 348–357.

Goldman-Rakic, P.S., Friedman, H.R. (1991) The circuitry of working memory revealed by anatomy and metabolic imaging. In: *Frontal Lobe Function and Dysfunction* (Eds H.S. Levin, H.M. Eisenberg, A.L. Benton), pp. 72–91, Oxford University Press, Oxford.

Goldstein, G. (1986) The neuropsychology of schizophrenia. In: *Neuropsychological Assessment of Neuropsychiatric Disorders* (Eds I. Grant, K. Adams), pp. 147–171, Oxford University Press, Oxford.

Groenewegen, H.J., Berendse, H.W., Meredith, G.E., Haber, S.N., Voorn, P., Wolters, J.G., Lohman, A.H.M. (1991) Functional anatomy of the ventral, limbic system-innervated striatum. In: *The Mesolimbic Dopamine System: From Motivation to Action* (Eds P. Willner, J. Scheel-Kruger), pp. 19–59, Wiley, Chichester.

Hanes, K.R., Andrewes, D.G., Pantelis, C. (1995) Cognitive flexibility and complex integration in Parkinson's disease, Huntington's disease and schizophrenia. *Journal of the International Neuropsychological Society*, **1**, 545–553.

Hanes, K.R., Andrewes, D.G., Pantelis, C., Chiu, E. (1996) Subcortical dysfunction in schizophrenia: A comparison with Parkinson's and Huntington's disease. *Schizophrenia Research*, **19**, 121–128.

Harvey, C.A., Curson, D.A., Pantelis, C., Taylor, J., Barnes, T.R.E. (1996) Four behavioural syndromes of schizophrenia. *British Journal of Psychiatry*, **168**, 562–570.

Hemsley, D.R. (1982) Cognitive impairment in schizophrenia. In: *The Pathology and Psychology of Cognition* (Ed. A. Burton), pp. 169–203, Methuen, London.

Hikosaka, O., Sakamoto, M., Usui, S. (1989) Functional properties of monkey caudate neurones. I. Activities related to saccadic eye movements. *Journal of Neurophysiology*, **61**, 780–798.

Hurwitz, T.A., Clark, C. (1990) Response to editor on Warner et al. *Biological Psychiatry*, **27**, 458.

Hurwitz, T., Kopala, L., Clark, C., Jones, B. (1988) Olfactory deficits in schizophrenia. *Biological Psychiatry*, **23**, 123–128.

Isseroff, R.G., Stoler, M., Ophir, D., Lancet, D., Sirota, P. (1987) Olfactory sensitivity to androstenone in schizophrenic patients. *Biological Psychiatry*, **22**, 922–925.

Jones-Gotman, M., Zatorre, R.J. (1988) Olfactory identification deficits in patients with focal cerebral excision. *Neuropsychologia*, **26**, 387–400.

Joyce, E.M., Collinson, S.L., Crichton, P. (1996) Verbal fluency in schizophrenia: Relationship with executive function, semantic memory and clinical alogia. *Psychological Medicine*, **26**, 39–49.

Kay, S.R., Fiszbein, A., Opler, L.A. (1987) The positive and negative syndrome scale (PANSS) for schizophrenia. *Schizophrenia Bulletin*, **13**, 261–276.

Kolb, B., Whishaw, I.Q. (1983) Performance of schizophrenic patients on tests sensitive to left or right frontal, temporal or parietal function in neurological patients. *Journal of Nervous and Mental Disorders*, **171**, 435–443.

Kopala, L., Clark, C. (1990) Implications of olfactory agnosia for understanding sex differences in schizophrenia. *Schizophrenia Bulletin*, **16**, 255–261.

Kopala, L., Clark, C., Hurwitz, T.A. (1989) Sex differences in olfactory function in schizophrenia. *American Journal of Psychiatry*, **146**, 1320–1322.

Laiacona, M., De Santis, A., Barbarotto, R., Basso, A., Spagnoli, D., Capitani, E. (1989) Neuropsychological follow-up of patients operated for aneurysms of anterior communicating artery. *Cortex*, **25**, 261–273.

Lewisohn, P.M., Zieler, J.L., Libet, J.L., Eyeberg, S., Nielson, G. (1972) Short term memory: A comparison between frontal and non-frontal right and left hemisphere brain damaged patients. *Journal of Comparative Physiological Psychology*, **81**, 248–255.

Lhermitte, F. (1986) Human autonomy and the frontal lobes. Part II: Patient behavior in complex and social situations: The "environmental dependency syndrome". *Annals of Neurology*, **19**, 335–343.

Lhermitte, F., Pillon, B., Serdaru, M. (1986) Human autonomy and the frontal lobes. Part I: Imitation and utilization behavior: A neuropsychological study of 75 patients. *Annals of Neurology*, **19**, 326–334.

Liddle, P.F. (1987a) The symptoms of chronic schizophrenia: A re-examination of the positive–negative dichotomy. *British Journal of Psychiatry*, **151**, 145–151.

Liddle, P.F. (1987b) Schizophrenic syndromes, cognitive performance and neurological dysfunction. *Psychological Medicine*, **17**, 49–57.

Liddle, P.F., Morris, D.L. (1991) Schizophrenic syndromes and frontal lobe performance. *British Journal of Psychiatry*, **158**, 340–345.

Liddle, P.F., Friston, K.J., Frith, C.D., Hirsch, S.R., Jones, T., Frackowiak, R.S.J. (1992) Patterns of cerebral blood flow in schizophrenia. *British Journal of Psychiatry*, **160**, 179–186.

Litvan I., Mohr, E., Williams, Gomez, C., Chase, T.N. (1991) Differential memory and executive functions in demented patients with Parkinson's disease and Alzheimer's disease. *Journal of Neurology, Neurosurgery and Psychiatry*, **54**, 25–29.

Malloy, P., Bihrle, A., Duffy, J., Cimino, C. (1993) The orbitomedial frontal syndrome. *Archives of Clinical Neuropsychology*, **8**, 185–201.

Maruff, P., Currie, J., Hay, D., Malone, V. (1995) Asymmetry in the covert orienting of visual attention in schizophrenia. *Neuropsychologia*, **33**, 1205–1223.

Maruff, P., Pantelis, C. Danckert, J., Smith, D., Currie, J. (in press) Deficits in the endogenous redirection of covert visual attention in chronic schizophrenia. *Neuropsychologia*.

Mega, M.S., Cummings, J.L. (1994) Frontal–subcortical circuits and neuropsychiatric disorders. *Journal of Neuropsychiatry and Clinical Neurosciences*, **6**, 358–370.

Mesulam, M.M. (1985) *Principles of Behavioral Neurology*, Davis, Philadelphia.

Mesulam, M.M. (1990) Large-scale neurocognitive networks and distributed processing for attention, language, and memory. *Annals of Neurology*, **28**, 597–613.

Mishkin, M. (1964) Perseveration of central sets after frontal lesions in monkeys. In: *The Frontal Granular Cortex and Behaviour* (Eds J.M. Warren, K. Akert), pp. 219–241, McGraw-Hill, New York.

Mishkin, M., Vest, B., Waxler, M., Rosvold, H.E. (1969) A re-examination of the effects of frontal lesions on object alternation. *Neuropsychologia*, **7**, 357–363.

Morice, R. (1990) Cognitive inflexibility and pre-frontal dysfunction in schizophrenia and mania. *British Journal of Psychiatry*, **157**, 50–54.

Morris, R.G., Rushe, T., Woodruffe, P.W.R., Murray, R.M. (1995) Problem solving in schizophrenia: A specific deficit in planning ability. *Schizophrenia Research*, **14**, 235–246.

Nelson, H.E. (1976) A modified card sorting test sensitive to frontal lobe defects. *Cortex*, **12**, 313–324.

Oscar-Berman, M. (1991) Clinical and experimental approaches to varieties of memory. *International Journal of Neurosciences*, **58**, 135–150.

Oscar-Berman, M., Zola-Morgan, S.M., Oberg, R.G.E., Bonner, R.T. (1982) Comparative neuropsychology and Korsakoff's syndrome. III. Delayed response, delayed alternation and DRL performance. *Neuropsychologia*, **20**, 187–202.

Oscar-Berman, M., McNamara, P., Freedman, M. (1991) Delayed-response tasks: Parallels between experimental ablation studies and findings in patients with frontal lesions. In: *Frontal Lobe Function and Dysfunction* (Eds H.S. Levin, H.M. Eisenberg, A.L. Benton), pp. 230–255, Oxford University Press, Oxford.

Owen, A.M., Downes, J.J., Sahakian, B.J., Polkey, C.E., Robbins, T.W. (1990) Planning and spatial working memory following frontal lobe lesions in man. *Neuropsychologia*, **28**, 1021–1034.

Owen, A.M., Roberts, A.C., Polkey, C.E., Sahakian, B.J., Robbins, T.W. (1991) Extra-dimensional versus intra-dimensional set shifting performance following frontal lobe excisions, temporal lobe excisions or amygdalo-hippocampectomy in man. *Neuropsychologia*, **29**, 993–1006.

Owen, A.M., James, M., Leigh, P.N., Summers, B.A., Marsden, C.D., Quinn, N.P., Lange, K.W., Robbins, T.W. (1992) Fronto-striatal cognitive deficits at different stages of Parkinson's disease. *Brain*, **115**, 1727–1751.

Owen, A.M., Roberts, A.C., Hodges, J.R., Summers, B.A., Polkey, C.E., Robbins, T.W. (1993) Contrasting mechanisms of impaired attentional set-shifting with frontal lobe damage or Parkinson's disease. *Brain*, **116**, 1159–1175.

Pakkenberg, B., Gundersen, H.J.G. (1989). New stereological method for obtaining unbiased and efficient estimates of total nerve cell number in human brain areas. Exemplified by the mediodorsal thalamic nucleus in schizophrenics. *Apmis*, **97**, 677–681.

Pantelis, C., Barber, F.Z., Barnes, T.R.E., Nelson, H.E., Owen, A.M., Robbins, T.W. (1996a) Intra- and extra-dimensional shift in patients with chronic schizophrenia. (MS in submission).

Pantelis, C., Barnes, T.R.E., Nelson, H.E. (1992) Is the concept of frontal–subcortical dementia relevant to schizophrenia? *British Journal of Psychiatry*, **160**, 442–460.

Pantelis, C., Barnes, T.R.E., Nelson, H.E., Robbins, T.W. (1993) The nature of dementia in schizophrenia. *Schizophrenia Research*, **9**, 184.

Pantelis, C., Barnes, T.R.E., Nelson, H.E., Tanner, S., Weatherley, L., Owen, A.M., Robbins, T.W. (1996b) Frontal–striatal cognitive deficits in patients with chronic schizophrenia (MS in submission).

Pantelis, C., Brewer, W.J. (1995) Neuropsychological and olfactory dysfunction in schizophrenia: Relationship of frontal syndromes to syndromes of schizophrenia. *Schizophrenia Research*, **17**, 35–45.

Pantelis, C., Curson, D. (1994) The assessment of social behaviour. In: *The Assessment of Psychoses. A Practical Handbook* (Eds T.R.E. Barnes, H.E. Nelson), pp. 135–154, Chapman & Hall, London.

Pantelis, C., Nelson, H.E. (1994) Cognitive functioning and symptomatology in schizophrenia. In: *The Neuropsychology of Schizophrenia* (Eds A. David, J. Cutting), pp. 215–230, Erlbaum, Hove, UK.

Pantelis, C., Egan, G., Pipingas, A., Maruff, P., O'Keefe, G., Velakoulis, D., Collinson, S., Chua, P. (1996c) Practice dependent alterations in activation of the anterior cingulate cortex during the Stroop task: A positron emission tomography study (MS in submission).

Pardo, J.V., Pardo, P.J., Janer, K.W., Raichle, M.E. (1990) The anterior cingulate cortex mediates processing selection in the Stroop attentional conflict paradigm. *Proceedings of the National Academy of Sciences USA*, **87**, 256–259.

Park, S., Holzman, P.S. (1992) Schizophrenics show spatial working memory deficits. *Archives of General Psychiatry*, **49**, 975–982.

Partiot, A., Jouvent, R., Dubois, B., Verin, M. et al (1992) Cortical dysfunction and schizophrenic deficit: Preliminary findings with the delayed reaction paradigm. *European Psychiatry*, **7**(4), 171–175.

Passingham, R. (1993) *The Frontal Lobes and Voluntary Action*, Oxford University Press, Oxford.

Potter, H., Butters, N. (1980) An assessment of olfactory deficits in patients with damage to prefrontal cortex. *Neuropsychologia*, **18**, 621–628.

Pribram, K.H., Mishkin, M. (1956) Analysis of the effects of frontal lesions in monkey. III. Object alternation. *Journal of Comparative Physiological Psychology*, **49**, 41–45.

Rafal, R.D., Henik, A. (1994) The neurology of inhibition. Integrating controlled and automatic processes. In: *Inhibitory Processes in Attention, Memory and Language* (Eds D. Dagenbach, T. Carr), pp. 1–50, Academic Press, San Diego.

Raine, A., Lencz, T., Reynolds, G.P., Harrison, G., Sheard, C., Medley, I., Reynolds, L.M., Cooper, J.E. (1992) An evaluation of structural and functional prefrontal deficits in schizophrenia: MRI and neuropsychological measures. *Psychiatry Research*, **45**, 123–137.

Rausch, R., Serafetinides, E.A. (1975) Specific alterations of olfactory function in humans with temporal lobe lesions. *Nature*, **255**, 557–558.

Robbins, T.W. (1990) The case for fronto-striatal dysfunction in schizophrenia. *Schizophrenia Bulletin*, **16**, 391–402.

Robbins, T.W. (1991) Cognitive deficits in schizophrenia and Parkinson's disease: Neural basis and the role of dopamine. In: *The Mesolimbic Dopamine System: From Motivation to Action* (Eds P. Willner, J. Scheel-Kruger), pp. 497–528, Wiley, Chichester.

Seidman, L.J., Talbot, N.L., Kalinowski, A.G., McCarley, R.W., Faraone, S.V., Kremen, W.S., Pepple, J.R., Tsuang, M.T. (1992) Neuropsychological probes of fronto-limbic system dysfunction in schizophrenia: Olfactory identification and Wisconsin Card Sorting performance. *Schizophrenia Research*, **6**, 55–65.

Serby, M., Larson, P., Kalkstein, D. (1990) Olfactory senses in psychoses. *Biological Psychiatry*, **28**, 829–830.

Shallice, T. (1988) *From Neuropsychology to Mental Structure*, Cambridge University Press, Cambridge.

Shallice, T., Burgess, P.W. (1991a) Higher-order cognitive impairments and frontal lobe lesions. In: *Frontal Lobe Function and Dysfunction* (Eds H.S. Levin, H.M. Eisenberg, A.L. Benton), pp. 125–138, Oxford University Press, Oxford.

Shallice, T., Burgess, P.W. (1991b) Deficits in strategy application following frontal lobe damage in man. *Brain*, **114**, 727–741.

Shallice, T., Burgess, P.W., Frith, C.D. (1991) Can the neuropsychology case-study approach be applied to schizophrenia? *Psychological Medicine*, **21**, 661–673.

Suddath, R.L., Casanova, M.F., Goldberg, T.E., Daniel, D.G., Kelsoe, J.R., Jr., Weinberger, D.R. (1989) Temporal lobe pathology in schizophrenia: A quantitative magnetic resonance imaging study. *American Journal of Psychiatry*, **146**, 464–472.

Suddath, R.L., Christison, G.W., Torrey, E.F., Casanova, M.F., Weinberger, D.R. (1990) Anatomical abnormalities in the brains of monozygotic twins discordant for schizophrenia. *New England Journal of Medicine*, **322**, 789–794.

Tranel, D., Damasio, H., Damasio, A.R., Brandt, J.P. (1995) Separate concepts are retrieved from separate neural systems: Neuroanatomical and neuropsychological double dissociations. *Society for Neuroscience Abstracts*, **21**, 588.4.

Velakoulis, D., Pantelis, C. (1996) What have we learned from functional imaging studies in schizophrenia? The role of frontal, striatal and temporal areas. *Australian and New Zealand Journal of Psychiatry*, **30**, 195–209.

Velakoulis, D., Pantelis, C., Cook, M.C., Murrie, V., Desmond, P.M., Tress, B.M., Brewer, W.J., Singh, B., Copolov, D. (1996) Bilateral hippocampal volume reduction in chronic schizophrenia on MRI volumetric analysis. *Schizophrenia Research*, **18**, 186.

Vogt, B.A., Gabriel, M. (1993) *Neurobiology of Cingulate Cortex and Limbic Thalamus*, Birkhäuser, Boston.

Vogt, B.A., Finch, D.M., Olson, C.R. (1992) Functional heterogeneity in cingulate cortex: The anterior executive and posterior evaluative regions. *Cerebral Cortex*, **2**, 435–443.

Warner, N.R., Peabody, C.A., Csernansky, J.C. (1990) Olfactory functioning in schizophrenia and depression. *Biological Psychiatry*, **27**, 457–467.

Watanabe, T., Niki, H. (1985) Hippocampal unit activity and delayed response in the monkey. *Brain Research*, **325**, 241–254.

Wechsler, D. (1987) *Wechsler Memory Scale – Revised*, Psychological Corporation, New York.

Weinberger, D.R. (1991) Anteromedial temporal–prefrontal connectivity: A functional neuroanatomical system implicated in schizophrenia. In: *Psychopathology and the Brain* (Eds B.J. Carroll, J.E. Barrett), pp. 25–43, Raven Press, New York.

Weinberger, D.R., Berman, K.F., Zec, R.F. (1986) Physiologic dysfunction of dorsolateral prefrontal cortex in schizophrenia. I. Regional cerebral blood flow evidence. *Archives of General Psychiatry*, **43**, 114–124.

Weinberger, D.R., Berman, K.F., Illowsky, B.P. (1988) Physiologic dysfunction of dorsolateral prefrontal cortex in schizophrenia. III. A new cohort and evidence for a monoaminergic mechanism. *Archives of General Psychiatry*, **45**, 609–615.

Weinberger, D.R., Berman, K.F., Suddath, R., Torrey, E.F. (1992) Evidence of dysfunction of a prefrontal–limbic network in schizophrenia: A magnetic resonance imaging and regional cerebral blood flow study of discordant monozygotic twins. *American Journal of Psychiatry*, **149**, 890–897.

Wykes, T., Sturt, E. (1986) The measurement of social behaviour in psychiatric patients: An assessment of the reliability and validity of the SBS schedule. *British Journal of Psychiatry*, **148**, 1–11.

17

The Neuropsychology and Neurophenomenology of Auditory Hallucinations

TONY NAYANI and ANTHONY DAVID

Anything one remembers is a repetition, but existing as a human being, that is being, listening and hearing is never repetition.

Gertrude Stein

INTRODUCTION

Neuropsychology in relation to psychopathology is in its infancy and the use of the term tends to obscure several important philosophical problems which demand acknowledgement if not resolution. All approaches to the problem of hallucinations must attempt to explain two fundamental features of this phenomenon: first, the unbidden, intrusive character of the hallucination; second, its non-self origin. Common sense draws us to conclude that these features may be two sides of the same coin, that is to say, it is because the hallucination *intrudes* into consciousness, that it is labelled as non-self or, because it feels non-self, that it must also be unbidden. This view may be mistaken and perhaps we should keep separate our consideration of these features.

Introspection suggests that the flow of consciousness contains much material that seems to occur without active intention or, perhaps more accurately, without the activity of intending. The sudden exclamation of the solution to a problem long since neglected or the revival of a memory without any apparent cause, are examples of these everyday happenings. Normal people are not persuaded that the occurrence of such a mental event, intrusive and unbidden though it may be, belongs to another person. It appears that all the experiences that an individual has of their mental phenomena carry an ineluctable sense of belonging to them. This labelling of experience is more tenuous when the connection between the

Schizophrenia: A Neuropsychological Perspective. Edited by C. Pantelis, H.E. Nelson and T.R.E. Barnes

mental event and the individual's narrative biography is remote: if, to one's irritation, one hears, with the mind's ear, the opening bars to Beethoven's fifth symphony again and again, in what sense is this experience owned? There was no active choosing to hear the tune, there seems to be little control over it and, although one accepts that this music is remembered, no explicit context for this memory can be found. Comparing this irritating form of musical memory with the quite distinct memory of hearing those same opening bars at a concert last summer, an important difference becomes apparent when the music is cloaked, in the latter case, in rich biographical detail (see Johnson et al, 1988a, 1988b, for related arguments). The absence of this narrative web may help in the understanding of how it is that some memories seem to occur in a particular, repetitive, immutable way. We will return to the subject of memory, context and the authorship of experience in a later section.

One might argue that the attribution of "self" arises *sui generis* from the function of memory although, in some cases, the context of the memory appears to be lost. How then should we regard those mental activities, acts of imagination, fantasy and creation, from which can arise, suddenly and without intention, mental events that seem to have no connection with memory? How do products of the imagination come to be accepted as belonging to self? In some circumstances the very effort that is expended in the process of imagining may inform this judgement, but what of the basis for this understanding in circumstances when the imagination yields mental objects unbidden? Of course, the experience of dreaming may demonstrate that in certain conditions precisely this realisation is surrendered (see Weiler et al, 1990 for an examination of this issue). We will again touch upon the subject of fantasy and imagination and their relation to the hallucination at a later point.

Returning now to the relation of the qualities of intrusiveness and alien attribution, consider the problem posed by Parkinson's disease: the experience of the patient who suffers the rigidity and tremor caused by this organic disturbance is expressed as impediment that happens to him. Compare this complaint with the psychotic patient who describes the inability to move his arm because the Martians are controlling his body (a passivity experience) and yet can recognise that the rigidity caused by his neuroleptic medication is a completely distinct experience. Tourette's syndrome (see Friedhoff & Chase, 1982) provides a model of a disease where, unlike rigidity and tremor, *mental events* (unverbalised coprolalia) occur which bear a striking resemblance to the reports of insulting pseudo-hallucinations in psychotic patients. A remarkable difference between the psychotic and the Tourette patient is that the experience of the coprolalia, whilst unbidden and intrusive, is not felt to originate from another. It is important to realise that there is no intuitive difficulty in accepting a physical explanation for certain types of intrusive mental events, such as the expletives of coprolalia, as long as a "self" label comes attached to them, just as it is possible to accept that the tremor of the Parkinsonian patient is caused by an imbalance of neurotransmitters in the brain, because the tremor feels to the patient that it *belongs* to him.

The curious double orientation of the psychotic who might vigorously protest the reality of his hallucination and yet behave as though it is not quite as real as the experience of lunch queues and housing benefits, is a source of interest to the clinician who attempts to capture this paradox by describing the degree of insight that a patient possesses (David, 1990). Similarly, the judgement of the reality of the hallucination is not straightforward. Aggernaes (1972) described a series of criteria that should be satisfied to support this verdict, including judgements of sensation, independence of experience, and so on. Applying these measures to a group of hallucinating patients, Aggernaes found that most hallucinations were found to satisfy the majority of these criteria with the notable exception of "publicness" which only 15 of the 45 hallucinations fulfilled. Publicness refers to the feature of an experience which implies that any other normal person could share the sensation that is being described if they possess the appropriate sensory faculty. The implications seem clear: if the hallucinating patient can be said to have radically mistaken the authorship of his voices, describing as belonging to others what clearly arises from self, it remains true that the same patient may readily concede that the *voices are his*, that they belong in some sense to him, and that they are private. In short, if the hallucinator misattributes the source of his experiences, he does not disown them.

The question now is whether it can be said that the hallucinator *owns* his voices in the same way that the patient with Parkinson's disease *owns* his tremor, or the sufferer of Tourette's syndrome might be said to *own* his coprolalia? We hear the explicit repudiation of the psychotic that his hallucinations arise from him. The hallucinator's sense of possession of his voices must have a different source, as it seems to represent a different form of ownership. This source may lie in the deep and subtle *intimacy* that is described in the relationship that exists between the hallucinator and his voice. This sense of intimacy has two obvious components: it springs from the patient's knowledge about his hallucinations, for example, its characteristic prosodic form. However, it also seems to originate from the sense that the *voice knows the patient*, his thoughts, plans and secrets. A recently completed survey of the verbatim reports of hallucinations (Nayani and David, 1996) testifies to this sense of intimacy. Voices were often found to comment on the patient's actions, thoughts and intentions, and many patients spontaneously complained of a sense of having lost all sense of privacy to the importunate voices.

Having considered intrusiveness, unintendedness, alien attribution and intimacy as features of hallucinations which merit attention we now turn to *intention* (see Frith, 1987). If a patient initiates a conversation with his/her voice and can summon it, then the patient might be said to be influencing the occurrence of the hallucination. Can this apparent influence be equated with intention? If one accepts this equivalence, it would lead to the curious position of accepting that an individual might be capable of giving intention to something that is otherwise apprehended as alien. However, if we refute this argument, then we must accept that between the poles of mental events that seem unbidden and those that appear to be intended, there might lay a grey territory of mental phenomena that are neither one nor the other. In the context of a dialogue with an hallucinated voice, features of unintendedness and intrusiveness become less convincing, whilst alien attribution and intimacy becomes even more so. The explanation of non-self attribution seems to exhaust the potential that purely neurological accounts of mental events can provide. Some form of psychological expression is required to explain this phenomenon.

In this review, we attempt to address the types of problems that hallucinations pose, in form and content (see Sims, 1988), to which we have alluded. What makes these events happen and why are they apprehended as alien? Why do patients describe these hallucinations in intimate terms? How is it that some patients seem able to conduct dialogues with their voices? Why do many hallucinations have a repetitive, stereotypical form? Many of the accounts that follow may provide plausible explanations of the generation of mental fragments but they may fail to convince that the essential nature of the hallucination, the curious admixture of the intimate and the alien and the unbidden and the controlled, has been adequately addressed.

In mapping the boundaries of what might be called "neurophenomenology", this chapter borrows from "Theory Dualism" (Churchland, 1988) the idea that mental states and processes are states in the nervous system, but that psychology offers an autonomous parallel level of explanation. In addition, it is assumed that it is best to understand abnormal mental events as arising from the distortion and deviation of normal psychological processes; this is a position long fostered by psychologists but challenges the categorical, disease orientated models of psychiatrists. The deliberate focus of this article on a symptom as opposed to a syndrome echoes the recent proposition (Costello, 1992; David, 1993) that such an approach is more likely to yield profitable understanding.

This chapter is divided into five main sections. In the first, comments about phenomenology and the occurrence of auditory hallucinations in normal people are offered. The second section concentrates on neurological research, whereas section three entails a discussion of the possible significance of speech mechanisms in the genesis of this phenomenon. Section four brings the focus of psychological models and, finally, in section five a theoretical model linking memory and affect is proposed.

PHENOMENOLOGY

Auditory hallucinations, of which strictly speaking verbal hallucinations are a form, are important and common features of mental illness; their occurrence is often thought to signify the presence of psychotic or schizophrenic illness (Goodwin, 1971). Slade & Bentall (1988) using data accumulated from 16 reports, yielding 2924 cases of schizophrenia, found a prevalence of 60.2%. In comparison, in an international survey, Wing et al (1974) established that 74% of patients with schizophrenia suffered this symptom.

Classical psychiatric teaching makes much of the discrimination of form and content in assessing verbal hallucinations. The location of the source and grammatical form of address (Schneider, 1959) are features of form which are thought to carry particular weight. The explicit content (Larkin, 1979) of the hallucination is generally given less attention, although judgements of mood congruence, in for instance PSE 10 (World Health Organisation, 1992), are required in most diagnostic interviews. Psychodynamically flavoured accounts make more of the unpleasant and victimising content of so many hallucinations and Freud (1926) proposed that they represent the defensive projection of subconscious wishes and desires, these being unacceptable by virtue of content to the conscious mind. This account encounters difficulty in encompassing the sheer banality, neither offensivenor anodyne, of the third person commentaries of the schizophrenic patient, when it is difficult to discern what wish or desire could cause such a dramatic rejection.

Clinical experience shows that these phenomenological descriptions are not wholly stable and that the subjective report of the voice may vary in response to mood, medication and the interest shown by others. Folk psychology (Rosenthal, 1986) studies the form of such descriptions in their natural habitat, the patient's mind. The folk psychologist might ask what is it that is lost when such statements are subject to the refinements of clinical description? In a similar vein, Jaynes (1979) argued that the tendency to hallucinate is determined by the way people think of their own thoughts, a determination that is grounded in a specific historical and cultural milieu; this determination led to the promotion of the belief amongst ancient peoples that they were being addressed by the gods. A dimensional perspective of phenomenology places many of the discriminations beloved by the textbooks along continua; thus, the location of the voice, internal or external, would indicate one such axis. Some support for this comes from patient's own ratings of hallucinations (Junginger & Frame, 1985). If the dimensional view is correct, one would predict the occurrence of this phenomenon in the normal population, in forms or by virtue of content, that may differ from those of the clinical population.

In 1894, 17,000 adults were interviewed for the Sidgewick Study of psychic phenomena. This remarkable endeavour yielded data, amongst other things, about the prevalence of hallucinations in this sample. A comparison of this data with results from the vast Epidemiological Catchment Area (ECA) Program was recently presented by Tien (1991). The ECA study found a prevalence of hallucinations (all modalities) of at least 10–15% with an annual incidence of 4–5%; these rates were very similar to those found a century earlier. The age peak for hallucinations in males (25–30 years) was earlier than females (40–50 years) a finding which neatly mirrors the gender profile of the schizophrenic illnesses.

Much higher rates of hallucinations in subjects presumed to be normal were given by Posey and Losch (1983). In their study of college students, an astonishing 71% admitted to hallucinating voices whilst awake. The study of Rees (1971) of the hallucinations of widowhood testified strongly to the tendency of otherwise healthy people to hallucinate in particular contexts. In this study, almost half the subjects experienced these phenomena, although visual hallucinations were slightly more common than auditory. Rees concluded that such hallucinations are a normal, perhaps helpful, part of grief.

In summary, the expedience and familiarity of traditional phenomenological discriminations may obscure important perspectives. Eschewing a categorical approach and placing hallucinations along dimensions encourages us to seek their cause amongst normal neuropsychological mechanisms (see Claridge, 1987) and broadens the horizons of the enquiry from the confines of the clinic.

NEUROLOGICAL MODELS

BRAIN STIMULATION AND EPILEPSY

The rationale that inspired the brain stimulation experiments of Penfield and his co-workers (Penfield & Perot, 1963) was beguilingly simple: if mental events are caused by electrical brain events, then electrical stimulation of specified brain regions may tell us which mental events reside where. Sadly, mental phenomena proved to be recalcitrant. Of 520 stimulations of the temporal lobes, only 40 resulted in the experience of "hallucinations". A closer scrutiny of these phenomena reveals that the majority would not satisfy modern criteria for auditory hallucinations, although some may be described as dissociative hallucinations (Wing et al 1974). Penfield et al did describe illusions of recognition in a number of patients, such as *déjà vu* phenomena and strange affect laden distortions, of sadness, fear or loneliness. The *déjà vu* experience was particularly associated with right temporal stimulations. Halgren et al (1978) performed 3495 deep stimulations of the temporal lobes in 36 epileptic subjects. No formed hallucinations occurred, though memory-like episodes were recorded in three. Although these results were disappointing, the repetitive, stereotypical quality of many auditory hallucinations leads one to conclude that they are remembered and reactivated in some sense (this feature is particularly evident when the same voice is resuscitated at different episodes of illness). Perhaps then, Penfield's view that he was causing, with the stimulations, a replaying of a record of experience may have some merit after all and we will return to this theme in the section concerning memory and affect (see Gloor, 1990 for an updated view of this research).

Psychotic disturbance occurring in the post-ictal period, or in the context of long-standing epilepsy, is well recognised (Blumer, 1984; Trimble, 1990; So et al, 1990). On the whole hallucinations do not seem to be a feature of seizures as such. A study by Currie et al (1981) of a group of 666 patients with epilepsy showed that 16% had experienced auditory-sensory disturbances during their attack, but these were much more likely to be phenomenologically crude rather than elaborate. An interesting case of a patient who experienced hallucinations during the aura of epilepsy caused by an arteriovenous malformation was described by De Reuck et al (1989). Using positron emission tomography (PET), a decrease in the blood flow and oxygen metabolism was demonstrated behind the left insular region.

Brain tumours are only rarely associated with hallucinations (Hécaen & Ropert, 1959). In a study of 61 tumours of the temporal lobe, Gal (1958) reported no instances. Tanabe et al (1986) did, however, describe the occurrence of voices coming from the right ear in a patient with a left temporal gyrus infarction. These occurred in association with transient aphasia and were characterised as the voice of a female TV announcer, a description with a more psychotic feel than most in the literature. Unilateral hallucinations appear more likely to be associated with an underlying brain abnormality (Bergman, 1965), although these are not common in schizophrenia (Gruber et al, 1984; Bracha et al, 1985).

The association of hallucinations with ear disease is established (Morel, 1936; Gordon, 1987) but the finding of an association of ear disease with musical hallucinations is particularly intriguing. Keshavan et al (1992) found the latter association in 38 out of 59 cases. Sensory deficits are of course more common amongst elderly subjects and seem to be particularly so among the elderly paranoid. The tendency to misinterpret sensations is promoted by sensory deprivation (Zuckerman & Cohen, 1964) and most neuropsychological explanations of this phenomenon (West, 1975) postulate that, in conditions of low or reduced environmental stimulation, the seepage into consciousness of perceptual traces of old experiences occurs and that these are then experienced as hallucinations.

THE CEREBRAL HEMISPHERES

In 1874, Hughlings Jackson observed that amongst those severely aphasic patients who had lost most of their propositional speech, many still retain the capacity to speak "automatically" with overlearned phrases and phatic utterances. Smith (1966) described a patient who had his left hemisphere removed in order to treat a malignant tumour; he was left hemisphere dominant preoperatively. Following this operation he lost most of his expressive speech but was still able to utter expletives or emotionally charged stock phrases. These particular forms of speech share the feature that they do not require the translation of concept into language (Van Lancker, 1975). Jackson's contention that such non-propositional speech may originate in the right cerebral hemisphere found support in the report by Smith (see also Kinsbourne, 1971; Basso et al, 1989; Coltheart et al, 1987). Experimental evidence for this view comes from studies of the processing of emotional words by the right hemisphere (Ley, 1984). Of potential interest is the similarity of these words to the content of many hallucinations (Hill, 1936). Also noteworthy is the superior capacity of this hemisphere to process prosody (Ross, 1981) and such pragmatic functions as the appreciation of humour, metaphor and intended meaning (Gardner et al, 1983).

Cutting (1990) argues that if the right hemisphere is not functioning properly, errors in the interpretation of the prosodic components of thought and its grammatical form, may lead the left hemisphere to conclude incorrectly that the patient's thoughts are voices speaking to him. This ingenious theory tackles in a forthright manner the alien quality of the hallucination but does not address the characteristic content, such as the prolific abuse and menace. Neither does it explain how patients are able to converse fluently with their voices in private internal speech. Thus, it is difficult to imagine how such a misattribution of thought due to tonal and grammatical error could support this activity without completely muddling the patient.

In contrast there are those who nominate the left cerebral hemisphere as the locus of disturbance in schizophrenia. Flor-Henry (1969) proposed such a link with evidence showing that psychotic-like symptoms were more likely to be related to left temporal foci in epileptics. Neuropsychological support for this view was provided in a study by McKay et al (1981) in which groups of hallucinating patients (auditory and visual) were compared with non-hallucinating patients on a variety of standard neuropsychological measures. They found some evidence for left frontal lobe impairment in the auditory hallucinators but not in the other groups. The computerised tomography (CT) study of Takahashi et al (1981) demonstrated an association of hallucinations with left temporal cortical atrophy.

Finally, in this context it is worth remembering the split-brain experiments summarised in Sperry (1968). The demonstration of apparently autonomous function of the two hemispheres in his subjects did much to further our understanding of the lateralisation of function in the brain. It also provoked important debate about the unity of consciousness and the nature of identity, questions that were touched upon in the introduction of this chapter. Sperry talked of "two free wills in one cranial vault" which raises the bizarre possibility of a dialogue between them. The elegant experiments of MacKay & MacKay (1972) on these subjects seemed to demonstrate that such a conversation is in a sense possible, although he distanced himself from the radical notion of two consciousnesses and offered instead the explanation that what was seen was one person prone "to show a peculiar form of absent-mindedness". Parfit (1987) expressed this idea differently: we are all aware at any moment of several different experiences; the split brain patient is distinguished in having two such states of awareness, but we do not need to concede the presence of two egos to make this judgement. This subtle argument is germane to our consideration of hallucinations and may help us understand how alien attribution of verbal fragments can occur (see also Nasrallah, 1985) although the extent to which the right hemisphere can support language is much debated (Zaidel, 1985).

NEUROIMAGING

The contribution of the early CT scanning projects in reviving the search for the cause of psychosis in the substrate of the brain itself has now passed into received wisdom. The finding of cortical atrophy and increased ventricular size in patients with schizophrenia (Johnstone & Crow, 1976) did much to quicken the collective pulse of those who believed that, in time and with more complex imaging techniques, the brain would finally yield its secrets to the eye. The success of this approach has been in the main confined to general statements about abnormalities in the gross brain architecture of broadly defined patient groups. Less successful has been the quest reliably to link specific symptoms or phenomenological items with localised brain abnormality, although the association of ventricular enlargement with negative symptoms has been recorded (Andreasen et al, 1982). Owens et al (1985) found a negative correlation between ventricular–brain ratio and auditory hallucinations. The crude but tempting conclusion is that the activity of hallucinating may require relatively intact cerebral substrate.

Magnetic resonance imaging (MRI) offers the opportunity to image the brain in living subjects with greater resolution than CT (see also Bilder and Szeszko, chapter 14). A recent study using this new technology (Young et al, 1991) found that ventricular enlargement and cerebral atrophy were related to the severity of symptoms in general. However, the findings of abnormalities in the structures of the limbic system, which they describe in the schizophrenic group, may be germane to the consideration of memory and affect function that we offer in a later section. Barta et al (1990) reported a reduction in volume of the left superior temporal gyrus and amygdala in schizophrenic subjects which correlated highly with their report of hallucinations. Excluding the single non-hallucinator from this calculation weakens the reported correlation, which falls from $r = 0.7$ to $r = 0.54$ (David & Lucas, 1992).

Single-photon emission tomography (SPET) and PET represent important advances in the study of mind/brain function, while remaining mostly faithful to the spirit of the project of localisation (see also Liddle, chapter 15). However, researchers using these tools have had to acknowledge the frustrating effects of confounders such as anticipation and anxiety on indices of mind/brain function. Globally the results of a decade of PET scans have been contradictory. The conflicting results owe as much to the problems of patient selection and symptom incongruence as to the limitations of the technology itself. The three main regions that have been nominated as sites of disturbance in schizophrenia are the frontal lobes, basal ganglia and the temporal lobes (Buchsbaum, 1990).

A SPET study of Musalek et al (1989) compared tactile and auditory hallucinators. In this study, both groups demonstrated abnormally low frontal activity and higher basal regional cerebral blood flow (rCBF). In addition, those with auditory hallucinations manifested increased flow in the amygdala, hippocampus and parahippocampus bilaterally. Our state of ignorance is such that it is difficult to know how to begin interpreting such a result. Mindful of the quagmire of confounders, a SPET study conducted by McGuire et al (1993) scanned individuals in both hallucinating and non-hallucinating states; results have shown increased flow in left frontal and lateral temporal lobe during the hallucination.

Other studies reveal conflicting results. For instance, Mathew et al (1982) report inverse correlations between the experience of the hallucination and blood flow in the left parietal and temporal lobes as well as the right temporoparietal and occipital regions. Volkow et al (1987) described a positive correlation between this symptom and right temporal glucose metabolism. Notardonato et al (1989) also found a right sided abnormality in a patient with left sided hallucinations while Matsuda et al (1988) demonstrated a left sided accumulation of a blood-flow tracer with SPET. Cleghorn et al (1990) found a high correlation of hallucinations and activity in the anterior cingulate region but Weiler et al (1990) showed diminished activity in the left caudate. An older functional measure, the electroencephalogram (EEG) has failed to reveal reliable correlates of auditory hallucinations in patients with schizophrenia (Sem-Jacobsen et al, 1955; Stevens & Livermore, 1982).

Magnetoencephalography (MEG) is a new technique that can show neural activity beneath the skull. Unlike the EEG, which detects both radial and tangential currents, the MEG is sensitive to tangential currents only, which means the results reflect pyramidal cell activity in the main. An interesting study (Tiihonen et al, 1992) using this technology was conducted with two hallucinating patients. This study showed that small response delays occurred during the hallucination in the auditory cortex, results that resemble the effects of real sounds. The authors conclude by suggesting that the hallucination may arise from dysfunctions in the circuits serving auditory memory particularly those that run between the mesial temporal lobe and the auditory cortex.

There are conceptual difficulties inherent in the neuroimaging project: it is difficult to believe that a mental event such as an hallucination is actually localised in a fixed mind/brain relation in a region of the cerebrum, and has yet to find vindication from this approach. However, if there are complex and possibly irreducible functions of the mind/brain, it remains plausible to propose structural models of these functions, employing principles of localisation in the phrenological sense. For instance, the finding of increased basal ganglia activity in subjects with obsessional disorder (OCD) led Baxter et al (1989) to suggest that orbital cortical overactivity may overwhelm the integrative function of the caudate. We might mention that the perseverating and intrusive character of hallucinations bears a striking resemblance to the phenomena of the obsessional patient and the finding of increased activity of the globus pallidus in untreated patients with schizophrenia (Early et al, 1987) is interesting in this context.

The neurologically informed studies of hallucinations have become more sophisticated in recent years. This change reflects the emergence of new technologies that permit the observation of mind/brain activity *in vivo* and which may represent an important advance over the older structure-oriented techniques. Caution, however, is warranted and springs from an understanding that the mind/brain probably differs from other physiological systems in being less accommodating than most to the spartan rigours of the reductionist paradigm. Systemic models of mind/brain function find support from the emerging cognitive sciences and it is likely that in the near future such models may be employed to generate testable hypotheses, whilst encouraging us to think of the mind/brain in fresh ways.

SPEECH MECHANISMS

Verbal hallucinations are experienced by the subject as speech acts, usually but not necessarily, addressed to the subject. This glib observation has two arresting implications. Firstly, if verbal hallucinations are meaningful words, then those neuropsychological mechanisms that are thought to subserve speech generation and reception are likely to be active during the hallucination. Secondly, as the capacity to internalise language leading to the production of inner speech is probably universal, there exists already a process that can, amongst other things, generate private messages (thoughts) which implies that the owner of these thoughts must be both author and recipient of the message. This dual role resembles the problem posed by the hallucination (Johnson, 1978), that is, how is it that an individual can generate mental events that feel alien? Perhaps by studying the nature of inner speech mechanisms, we may determine the psychological roots of the attitude that enables us to speak to ourselves. We must voice a caveat that, although auditory hallucinations are often heard as "voices", other forms of this phenomenon, such as music, whistles or the sound of machinery, are not infrequently encountered; therefore, those models that propose disturbances of inner speech as being of primary importance in the generation of the hallucination, cannot encompass alone all hallucinatory experiences. Furthermore, psychologists that work in the field of linguistics emphasise that language as an activity deserves to be placed firmly in the context of social interaction, that the speech act is but one of many avenues that are exploited during the communication. Althuser (1971) quotes, for example, the case of profoundly deaf schizophrenics who describe their "voices" as acts of communication in sign language. In a similar way, accepting that the language of gesture exists as a distinct channel of meaning (Ekman & Friesen, 1969) may help us to understand the symptom of delusion of reference (Wing et al, 1974) as a disturbance of this gestural system of communication.

INNER SPEECH AND THOUGHT

Egocentric speech (Piaget, 1926) is speech that is not addressed or adapted to any listener but is produced for the satisfaction of the individual him/herself. Such speech is particularly prevalent among children aged 5–6 years but it declines rapidly with age. Piaget (1926) characterised this phenomenon as speech lacking social or communicative function, functions that would be assembled with developmental time. Vygotsky (1962) took a more positive view. He regarded egocentric speech as having an important function in its own right, namely that of cognitive self-guidance. Thus, Vygotsky's view was that on its disappearance from the child, egocentric speech re-emerges as thought in the adult. An intermediate position was proposed by Flavell & Beach (1966), who argued on the basis of experiments conducted on young children, that both views of the significance of private speech contain elements of truth but that neither view exhausts the range of phenomena observed. Klein (1963) suggested that one of these functions may be affect expression. Most adults admit to speaking to themselves from time to time but the spontaneous verbalisation of the inner dialogue is especially likely to occur if suddenly emotionally aroused, for example, by pain.

Neuroimaging data lend support for the classical neurological expectations of activity during speech. For example, Ingvar & Schwartz (1974) showed left anterior increases of cerebral blood flow. Inner speech has only recently been specifically studied using the PET technology (Chetkow et al, 1991). However, work by Petersen et al (1988) and Wise et al (1991) on word recognition tasks showed that phonological coding leads to the activation of the temporal cortices bilaterally and the temporoparietal cortex on the left. Speech leads to the activation of the peri-sylvian regions bilaterally and the left prefrontal area.

The existence of models describing the relation of inner speech, short-term memory and psycholinguistic processes, such as rehearsal, have been used to explore the relationship of inner speech to hallucinations. The repetition of empty phrases and words (e.g. "the, the, the") serves to occupy inner speech in a condition called articulatory suppression (Baddeley & Lewis, 1981). Short-term memory is affected by such a process, for instance, the serial recall span of short words is impaired (Baddeley, 1986). We may therefore ask: do hallucinations occupy this rehearsal system? If they do then we would expect that the effect of experiencing an hallucination would be similar to the effect of artificially occupying this system with articulatory suppression. Early studies (David & Lucas, 1993) seem to indicate that this does not happen. Perhaps this is not so surprising as it is perfectly possible to repeat empty phrases to oneself whilst reading or listening to language without any loss of understanding. It is also clear from the anecdotal reports of patients' descriptions of their hallucinations that they can, in some cases, disattend from the hallucination which may continue "in the background". Distraction techniques (Margo et al, 1981) for the treatment of hallucinations probably utilise similar mechanisms.

The implication of these observations is that hallucinations may enjoy a degree of autonomy that frees them from the constraints of the purposeful speech mechanisms that are employed to speak and to speak inwardly (Sedman, 1966). This conclusion is easier to concede if the hallucination is viewed as a phenomenon that is essentially passively received, say by the activation of memory traces, rather than actively constructed.

SUBVOCALISATION AND UNINTENDED SPEECH

Subvocalisation refers to the covert activity of the musculature of speech which, some argue, accompanies inner speech acts and, by implication, acts of hallucination. Gould (1948, 1949) proposed in a series of studies that hallucinations do indeed lead to increased rates of subvocal activity as detected by lip and chin electromyographic (EMG) recordings. These early reports have been replicated in later studies (Inouye & Shimizu, 1970; Green & Preston, 1981) although the precise implication of this observation remains opaque (Green & Kinsbourne, 1990). Is this phenomenon a form of motor overflow, an epiphenomenon of the hallucination itself, a non-specific effect such as anxiety or tension, or is it specifically related to articulation? In favour of the last account are the descriptions of amplifications of the throats of patients who are hallucinating (Gould, 1949; Green & Preston, 1981) when subaudible speech is rendered audible and found to match the patient's own account of the hallucination. The authors of this review are attempting to reproduce these findings in a study of hallucinators using extremely sensitive laryngographic instruments which we hope might confidently distinguish the types of peri-oral movements described in some studies, from the specific subvocalisations which must originate in the larynx if, when amplified, they reveal actual speech.

The Freudian slip is a common enough experience and was adduced by Freud in 1901 to demonstrate the concurrent existence of two different intentions, the one conscious and the other unconscious. This view has not gone unchallenged. Ellis (1980) argued that such errors could arise simply from mechanical breakdowns in the speech production processes. Another familiar sensation is the tip-of-the-tongue phenomenon when the speaker gropes for a word that they know and wish to use (Brown & McNeil, 1966) but which remains tantalisingly remote. These two phenomena serve to demonstrate a single important idea, that speech is planned and that this planning seems to occur at several different levels (Dell, 1986).

Borrowing such ideas as these from psycholinguistics, Hoffman (1986) suggests an ingenious hypothesis to explain the genesis of hallucinations as a particular species of speech planning error. He proposes that the speech disorder that characterises schizophrenia (formal thought disorder) arises from a disturbance in the discourse planning (see also McGrath, chapter 10). This external and observable symptom is mirrored by disruptions of the internal planning system that is responsible for the production of thought, or verbal imagery as he prefers to call it. The disruption of this system causes the production of unintended internal speech and it is these verbal imagery fragments that are experienced as the hallucination.

There are notable difficulties with this otherwise attractive theory, not least of which is the poor correlation of speech disorder and the symptom of hallucinations (Marengo & Harrow, 1985; see also Liddle, chapter 15). An additional and related criticism is that the syntactical and semantic organisation of the hallucination itself is seldom deranged: why should a general disturbance of discourse planning, which can produce frankly disordered speech, spare the hallucination? (see Leudar et al, 1994, for experimental approaches to these questions).

For the sake of completeness, we should also mention the ideas of Frith (1979; see also Cahill and Frith, chapter 18). Frith claimed that during the process of listening to the speech of another, numerous hypotheses are spontaneously generated about the meaning of what is being said. Under normal circumstances, only the real one comes into consciousness, while in the hallucinator the threshold that determines this entry is reduced and the result is the emergence of other alternative meanings into consciousness which are then experienced as hallucinations. Why such meanings should be rendered explicitly into the prosodic form of the voice of another person remains unanswered.

Following Gray et al (1991), Frith & Done (1988) propose a neuropsychological model to explain a range of psychotic phenomena that bestows a monitoring function on the hippocampus. This region is fed information about intended actions from the prefrontal cortex, the site of their initiation, by way of the cingulate and parahippocampus: they argue that disruptions to these connections cause the characteristic symptoms of the psychotic.

PSYCHOLOGICAL PERSPECTIVES

In this section we review several psychological theories of hallucinations including ones that rely on disorders of imagery in the psychotic, attribution error and poor reality discrimination.

IMAGERY IN THE PSYCHOTIC

> The young French girl, and she could have been no older than nine or ten years, approached her mother weeping: "Maman", she cried, "It is not fair, Jean-Paul has gone to the fair with Maria," she raised her voice and stamped her foot, "and I too will go to the fair!"

We can all summon voices into our heads; in the case of the young French girl, you should have created a voice quite distinct from your own (we assume) and possibly one that you have not previously encountered. The remarkable facility of mental imagery has provided a point of departure for those interested in the nature of the hallucination.

Imagery research has a long and distinguished pedigree beginning with Aristotle who regarded imagery as the principal medium of thought. In the twentieth century, the advent of behaviourism led to neglect of this area until it was resurrected as a legitimate enquiry by scientists who became interested in the role of imagery in problem solving, sensory deprivation and the effects of the psychomimetic drugs (see Eysenck, 1990, for a thoughtful review). Attempts to localise the imagery processes in the cerebral hemispheres have produced some significant findings. For example, experiments on split-brain patients (Farah, 1988) demonstrate that the left hemisphere may contain the mechanisms of imagery generation whereas the right probably holds many of the components of imagery. Kosslyn (1987) has also nominated the left hemisphere as the site of generation of images, particularly part-images. However, exploring further the different types of image processing that the two hemispheres may be specialised to perform, led David & Cutting (1992) to propose that the left hemisphere may be programmed to produce semantic and categorical distinctions about presented material, whereas the right hemisphere may be specialised in spatial coordination. They found that visual but not auditory hallucinations appeared to be related to the impaired left hemisphere imagery functions (David & Cutting, 1993). A SPET study by Goldenberg et al (1991) looked at the effects of imaging tasks on cerebral blood flow. They showed increased flow in the hippocampi and the right inferior and superior temporal regions.

Could hallucinations represent the outpourings of especially vivid and intense mental images? Early studies (e.g. Cohen, 1938) failed to find any association between the mode that individuals habitually use to think with and the mode of the hallucination. Again Roman & Landis (1945), using a structured interview of their subjects with special emphasis on the intensity of experienced images, found no evidence to support the view that hallucinators are particularly prone to vivid imagery. Finally, Seitz & Molholm (1947) replicated these findings but concluded that auditory hallucinators may not only employ less auditory imagery, but that they may actually experience a relative deficiency of use in this mode of imagery. From this observation, about the occurrence of imagery in non-preferred modes, led the hypothesis that the imagery that does occur may be so unfamiliar to the subject that he might tend to misinterpret the source of his experiences as arising from the outside.

Reviving the question of vividness, Mintz & Alpert (1972) asked hallucinators to rate their belief about whether the record "White Christmas" had been played following suggestion. They found support for the notion that hallucinators do experience more vivid images than normal subjects. However, a study by Brett & Starker (1977), which explored the relationship between the report of vividness of mental images and the content of the stimuli used to provoke them, found that no difference in imagery vividness was seen between the hallucinating and control groups, but hallucinators reported less vivid images for emotional material. They speculated that the basic machinery of image construction is intact in the hallucinating patient but is prone to disruption by emotion. A similar approach employing more strictly defined clinical categories was taken by Starker & Jolin (1982). Again comparing hallucinators and controls on tests of volitional imagery, these investigators discovered little evidence to support the vividness model and found themselves on the verge of endorsing the imagery deficit model of hallucination genesis. They hesitated, arguing that most of the research on imagery had been conducted using volitional prompts, such as asking of patients that they imagine particular sounds. They speculated that such investigations may not adequately capture the range of phenomena that are expressed as the "spontaneous imagery/fantasy" life of the patient and which may be of importance in our consideration of hallucinations.

Research in this area is notoriously difficult to conduct, but Starker and John may have a point. There is a problem in arguing that a patient who is hearing voices can be shown on measures of imagery to have a relative inability to form auditory images. The patient is surely producing voices that arise from his/her imagination which not only feel real but seem to have an identity of their own. How many normal people can generate such cogent images? We may also choose to theorise that this same capacity may lead to the relative impoverishment of other imagery systems in producing more conventional images in other, say, experimental contexts. It is, however, equally problematic to argue that in order to be believed the hallucination must be vivid. Phenomenological features of vividness, such as clarity of loudness, cannot in themselves persuade a subject to accept the reality of the image. Consider the example of the patient who believes that there is a man who follows him and makes sarcastic remarks in the softest of whispers, not all of which are audible. Compare this with the grotesque and mesmerising images that can occur following the ingestion of an hallucinogen, but where the subject retains a firm understanding that these hallucinations represent the effects of the drug and are not real.

Conventional wisdom, and clinical phenomenology, tells us that experiences, true or false, are one thing but beliefs about the nature of these experiences are quite another. Perhaps this is the wrong way to look at these matters: the belief, "I am being followed by a person who mutters barely audible vulgarities", may be no less compelling or persuasive than the effects of more striking experiences. This argument challenges an important prejudice that is common place in clinical teaching (Maher, 1974), the assumption that delusions often arise from hallucinations, in a linear sequence. Indeed, this view threatens the phenomenological distinction of false percepts (hallucinations) and false beliefs (delusions): for is there any difference between saying of a patient "he believes falsely that another person is speaking" and the description, "this patient holds the false belief that another person is speaking"? This is not to say that recording phenomenological experience in these discrete categories is not useful; rather it is to emphasise the point that distinctions that are made in the clinical process may not necessarily correspond to underlying neuropsychological processes.

In summary, the relation of the hallucination to the mental image provides an interesting approach to the study of this phenomenon. Wider debates have questioned the very status of the image in our mental lives and have led to doubt over the value of this form of research. Methodological problems are inherent in this type of enquiry and are apparent in the research of imagery in hallucinating subjects. Largely neglected, the nature of imagination, creative thinking and the role of fantasy are subjects that may yield vital information on the generation of the hallucination.

REALITY MONITORING

In this, the second section of psychological models of hallucinations, we will briefly present an integrative model proposed by Slade & Bentall (1988). It can be shown that normal subjects are apt to confuse imaginary events and reality. The famous Perky (1910) effect demonstrates this tendency well. In an ingenious experiment, a group of subjects (trained introspectionists) were asked to imagine an object on a blank screen. They were not aware that the experimenter had arranged for the subtle back-projection of the same object onto the screen. All of the subjects failed to detect the projection of the object, reporting instead that the images that they had produced were unusually vivid. Errors of this type may represent a dysfunction in a particular system which represents metacognitive abilities. Flavell (1979) suggests that a disturbance of this metacognitive ability, the correct attribution of mental events to self or non-self, may be at the root of the hallucination. We will review some experimental data relating to this theory in the next section.

An important implication that relates to this outlook concerns the nature of perception. Many theorists (Gregory, 1972) emphasise that perception is an active, constructive process which combines external conditions relating to the stimulus with internal conditions relating to expectation, knowledge and inference. Some experimental evidence has accrued that hallucinators may be more likely to be influenced by context than normals (Hemsley, 1987) and may be intolerant of perceptual ambiguity. Fleminger (1992) argues that these "top-down" influences may be crucial in other psychotic phenomena especially delusional misidentification.

Less is known about the internal expectations of the psychotic that may drive the process of error, although the notion of mood congruence, in the description of hallucinations, seems indirectly to address this issue. Slade and Bentall argue convincingly that we should accept that the version of reality that we each hold results from a continuous process of judgement of reality discrimination. In order, therefore, to understand the psychotic patient's reality we must examine the processes that shape the judgements upon which he relies.

ATTRIBUTION ERROR

If hallucinations are regarded as thoughts that for some reason are not recognised by their authors as belonging to them, it is possible that these thoughts will come to be regarded as having an external origin. This novel approach requires that we accept the notion of familiarity with our own thoughts, a condition that would be dependent on a number of variables, for instance, attention and the tendency to monitor internal states at the expense of external reality. Heilbrun & Blum (1980) reported the results of an experiment guided by these considerations. They found that a group of hallucinators were less able to identify the words, meaning and grammatical style of their own expressed thoughts after a week had passed. The authors conclude with the proviso that lack of familiarity with lexical thought does not seem to be a sufficient explanation for the mislabelling of experience in the first place but it may be important in explaining the individual susceptibility to this symptom.

An additional study presented by Bentall et al (1991) is germane to this approach. The authors compared hallucinators with two groups of control subjects on a reality-monitoring task using paired associate responses which were re-presented to the subjects after a one week interval. The subjects were asked then to identify from lists of answers those which were the patient's own, as opposed to those that originated from the experimenter and those that were presented new. They also noted the difficulty of the association task, giving some measure of the cognitive effort that would be required to respond. The results were less than overwhelming: hallucinators were no less able than others to identify their own responses. However, the authors took heart from the finding that on high cognitive effort responses the hallucinated group were more likely to misattribute their answers to the experimenter. This finding they interpreted as showing that, in the face of uncertainty, hallucinators are more likely to attribute to external causes. There is a dissociation between this and the finding (Johnson et al, 1981) that normal subjects are generally better able to make the discrimination of self and non-self when the items under consideration are harder to generate. The affective connotation of words was not described in this experiment, which seems surprising as a salient feature of most hallucinated words is their striking emotiveness. The authors of this chapter are currently exploring the possible effects of affective valence on judgements of attribution in future experiments.

The attribution hypothesis bears a resemblance to the discourse planning error theory propounded by Hoffman (1986). There are difficulties with this approach, although the emphasis on errors of thinking, rather than errors of perception, provides a fresh perspective. Perhaps the most obvious problem is the fact that hallucinating patients do not themselves describe any confusion about the author-ship of their experiences, although to the observer, confused they obviously are. Most patients are quite sure that they are being addressed by another and, furthermore, they are usually quite explicit about the race, gender and disposition of these speakers. Even if one were to accept the silence of this theory about these prosodic and grammatical features, one would still require an explanation about the characteristic content of the hallucinations. One might ask, why should it be that certain types of thoughts, particularly frightening and abusive ones, are more likely to be misattributed than others? If in response to this question comes the proposition that these thoughts are most likely to be misattributed because they are the least acceptable to the subject, then it seems we are simply being drawn to a neo-Freudian model where misattribution as a mechanism comes to replace the psychodynamic concept of projection. Perhaps the merit of this approach lies elsewhere, for example, in understanding thought insertion, where clinical experience shows that patients do describe difficulties in discriminating the ownership of thought.

AFFECT, MEMORY AND HALLUCINATIONS

Ellis et al (1989) described an interesting neurological case that will preface this consideration of memory and affect. Following bilateral cerebrovascular accidents, the patient complained of persistent "natterings" plus musical fragments inside her head; she had been known to have a diminished short-term memory following a left thalamic haematoma, but these uncontrollable inner speech utterances began after a lesion in the right basal ganglia. The authors wondered whether the damage to her memory system resulted not only in lost capacity but also in an impaired ability to regulate its content, resulting in the intrusion of unwanted memory fragments, possibly from the right hemisphere, into consciousness. However, these experiences were not cast as alien in source nor did they carry affective connotations, so differing from the functional hallucinations that we have been concerned with.

The relation of affect and cognition has preoccupied psychologists and philosophers alike since ancient times. Modern conceptions of this relationship have arisen directly from the distinguished speculations of early psychological theorists of emotion, including James (1884), Cannon (1927) and Papez (1937). The recent focus on the roles of the amygdala and the hippocampus in mediating these processes can be traced to attempts to localise in the brain the dysfunction that characterises the Klüver–Bucy syndrome (Weiskrantz, 1956), where a gross disturbance of the link between behavioural response and sensory stimuli is observed, suggesting a contained disconnection of these processes that are responsible for bestowing affective connotation to stimuli. LeDoux (1992) argues persuasively that affect and cognition should be regarded as separate information processing systems. The pathways that connect the hippocampus and the amygdala, and which enable a free and direct flow of information between them, may be responsible for the affective (amygdala function) colour of cognitions (hippocampal function). Furthermore, LeDoux suggests that the amygdala may have an important although indirect role in the modulation of long-term memory organisation by attaching affective value to particular cognitions.

It is known that memory retrieval is influenced by mood (Blayney, 1986). As mentioned earlier, the pervasive quality of mood states provides a rich context for the processes entailed in the judgement of reality, but it is also likely that an important component of this context takes the form of automatically retrieved memories, memories that are congruent with the mood state and which serve to reinforce it. However, the functions of affect in providing contextual cues for the emergence of memories are complex. Tranel & Damasio (1985) report the case of a patient who suffered profound global amnesia due to destruction bilaterally of his mesial temporal lobes. Having lost the ability to learn new information about people, including their names or biographical details, the patient was still able to classify people into "good" and "bad" after they had been systematically paired with affect valencies, although he had no access consciously to information that could guide this choice.

A striking and enigmatic feature of memory is the sense of familiarity that accompanies the recognition of an experience which has been previously encountered. The experience of *déjà vu* indicates that this sense of the familiar is itself prone to abnormality when it is incorrectly bestowed on novel circumstances. It is worth reminding ourselves that the notion of familiarity seems to involve the ownership of experience as a manifestation of self, expressed as a continuity in time. Therefore, the association of *déjà vu* with other disorders relating to the experiences of self, including derealisation and depersonalisation (Bingley, 1958), is not surprising and the relation of these unusual experiences to putative disorders of the temporal lobes is pertinent to our argument. If the mechanisms that generate our sense of familiarity apply to external experiences, then do they also operate in the experience of internal events such as images, thoughts and memories? This idea was alluded to in the section dealing with attribution theory: there we suggested that the faulty self-attribution mechanism for hallucinations seems to founder because there is no compelling reason to believe that such a fault would give rise to the experience of a thought in the voice of another person. We may now revive this theory but recast it to accommodate this singular feature of verbal hallucinations.

Let us imagine that owing to the presence of a pervasive disturbance of mood, such as paranoia, the psychotic patient is apt to retrieve certain memories which would be congruent with this state, memories for instance of being menaced, abused or threatened by other people. Let us suppose that the psychotic patient is prone to a *specific disturbance of the mechanisms of familiarity* which would normally come to be engaged when these memories pierce into consciousness. The subjective experience of the memory would radically alter so that the memory would no longer be recognised as a memory: the psychological meta-organisation that allows us correctly to label our mental events would be deranged. Spoken instances of threats, menace or abuse would be experienced as *the voices of other people*, the patient would feel himself addressed by them and he would describe the experience as issuing from these others *in the present* rather than correctly placing them as instances of having being spoken to *in the past*.

Thus, the hallucination may represent a disturbance of those functions that serve to bind memories into their appropriate context, which in the case of a memory, implies a relationship between the mental event, time and self. Since we have argued that verbal hallucinations may represent mis-remembered 'voices, the peculiar and characteristic prosodic form of the verbal hallucination, experienced as the voice of another person, is explained. In addition, the striking content, frequently of disturbing material, can be understood as the selective activation of disturbing mood-congruent memory traces. Again, the intrusive quality of the hallucination and its unbidden nature are seen as features of these automatically retrieved memory traces. Finally, the alien quality of the hallucination which vexed us in the introductory section is now seen as a red herring: the patient who hears voices is *correctly* reporting that he hears the voice of other people, he simply mistakes the context of time (present for past) and intention (present threat rather than remembered menace).

An important objection to this theory of hallucinations concerns the fact that the majority of hallucinated voices are not recognised by the patient as belonging to any person that he/she can identify. Even if, as we have argued, the familiarity of memory is lost, there is no reason to believe that all processes of recognition of the *content* of the memory will be also lost. If these voices do not originate from the remembrance of words spoken in reality, it follows that they may represent the products of the hallucinator's imagination. It is possible that these voices represent the personification of figures that have been created by the individual in imagination. These imaginings, one conjectures, highly charged with affect, come to dwell as memories only to be reactivated in times of emotional arousal (see Cooklin et al, 1983). Apart from fantasy thinking, it is also possible that these voices are conveyed to the individual, probably during early development, by the popular culture (e.g. cinema and television). Therefore, even if we were to ignore the capacity of the mind to generate voices *de novo*, it is clear that if only a fraction of the thousands of voices that an individual hears during his/her development are remembered, then an ample reservoir of potential hallucinations exists. Taking this argument further, it seems that of these many thousands of heard voices, the most likely to be remembered would be those that carry an emotional charge, such as fear. Therefore, emotive memory may be prone to selective bias.

If we return now to the psychotic patient who finds himself mis-remembering the spoken threats and intimidations of figures from the past, or derived from past imaginings, or even remembered from the various media of culture, the experience of misconstruing these memories as real happenings, occurring in his/her present, may reinforce his mood state and increase the likelihood of the further automatic intrusions of congruent memory fragments; again these would be perceived as the occurrence of yet more voices. This brings us to another feature of this model. If we accept that a memory can be misconstrued, in the way that we have suggested, as a real event happening to the patient, then it is likely that the *perception of this hallucination* will also come to be laid down into the patient's memory store as an instance of a voice addressing the patient and, at a future time, if subject to the forces that cause its automatic retrieval and mis-remembering, will re-emerge into consciousness as an hallucination again. A *stable cycle* is thereby created which may help to explain the persistence of this form of psychotic feature, not only within a single episode of illness, but also across different illness episodes.

Can this model help us to understand how hallucinators seem to speak to their voices and establish with them a sense of intimacy? If we accept the basis of the stable cycle just described, the implication of a dynamic system that corresponds between memory, falsely construed experience of memory and new memory, could, one imagines, under certain circumstances become *unstable*. Under these conditions, instead of ensnaring single misremembered items in a vicious cycle, it would be possible for the hallucination (mis-remembered voice) to stimulate, by association, other related memory items. These too would emerge in consciousness and would be mis-construed in turn, in the way that we have described, as real voices. Again, some of these new voices may become established in a stable cycle, whereas others might stimulate fresh instances of instability. In this way a rich array of hallucinations would appear to consciousness *in sequence*. If the patient were able to learn how to interrupt this process by inserting his own voice or thought into the cycle, it might then be possible for him to use his actively intended speech as a prompt for a memory (mis-remembered, of course, as a hallucination): a conversation of sorts is the result. Again, each of these instances of new hallucinations would serve to add detail to the original hallucinatory scheme and with time a sense of intimacy would emerge. If this model is correct, one would predict that hallucinations would appear to *accumulate* following each illness episode. This prediction appears to be upheld by our verbatim hallucinations research (Nayani and David, 1996) where both a progression was seen in terms of hallucination complexity in successive episodes of illness and a hierarchy of hallucinations was observed, with the most elemental (vulgar swear words in the main) being the most frequently encountered.

In summary, the verbal hallucination may represent the activation of memory traces by automatic, preconscious processes which are dictated by the advent of pervasive distortions of judgement caused by mood states. We suggest that the psychotic patient may be prone to a particular dysfunction of those processes involved in the construction of a sense of familiarity that accompanies memory retrieval. In consequence, the occurrence of memory fragments of, for example, hostile or abusive speech directed at the patient from the past and deriving either from real events, imagination or by way of the various media of fantasy, come to be perceived by the patient, shorn of their familiar binding contexts of time, place and ownership. These mis-remembered memories feel as though they are real events, occurring in the present and issuing from real people with malicious intent directed at the patient. Finally, we would suggest that the pathways that connect the hippocampus and the amygdala, which may be involved in the affective valence given to experiences, are perhaps implicated in this form of psychotic disturbance (see Gloor et al, 1982). These connections are important mediators of the organisation of long-term memory stores and, by dint of their function of affective coding, retrieval mechanisms. Emerging descriptions of abnormalities of the structure of the limbic region in patients with schizophrenia (e.g. Young et al, 1991; see also Bilder and Szeszko, chapter 14) seem to support the proposal that future neuropsychological investigations might profit by focusing on the activities of this region.

CONCLUSION

This review of neuropsychological perspectives on the problem of hallucinations has covered a considerable amount of territory in only a short space. Inevitably, such a condensation is costly in terms of subtlety and justice to the authors whose papers were mentioned. It is hoped that some general points will have emerged from this discussion which may serve to focus consideration about this problem in the future:

1. The commonsense association of intrusiveness and alien attribution of hallucinations must be reconsidered: not all unbidden mental events are alien in feel and not all hallucinations are unbidden.
2. Other phenomenological features that we have delineated include: intimacy, repetitiveness, and affect-loading. Not all hallucinations share all these characteristics but the majority may do.
3. The emerging disciplines of neuropsychology and neurophenomenology are yet in the process of finding a natural vocabulary of expression to span the differences between the neuro-biased and psyche-biased approaches to their subject matter. Brain-based accounts have, so far, proved inadequate in explaining hallucinations.
4. The categorical perspective favoured in clinical practice and the use of conventional cross-sectional diagnostic schemes may mislead the investigator by obscuring differences between groups of hallucinations which may be of theoretical interest.
5. The postulated disturbances of "reality impairment" that may lie at the root of the hallucinator's problem demands the explicit description of contextual determinants. This will include not only psychophysiological measures, like arousal, but also the construction of narrative reports which should serve to impress us that, for the hallucinator, the voices are usually meaningful at various levels.
6. Neurologist and psychologist are alike in avoiding, for the most part, certain subjects of inquiry: the role of fantasy, the capacities of the imagination, and the relation that these may have to psychotic processes. A science of such processes, if developed, will play a role in the understanding of the psychotic experience.
7. The tentative model that we have sketched in the section on memory and affect attempts to combine dynamic conceptions of brain function with the phenomenological constraints that are suggested by the subjective report of the hallucination. Implied by this model are assumptions that the products of mind/brain activity will be captured only by systemic models of function which can accommodate the complex and manifold interactions of mental events and processes.

REFERENCES

Aggernaes, A. (1972) The experienced reality of hallucinations and other psychological phenomena: An empirical analysis. *Acta Psychiatrica Scandinavica*, **48**, 220–238.
Althuser, K.Z. (1971) Studies of the deaf: Relevance to psychiatric theory. *American Journal of Psychiatry*, **127**, 1521–1526.

Andreasen, N.C., Olsen, S.A., Dennert, J.W. (1982) Ventricular enlargement in schizophrenia: Relationship to positive and negative symptoms. *American Journal of Psychiatry*, **139**, 297–302.

Baddeley, A.D. (1986) *Working Memory*, Oxford University Press, Oxford.

Baddeley, A.D., Lewis, V.J. (1981) Inner active processing in reading: The inner voice, the inner ear and the inner eye. In: *Interactive Process in Reading* (Eds A.M. Lesgold, C.A. Perfetti), Erlbaum, Hillsdale, NJ.

Barta, P.E, Pearlson, G.D, Powers, R.E., Richards, S.S., Tune, L.E. (1990) Auditory hallucinations and smaller superior temporal gyral volume in schizophrenia. *American Journal of Psychiatry*, **147**, 457–462.

Basso, A., Gardelli, M., Grassi, M.P., Mariotti, M. (1989) The role of the right hemisphere in recovery from aphasia: Two case studies. *Cortex*, **25**, 555–566.

Baxter, L.T., Thompson, J.M., Phelps, M.E. (1988) Trazodone treatment response in obsessional compulsive disorder correlated with shifts in glucose metabolism in the caudate nuclei. *Psychopathology*, **20**, 114–122.

Bentall, R.P. (1990) The illusion of reality: A review and integration of psychological research on hallucinations. *Psychological Bulletin*, **107**, 82–95.

Bentall, R.P., Baker, G.A., Havers, S. (1991) Reality monitoring and psychotic hallucinations. *British Journal of Clinical Psychology*, **30**, 213–222.

Bergman, P.S. (1965) Unilateral auditory hallucinations. *Transactions of the American Neurological Association*, **90**, 226–227.

Bingley, T. (1958) Mental symptoms in temporal lobe epilepsy and temporal gliomas. *Psychiatrica et Neurologica Scandinavica*, **33** (Suppl. 120), 1–151.

Blumer, D. (1984) *Psychiatric aspects of epilepsy*, American Psychiatric Press, Washington, DC.

Blayney, P.H. (1986) Affect and memory: A review. *Psychological Bulletin*, **99**, 229–246.

Bracha, H.S., Cabrera, F.J., Karson, C.N., Bigelow, L.B. (1985) Lateralization of visual hallucinations in chronic schizophrenia. *Biological Psychiatry*, **20**, 1132–1136.

Brett, E., Starker, S. (1977) Auditory imagery and hallucinations. *Journal of Nervous and Mental Disease*, **164**, 394–400.

Brown, R., McNeil, D. (1966) The "tip of the tongue phenomenon". *Journal of Verbal Learning and Verbal Behaviour*, **5**, 325–337.

Cannon, W.B. (1927) The James-Lange theory of emotions: A critical examination and an alternative theory. *American Journal of Psychology*, **39**, 106–124.

Chetkow, H., Bub, D., Evans, A., Meyer, E., Merrit, S. (1991) Functional activation of frontal cortex in subvocalisation. *Neurology*, **41** (Suppl. 1), 300.

Churchland, P.S. (1988) Reduction and the neurobiological basis of consciousness. In: *Consciousness in Contemporary Science* (Eds A.J. Marcel, E. Bisiach), Oxford University Press, Oxford.

Claridge, G. (1987) "The schizophrenias as nervous types" revisited. *British Journal of Psychiatry*, **151**, 735–743.

Cleghorn, J.M., Garnett, E.S., Nahmias, C., Brown, G.M., Kaplan, R.D., Szechtman, H., Szechtman.B., Franco, S., Dermer, S.W., Cook, P. (1990) Regional brain metabolism during auditory hallucinations in chronic schizophrenia. *British Journal of Psychiatry*, **157**, 562–570.

Cohen, I.H. (1938) Imagery and its relation to schizophrenia symptoms. *Journal of Mental Science*, **84**, 284–346.

Coltheart, M., Patterson, K., Marshall, J.C. (1987) *Deep Dyslexia* (2nd edn), Routledge & Kegan Paul, London.

Cooklin, R., Sturgeon, D., Leff, L. (1983) The relationship between auditory hallucinations and spontaneous fluctuations of skin conductance in schizophrenia. *British Journal of Psychiatry*, **142**, 47–52.

Costello, C.G. (1992) Research on symptoms versus research on syndromes: Arguments in favour of allocating more time to the study of symptoms. *British Journal of Psychiatry*, **160**, 304–309.

Currie, S., Heathfield, K.W.G., Henson, R.A., Scott, D.F. (1971) Clinical course and prognosis of temporal lobe epilepsy: A survey of 666 patients. *Brain*, **92**, 173–190.

Cutting, J. (1990) *The Right Cerebral Hemisphere and Psychiatric Disorders*, Oxford University Press, Oxford.

David, A.S. (1990) Insight and psychosis. *British Journal of Psychiatry*, **156**, 798–808.

David, A.S. (1993) Cognitive neuropsychiatry? *Psychological Medicine*, **23**, 1–5.

David, A.S., Cutting, J.C. (1992) Categorical-semantic and spatial-imagery judgements of non-verbal stimuli in the cerebral hemispheres. *Cortex*, **28**, 339–351.

David, A.S., Cutting, J.C. (1993) Visual imagery and visual semantics in the cerebral hemispheres in schizophrenia. *Schizophrenia Research*, **8**, 263–271.

David, A.S., Lucas, P.A. (1992) Neurological models of auditory hallucinations. In: *Delusions and Hallucinations in Old Age* (Eds C. Katona, R. Levy), pp. 57–83, Gaskell, London.

David, A.S., Lucas, P.A. (1993) Auditory–verbal hallucinations and the phonological loop: A cognitive neuropsychological study. *British Journal of Clinical Psychology*, **32**, 431–441.

Dell, G.S. (1986) A spreading-activation theory of retrieval in sentence production. *Psychological Review*, **93**, 283–321.

De Reuck, J., Van Aken, J., Van Langdegem, S., Vakaet, A. (1989) Positron emission tomography studies of changes in cerebral blood flow and oxygen metabolism in arteriovenous malformation of the brain. *European Neurology*, **29**, 294–297.

Early, T.S., Reinman, E.M., Raichle, M.E. (1987) Left globus pallidus abnormality in never-medicated patients with schizophrenia. *Proceedings of National Academy of Sciences*, **84**, 561–563.

Ekman, P., Friesen, W.V. (1969) The repertoire of non-verbal behavior: Categories, origins, usage and coding. *Semiotica*, **1**, 49–98.

Ellis, A.W. (1980) On the Freudian theory of speech errors. In: *Errors In Linguistic Performance, Slips of the Tongue, Ear, Pen and Hand* (Ed. V. Fromkin), Academic Press, New York.

Ellis, A.W., Young, A.W., Critchley, E.M.R. (1989) Intrusive automatic or nonpropositional inner speech following bilateral cerebral injury. *Aphasiology*, **3**, 581–585.

Eysenck, M.W. (1990) *Cognitive Psychology: A Students Handbook*, Erlbaum, Hove, UK.

Farah, M.J. (1988) Visual and spatial mental imagery: Dissociable systems of representation. *Cognitive Psychology*, **20**, 205–254.

Flavell, J.H. (1979) Metacognition and cognitive monitoring. *American Psychologist*, **34**, 906–911.

Flavell, J.H., Beach, D.R. (1966) Spontaneous verbal rehearsal in a memory task as a function of age. *Problems of Psychology*, **1**, 26–35.

Fleminger, S. (1992) Seeing is believing: The role of preconscious perceptual processing in delusional misidentification. *British Journal of Psychiatry*, **160**, 293–304.

Flor-Henry, P. (1969) Psychosis and Temporal Lobe Epilepsy. *Epilepsia*, **10**, 363–395.

Freud, S. (1901) *The Psychopathology of Everyday Life*, Penguin, Harmondsworth, 1975.

Freud, S. (1926) Metapsychological supplement of theory of dreams. In: *Collected Papers* (Vol. 4), Hogarth Press, London.

Friedhoff, A.J, Chase, T.N. (1982) Gilles de la Tourette syndrome. In: *Advances in Neurology* (Vol 35), Raven Press, New York.

Frith, C.D. (1979) Consciousness, information processing and schizophrenia. *British Journal of Psychiatry*, **134**, 225–235.

Frith, C.D. (1987) The positive and negative symptoms of schizophrenia reflect impairments in the perception and initiation of action. *Psychological Medicine*, **17**, 631–648.

Frith, C.D., Done, D.J. (1988) Towards a neuropsychology of schizophrenia. *British Journal of Psychiatry*, **153**, 437–443.

Gal, P. (1958) Mental symptoms in cases of tumor of the temporal lobe. *American Journal of Psychiatry*, **115**, 157–160.

Gardner, H., Brownell, H.H., Wapner, W., Michelow, D. (1983) Missing the point: The role of the right hemisphere in the processing of complex linguistic material. In: *Cognitive Processing in the Right Hemisphere* (Ed. E. Perecman), pp. 169–191, Academic Press, New York.

Gloor, P. (1990) Experiential phenomena of temporal lobe epilepsy. *Brain*, **133**, 1673–1694.

Gloor, P., Olivier, A., Quesney, L.F., Andermann, F., Horowitz, S. (1982) The role of the limbic system in experiential phenomena of temporal lobe epilepsy. *Annals of Neurology*, **12**, 129–144.

Goldenberg, G., Podreka, I., Steiner, M., Franzen, P, Deeke, L. (1991) Contributions of occipital and temporal brain regions to visual and acoustic imagery: A SPECT study. *Neuropsychologia*, **29**, 695–702.

Goodwin, D. (1971) Clinical significance of hallucinations in psychiatric disorders. *Archives of General Psychiatry*, **24**, 76–80.

Gould, L.N. (1948) Verbal hallucinations and activity of vocal musculature. *American Journal of Psychiatry*, **105**, 367–372.

Gould, L.N. (1949) Auditory hallucinations and subvocal speech. *Journal of Nervous and Mental Disease*, **109**, 418–427.

Gordon, A.G. (1987) Letter to the editor. *Acta Psychiatrica Scandinavica*, **75**, 664–668.

Gray, J.A., Feldon, J., Rawlins, J.N.P., Hemsley, D.R., Smith, A.D. (1991) The neuro-psychology of schizophrenia. *Behavioral and Brain Sciences*, **14**, 1–84.

Green, M.F., Kinsbourne, M. (1990) Subvocal activity and auditory hallucinations: Clues for behavioral treatments? *Schizophrenia Bulletin*, **16**, 617–625.

Green, P., Preston, M. (1981) Reinforcement of vocal correlates of auditory hallucinations by auditory feedback: A case study. *British Journal of Psychiatry*, **139**, 204–208.

Gregory, R.L. (1972) Seeing as thinking. *Times Literary Supplement*, June 23.

Gruber, L.N., Mangat, B., Balminder, S., Abou-taleb, H. (1984) Laterality of auditory hallucinations in psychiatric patients. *American Journal of Psychiatry*, **141**, 586–588.

Halgren, E., Walter, R.D., Cherlow, D.G., Crandall, P.H. (1978) Mental phenomena evoked by human electrical stimulation of the human hippocampal formation and amygdala. *Brain*, **101**, 83–117.

Hécaen, H., Ropert, R. (1959) Hallucinations auditives au cours de syndromes neurologiques. *Annales Médico-Psychologiques*, **1**, 257–306.

Heilbrun, A.B., Blum, N.A.(1980) Impaired recognition of self-expressed thoughts in patients with auditory hallucinations. *Journal of Abnormal Psychology*, **89**, 728–736.

Hemsley, D.R. (1987) An experimental psychological model for schizophrenia. In: *Search for the Causes of Schizophrenia* (Eds H. Hafner, W. Gattaz, W. Janzaric), pp. 179–188, Springer-Verlag, Heidelberg.

Hill, J.M. (1936) Hallucinations in psychosis. *Journal of Nervous and Mental Disease*, **83**, 402–421.

Hoffman, R.E. (1986) Verbal hallucinations and language production processes in schizophrenia. *The Behavioral and Brain Sciences*, **9**, 503–548.

Ingvar, D.H., Schwartz, M.S. (1974) Blood flow patterns induced in the dominant hemisphere by speech and reading. *Brain*, **96**, 274–288.

Inouye, T., Shimizu, A. (1970) The electromyographic study of verbal hallucinations. *Journal of Nervous and Mental Disease*, **151**, 415–422.

Jackson, J.H. (1874/1932) *Selected Writings of John Hughlings Jackson* (Vol. 2) (Ed. J. Taylor), Hodder & Stoughton, London.

James, W. (1884) What is emotion? *Mind*, **9**, 188–205.

Jaynes, J. (1979) *The Origins of Consciousness in the Breakdown of the Bicameral Mind*, Houghton-Mifflin, Boston.

Johnson, F. (1978) *The Anatomy of Hallucinations*, Melson Hall, Chicago.

Johnson, M.K., Foley, H.J., Foley, M.A. (1981) Cognitive operations and decision bias in reality monitoring. *American Journal of Psychology*, **91**, 37–64.

Johnson, M.K., Foley, M.A., Suengas, A.G., Raye, C.L. (1988a) The phenomenal characteristics of memories for perceived and imagined autobiographical events. *Journal of Experimental Psychology: General*, **117**, 371–376.

Johnson, M.K., Foley, M.A., Leach, K. (1988b) The consequence for memory of imagining in another person's voice. *Memory and Cognition*, **16**, 337–342.

Johnstone, E., Crow, T.J. (1976) Cerebral ventricular size and cognitive impairment in chronic schizophrenia. *Lancet*, **ii**, 924–926.

Junginger, J., Frame, C.L. (1985) Self-report of the frequency and phenomenology of verbal hallucinations. *Journal of Nervous and Mental Disease*, **173**, 149–155.

Keshavan, M.S., David, A.S., Steingard, S., Lishman, W.A. (1992) Musical Hallucinations: A review and synthesis. *Neuropsychiatry, Neuropsychology and Behavioral Neurology*, **3**, 211–223.

Kinsbourne, M. (1971) The minor cerebral hemisphere as a source of aphasic speech. *Archives of Neurology*, **25**, 302–306.

Klein, W.L. (1963) *An investigation of the spontaneous speech of children during problem solving.* PhD dissertation, Rochester, New York.

Kosslyn, S.M. (1987) Seeing and imagining in the cerebral hemisphere: A computational approach. *Psychological Review*, **94**, 148–175.

Larkin, A.R. (1979) The form and content of schizophrenic hallucinations. *American Journal of Psychiatry*, **136**, 940–943.

LeDoux, J.E. (1992) Brain mechanisms of emotion and learning. *Current Opinion in Neurobiology*, **2**, 191–197.

Leudar, I., Thomas, P., Johnston, M. (1994) Self-monitoring in speech production: Effects of verbal hallucinations and negative symptoms. *Psychological Medicine*, **24**, 749–761.

Ley, R.G. (1984) Right hemispheric processing of emotional and imageable words. In: *International Review of Mental Imagery* (Ed. A. Sheikh), pp. 191–203, Academic Press, London.

MacKay, D.M., MacKay, V. (1972) Explicit dialogue between left and right half systems of split brains. *Nature*, **295**, 690–691.

Maher, B. (1974) Delusional thinking and perceptual disorder. *Journal of Individual Psychology*, **30**, 98–113.

Marengo, J., Harrow, M. (1985) Thought disorder a function of schizophrenia, mania or psychosis. *Journal of Nervous and Mental Disease*, **173**, 35–41.

Margo, A., Hemsley, D.R., Slade, P.D. (1981) The effects of varying auditory input on schizophrenic hallucinations. *British Journal of Psychiatry*, **139**, 122–127.

Mathew, R.J., Duncan, G.C., Weinman, M.L., Barr, D. (1982) Regional cerebral blood flow in schizophrenia. *Archives General Psychiatry*, **39**, 1121–1124.

Matsuda, H., Gyobu, T., Masayasu, I., Hisada, K. (1988) Increased accumulation of N-isopropyl-(I-123) p-iodoamphetamine in the left auditory area in a schizophrenic patient with auditory hallucinations. *Clinical Nuclear Medicine*, **13**, 53–55.

McGuire, P.K., Shah, G.M.S., Murray, R.M. (1993) Increased blood flow in Broca's area during auditory hallucinations in schizophrenia. *Lancet*, **342**, 703–706.

McKay, S.E., Golden, C.J., Scott, M. (1981) Neuropsychological correlates of auditory and visual hallucinations. *International Journal of Neurosciences*, **15**, 87–94.

Mintz, S., Alpert, M. (1972) Imagery vividness, reality testing and schizophrenic hallucinations. *Journal of Abnormal Psychology*, **79**, 310–316.

Morel, F. (1936) Des bruits d'oreille des bourdonnements des hallucinations auditives élémentaires, communes et verbales. *Encephale*, **31**, 81–95.

Musalek, M., Podreka, I., Walter H., Suess, E., Passweg, V., Nutzinger, D., Strobl, R., Lesch, O.M. (1989) Regional brain function in hallucinations: A study of regional cerebral blood flow with 99M Tc HMPAO-SPECT in patients with auditory hallucinations, tactile hallucinations and normal controls. *Comprehensive Psychiatry*, **30**, 99–108.

Nasrallah, H.A. (1985) The unintegrated right cerebral hemispheric consciousness as alien intruder. *Comprehensive Psychiatry*, **26**, 273–282.

Nayani, T., David, A.S. (1996) The auditory hallucination: a phenomenological survey. *Psychological Medicine*, **26**, 177–189.

Notardonato, H., Gonzalez-Avilez, A., Van Heertum, R.L., O'Connell, R.A., Yudd, A.P. (1989) The potential value of serial cerebral SPECT scanning in the evaluation of psychiatric illness. *Clinical Nuclear Medicine*, **14**, 319–321.

Owens, D.G., Johnstone, E.C., Crow, T.J., Frith, C.D., Jagoe, J.R., Kreel, L. (1985) Lateral ventricular size in schizophrenia: Relationship to the disease process and its clinical manifestations. *Psychological Medicine*, **15**, 27–41.

Papez, J.W. (1937) A proposed mechanism of emotion. *Archives of Neurology and Psychiatry*, **79**, 217–224.

Parfit, D. (1987) Divided minds and the nature of persons. In: *Mindwaves* (Eds C. Blakemore, D. Greenfield), Blackwell, Oxford.

Penfield, W., Perot, P. (1963) The brain's record of auditory and visual experience: A final summary and conclusion. *Brain*, **86**, 595–696.

Perky, C.W. (1910) An experimental study of the imagination. *American Journal of Psychology*, **21**, 422–452.

Petersen, S.E., Fox, P.T., Posner, M.I., Mintum, M., Raichle, M.E. (1988) Positron emission tomographic studies of the cortical anatomy of single-word processing. *Nature*, **331**, 585–589.

Piaget, J. (1926) *The Language and Thought of the Child*, Routledge & Kegan Paul, London.

Posey, T.B., Losch, M.E. (1983) Auditory hallucinations of hearing voices in 375 normal subjects. *Imagination, Cognition and Personality*, **2**, 99–113.

Rees, D.W. (1971) The hallucinations of widowhood. *British Medical Journal*, **4**, 37–41.

Roman, R., Landis, C. (1945) Hallucinations and mental imagery. *Journal of Nervous and Mental Disease*, **102**, 327–331.

Rosenthal, D. (1986) Two concepts of consciousness. *Philosophical Studies*, **49**, 329–359.

Ross, E.D. (1981) The aprosodias: Functional–anatomic organization of the affective components of language in the right hemisphere. *Archives of Neurology*, **36**, 144–148.

Schneider, K. (1959) *Clinical Psychopathology*, Grune & Stratton, New York.

Sedman, G. (1966) Inner voices: Phenomenological and clinical aspects. *British Journal of Psychiatry*, **112**, 485–490.

Seitz, P.F., Molholm, H.B. (1947) Relation of mental imagery to hallucinations. *Archives of Neurology and Psychiatry*, **57**, 469–480.

Sem-Jacobsen, C.W., Petersen, M.C., Lazarte, J.A., Dodge, H.W. (1955) Intracerebral electrographic recordings from psychotic patients during hallucinations and agitation. *American Journal of Psychiatry*, **112**, 278–288.

Sims, A. (1988) *Symptoms in the Mind: An Introduction to Descriptive Phenomenology*, Ballière Tindall, London.

Slade, P.D., Bentall, R.P. (1988) *Sensory Deception: A Scientific Analysis of Hallucinations*, Croom-Helm, London.

Smith, A. (1966) Speech and other functions after left (dominant) hemispherectomy. *Journal of Neurology and Psychiatry*, **49**, 159–187.

So, N.K., Savard, G., Andermann, F., Olivier, A., Quesney, L.F. (1990) Acute postictal psychosis: A stereo EEG study. *Epilepsia*, **31**, 188–193.

Sperry, R.W. (1968) Hemisphere disconnection and unity in conscious awareness. *American Psychologist*, **23**, 723–733.

Starker, S., Jolin, A. (1982) Imagery and Hallucinations in schizophrenic patients. *Journal of Nervous and Mental Disease*, **170**, 448–450.

Stevens, J.R., Livermore, A. (1982) Telemetered EEG in schizophrenia: Spectral analysis during abnormal behaviour episodes. *Journal of Neurology, Neurosurgery and Psychiatry*, **45**, 385–395.

Takahashi, R., Inabe, Y., Inanaga, K. (1981) *CT scanning and the investigation of schizophrenia*. Third World Congress of Biological Psychiatry, Stockholm (cited by Flor-Henry, 1986).

Tanabe, H., Sawada, T., Asai, H., Okuda, J., Shiraishi, J. (1986) Lateralisation phenomenon of complex auditory hallucinations. *Acta Psychiatrica Scandinavica*, **74**, 178–182.

Tien, A.Y. (1991) Distributions of hallucinations in the population. *Journal of Social Psychiatry and Psychiatric Epidemiology*, **26**, 287–292.

Tiihonen, J., Hari, R., Naukkarinen, H., Rimon, R., Jousmaki, V., Kajola, M. (1992) Modified activity of the human auditory cortex during auditory hallucinations. *American Journal of Psychiatry*, **149**, 255–257.

Tranel, D., Damasio, A.R. (1985) Knowledge without awareness: An autonomic index of facial recognition by prosopagnosics. *Science*, **228**, 1453–1454.

Trimble, M.R. (1990) First-rank symptoms of Schneider: A new perspective? *British Journal of Psychiatry*, **156**, 195–200.

Van Lancker, D. (1975) Heterogeneity in language and speech: Neurolinguistic studies. *UCLA Working Papers in Phonetics*, no. 29.

Volkow, N.D., Wolf, A.P., Van Gelder, P., Brodie, J.D., Overall, J.E., Cancro, R., Gomez-Mont, F. (1987) Phenomenological correlates of metabolic activity in 18 patients with chronic schizophrenia. *American Journal of Psychiatry*, **144**, 151–158.

Vygotsky, L.S. (1962) *Thought and Language*, MIT Press, Cambridge, MA.

Weiler, M.A., Buchsbaum, M.S., Gillin, J.C., Tafalla, R., Bunney Jr, W.E. (1990) Explorations in the relationship of dream sleep to schizophrenia using positron emission tomography. *Neuropsychobiology*, **23**, 109–118.

Weiskrantz, L. (1956) Behavioral changes associated with the ablation of the amygdaloid complex in monkeys. *Journal of Comparative Physiology and Psychology*, **49**, 381–391.

West, D.J. (1948) A mass observation questionnaire on hallucinations. *Journal of the Society for Psychical Research*, **34**, 187–196.

West, L.J. (1975) A clinical and theoretical overview of hallucinatory phenomena. In: *Hallucinations: Behaviour, Experience and Theory* (Eds J. Seigel, L.J. West), Wiley, New York.

Wing, J.K., Cooper, J.E., Sartorius, N. (1974) *Measurement and Classification of Psychiatric Symptoms*, Cambridge University Press, Cambridge.

Wise, R., Chollet, F., Hadar, U., Friston, K., Hoofner, E., Frackowiak, R. (1991) Distribution of cortical neural networks involved in word comprehension and word retrieval. *Brain*, **114**, 1805–1817.

World Health Organisation (1992) *Schedules for Clinical Assessment in Neuropsychiatry* (SCAN), WHO, Geneva.

Young, A.H., Blackwood, D.H.R., Roxborough, H., McQueen, J.K., Martin, M.J., Kean, D. (1991) A magnetic resonance imaging study of schizophrenia. *British Journal of Psychiatry*, **158**, 58–165.

Zaidel, E. (1985) Language in the right hemisphere. In: *The Dual Brain* (Eds D.F. Benson, E. Zaidel), Guilford Press, New York.

Zuckerman, M., Cohen, N. (1964) Source of reports of visual and auditory sensations in perceptual isolation experiments. *Psychological Bulletin*, **62**, 1–20.

18

A Cognitive Basis for the Signs and Symptoms of Schizophrenia

CONNIE CAHILL and CHRIS FRITH

A FRAMEWORK FOR LINKING THE SIGNS AND SYMPTOMS OF SCHIZOPHRENIA

Eighty years on from Bleuler's (1911) coining of the term "schizophrenia" it seems that the concept still remains largely beyond our intellectual and technological grasp. Heterogeneity in the clinical presentation continues to throw up the question of whether or not the concept represents a discrete entity. The discovery of the "neuroleptic" drugs in the early 1950s has failed to produce a return in respect of our understanding of the biological substrate of the disorder. This chapter represents an attempt to come to an understanding of the signs and symptoms characteristic of schizophrenia through the application of the discipline of cognitive neuropsychology. Within this conceptual framework we propose that these signs and symptoms may be construed as reflecting abnormalities in the functioning of a small subset of cognitive processes. Rather than treating the disorder as a unitary concept, we suggest that focusing on individual signs and symptoms in their own right may prove a more efficient approach to understanding what is, or what is meant by, "schizophrenia".

THE COGNITIVE APPROACH

The basic building blocks of cognitive models are cognitive representations and processes. In general, a representation "is a theoretical object that bears an abstract resemblance to something outside itself . . . there is an isomorphism between the representation and the thing that is represented" (Baars, 1988, p. 44).

Schizophrenia: A Neuropsychological Perspective. Edited by C. Pantelis, H.E. Nelson and T.R.E. Barnes
© 1996 John Wiley & Sons Ltd

Cognitive representations therefore amount to theoretical constructs which refer to information that is coded in the brain. Cognitive processes correspond to changes in these representations. These processes underlie behaviour and experience and are described in computational or psychological terms. In putting forward theories of the signs and symptoms of schizophrenia we attempt to specify the cognitive representations and processes which could give rise to these phenomena. However, modelling schizophrenic symptoms in abstract information-processing terminology is not simply an end in itself: it is a means to an end. That end being to identify the brain processes which give rise to the symptoms of schizophrenia. Testing the validity of our model, therefore requires us to do more than test hypotheses generated by the model and assess its compatibility with other models. Ultimately, we wish to say something about how these models relate to the structure in which they operate: this implies saying something about the brain.

From the cognitive perspective, the brain and nervous system provide the medium through which the organism interacts with the environment via serial and parallel processing of information, which results in conscious experience and the organisation and control of behaviour. In the final analysis, therefore, cognitive neuropsychology has to explain how its information-processing models are realised in brain function.

In this chapter we suggest possible cognitive models for the signs and symptoms of schizophrenia, assess the evidence for these models and put forward explanations for how these models could map onto, or be actualised in, brain processes.

SIGNS AND SYMPTOMS

Persons to whom the diagnosis of schizophrenia could be applied may have very different clinical presentations. The variety in symptomatology is hinted at in the five "types" of schizophrenia specified in DSM-III-R (APA, 1987), that is, "catatonic", "disorganised", "paranoid", "undifferentiated", and "residual". For a cognitive theory of schizophrenia to "get off the ground" we have to put some conceptual order on this apparent behavioural chaos. This requires searching for some underlying abnormality (or set of abnormalities), which can account for, and accommodate, the diversity in symptomatology. There are two basic approaches to this problem, one empirically based, one theoretically based.

Liddle's correlational analysis of different symptoms in schizophrenia is a good example of the former (Liddle, 1987; see Liddle, chapter 15). This analysis suggested a segregation of symptoms into three clusters: "reality distortion" – primarily auditory hallucinations and delusions; "disorganisation" – inappropriate affect, formal thought disorder and poverty of speech content; "psychomotor poverty" – blunting of affect, poverty of speech, decreased spontaneous movement.

The theoretical approach, on the other hand, seeks to classify or organise the various symptoms along conceptual lines. A popular categorisation, suggested by Crow (1980) distinguishes "positive" and "negative" signs and symptoms. "Positive" symptoms are so called because they are present in psychosis; they are additional to usual behaviours or experiences. Examples of "positive" symptoms

Table 18.1. Classification of the signs and symptoms of schizophrenia according to Frith (1992)

Abnormal behaviour:	Negative signs	Positive signs
	Poverty of speech Social withdrawal Flattening of affect	Incoherence Incongruity of affect
Abnormal experience: (positive symptoms)	Of self	Of others
	Thought broadcast Delusions of control	Delusions of reference Paranoid delusions

include hallucinations and delusions. "Negative" symptoms are distinguished by representing an absence of a behaviour or experience, for example, flattening of affect, poverty of speech or social withdrawal.

Most importantly, as Arndt et al (1991) have pointed out, this theoretical distinction is backed up by empirical reasons for dividing symptoms along these lines; the two categories for instance demonstrate independence and a divergence of relations with other variables, such as outcome. Indeed, Crow proposed that the classification reflected differences in disease processes, "positive" symptoms being associated with dopamine overactivity while "negative" symptoms are associated with structural brain changes.

These kinds of theoretical classificatory systems are useful in that they not only have the potential to broaden our understanding, but they also stimulate the production of testable hypotheses and ever more precise models. Frith (1987) for example, developed a more comprehensive model which could resolve some of the problems inherent in Crow's (1980) formulation. He proposed that the distinction between "positive" and "negative" signs and symptoms, could be made more precise by a classification along the lines of observable signs versus experiential symptoms. This, he suggested, would provide a more clear-cut dimension that was easier to work with. This distinction can also reveal something about the nature of the deficits underlying schizophrenia. Frith's classification of the signs and symptoms of schizophrenia is detailed in Table 18.1.

Following this classification, Frith (1992) further proposed that three classes of cognitive dysfunction can account for the major signs and symptoms of schizophrenia: (i) disorders of willed action (ii) deficits in self-monitoring, and (iii) deficits in inferring the mental states of others.

COGNITIVE MODELS OF THE SIGNS AND SYMPTOMS

DISORDERS OF WILLED ACTION (ABNORMAL SIGNS)

William James (1890) defined willed action as "an action that we consciously and deliberately choose from among a number of possibilities". It stands in contrast

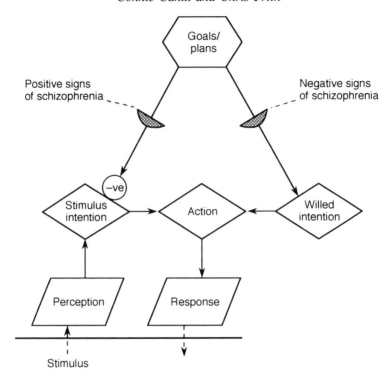

Figure 18.1. The two routes to action. Two routes: (i) Stimulus-driven action: stimulus perception
– stimulus-driven intention – action; (ii) willed action: goals/plans – willed intention – action.
Two disconnections are shown: (i) goals fail to generate intentions producing "negative" features
(e.g. poverty of action); (ii) goals fail to inhibit stimulus-driven actions producing "positive" features (e.g. incoherence of action, perseveration)

to another class of action familiar to us, that is action of an automatic nature.
Evidence for automatic action can be found in the slips of action, familiar to us
all, whereby we find ourselves engaging in an unintended – though often highly
overlearned and context-appropriate – act (such as driving to a friends previous
address). Typically, in these instances one's mind is preoccupied with some other
thought (Reason, 1984).

Frith (1987) outlines a general model of action, which incorporates both these
types of action, and details how a number of signs and symptoms of schizophrenia may reflect dysfunctions in this action system (see Figure 18.1). Central
to the analysis, are the two routes to action: one stimulus-driven (i.e. automatic),
one internally driven (i.e. self-initiated or "willed").

We propose that patients with "negative" signs, specifically poverty of action
and poverty of speech, have a specific deficit concerning the production of
"internally generated", or "willed", action. They do, however, remain capable of
stimulus-driven responses.

How this problem will manifest itself will depend on the kind of response that is acceptable in the circumstances. It is suggested that a breakdown in the ability to generate action internally can result in three distinct patterns of behaviour. In the first case, the person does nothing, that is, they fail to emit spontaneous behaviour. Second, stimulus-driven responses may be elicited, though they may be inappropriate in the particular context. This is what Luria (1973) described as "inert stereotypies". Finally, they can simply repeat previous actions, though again, they are likely to be inappropriate in a new context. Thus, the same underlying deficit can give rise to different observable behaviours. These kinds of behaviour patterns are seen in schizophrenic patients and would be considered indicators of "negative" signs. DSM-III-R for example, refers to "reduction in spontaneous movements and activity" and "excited motor activity, apparently purposeless" (1987, p. 117).

Supporting Evidence

There is a long history of experimental research suggesting that patients with schizophrenia can be "captured" by the immediate details of stimuli, even when the resultant response is inappropriate in the wider context (e.g. Salzinger et al, 1978). This kind of behaviour reflects a deficit in "willed" action. Unfortunately, the thrust of schizophrenia research in the past has been to study schizophrenic patients as a group, with little or no attempt at a finer-grain analysis relating symptom profile to patterns of performance.

Frith & Done (1983) went some way towards this in their analysis of stereotypy in patients with schizophrenia and consequently were able to report differential performance in patients with "positive" and "negative" symptoms. In their task, a two-choice guessing paradigm, subjects are presented with two filled-in squares on a computer monitor. They are told that one of the squares conceals a cross and their task was to guess or work out where the cross would be on each trial. Feedback as to the correct location is given after each choice is made. Normal subjects typically respond with a random sequence (i.e. "left"s and "right"s). Stereotyped behaviour is defined as occurring when the current response made by the subject can be predicted from their previous responses; typically, it takes the forms of perseveration (i.e. L,L,L,L,) or regular alternations (i.e. L,R,L,R,L,R,L). Frith and Done found the performance of chronic schizophrenic subjects with negative signs to be characterised by perseverative responses, while alternations were seen in patients with negative signs at an earlier stage of the illness. Similar results have been obtained by Lyon et al (1986).

Clearly, this is a task in which the subject has minimal help in choosing the next response and is therefore highly dependent upon their defining the output. As such it is very much an "internally generated"/"willed" response mode, and the results (cited above) point towards a link between "negative" signs and problems in the control of "internally generated"/"willed" action.

As noted above, the theory also predicts that these same subjects, that is, patients exhibiting poverty and perseveration, would not have difficulties with stimulus-driven behaviour. Ironically, Frith obtained data in support of this while making a second attempt on eliciting stereotyped behaviour in another version of the above task. In the new version, the subject has to dodge "enemy" space ships. Again the subject has a choice – to go left or right. If the "wrong" choice is made there is a collision and explosion, whereas if the "correct" choice is made the ship passes by harmlessly. Interestingly, it became apparent that in this new version of the task the behaviour of both patients and controls is strongly influenced by the outcome of the previous trial. If a collision occurred in a trial the subject would go in the opposite direction on the next trial and, conversely, if there was no collision they would dodge in the same direction. Thus, the new version of the task became a test of stimulus-driven behaviour as the outcome of the previous trial determined the response emitted in the current trial. Consistent with his theory, Frith found that schizophrenic patients exhibiting negative signs showed the normal stimulus-elicited pattern of performance, even though the same patients showed perseverative behaviour on the original two-choice guessing task.

The model proposed here is consistent with Shallice's (1988) more general cognitive model of how actions are selected and executed. In fact this model was developed to explain the kinds of behaviours observed in patients with frontal lobe lesions. According to this theory, actions may be emitted either as a direct result of a process he terms "contention scheduling", or as a result of the action of a "Supervisory Attentional System" (SAS). "Contention scheduling" refers to the process whereby actions triggered by environmental stimuli compete for access to the execution system, purely on the basis of level of activation. This system is therefore only capable of what has been termed stimulus-driven action. In the absence of environmental signals no behaviour is emitted, or perseveration may occur. Such a "low-level" system is capable of exhibiting relatively complex behaviours so long as they have been completely specified by the environment or context. It is the SAS component of Shallice's model which allows for the initiation of action that is not entirely specified by the environmental input. This corresponds to "willed actions" in terms of the model above. The SAS in effect modulates the "contention scheduling" system; it can modify the strengths of the competing actions, activate a particular system in the absence of an appropriate stimulus, suppress automatic responses and most importantly, generate actions in situations for which no routine act exists. Thus, in terms of this model "negative" signs could arise as a result of a failure in the SAS: leaving the patient capable of emitting only stimulus-driven behaviour.

DEFICITS IN SELF-MONITORING

Any explanation of schizophrenia must, at some point, account for the "1st rank" (Schneider, 1959) symptoms of auditory hallucinations, thought insertion and thought withdrawal. Frith (1987) proposes that a number of these symptoms may share the one cognitive basis, namely, a deficit in self-monitoring.

The self-monitoring system described by Frith is a hypothetical process the function of which is to discriminate events which are internally generated from those which are external in origin. It can operate at two levels: First, the relationship between actions and external events is monitored in order to distinguish

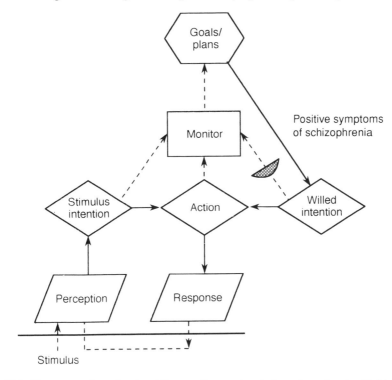

Figure 18.2. The monitoring of action. The monitor receives information about willed intentions, stimulus intentions and selected actions. One disconnection is shown: When information concerning willed intentions is unavailable to the monitor, actions are not felt to be under the subject's control. This experience may be expressed in the form of a delusion of control

events caused by our own actions and those which result from the actions of other agents; second, intentions to act are monitored so that we may distinguish "willed" actions (i.e. those resulting from our own goals and plans) and "stimulus-driven" actions (i.e. automatic responses to external stimuli). Such monitoring is essential if we are to have awareness of the causes of our actions. Figure 18.2 illustrates how this monitoring system relates to the model of action presented in Figure 18.1. According to this model, schizophrenic patients' misattribution of their own "willed" actions to outside agents represents a failure of the self-monitoring mechanism.

Hallucinations: A Failure of Self-monitoring

Hallucinations may occur in any of the five senses and also with somatic sensation. However, we will concern ourselves with auditory verbal hallucinations, the most common form of hallucination reported in schizophrenia. Before coming to hallucinations proper, however, it is important to consider the differential diagnosis of hallucination, which distinguishes illusions from pseudohallucinations. Illusions were separated phenomenologically from hallucinations by Esquirol (1838). He described illusions as transformations of perceptions, engendered by a confluence of the subject's fantasy and natural perception.

Pseudohallucinations, described by Kandinskii (1890) as a separate form of perception from true hallucination, are in general recognised by the subject as having no external correlate. Though the image may seem to be reasonably well defined it is always located in subjective space and perceived with the "inner eye" or "inner ear" (Sims, 1988). The distinguishing feature of a true hallucination, therefore, is that it is experienced subjectively as similar to a normal percept. Typically, patients do not doubt the reality of their hallucinatory percepts.

These phenomenological distinctions clearly suggest that hallucinations are not simply misperceptions; that is to say they are not derived from external stimuli. Indeed, research examining auditory discrimination and bias in schizophrenic subjects generally supports this view. For example, Done & Frith (in preparation) used a lexical decision task to test the hypothesis that any bias must be towards perceiving sounds as words, and should be most apparent when the sounds are most word-like. Subjects had to decide whether or not computer-generated phoneme strings – some real words, some word-like – were in fact real words. They found no evidence to indicate schizophrenic patients with hallucinations had a bias for perceiving non-words as words. On the other hand, Bentall & Slade (1985) obtained results to the opposite effect. They asked their subjects to listen to auditory stimuli, half of which were noise and half were the word "who". Hallucinating patients frequently claimed to hear the word "who" in the "noise" trials as well as in the "signal" trials.

It would seem that we can safely conclude that hallucinations are entirely internal in origin but somehow they are experienced as being external. This kind of experience can be accounted for by the model above in terms of a failure of the verbal self-monitoring system. According to this explanation, hallucinations can arise when that system, which normally identifies an internally generated verbal stimulus as such, fails to do so. The subjective experience of such an event would be of a verbal experience not initiated by the patient. That is to say the experience would lack the usual, "normal" "feeling of intendedness" associated with a willed act.

This theoretical explanation of hallucinations belongs to the tradition which considers that hallucinations result from a failure of some form of "reality discrimination" (see for example, Bentall et al, 1991; Heilbrun, 1980; Sarbin, 1967). In a similar vein, Hoffman (1986) proposed that hallucinators might wrongly infer that "unintended" subvocalisations originate from an external source and would therefore experience them as auditory hallucinations. This deduction is based on Hoffman's more general hypothesis that schizophrenics suffer from a disorder of discourse planning (Hoffman et al, 1982). Such a disorder he argues would give rise to "unintended subvocalisation" which, by virtue of being unintended, would be classified as alien. It is reassuring to find that these theories have much in common with that presented here (see also Nayani and David, chapter 17).

However, this formal model needs raw material with which to work. An obvious candidate is "inner speech", that is, verbal thought or subvocalisation. Kandinskii (1890) was the first to suggest that there might be a relationship between inner speech and hallucinations. Since then a number of investigators have formulated theories based on such a link. Johnson (1978), for example, argued that a disorder of the inner speech mechanism might lead to the misattribution of verbal thought to an external source.

Supporting Evidence

Experimental studies of these kinds of hypotheses have understandably focused on the possible role of subvocalisation in the experience of hallucinations. For example, Gould (1949) investigated a schizophrenic patient who experienced hallucinations almost continuously. This patient had been observed to make barely audible sounds in her nose and mouth. Gould amplified these sounds and found them to be whispered speech which was qualitatively different from the patients usual whispers yet similar, in terms of content, to the patients hallucinations. He concluded that the subvocal speech provided the basis for this patient's hallucinations.

More convincing data was provided by Inouye & Shimizu (1966), who recorded activity from four speech muscles in nine patients with schizophrenia. The patients were required to press a switch whenever they experienced an hallucination. Significantly more vocal activity was recorded at this time compared to the time period when they were simply asked to press the switch on a random basis. However, these data are merely correlational and Lindsley (1963) has argued that the vocalisations in fact represent patients responding to their hallucinations. Bick & Kinsbourne (1987) therefore attempted to examine the question experimentally. These investigators argued that getting hallucinating patients to engage in a mouth opening manoeuvre would occupy the speech musculature and, consequently, hallucinations would no longer be possible. The results did appear to support this notion. However, Green & Kinsbourne (1989) failed to replicate these results, though they did find that humming significantly reduced the time spent hallucinating.

However, it is also possible for sub-vocal speech to occur in the absence of any detectable sound or muscle activity. Take for instance, the "articulatory loop" of Baddeley (1986). This loop is primarily used for the temporary, short-term storage of verbal material. Baddeley contends that this loop relies on "central speech control codes which appear to be able to function in the absence of peripheral feed-back" (1986, p. 107). Baddeley & Lewis (1981) elaborated on this further by proposing that the phonological coding of visually presented material depends on two processes: the inner voice and the inner ear. The inner voice corresponds to the articulatory loop requiring subvocal speech, whilst the inner ear holds some form of acoustic image. Based on this model, Frith (1992) has suggested that if hallucinations result from an abnormality of these central speech processes, then hallucinations should interfere with tasks involving phonological coding (and vice versa). They would also have differential effects on verbal and visual digit span. Preliminary tests of this hypothesis are reported by David (1994).

One experimental paradigm which comes close to being able to test the hypotheses concerning self-monitoring is that described by Johnson & Raye (1981) as a test of "reality monitoring". This paradigm was applied by Bentall et al (1991), who asked hallucinating psychiatric patients, patients with delusions but no history of hallucinations and normal controls to generate answers to "easy" or "difficult" clues (e.g. "Think of a type of dwelling beginning with the letter H" . . . "Think of a fruit beginning with the letter T") and to listen to low or high probability paired associates (e.g. "A country – Norway" ... "A type of footwear – shoe"). After a period of 1 week the subjects were presented with a list in which their answers to the clues were mixed with the associates and with words not previously presented. Their objective was to identify the source of each item, that is, "self", "presented by the experimenter" or "new". Bentall and colleagues had predicted that hallucinators would misattribute more of their thoughts to the experimenter than the controls. However, only one difference emerged between hallucinators and controls: when errors were examined the hallucinators attributed more self-generated high cognitive effort words to the experimenter. Bentall and co-workers suggested this reflected a bias in the hallucinators towards attributing an event to an external source rather than to themselves in cases where they are uncertain.

In the light of the theory proposed here, we would suggest that high cognitive effort items are, under normal conditions, associated with relatively high "feeling of intendedness". It is presumably some trace of this component which is accessed by this task. However, if the system underlying this function is compromised from the outset (what one might call the encoding stage), hallucinators will have little or no such trace to draw on when asked to decide whether an item was self-generated or not.

Delusions of Control: A Failure of Self-monitoring

Sometimes called "passivity phenomena", delusions of control are characterised by the expression of a belief that one's behaviour is not under one's own control but is in some way affected by other agents. The reports are classified as delusions because they appear to reflect an abnormal belief. However, it is also possible that the primary disturbance is an abnormal experience. That patients can only describe these experiences in the vaguest terms, or at the highest level (that is as a belief), may be explained by the fact that many experiences are exceedingly difficult to describe. (As an exercise one might try to describe the experience of the tip-of-the-tongue phenomena.) We have over time developed vocabularies or expressions for common, normal experiences, but the schizophrenic patient has to try to come up with verbal expressions to describe the most abnormal and novel experiences. Not surprisingly, there is great temptation for the busy psychiatrist to help him/her along in their efforts, by providing the vocabulary which has evolved in psychiatry.

Frith (1992) has argued that the impairment which gives rise to these phenomena is fundamentally the same as that underlying hallucinations. Here too internally generated action is misattributed to a foreign agent, representing a failure of that process which labels actions as either internal or external in origin.

This explanation of certain "positive" symptoms stands in contrast to that for "negative" signs: "negative" signs arise from a complete failure of the mechanism for "willed" actions, whereas, in the case of "positive" symptoms actions are "internally generated" but there is a failure in the mechanism for monitoring the origin of these acts.

Supporting Evidence

At least two experiments have found evidence of faulty monitoring in schizophrenia (Malenka et al, 1982; Frith & Done, 1989). Both these studies examined error correction, with particular attention being paid to correction in the absence of the usual (visual) feedback. It is known that normal subjects can make very rapid error corrections in a situation in which external feedback is absent (Rabbitt, 1966; Megaw, 1972). This may be achieved through the monitoring of intentions, so that subjects can be aware that an intended response was wrong after that response has been initiated, but before the consequences of that response are visible.

Malenka and colleagues (1982) found that schizophrenic subjects were less likely than normal and alcoholic people to correct their errors in the absence of visual feedback. In a very similar task disguised as a video game (Frith & Done, 1989) confirmed that acute schizophrenic patients corrected their errors normally when visual feedback was supplied but often failed to do so when the same feedback was absent. Most notable, was the observation that this deficit was restricted to patients with passivity experiences.

Mlakar (et al, 1994) used a different technique to study central monitoring of actions in schizophrenic subjects. This paradigm required subjects to copy simple geometric designs onto a computer screen via either a joystick or direction keys. In one condition, the "feed-back" condition, the results of their movements appeared on the VDU, while in the second – "self monitor" – condition there was no such display. They found that schizophrenic patients with first rank symptoms were much more impaired than other schizophrenic patients in the "self monitor" condition.

DEFICITS IN INFERRING THE MENTAL STATES OF OTHERS

We have already referred to a deficit in monitoring one's own mental processes. We will now refer to a deficit in inferring the mental states of other individuals, which Frith (1992) suggests may account for a different set of "positive" symptoms, including paranoid delusions, delusions of reference and third person auditory hallucinations.

Evidence for a discrete cognitive system for such a function comes from two sources: developmental psychology and recent research on autism. The ability to represent the intentions and beliefs of other people has been extensively studied by developmental psychologists (Astington & Gopnik, 1991). This ability it seems does not emerge until four years of age and is crucial for the development of a "theory of mind". It is this ability which has been found lacking in autism (Baron-Cohen et al, 1985). Without this ability the young child, and the autistic child, cannot handle the possibility that another person has a false belief. Such a child is also incapable of deliberate lying or deception.

However, because the onset of schizophrenia typically occurs in early adulthood, whereas autism is almost certainly present from birth, we would expect that the failure of such a system would lead to qualitatively different behavioural abnormalities in the two conditions.

Paranoia

One must assume (given the lack of evidence to the contrary) that adult schizophrenic patients, in contrast to autistic children or adults, have experienced relatively normal early cognitive development. As a consequence, they will continue trying to use this ability. However, if their ability to represent the contents of other people's minds is compromised they are likely to make errors in their assessments of the intentional states of others. Should they find that they are completely unable to "read" or infer others intentions, they may start to believe that people are deliberately behaving in such a way as to disguise their thoughts or feelings; they may indeed come to the conclusion that there is a conspiracy against them.

Ideas of Reference

Frith (1992) proposes that abnormalities in the recognition of ostensive signals in communication, a subset in the repertoire of behaviours which enables one to infer the mental states of others, can account for a "positive" symptom known as "delusion of reference". The characteristic feature of this symptom is that patients falsely believe that events have special significance for them. In some cases this refers to things other people have said. A well-known example is the patient who believes that verbal output from the television or radio has some special meaning for her/him. Ostensive signals indicate that a person wishes to initiate a communication (Sperber & Wilson, 1986). Were patients to see ostensive signals where none existed, one would have a basis for the kind of delusion described here. Patients would be expecting a communication and the usual, normal processes of understanding a communication would be brought into play.

At this point we would predict that one of two things may happen, depending on the patients state of mind. If this experience occurs in the context of a relatively "normal" belief system, the patient may experience what is termed "delusional mood". That is, he comes to believe that something strange is going on, yet he is not quite sure what. Further down the line, were a patient to hold abnormal beliefs, these are likely to get drawn into his interpretation of this experience, giving rise to the often bizarre meanings which feature in these particular kinds of delusions.

Third Person Auditory Hallucinations

The theoretical account given for the failure of "mind reading" in autism is based on a distinction between two kinds of mental (cognitive) representations: "first order" (or "primary") representations and "second order" (or "meta-") representations. Primary representations correspond to literal representations of the world; they represent the physical environment in as accurate and faithful a way as possible. Perceptions are an example of such representations. Meta-representations refer to knowledge about the more basic primary representations. Their function would seem to be to enable us to manipulate the primary representations. Meta-representations therefore are always characterised by having at least two components – a content component and a functional component. Thus, while "I know the sky is blue" and "You believe the sky is blue" both have the same content (i.e. "the sky is blue"), their form is different. This distinction is central to Frith's (1992) explanation of third person auditory hallucinations.

Frith proposes that the content component of the whole proposition may become detached, forming a free-floating notion, which may be experienced as a third person auditory hallucination. So, for example, were a patient ("X") to hold the proposition "my mother thinks 'X is a wretched nuisance'", when he thinks of his mother, the statement "X is a wretched nuisance" may come into his mind.

As yet there is no experimental evidence in support of the idea that some schizophrenic symptoms arise because of abnormalities in processes by which the mental states of others are inferred. However, a wide range of techniques have been developed for studying these processes in children. A number of studies are currently under way in which these techniques are being adapted for use with schizophrenic subjects. For example, in the study by Frith & Corcoran (1996) subjects had to make inferences about the mental states of characters in stories. Patients in remission had no problems with this task, but patients with paranoid delusions had specific difficulties with making such inferences.

Language Disorders in Schizophrenia

In her classic study of schizophrenic language Andreasen (1979) identified many abnormal features of schizophrenic verbal behaviour including: "poverty" of speech, derailment, loss of goal, perseveration, tangentiality and incoherence. Indeed, disorders of language and speech are well documented, and probably the most-researched aspect of behaviour in schizophrenia (see McGrath, chapter 10). It is also one of the more problematic symptoms, involving as it does one of the most long-standing unresolved issues in psychology (and philosophy), that is the nature of the relationship between language and thought. Thus, the abnormal speech observed in schizophrenia is frequently labelled "thought disorder". However, this assumption remains unproven, and we would emphasise that language is not simply the expression of thoughts, rather it is the expression of thoughts in a manner designed to communicate these thoughts to others.

There is now a considerable body of evidence which suggests that the deficit in the language domain in schizophrenia is confined to the level of speech output, receptive functions remaining intact (with the single exception perhaps of ideas of reference) (see Cohen, 1978; Andreasen et al, 1985; Frith & Allen, 1988; McGrath, 1991). Cohen (1976) elegantly demonstrated the contrast in receptive and expressive verbal abilities of schizophrenic subjects. He asked volunteers to describe a coloured disk in such a way that a listener would be able to identify that disk in an array of different disks. The results were very clear: communication failed only when it was a schizophrenic patient who was describing the disk. The same patient, however, has no difficulty in using the description provided by the normal volunteer.

We propose that, as with other symptom groups, such as delusions, the general classification belies a heterogeneity which may yield to understanding when a finer analysis is applied. We suggest that there are disorders of language corresponding to each of the abnormalities we have discussed in this chapter so far.

Thus, a failure to suppress inappropriate associations, reflecting a general impairment in "willed" actions, may well explain the derailment, distractible speech and clanging components of schizophrenic speech output. Incoherence and "loss of goal" on the other hand, may reflect a general failure to edit speech as a result of a failure to monitor internally what is to be spoken. In this case, patients would only be able to monitor their speech via peripheral feedback, that is, after they had spoken. Leudar and colleagues (1994) have found some evidence of this in studying "self-repair" in the communications of patients with schizophrenia. Though patients used self-repair as often as controls, in many cases their attempts were inadequate and did not actually improve the quality of the communication.

Cohen's reports (cited above) would also be consistent with such an analysis. He observed that his patients did not simply or rapidly emit a nondiscriminating response and then stop. Rather, he wrote: "There is a futile, but still persisting struggle to communicate adequately."

Finally, patients may fail in communication because of the third class of cognitive dysfunction referred to above, that is because of a difficulty in taking into account the knowledge of the listener in constructing their output. Rutter (1985) noted this feature in his analysis of conversations between schizophrenic patients and nurses as a problem in "the social process of taking the role of the other". This may be expressed at the syntactical level by the lack of sufficient use of what Rochester & Martin (1979) termed cohesive ties and referents. The function of these syntactical elements is to increase efficiency in communication – primarily by reducing reiteration of information already known to the listener. Frith & Allen (1988) reported that schizophrenic patients frequently fail to use such referents correctly.

BRAIN SYSTEMS UNDERLYING THESE COGNITIVE DEFICITS

Having produced cognitive theories concerning the signs and symptoms of schizophrenia it is incumbent upon us to suggest how these theories might be expressed in terms of brain function. Three deficits have been put forward to explain a variety of symptoms characteristic of schizophrenia. We have attempted to explain these deficits in terms of more general systems, namely, "action" systems, "self-monitoring" systems, "meta-representational" systems. Because these are new theories and have not yet been examined directly in patients we will draw on research in the fields of clinical neuropsychology and animal behaviour. As data relevant to the inferencing of mental states is as yet limited this section will be confined to a discussion of the action and "self-monitoring" systems (but see Fletcher et al, 1995).

The Regulation of Action

Central to the theses is a distinction between "willed" and "stimulus-driven" action. Gary Goldberg (1985) has reviewed the evidence for a physiological basis for two such action routes, that is, one stimulus-driven, one internally driven. He suggests that there is a medial system for "willed" actions and a lateral system for stimulus-elicited actions. He argues that the main structures involved in willed actions are dorsolateral prefrontal cortex, anterior cingulate, supplementary motor area (SMA) and basal ganglia, and makes the point that the SMA in particular, has an important role to play in "the development of the intention-to-act and the specification and elaboration of action through its mediation between medial limbic cortex and primary motor cortex". This formulation is broadly consistent with Passingham's (1987) experimental work on the control of action in monkeys.

It is also worth noting the work of Alexander et al (1986) concerning their generalised schema of basal ganglia–thalamocortical loops. This conceptual framework of segregated functional circuits identifies, amongst others, a "motor loop" in which multiple overlapping corticostriate inputs from motor and somato-sensory areas project to the putamen, thence to the globus pallidus and substantia nigra, and finally, to the ventrolateral nucleus of the thalamus from which fibres project back to SMA (see also Pantelis and Brewer, chapter 16).

There is strong evidence implicating changes in reaction time performance to the operation of frontal–striatal circuitry (Goldberg, 1985; Alivisados & Milner, 1989) and significantly, these deficits have been attributed to impairments in the mechanism by which stimuli of internal origin activate behaviour (Brown & Marsden, 1988; Robbins & Brown, 1990; cited in Robbins 1991).

For a model of stimulus-driven action we draw upon the work of Glickstein & Stein (1991), who have formulated a theory of stimulus-driven behaviour to account for what they call "paradoxical" movement in Parkinson's disease. This refers to the astonishing ability of motorically disabled Parkinson's disease patients to perform rapid, accurate and even skilled movements under certain, often intensely emotional circumstances, such as, responding to a fire alarm. They suggest that this may be explained by the fact that visual pathways relaying information regarding rapidly moving targets project directly to the cerebellum via the pontine nuclei, bypassing the basal ganglia system. Furthermore, they point out that in addition to visual input that there are also somatosensory and auditory projections to the cerebellum via the pontine nuclei.

With the advent of functional brain imaging it has become possible to examine experimentally the neurological substrates of the various classes of motor responses. Frith and colleagues (1991), for instance, designed an experiment using the positron emission tomography (PET) technique, with the aim of explicating the different brain systems involved in "stimulus-driven" and "willed" actions. Three conditions (i.e. activations) were employed: "shadowing" – subjects simply repeat words read out loud to them as they heard them; "opposites" – subjects are required to say the opposite word to that said to them, for example, "hot – cold"; "verbal fluency" – subjects respond with a word beginning with the letter 'F' when they hear the word "next". These three tasks differ in the degree to which the responses required of the subject are specified or limited by the stimulus. Responses in the "shadowing" condition are clearly entirely determined by the input and are therefore considered "stimulus-driven". This is also the case to some extent in the "opposites" condition. Although the task does require semantic analysis, it is still the case that the responses are largely determined by the input as the stimuli chosen were all highly associated with single unambiguous opposites. By contrast, in the "verbal fluency" condition responses are minimally specified. This task was associated with activation of the left dorsolateral prefrontal cortex (DLPFC) and anterior cingulate and a reduction of regional cerebral blood flow in superior temporal areas. It was concluded that a particular area of DLPFC is activated when responses have not been sufficiently specified or constrained by the stimulus.

Thus, animal and human experimental data point towards a significant role for the frontal cortex in the generation of "willed" action. This is consistent with our knowledge of frontal lobe functions based on observations and data obtained from clinical neurological cases. "Clinical wisdom", for instance, distinguishes two personality syndromes: The "dorsolateral", "pseudoretarded" or "pseudode-pressed" group, characterised by apathy, lethargy and lack of spontaneity; and the "orbitofrontal" "pseudopsychopathic" group, displaying sexual disinhibition, increased motor activity and inappropriate social and personal behaviour (see Stuss & Benson, 1983). Disorders of "willed" action, reflected in the inability to generate new or appropriate actions also feature in more controlled tests of cognitive functioning in these individuals. Milner's (1964) classic paper demon-strating perseverative behaviour on the Wisconsin Card Sorting Test in patients with dorsolateral prefrontal damage is one such example. A most informative neurological condition for our purposes is the "alien hand" syndrome. This syndrome, first reported by Goldstein (1908), is characterised by the patient's experience of movement of their hand without the feeling of having intended it to move. Frequently, the movements of the "alien" hand are contrary to the patient's intentions and the normal hand acts to restrain the "alien" one. It is notable that the kinds of movements performed by the "alien" hand are often "stimulus-driven", for example, on seeing a cup on a table the patient automati-cally reaches for it. Frith (1992) has suggested that these kinds of actions are not normally accompanied by a "feeling of intendedness". Such a feeling occurs only when an action is deliberately permitted, that is, in a situation where it could have been deliberately suppressed. Patients with the "alien hand" syndrome appear to have suffered damage to that part of the brain which normally permits or suppresses, stimulus-elicited actions. Therefore, the identification of the neuro-pathological substrate of this syndrome as either medial frontal or callosal (Feinberg et al, 1992) represents further support for the notion of a frontal neuro-physiological basis for "willed" action.

"Self-monitoring" Systems

Central to the account of "positive" symptoms is the notion of a system which distinguishes self-generated actions from those of external origin. We must now ask, is this a viable model in terms of brain function?

That the experience of an intention to act represents a distinct cognitive function capable of being mapped onto a discrete brain system seems, at first sight, an improbable proposition. In fact the notion of the existence of some physiological system capable of mediating this kind of function has been around for quite some time in the form of the concept of "corollary discharge". The phenomenon was first described as "intensity of the effort of will" by von Helmholtz (1866) following his observation that one is able to distinguish between movement on the retina due to movement in the world from movement due to our own, that is self-initiated, eye movements. This later came to be conceptualised as a feed-forward or internal feedback system (see Evarts, 1971; McKay, 1966), though precisely how this is achieved is still a matter of considerable debate. An explanation along the lines suggested here would posit that an input into an effector mechanism could be used to monitor our intention to move our eyes; the information in the input would be used in the calculation of displacement and compensation. Interestingly, Feinberg (1978) suggested that monitoring mechanisms like "corollary discharge" apply not only to overt movements of limbs and eyes but also to covert actions such as thinking. In this case the corollary discharges accompanying these higher order functions would "correspond to nothing less than the experience of will or intention".

Furthermore, recent research in neuropsychology also suggests that this notion is not as far-fetched as it may seem. The well-documented neuropsychological case studies reporting dissociations between access or use of information and subjective awareness, that is consciousness, of that information have shown that understanding entirely subjective experiences in terms of their functional brain correlates is, at the very least, a legitimate enterprise (Milner & Rugg, 1992). These studies of consciousness are requiring ever more detailed analyses of what is meant by consciousness in various specific situations and some of these analyses are not unlike those offered above. For instance, Frith (1992) considers that the "feeling of intention" to act is akin to Bauer's (1984) "feeling of familiarity". Bauer suggests that the loss of such a function can explain the dissociation between face identification and face recognition reported in a number of cases of prosopagnosia (see, for example, De Haan et al, 1987). He also suggests that each of these functions could be mediated by different pathways (see also Ellis and Young, chapter 19).

Our task therefore is to delineate a possible physiological mechanism for the "feeling of intendedness". Recent work by Fried et al (1991; cited in Kiyoshi,

1992) indicates this may be a function of the supplementary motor area. In a systematic stimulation study in patients with intractable seizures, arrays of surface electrodes placed on the medial surface of the cerebral cortex dorsal to the cingulate sulcus were used to examine the issue of somatotopy in human SMA. They report that preliminary sensations of the "urge" to perform a movement, or an anticipation that some movements were about to occur, were elicited. They propose therefore that the human SMA is involved in the intention to perform a motor activity. Clearly, they also observed a specific feeling associated with this intention.

Unfortunately, human case studies severely limit our making advances in delineating discrete anatomical systems involved in cognitive constructs. In this situation we must consult the literature on animal studies to provide us with more detailed and reliable information.

At the most basic level, the "self-monitoring" system is necessary to enable us to distinguish between events which have been caused by our own actions, as opposed to those which have external causes. It is significant, therefore, that Robinson & Wurtz (1976) identified cells in the superficial layer of the superior colliculus of the rhesus monkey which can apparently distinguish between real and self-induced movement, as relayed in the visual system. These cells respond to rapid stimulus movements, but do not respond when the monkey moves his eye past a stationary stimulus. This is in marked contrast to the functioning of cells in the striate cortex which do not respond differentially in this manner to stimulus movement. These investigators concluded that the input to the superior colliculus that permits the detection of real stimulus movement is a "corollary discharge" from some part of the oculomotor system and they tentatively identify the frontal eye field as the most likely source of this information.

Ploog (1979) has suggested that a similar system permits the monkey to distinguish self-generated and externally produced vocalisations. In support of this, Müller-Preuss (1978) identified cells in the auditory cortex of the squirrel monkey which respond to loudspeaker transmitted vocalisations, but not to self-produced vocalisations. Ploog argues that this could be achieved through an inhibition of these cells initiated during self-produced calling. This formulation is consistent with the theory advanced by Müller-Preuss & Jürgens (1976) to the effect that the cingulate cortex is the source of "willed" vocalisations. These investigators demonstrated the existence of connections from this structure not only to the monkey analogue of Broca's area, but also auditory association areas associated with speech perception (Brodmann's area 22).

Clearly, these animal studies also have their particular limitations. They do not, for instance, permit us to study subjective experiences, such as the feeling of intention. They do, however, strongly suggest that the "internal origin/external origin" dimension to events or actions may well be realised in brain organisation and function. Furthermore, they are consistent with the human data in implicating anterior brain structures (in these cases the frontal eye fields and anterior cingulate cortex) as possible sources of "corollary discharges" which may be responsible for distinguishing self-generated from externally generated perceptions.

IN CONCLUSION: A UNIFIED THEORY OF "POSITIVE" AND "NEGATIVE" SYMPTOMS

We are provided with the possibility of developing a general theory of the wide range of signs and symptoms reported in schizophrenia by the fact that there are two recurring features in the speculations presented above. First, the repeated references to the more anterior brain structures (in particular the prefrontal cortex) and second, the distributed nature of the systems (see Figure 18.3).

The anatomically oriented data we have reviewed appears to support the notion of a special role for the anterior brain structures in the initiation of willed actions. However, it is also the case that the anterior structures are merely functional

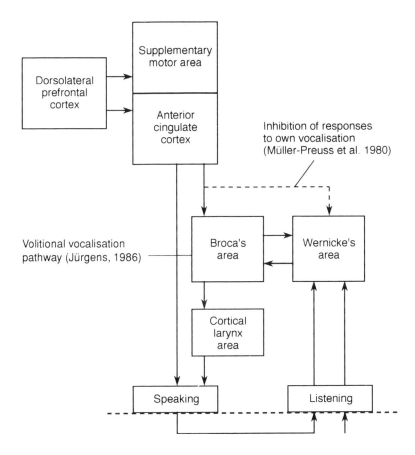

Figure 18.3. A possible brain system underlying various aspects of vocalisations. Damage to the "volitional vocalisation system" (Jürgens, 1986) might lead to negative features like poverty of speech. Damage to the "corollary discharge" from anterior cingulate to Wernicke's area (Müller-Preuss et al, 1980) might lead to auditory hallucinations, since responses to self-generated vocalisations would no longer be suppressed

components of more complex cortico-subcortical loop systems. Furthermore, anatomical studies have shown many reciprocal connections between prefrontal cortex and various other areas of association cortex. Such a system could provide the basis for a range of "self-monitoring" systems.

"Negative" signs and symptoms are hypothesised as representing a failure in a particular branch of the willed action system. This kind of deficit is generally readily observable in the reduced, or repetitive, or inappropriate behaviour of the patient. The most likely candidate as the brain structure with the most significant input into this function would appear to be the supplementary motor area and the anterior cingulate cortex. "Self-monitoring" – the labelling of internally generated actions as such – may be considered a sub-component of the willed action system. The failure of self-monitoring described above may be explained by a disconnection of (as yet unidentified) frontal structures (whose role it is to send "corollary discharges" to the relevant posterior structures) from their target structures (see McGuire et al, 1995; Friston & Frith, 1995). This results in the abnormal experience of one's behaviour lacking a feeling of being intended.

It is a prerequisite of this hypothesis that those structures responsible for the initiation of "willed" actions are intact. This formulation would therefore seem to imply that persons experiencing "negative" symptoms could not also experience "positive" symptoms. Were no "willed" action initiated there would be no actions to misattribute to an external agent. However, it is possible that we are not dealing with an "all or nothing" dysfunction. It is likely for instance that these systems would be modulated by neurotransmitter interactions which may be subject to significant alterations in function.

More realistically, however, we might have to accept that our best efforts at understanding the signs and symptoms of schizophrenia fall more than a little short of the mark. To think otherwise would probably amount to a delusion. We remain convinced however that the particular approach adopted here, that is a cognitive neuropsychological approach, is one which offers promise. It has distinct advantages: it requires one to think in terms of underlying cognitive processes; it facilitates the generation of testable hypotheses; it challenges one to make an attempt to understand how hypothetical cognitive processes might be effected in brain function. Understanding schizophrenia is going to require all this and more.

REFERENCES

Alexander, G.E., DeLong, M., Strick, P.E. (1986) Parallel organisation of functionally segregated circuits linking basal ganglia and cortex. *Annual Review of Neuroscience*, **9**, 357–381.

Alivisados, B., Milner, B. (1989) Effect of temporal or frontal leucotomy on the use of advance information in a choice reaction time task. *Neurospsychologia*, **27**, 495–503.

American Psychiatric Association (1987) *Quick Reference to the Diagnostic Criteria from DSM-III-R*, APA, Washington, DC.

Andreasen, N.C. (1979) Thought, language, and communication disorders: I. Clinical assessment, definition of terms, and assessment of their reliability. *Archives of General Psychiatry*, **36**, 1315–1321.

Andreasen, N.C., Hoffman, R., Grove, W.M. (1985) Mapping abnormalities in language and cognition. In: *Controversies in Schizophrenia: Changes and Constancies* (Ed. A. Alpert), Guilford Press, New York.

Arndt, S., Alliger, R.J., Andreasen, N.C. (1991) The distinction of positive and negative symptoms: The failure of the two-dimensional model. *British Journal of Psychiatry*, **158**, 317–322.

Astington, J.W., Gopnik, M. (1991) Theoretical explanations of children's understanding of mind. *British Journal of Developmental Psychology*, **9**, 7–31.

Baars, B.J. (1988) *A Cognitive Theory of Consciousness*, Cambridge University Press, Cambridge.

Baddeley, A. (1986) *Working Memory*, Oxford University Press, Oxford.

Baddeley, A., Lewis, V.J. (1981) Inner active processes in reading: The inner voice, the inner ear and the inner eye. In: *Interactive Processes in Reading* (Eds A.M. Lesgold, C.A. Perfetti), Erlbaum, Hillsdale, NJ.

Baron-Cohen, S., Leslie, A.M., Frith, U. (1985) Does the autistic child have a "theory of mind"? *Cognition*, **21**, 37–46.

Bauer, R.M. (1984) Autonomic recognition of names and faces in prosopagnosia: A neuropsychological application of the Guilty Knowledge Test. *Neuropsychologia*, **22**, 457–469.

Bentall, R.P., Baker, G.A., Havers, S. (1991) Reality monitoring and psychotic hallucinations. *British Journal of Clinical Psychology*, **30**, 213–222.

Bentall, R.P., Slade, P.D. (1985) Reality testing and auditory hallucinations: A signal detection analysis. *British Journal of Clinical Psychology*, **24**, 159–169.

Bick, P.A., Kinsbourne, M. (1987) Auditory hallucinations and subvocal speech in schizophrenic patients. *American Journal of Psychiatry*, **155**, 222–225.

Bleuler, E. (1911) *Dementia or the Group of Schizophrenias* (translated by J. Zinkin, 1950), International Universities Press, New York.

Brown, R.G., Marsden, C.D. (1988) Internal versus external cues in the control of attention in Parkinson's disease. *Brain*, **111**, 323–345.

Cohen, B.D. (1976) Referent communication in schizophrenia: The perseverative chaining model. *Annals of the New York Academy of Sciences*, **270**, 124–141.

Cohen, B.D. (1978) Referent communication disturbances in schizophrenia. In: *Language and Cognition in Schizophrenia* (Ed. S. Schwartz), Erlbaum, Hillsdale, NJ.

Crow, T.J. (1980) Molecular pathology of schizophrenia: More than one disease process? *British Medical Journal*, **280**, 66–68.

David, A.S. (1994) The neuropsychological origin of auditory hallucinations. In: *The Neuropsychology of Schizophrenia* (Eds A.S. David, J.C. Cutting), pp. 269–313, Lawrence Erlbaum, Hove, UK

De Haan, E.H.F., Young, A., Newcombe, F. (1987) Face recognition without awareness. *Cognitive Neuropsychology*, **4**, 385–415.

Esquirol, J.E.D. (1838) *Les Maladies Mentales*, Baillière, Paris.

Evarts, E.V. (1971) Feedback and corollary discharge: A merging of the concepts. *Neurosciences Research Program Bulletin*, **9**, 86–112.

Feinberg, I. (1978) Efference copy and corollary discharge: Implications for thinking and its disorders. *Schizophrenia Bulletin*, **4**, 636–640.

Feinberg, T.E., Schindler, R.J., Flanagan, N.G., Haber, L.D. (1992) Two alien hand syndromes. *Neurology*, **42**, 19–24.

Fletcher, P., Happé, F., Frith, U., Baker, S.C., Dolan, D.J., Frackowiak, R.S.J., Frith, C.D. (1995) Other minds in the brain: a functional imaging study of "theory of mind" in story comprehension. *Cognition*, **57**, 109–128.

Freid, I., Katz, A., McCarthy, G., Sass, K.J., Williamson, P., Spencer, S.S., Spencer, B.D. (1991) Functional organisation of human supplementary motor cortex studied by electrical stimulation. *Journal of Neuroscience*, **11**, 3656–3666.

Friston, K.J., Frith, C.D. (1995) Schizophrenia: A disconnection syndrome? *Clinical Neuroscience*, **3**, 89–97.

Frith, C.D. (1987) The positive and negative symptoms of schizophrenia reflect impairments in the perception and initiation of action. *Psychological Medicine*, **17**, 631–648.

Frith, C.D. (1992) *Cognitive Neuropsychology of Schizophrenia*, Erlbaum, Hove, UK.

Frith, C.D., Allen, H.A. (1988) Language disorders in schizophrenia and their implications for neuropsychology. In: *Schizophrenia: The Major Issues* (Eds P. Bebbington, P. McGuffin), Heinemann, Oxford.

Frith, C.D., Corcoran, R. (1996) Exploring "theory of mind" in people with schizophrenia. *Psychological Medicine*, **26**, 521–530.

Frith, C.D., Done, D.J. (1983) Stereotyped responding by schizophrenic patients on a two-choice guessing task. *Psychological Medicine*, **13**, 779–786.

Frith, C.D., Done, D.J. (1989) Experiences of alien control in schizophrenia reflect a disorder in the central monitoring of action. *Psychological Medicine*, **19**, 359–363.

Frith, C.D., Friston, K.J., Liddle, P.F., Frackowiak, R.S.J. (1991) Willed action and the prefrontal cortex in man: A PET study. *Proceedings of the Royal Society of London, Series B*, **244**, 241–246.

Glickstein, M., Stein, J. (1991) Paradoxical movement in Parkinson's disease. *Trends in Neurosciences*, **14**, 480–482.

Goldberg, G. (1985) Supplementary motor area structure and function: Review and hypotheses. *Behavioural and Brain Sciences*, **8**, 567–616.

Goldstein, K. (1908) Zur Lehre der motorischen Apraxie. *Journal für Psychologie und Neurologie*, **11**, 169–187.

Gould, L.N. (1949) Auditory hallucinations and subvocal speech. *Journal of Nervous and Mental Disease*, **109**, 418–427.

Green, M.F., Kinsbourne, M. (1989) Auditory hallucinations in schizophrenia: Does humming help? *Biological Psychiatry*, **25**, 633–635.

Heilbrun, A.B. (1980) Impaired recognition of self-expressed thought in patients with auditory hallucinations. *Journal of Abnormal Psychology*, **89**, 728–736.

Hoffman, R.E. (1986) Verbal hallucinations and language production processes in schizophrenia. *The Behavioural and Brain Sciences*, **9**, 503–548.

Hoffman, R.E., Kirstein, L., Stopek, S., Cicchetti, D. (1982) Apprehending schizophrenic discourse: A structural analysis of the listener's task. *Brain and Language*, **15**, 207–233.

Inouye, T., Shimizu, A. (1966) The electromyographic study of verbal hallucinations. *Psychophysiology*, **3**, 73–80.

James, W. (1890) *The Principles of Psychology*, Macmillan, London.

Johnson, F. (1978) *The Anatomy of Hallucination*, Nelson Hall, Chicago.

Johnson, M.K., Raye, C.L. (1981) Reality monitoring. *Psychological Review*, **88**, 67–85.

Jürgens, U. (1986) The squirrel monkey as an experimental model in the study of cerebral organisation of emotional utterances. *European Archives of Psychiatry and the Neurological Sciences*, **236**, 4043.

Kandinskii, V. (1885) Kritische und klinische. Betrachtungen im Gebeite der Sinnestanschangen.

Kandinskii, V. (1890) *O Psuedogallucinaciyach*, St Petersburg.

Kiyoshi, K. (1992) Somatotopy in the human supplementary motor area. *Trends in Neurosciences*, **15**, 159–160.

Leudar, I., Thomas, P., Johnston, M. (1994) Self-monitoring in speech production: Effects of verbal hallucinations and negative symptoms. *Psychological Medicine*, **24**, 749–761.

Liddle, P. (1987) The symptoms of chronic schizophrenia: A re-examination of the positive–negative dichotomy. *British Journal of Psychiatry*, **151**, 145–151.

Lindsley, O.R. (1963) Direct measurement and functional definition of vocal hallucinatory symptoms. *Journal of Nervous and Mental Disease*, **136**, 293–297.

Luria, A.R. (1973) *The Working Brain*, Basic Books, New York.

Lyon, N., Mejsholm, B., Lyon, M. (1986) Stereotyped responding by schizophrenic patients: Cross-cultural confirmation of perseverative switching on a two-choice guessing task. *Journal of Psychiatric Research*, **20**, 137–150.

Malenka, R.C., Angel, R.W., Hampton, B., Berger, P.A. (1982) Impaired central error correcting behaviour in schizophrenia. *Archives of General Psychiatry*, **39**, 101–107.

McGrath, J. (1991) Ordering thoughts on thought disorder. *British Journal of Psychiatry*, **158**, 307–316.

McGuire, P.K., Silbersweig, D.A., Wright, I., Murray, R.M., David, A.S., Frackowiak, R.S.J., Frith, C.D. (1995) Abnormal inner speech: a physiological basis for auditory hallucinations. *Lancet*, **346**, 596–600.

McKay, D.M. (1966) Cerebral organisation and the control of action. In: *Brain and Conscious Experience* (Ed. J.C. Eccles), Springer-Verlag, New York.

Megaw, E.D. (1972) Directional errors and their correction in a discrete tracking task. *Ergonomics*, **15**, 633–643.

Milner, A.D., Rugg, M.D. (Eds) (1992) *The Neuropsychology of Consciousness*, Academic Press, London.

Milner, B. (1964) Some effects of frontal lobectomy in man. In: *The Frontal Granular Cortex and Behaviour* (Eds J.M. Warren, K. Akert), McGraw Hill, New York.

Mlakar, J., Jensterle, J., Frith, C.D. (1994) Central monitoring deficiency and schizophrenic symptoms. *Psychological Medicine*, **24**, 557–564.

Müller-Preuss, P. (1978) Single unit responses of the auditory cortex in the squirrel monkey to self-produced and loudspeaker transmitted vocalisations. *Neuroscience Letters*, Suppl. 1, S.7.

Müller-Preuss, P., Jürgens, U. (1976) Projections from the "cingular" vocalisation area in the squirrel monkey. *Brain Research*, **103**, 29–43.

Müller-Preuss, P., Newman, J.D., Jürgens, U. (1980) Evidence for an anatomical and physiological relationship between the "cingular" vocalisation area and the auditory cortex in the squirrel monkey. *Brain Research*, **202**, 307–315.

Passingham, R.E. (1987) Two cortical systems for directing movement. In: *Motor Areas of the Cerebral Cortex. CIBA Foundation Symposium 132*, Wiley, Chichester.

Ploog, D. (1979) Phonation, emotion, cognition: With reference to the brain mechanisms involved. In: *Brain and Mind. CIBA Foundation Symposium 69*, Elsevier, North-Holland.

Rabbitt, P.M.A. (1966) Error-correction time without external signals. *Nature*, **212**, 438.

Reason, J.T. (1984) Lapses of attention. In: *Varieties of Attention* (Eds R. Parasuraman, R. Davies, J. Beatty), Academic Press, Orlando, Fla.

Robbins, T.W. (1991) Cognitive deficits in schizophrenia and Parkinson's disease: Neural basis and the role of dopamine. In: *The Mesolimbic Dopamine System: From Motivation to Action* (Eds P. Willner, J. Scheel-Kruger), Wiley, Chichester.

Robbins, T.W., Brown, V.J. (1990) The role of the striatum in the mental chronometry of action: A theoretical review. *Reviews in the Neurosciences*, **2**, 181–213.

Robinson, D.L., Wurtz, R.H. (1976) Use of an extra-retinal signal by monkey superior colliculus neurones to distinguish real from self-induced movement. *Journal of Neurophysiology*, **39**, 852–870.

Rochester, S., Martin, J.R. (1979) *Crazy Talk: A Study of the Discourse of Schizophrenic Speakers*, Plenum Press, New York.

Rutter, D.R. (1985) Language in schizophrenia: The structure of monologues and conversations. *British Journal of Psychiatry*, **146**, 399–404.

Salzinger, K., Portnoy, S., Feldman, R.S. (1978) Communicability deficit in schizophrenics resulting from a more general deficit. In: *Language and Cognition in Schizophrenia* (Ed. S. Schwartz), Erlbaum, Hillsdale, NJ.

Sarbin, T.R. (1967) The concept of hallucination. *Journal of Personality*, **35**, 359–380.

Schneider, K. (1959) *Clinical Psychopathology*, Grune & Stratton, New York.

Shallice, T. (1988) *From Neuropsychology to Mental Structure*, Cambridge University Press, Cambridge.

Sims, A. (1988) *Symptoms in the Mind: An Introduction to Descriptive Psychopathology.* Baillière Tindall, London.

Sperber, D., Wilson, D. (1986) *Relevance: Communication and Cognition*, Blackwell Scientific, Oxford.

Stuss, D.T., Benson, D.F. (1983) Frontal lobe lesion and behavior. In: *Localization in Neuropsychology*, Academic Press, New York.

von Helmholtz, H. (1866) *Handbuch der Physiologischen Optik*, Voss, Leipzig.

19

Problems of Person Perception in Schizophrenia

HADYN D. ELLIS and ANDREW W. YOUNG

INTRODUCTION

Kraepelin (1913/1919) suggested that in dementia praecox "perception is not usually lessened". There is, however, a small literature on deficits in sensory perception in schizophrenia. It would appear that the kinds of flagrant impairment commonly encountered in neurological patients with posterior cerebral damage do not occur; that is to say, patients with schizophrenia are able to see, hear and touch, and objects can be identified, sounds can be understood and so on. There are though some forms of perceptual abnormality. Hallucinations form an obvious example. Although hallucinations can in general be considered to result from a misattribution of an internal state to an external source, and hence as a defect in "reality monitoring" (Bentall & Slade, 1985; Slade & Bentall, 1988; Bentall et al, 1991), they can none the less be interpreted as unequivocal perceptual experiences as is shown by the following interview reported by Ames (1984) of a man who had shot himself in the head in order to get rid of a phantom head which talked to him (his dead wife's gynaecologist). He was questioned about the two heads:

Q: Could you see the other head?
A: Yes.
Q: You felt it, or you could see it?
A: I could see it.
Q: And the voices were coming from the other head?
A: From that head and my own head too.
Q: Whose voice was it?
A: It was the voice of my wife's doctor.

Schizophrenia: A Neuropsychological Perspective. Edited by C. Pantelis, H.E. Nelson and T.R.E. Barnes
© 1996 John Wiley & Sons Ltd

Such evidence of hallucinatory perception of bicephaly is a vivid illustration of just how strong such an erroneous perceptual experience can be. No less bizarre are a set of phenomena, largely associated with failures by patients with schizophrenia correctly to perceive information about other people's identity. These phenomena are referred to as delusional misidentification (DMI) but include other types of failure of interpretation.

PERCEPTIONS AND DELUSIONS

The central thesis of this chapter is that delusions concerning people – who they are and what intentions/moods they currently have – are founded upon impairments at different points within the face processing system. This view is predicated on the assumption that an adequate model of normal function should also be able to account for the patterns of abnormality which can arise from malfunction of the system (Young, 1992). This assumption is widely used in neuropsychology (A. Ellis & Young, 1988), but it is much less common in psychiatry. Some would argue that psychiatric symptoms are so bizarre that there are no parallels to be drawn between normal and abnormal function; a view we explicitly reject. Shortly we shall outline what the organisation of the normal face processing system may look like, but before doing so we shall attempt to justify further the philosophical and scientific basis of our own belief.

One of the theorists with whom we have much in common is Brendan Maher (1974, 1988). He has long argued that delusions in general are the result not of faulty reasoning but instead arise from distortions in sensory input such that the illusory perceptual evidence elicits a rational explanation, given the available sensory information.

So if "a delusion is a hypothesis designed to explain unusual perceptual phenomena and developed through the operation of normal cognitive processes" (Maher, 1974, p. 103) why does the patient not check the data and correct the hypothesis? As Nathan (1967) observed, we all experience perceptual errors from time to time but we do not develop delusional beliefs as a result. According to Maher (1974) it is the intensity or vividness of schizophrenic perceptual abnormalities that provides the key. He invokes, for example, the work of McGhie & Chapman (1961) which suggests a perceptual or attentional problem in schizophrenia leading to a difficulty in distinguishing figure from ground and in avoiding being overwhelmed by a flood of sensory excitation. This is perhaps the weakest part of Maher's position. Whilst we accept that patients with schizophrenia need not be irrational in a formal, logical sense, we prefer to explore the idea that delusions, and delusional misidentification in particular, reflect an interaction of deficits in which perceptual error is coupled with an impaired attributional mechanism or decision-making system. This will be briefly explored after we have outlined our own approaches to delusional misidentifications and to other problems in perceiving information from faces.

A MODEL OF NORMAL FACE PROCESSING

In the last 10 years a number of theorists have offered theoretical models of how normal individuals extract identity, expression and communication information from faces (e.g. Hay & Young, 1982; Ellis, 1983, 1986; Rhodes, 1985). The most widely used variant of these "functional models" is the one advanced by Bruce and Young (1986). This model is currently undergoing modification and amplification (Bruce et al, 1992; Burton et al, 1990; Young & Bruce, 1991) but the original and unrevised form is perfectly suitable for the present exercise of examining perceptual errors and delusions involving faces.

Figure 19.1 is a diagrammatic representation of Bruce and Young's model. It depicts the flow of facial information and indicates those components that are linked in a sequential order and those that function independently in parallel. Basically, the route to identity involves a series of sequentially organised components, while satellite systems for determining non-identity information are represented as a set of parallel processes which individually establish expression, categorical information such as age, sex and race and a final component that seems to play an integral part in understanding oral communications by lip-reading.

There are numerous sources describing in detail each of these components of the face processing system (see Bruce, 1988; Young & Ellis, 1989). Here we shall merely outline some of the more persuasive evidence arising from studies of neurological patients with specific face-processing impairments. Central to an appreciation of this type of evidence is the acceptance of the explanatory potential of dissociable impairments (A. Ellis & Young, 1988; Shallice, 1988; see also Goldstein, chapter 3). That is, patients have been described who are unable to identify people by face but can interpret expressions (Bruyer et al, 1983; Tranel et al, 1988); others have been unable to do the latter but are unimpaired in the former (Bornstein, 1963; Kurucz & Feldmar, 1979; Kurucz et al, 1979); and another dissociation has been described between deficits affecting lip-reading or the identification of faces and facial expressions (Campbell et al, 1986). As yet, however, there has not been a description of a patient whose deficit is in extracting categorical information such as age or sex from faces, but who can determine identity.

The occurrence of such dissociable impairments reinforces many other sources of information that favour models such as Bruce & Young's (1986). In the following sections we shall examine different kinds of impairment in person perception by patients with schizophrenia. It will soon become apparent that, while we favour a broadly organic approach to understanding these impairments, for the moment we distinguish between the manifestations of psychiatric impairments and those arising from unequivocal neurological disorders. In doing so, however, we have no wish to weaken our avowedly mechanistic scientific philosophy: instead we are determined to help establish what has recently been termed a cognitive neuropsychiatric approach to understanding certain phenomena of schizophrenia (Ellis, 1991; David, 1993; Ellis & de Pauw, 1994). The study of psychiatric patients with different types of breakdown in person recognition, as we shall demonstrate, may be more clearly understood within the theoretical

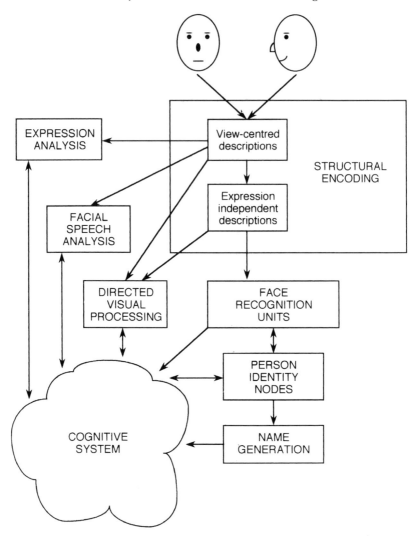

Figure 19.1. Bruce & Young's (1986) functional model for face recognition

framework of normal face processing, and the resulting observations may themselves help to modify the theory. This reciprocity is an important factor which parallels that found in the better-established field of cognitive neuro-psychology (Coltheart, 1984; Caramazza, 1992).

We first applied the above principles to the study of delusional misidentification a few years ago (Ellis & Young, 1990). Here we shall not only necessarily retrace our footsteps but we shall extend our original exposition beyond the route to identity to include similar interpretations of expression and lip-reading.

The following review is structured around five kinds of problem involving person perception that have attracted clinical and scientific interest. These are: three of the DMIs – intermetamorphosis, the Frégoli delusion, and the Capgras delusion; together with failures in the recognition of emotional expression; and problems in lip-reading. Each topic will be dealt with separately but in relation to the face recognition model shown in Figure 19.1.

Our primary concern will be with delusional misidentification. This is often considered to be an unusual and uncommon psychiatric phenomenon, and there has been much discussion as to whether the different forms of delusional misidentification can be separated into distinct syndromes (Enoch & Trethowan, 1991). However, delusional misidentification is probably more common than was once thought (Förstl et al, 1991a, 1991b) and a corollary of our position is that each type of delusion is worth investigating as an interesting *symptom* in its own right. Again, this symptom-based approach is at present more common in neuropsychology, but it has recently found persuasive advocates in clinical psychology and psychiatry (Bentall, 1991; Costello, 1992). Delusional misidentification thus forms a useful testing ground for this approach, which may well be much more widely applicable to other types of delusion.

INTERMETAMORPHOSIS

Courbon & Tusques (1932) reported the first account of intermetamorphosis or the delusional belief that others have changed to an appearance exactly like someone else's. Sylvie G., a 49-year-old woman with an 8-year psychiatric history, reported that objects and animals she owned had been altered. Two of her young chickens, for example, had become old; her new coat had been replaced by one that was worn and ripped; and children in the street could look just like her son ". . . dressed in the same way, with the same nose, the same rosy face, the same small mouth".

The patient then began to believe that her husband could become physically and psychologically transformed. "In a second my husband is taller, smaller or younger. It's the individual into which he is transformed that lives, that is in his skin, that moves . . . It was not a simple change but a complete transformation." On one occasion Sylvie G.'s husband, an electrician, was transformed into a Mr Pannier when there was an interruption to the power supply. Mr Pannier, unlike her husband, was not an electrician and so he could not repair it but, happily, her husband retransformed in time to sort things out. Interestingly, she claimed that during any of his transformations her husband's hand, which had had a finger amputated, and his eye colour did not change. When others took on the appearance of her son she relied upon the large size of his feet and the habitual muddiness of his shoes to determine whether or not she was truly confronted with him or someone else who had become transformed to look like him.

Courbon & Tusques' (1932) description of their patient's beliefs suggests that intermetamorphosis may involve attending excessively to details at the expense of the whole, which has been considered something of a general tendency for patients with schizophrenia (Bemporad, 1967). This might be thought to be the basic malfunction, or it may form part of a process that supports the intermetamorphosic experience, insofar as excessive attention to details will allow the patient to think that the appearance of the (unattended) whole is somehow different whilst simultaneously minimising the possibility of noticing that the person's appearance has not really changed.

Since the report by Courbon and Tusques there have been relatively few similar cases. Bick (1986) reviewed two cases reported since 1932 (Malliaras et al, 1978; Christodoulou, 1975) before describing one of his own. This patient, a 42-year-old woman diagnosed as suffering from paranoid schizophrenia 15 years earlier, during a hospital interview suddenly expressed the belief that the doctor was her Uncle Henry. Following treatment with haloperidol over two days, the patient's intermetamorphosis remitted. As with the patients described by Malliaras et al (1978) and Christodoulou (1975), Bick's patient was found to have an abnormal EEG, indicating temporal lobe dysfunction.

The largest study of intermetamorphosis has been carried out by Young et al (1990), who recently reported three cases. The first was a 29-year-old man who mistook his mother for his brother and believed his psychiatrist to be a woman he had met a year earlier in a casino. During a subsequent relapse he attacked a shopkeeper whom he mistook for a famous snooker player. The second case also a 29-year-old man, attacked his mother because he claimed that when she put her spectacles on she acquired the appearance of a neighbour he disliked. This transformation happened instantly, as did that of his father, who became someone he believed had been spying on him. The third case was a 30-year-old man who had become infatuated by a woman whom he "saw" wherever he went. He even mistook his own mother for the woman and began to see in others resemblances with her parents.

In the third of the cases described by Young et al (1990) there were clear EEG abnormalities (indeed a prior record of temporal lobe epilepsy existed). The first case was a man who, at the age of 17, had received a head injury after being struck by a car. In the second case there was no obvious evidence of any brain injury, though the patient would not allow neurological investigations to be carried out.

Ellis & Young (1990) argued that intermetamorphosis is the result of some kind of malfunctioning at the Face Recognition Units (FRUs) stage shown in Figure 19.1. That is to say, the wrong recognition unit responds to the seen face. The reason why the system should develop such a fault is open to further speculation. Possibly, certain face recognition units become hypersensitive so that they are activated by input which, normally, would excite a different face recognition unit.

Ellis & Young (1990) pointed out that if this general position is correct, then faces that are physically similar to the falsely recognised person's are most likely to produce the inappropriate response. The second corollary to their theory is that voices should not appear to alter as the face changes, because voice recognition is assumed to be subserved by an independent module which converges at the level of the person identity node stage – but not beforehand. Neither prediction has yet been tested, but the fact that clear and readily falsifiable predictions can be derived shows the benefits of linking observations to an explicit model.

FRÉGOLI DELUSION

The Frégoli delusion differs from intermetamorphosis because it does not involve an underlying change in physical appearance: instead the patient insists that familiar persons disguise themselves as others. The disorder was named after Leopoldo Frégoli, the Italian mimic, who was well known in France during the early part of this century.

The first description of this delusion was given by Courbon & Fail (1927), when they reported a 27-year-old woman who developed the belief that the actresses Robine and Sarah Bernhardt were disguising themselves as other people in order to make her masturbate and do other things she did not want to do.

The distinction between intermetamorphosis and the Frégoli delusion is a fine one because Courbon & Tusques (1932) included both physical and psychological change in their definition of intermetamorphosis, though this is often ignored in the literature. The symptoms of the Frégoli patient given by Courbon & Fail (1927) also included physical alterations. She perceived in actors playing alongside Robine members of her own family. In the more recent literature the two delusions are sometimes confused which poses a nosological difficulty that has yet fully to be resolved. Young et al (1990) attempted to distinguish the two delusions empirically by administering a battery of face processing tests to a patient previously diagnosed by de Pauw et al, (1987) as displaying the Frégoli delusion, and comparing the results with the three cases of intermetamorphosis mentioned earlier.

The patient with the Frégoli delusion was a 66-year-old woman, GC, who had suffered a right sided temporoparietal infarct. She believed her cousin (the father of her only child) was harassing her in the guise of others. On formal tests designed to measure face processing abilities, GC was impaired in ability to identify and name famous faces and to identify faces disguised with false beards, wigs, etc. She also showed a significant discrepancy between her good recognition memory for words and her poor recognition memory for faces (Warrington, 1984). None of the intermetamorphosis patients was impaired on the disguise test, although one was poor at identifying famous faces and two had problems in naming them and in recognition memory for faces. All of the patients showed normal recognition memory for words.

A second patient with the Frégoli delusion has also been found to show impaired performance on our disguise test (Wright et al, 1993). In this case the Frégoli delusion was associated with erotomania (also referred to as de Clérambault's syndrome), the delusional belief that someone (usually of higher social standing) is in love with the patient (Enoch & Trethowan, 1991). Although she manifested other delusional beliefs, the Frégoli and erotomanic delusions dominated the clinical picture.

This patient was a 35-year-old, divorced, unemployed woman with a history of chronic paranoid schizophrenia. She believed that she was the girlfriend of Erik Estrada (an American actor and pin-up), with whom she communicated across the Atlantic via telepathy. She also believed that Erik Estrada visited her home city regularly, disguised as acquaintances or her current boyfriend. She stated that she knew her actual boyfriend was Erik Estrada in disguise because of the absence of a previous scar on his face. She was convinced that Erik Estrada was in love with her and that he planned to marry her one day.

Her pattern of impairment on face processing tests was closely comparable to that found for GC. Both patients were impaired at recognising familiar faces, matching disguised faces, and showed poorer recognition memory for faces than words. Although an EEG suggested bilateral abnormalities for the second patient, whereas GC had suffered right cerebral infarction, these face processing impairments point toward involvement of the right cerebral hemisphere, which has been noted as a feature in other cases of erotomania and delusional misidentification (Barton & Barton, 1986).

A more comprehensive battery of relevant tests, however, may be necessary to support the distinction between intermetamorphosis and the Frégoli delusion. On the assumption that such a division is merited, Ellis & Young (1990) suggested that a possible functional site for the latter is the Person Identity Nodes (PINs) shown in Figure 19.1, and their interaction with the cognitive system, which can be thought of here as fulfilling a principal decision-making role.

Ellis & Young (1990) argued that particularly significant PINs may become hyperactive, so that they may become activated even when inappropriate input arrives from the FRU stage. Thus the unit corresponding to person X may be excited within the FRU but instead of the corresponding PIN for person X being subsequently triggered the node for person Y may become activated. This is obviously closely related to our account of intermetamorphosis, which involved a similar problem at the FRU level. The difference is that PINs also serve voice and other inputs that identify people, so that if the problem is correctly located at this level we would expect that the same errors will occur to voices, and this would be worth exploring.

We can speculate as to the mechanism of this hyperactivity by suggesting that strong interpersonal feelings are involved which create pervasive top-down influences. Hay & Young (1982) had noted that top-down influences on recognition must exist; for example, if we are expecting to meet person X, then we will think that we have seen and recognised them on the basis of much less evidence than if we do not expect them. Many everyday errors are of this type, but they are usually quickly corrected (Young et al, 1985); even so, there are rare occasions when we have to apologise after greeting a stranger. In Frégoli cases, though, inconsistent evidence proves insufficient to alter the misidentification; even though the patients can see that it is not X, they account for the discrepancy by proposing a disguise that is sufficiently clever to fool others. As Ellis & Young (1990) emphasised, this must involve impaired decision mechanisms, which means it may well be more than a coincidence that Frégoli patients are poor at disentangling the effects of disguise.

Fleminger (1992) has argued persuasively that such expectations may be quite generally involved in delusional misidentification, and they certainly seem to have a potentially dominant role in accounting both for intermetamorphosis and for the Frégoli delusion.

If an impairment at the PIN stage underlies the Frégoli delusion and one at the FRU stage underlies intermetamorphosis then it follows from the Bruce & Young (1986) model that voices should be able to trigger the delusion in the former but not in the latter because FRUs do not receive vocal input but PINs do. The advantage of working with a cognitive framework such as the one we are using here is thus that it again enables sharp distinctions to be made and facilitates clear predictions for future work. Although these have yet to be confirmed they may serve to guide clinical observations, which so far form the basis for our knowledge of the DMSs.

The functions of the PIN system have been recently redefined and clarified by Burton et al (1990) in their simulation of the Bruce & Young (1986) model using an interactive activation and competition (IAC) connectionist architecture. It will be interesting to see in future whether this IAC simulation of the normal face processing system can provide a working computer model of DMS; it has already achieved a notable success in providing a simple explanation for some prosopagnosic patients being able covertly to recognise faces (Burton et al, 1991).

CAPGRAS DELUSION

The most commonly observed form of delusional misidentification is the Capgras delusion, first systematically described by Capgras & Reboul-Lachaux in 1923 but reported much earlier in Germany (Kahlbaum, 1866). The essential feature of the Capgras delusion is the belief that others including animals and objects, usually, but not necessarily, close to the patient have been replaced by doubles, robots, etc. Thus, unlike intermetamorphosis, the perceptual impairment is subtle. People's appearance may seem physically altered in small detail but the usual feeling described by patients is that, although the person, animal or object before them looks like their spouse or whomever, they know that they are really someone or something else.

Although most patients manifesting the Capgras delusion suffer from paranoid schizophrenia, it can arise in the clinical setting of depression, dementia, AIDS-related encephalopathy, diabetes, stroke, and other forms of cerebral dysfunction. In fact it is common with brain-imaging techniques to find evidence of structural brain pathology (MacCallum, 1973; Joseph, 1986). There may well be accompanying psychopathology to the Capgras delusion (Berson, 1983) but, as Ellis & de Pauw (1994) have argued, there are many resemblances to reduplicative paramnesia (Pick, 1903; Alexander et al, 1979) which has conventionally been regarded as a purely neurological disorder.

The importance of an organic component in the production of the Capgras delusion has been supported by findings that Capgras patients perform poorly on standard neuropsychological tests of face recognition. For example, Shraberg & Weitzel (1979) found that two Capgras patients made more errors on the Benton

Test of Facial Recognition (Benton et al, 1983) than did normal or schizophrenic controls. Wilcox & Waziri (1983) and Morrison & Tarter (1984) also noted impairment on the Benton test in their Capgras patients, and Luaute et al (1978) and Tzavaras et al (1986) found impairments on the face matching test devised by Tzavaras et al (1970). Lewis (1987) and Crichton & Lewis (1990) also reported poor recognition memory for faces.

These reports of impairment on neuropsychological tests of face processing in Capgras patients have mostly relied on tests of unfamiliar face matching. Both the Benton Test of Facial Recognition (Benton et al, 1983) and Tzavaras et al's (1970) test require subjects to match photographs of faces of unfamiliar people, by picking out those that are pictures of the same person. As we have explained, however, neuropsychological impairments can affect face processing in a number of dissociable ways. Hence, it will be important in future work to test a wider range of face processing abilities in ways capable of pinpointing which abilities are impaired and which intact, rather than relying on a single test. This is now done routinely in neuropsychological investigations (Bruyer et al, 1983; Young & Ellis, 1989).

Ellis & de Pauw (1994) have argued that the Capgras delusion may be best understood by applying techniques borrowed from cognitive neuropsychology (Coltheart, 1984). They coined the term *cognitive neuropsychiatry* to indicate a difference in emphasis, if not in conceptual substance, between the two. Cognitive neuropsychiatry is the interplay between cognitive modelling of processes such as face recognition and data derived from psychiatric patients who reveal specific disorders. The analysis of intermetamorphosis and Frégoli delusion by Ellis & Young (1990) is a good illustration of how this approach can be employed.

The use of a cognitive model to illuminate psychopathological phenomena is not a one-way process. As is abundantly clear with cognitive neuropsychology, the results derived from a patient population can usefully inform theorists and cause them to modify their models appropriately. This precept is demonstrated by the analysis of the Capgras delusion offered by Ellis & Young (1990). They suggested that the disorder could result from an impairment that may be considered as the mirror image of prosopagnosia, which is a profound inability to recognise previously familiar faces that can follow occipitotemporal brain injury (Bodamer, 1947; Bornstein, 1963; Hécaen, 1981). Recent work has revealed that, although prosopagnosics cannot consciously recognise faces, some show autonomic and behavioural responses that imply that at some level discrimination between the faces of known people and strangers has taken place (Bauer, 1984; Bruyer, 1991; de Haan et al, 1987; Sergent & Poncet, 1990; Tranel & Damasio, 1985; Young & de Haan, 1992).

Existing models of face recognition (e.g. Bruce & Young, 1986; Ellis, 1983, 1986) did not allow for such non-conscious registration of identity information and therefore could be considered deficient. Investigations of the Capgras delusion underline the need to consider the possibility that there may be multiple neurological routes to recognition, not all of which give rise to the conscious experience of the discrimination.

Ellis & Shepherd (1992) have argued that what may be missing in the perceptual experience of a patient with Capgras delusion looking at the face of someone significant to him or her is an accompanying sense of familiarity which may have an emotional valence. This hypothesis requires empirical support but, if found to be valid, it will emphasise the need for cognitive models of face recognition to include both an "identity" route and a "familiarity" route – much as Mandler (1980) suggested for all types of recognition. A commonly reported claim of Capgras patients is that people and things seem somehow strange or unfamiliar, and this is also found in other psychiatric and neurological conditions (Critchley, 1989; Sno & Linszen, 1990). We will need to pay more attention to distinguishing different kinds of familiarity, and especially those aspects which involve emotional and orienting reactions to people, things and events which have personal relevance (Van Lancker, 1991).

This is an elaboration of the suggestion made by Lewis (1987) and Ellis & Young (1990), that the basis of the Capgras delusion lies in damage to neuro-anatomical pathways responsible for appropriate emotional reactions to familiar visual stimuli. The delusion would then represent the patient's attempt to make sense of this puzzling change. However, this still leaves us with the question as to why they arrive at the seemingly extraordinary "impostors" hypothesis. Of particular interest in this respect are findings that people with persecutory delusions tend to attribute hypothetical negative events to external rather than internal causes (Candido & Romney, 1990; Kaney & Bentall, 1989). Persecutory delusions and suspiciousness are often noted in Capgras cases and may, therefore, contribute to the fundamental misinterpretation in which the patients mistake a change in themselves for a change in others (i.e. because altered affective reactions make people seem strange, they must have been "replaced").

Our hypothesis is thus that the Capgras delusion reflects an *interaction* of impairments at two levels. One set of contributory factors involve anomalous perceptual experience. The other factors lead to an incorrect interpretation of this. On this account, the Capgras delusion typically involves close relatives because these would normally produce the strongest reactions, and hence suffer the greatest discrepancy.

Since substantial parts of the pathways which imbue visual stimuli with affective significance are in close proximity to those involved in visual recognition, one would expect that few brain lesions will compromise emotional reactions to visual stimuli without also affecting other visual functions involved in recognition to some extent. Most Capgras patients will thus show defective face processing abilities because these are, for neuro-anatomical reasons, likely to co-occur with the fundamental problem in affective reactions.

Cutting (1990) as part of his general thesis relating psychotic states to right hemisphere pathology has advanced the view that the Capgras delusion arises from a general loss of ability to discriminate individuality. He derived this hypothesis from a more general stance on cerebral laterality in which the left hemisphere is held to perceive categories of information and the right to detect differences within categories. This idea has limited appeal since it seems to predict prosopagnosia rather than the Capgras delusion per se, but a link between right hemisphere deficit and impaired face perception in schizophrenia is worthwhile investigating. Magaro & Chamrad (1983) did find that patients with paranoid schizophrenia, when shown faces unilaterally (or bilaterally) in the left or right visual fields, were better at recognising faces presented to the right visual field – i.e. opposite to the normal asymmetry.

More recently Ellis et al (1993) examined the responses to lateralised and bilateral stimuli of three Capgras patients and three patients with paranoid schizophrenia. Contrary to earlier research by Magaro & Chamrad (1983), Ellis et al (1993) found that the latter group showed the normal left visual field advantage for matching pairs of faces. For the Capgras patients, however, the advantage was reversed. No such difference was found when line drawings of objects were used as stimuli (see Figure 19.2). These results support Cutting's view that the Capgras delusion is associated with right hemisphere abnormalities, but not his more general thesis that right hemisphere disorders underpin all types of schizophrenia.

The results from both groups of patients studied by Ellis et al (1993) indicated that the best face-matching performance was found for bilateral presentation. This observation is particularly significant because Joseph (1986) had speculated that the Capgras delusion may occur as a result of poor interhemispheric communication leading to the simultaneous activation of representations of faces in each hemisphere, unlike the normal state where, perhaps as a result of interaction between homologous sites, the unity of the person is preserved. The fact that the Capgras patients revealed fastest responses to bilaterally presented pairs of faces offers no support to a simple interpretation of Joseph's hypothesis.

PERCEPTION OF FACIAL EXPRESSIONS

Young et al (1990) gave the three patients with intermetamorphosis mentioned earlier a test of recognising facial expressions. This was based upon the work of Ekman & Friesen (1976): it comprised four examples of six emotions – happiness, sadness, surprise, fear, anger and disgust. The task required the patient to match the correct label with each of the 24 faces. Control data were obtained from men of comparable age. One of the patients, GS, was very poor at the task, scoring an average of 15 across two testing sessions (significantly less than the controls' mean of 22 correct). GS found the task difficult, not least because he insisted on being able to see "real" expressions behind the facial mask. Informal observation revealed him to have more difficulties in identifying negative compared with positive emotions.

The other two patients with intermetamorphosis had no difficulty matching facial expressions to verbal labels. This demonstrates the often-reported dissociation between processes underlying face recognition from those involved in the identification of facial expressions (Parry et al, 1991). The reported cases of double dissociation offer support for the notion that expression recognition and person identification are independently carried out. Having indicated that identification processes may be impaired in some patients with schizophrenia but simple expression identification skills can also be impaired or unaffected, we turn to the general issue of the ability in patients with schizophrenia to interpret the emotional state of others.

Deficits in the ability of patients with schizophrenia accurately to perceive facial

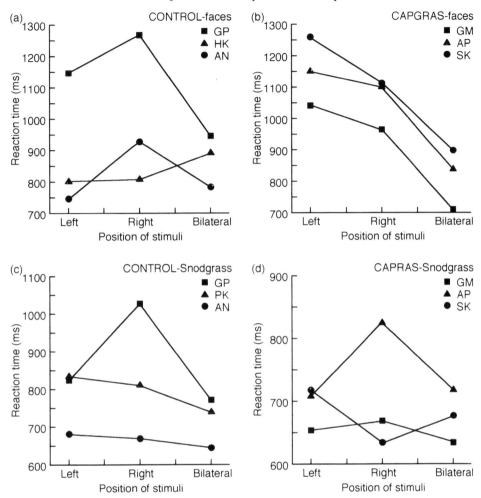

Figure 19.2. Graphs showing mean reaction times by three Capgras and three control patients shown pairs of faces and Snodgrass pictures (line drawings of objects) in LVF, RVF and bilaterally.

expressions have long been known (Shannon, 1970; Dougherty et al, 1974). They signal a breakdown in normal communicative skills: patients with schizophrenia who are unable to recognise the thoughts and intentions of others by perceiving changes in facial expression are clearly at a disadvantage in social interactions (Morrison et al, 1988 see also Cahill and Frith, chapter 18). It has often been reported that such patients have most difficulty in identifying negative emotional states (Pilowsky & Bassett, 1980) but it is often difficult to rule out either the influence of hospitalisation (Zuroff & Colussy, 1986) or the greater difficulty in perceiving negative affect (Ekman et al, 1972).

Novic et al (1984) also pointed to another possible artefact, viz. the fact that recognition of facial affect may be determined by more general face-processing skills. They found, for example, that 17 patients with chronic schizophrenia and 17 control subjects differed in their abilities to match facial expressions to a target expression; but that, when performance on a similar face identity matching task was used as a covariate, the difference was eliminated. Only when all test items were used, including those with poor discriminating power, was the schizophrenic subjects' poorer expression matching performance sustained after identity matching had been partialled out. Significantly, Novic et al (1984) found that negative affect expressions tended to be the ones that were most discriminating and they concluded that patients with schizophrenia may have more problems in interpreting these simply because they are more difficult.

Morrison et al (1988), when reviewing evidence implicating right hemisphere pathology in schizophrenia, proposed that, at least in some sub-categories of the illness, there may be consequent deficits in affect recognition, which is thought largely to involve right hemisphere structures (Ellis, 1983). They point out, however, the many methodological pitfalls in making the connection between right hemisphere pathology, schizophrenia and affect judgments; some of which we have already mentioned. Others include compatibility of the stimuli used in different studies and the task requirements as well as the ecological validity of using static photographs rather than moving faces which often display an expression quite briefly. Each of these present researchers with difficult problems and therefore it is unsurprising that any consensus has not yet emerged.

To eliminate some of these problems, Archer et al (1992) tested familiar face recognition, unfamiliar face matching, and expression analysis in groups of patients with schizophrenia, depressed patients, and control subjects using testing paradigms which relied entirely on a forced-choice procedure and thus involved (as far as possible) common task and response requirements. From previous studies, Archer et al (1992) distinguished the rival hypotheses of a generalised face-processing deficit, which would predict that the patients with schizophrenia would be impaired on all three tasks, and a dissociable impairment of expression analysis. Their results showed that the patients with schizophrenia were significantly impaired for all three tasks, which supports the generalised deficit hypothesis. Moreover, examination of the data from each of these twelve patients included in the study of Archer et al (1992) showed that not one of them revealed the pattern of impaired performance of the expression task and unimpaired performance of familiar face recognition and unfamiliar face matching tasks predicted by the hypothesis of a dissociable impairment of expression analysis. This does not mean that dissociable impairments of expression analysis do not occur in schizophrenia, but it does indicate that they are far from the norm.

LIP-READING

The face-processing model shown in Figure 19.1 contains a separate sub-module for lip-reading. As we mentioned earlier this is largely due to research by

Campbell and her colleagues (Campbell et al, 1986; Campbell, 1989) which revealed lip-reading to be dissociable from other face-processing tasks.

In a recent study Myslobodsky et al (1992) compared a group of patients with paranoid schizophrenia with a group of matched controls on a battery of lip-reading tests. These included tests used by Campbell et al (1986) which are sensitive to the influence of lip movements on speaker comprehension. The schizophrenics were as good as controls at recognising "visemes" (lip settings for 10 consonants). They were also just as susceptible to a blend illusion (McDonald & McGurk, 1976), where a sound is heard that does not correspond with the seen lip movements and a blend of the two is perceived. The schizophrenic group were also indistinguishable from controls in their ability to recognise words being silently spoken. In fact the only lip-reading test to elicit any difference between the groups involved the presentation of short sentences commonly used (e.g. "too good to be true").

Myslobodsky et al (1992) attributed the last finding to a deterioration in "sociocultural knowledge" among the patients with schizophrenia rather than to any impairment in lip-reading skills. They began their study with the assumption that lip-reading, being largely a left hemisphere activity, ought to be vulnerable in schizophrenia because of its putative association with left hemisphere pathology (Flor-Henry, 1976). They did not consider their data, however, as being consistent with Cutting's (1990) thesis that schizophrenia and other psychoses may originate from damage to right hemisphere functioning – which, if true, would lead one to predict that patients with schizophrenia should not show lip-reading dysfunctions.

OVERVIEW

In this chapter we have tried to illustrate how impairments in person perception in schizophrenia can be usefully considered within a general model of normal face processing. Not only may the classification of certain symptoms become more sharply defined by this operation, but principled explanations for them in whole or in part thus become available. For each of the five person perception symptom clusters associated with schizophrenia that we have considered here it is possible to appreciate the potential impact of what we have termed the cognitive neuropsychiatric approach.

Our own enthusiasm for the cognitive neuropsychiatric approach ought not to obscure the fact that it is based on a similar assumption to that made by Maher (1974, 1988) and others to account for all delusions, namely, that they occur as a result of perceptual information giving rise to erroneous data that the patient rationalises in the form of a delusion. What we have argued is that an understanding of several different categories of delusions and other failures involving person perception are interpretable by asserting that each disorder is the result of some kind of impairment within a complex set of cognitive structures that deal with facial information. As we pointed out earlier, however, to account fully for DMIs we also see the possible need to postulate some form of additional impairment in judgment or decision making which enables them to be sustained despite all other evidence to the contrary.

A rather similar conclusion, arrived at from another direction, was made by Benson & Stuss (1990). Over a number of years these researchers have developed a theory of delusions that concentrates upon the role of prefrontal structures in self-analysis. Applied to the Capgras delusion they would argue that, as a result of damage to these structures, there is a failure to monitor and disregard the delusion that someone has been replaced by an impostor. Although obviously concentrating on the judgment end of the process, they do acknowledge the need to posit some other sensory/cognitive malfunction as well as a failure of what they term self awareness. We, on the other hand, have emphasised the disordered detection of face familiarity (Ellis & Young, 1990) – but our ideas are not incompatible with those of Benson & Stuss (1990). Nor is an alternative theoretical analysis of the decision process in terms of attribution theory necessarily at variance with the notion that the critical judgmental aberration involves disordered self analysis. Young et al (1993) have discussed the possible role of attribution processes in the Capgras delusion and their social psychological approach could easily be married to the neurological ones forwarded by Benson and Stuss. It could be argued that, essentially, they offer the same argument at different levels of explanation.

Another point we wish to emphasise is that, although we have focused on problems in person perception displayed by sub-groups of patients with schizophrenia, some of the phenomena we have discussed are not restricted to this illness. These occur in other "idiopathic" psychoses as well as neurological conditions, and have been reported in acute, transient (and therefore reversible) disorders (Ellis & de Pauw, 1994). Such observations strengthen the already powerful case for interpreting many, if not most, psychopathological phenomena in part within an organic rather than a purely psychodynamic context.

Finally, it is worthwhile recapping the main conclusions we have drawn. The DMIs reviewed have each been tied to dysfunction within different parts of the normal face identification system: we claim intermetamorphosis to be associated with malfunctioning at the FRU stage, and the Frégoli delusion at the PIN stage. The Capgras delusion, however, may result from damage or disconnection within a neurological pathway signalling either emotional significance or familiarity. The impairments in the abilities of patients with schizophrenia to recognise the moods of others may arise from some sort of disorder within the expression recognition system, which many have argued involves right hemisphere structures. The lack of any deficit in simple tasks of lip-reading is also consistent (in a negative way) with the thesis that schizophrenia can be usefully understood as a manifestation of right cerebral hemisphere dysfunction. However, to develop this argument further is outside the scope of this chapter.

ACKNOWLEDGEMENTS

We should like to thank Karel de Pauw and Krystyna Szulecka for their thoughtful comments on an earlier draft of the chapter. The empirical work described in this chapter was supported by a NATO Collaborative Research Grant 1990/91 to Hadyn Ellis (Cardiff), Karel de Pauw (Doncaster), George Christodoulou (Greece) and Anthony Joseph (USA). Some of the theoretical ideas were developed with the assistance of an ESRC Programme Award (XC15250000) to the authors (with V. Bruce, I.G. Craw, A.W. Ellis and D.I. Perrett). The work described here is being pursued with grants from the Wellcome Trust and the EJLB Foundation.

REFERENCES

Alexander, M.P., Stuss, D.T., Benson, D.F. (1979) Capgras syndrome: A reduplicative phenomenon. *Neurology*, **29**, 334–339.

Ames, D. (1984) Self shooting of a phantom head. *British Journal of Psychiatry*, **145**, 193–194.

Archer, J., Hay, D.C., Young, A.W. (1992) Face processing in psychiatric conditions. *British Journal of Clinical Psychology*, **31**, 45–61.

Barton, J.L., Barton, E.S. (1986) Misidentification syndromes and sexuality. *Bibliotheca Psychiatrica*, **164**, 105–120.

Bauer, R.M. (1984) Autonomic recognition of names and faces in prosopagnosia: A neuro-psychological application of the guilty knowledge test. *Neuropsychologia*, **22**, 457–469.

Bemporad, J.R. (1967) Perceptual disorders in schizophrenia. *American Journal of Psychiatry*, **123**, 971–976.

Benson, D.F., Stuss, D.T. (1990) Frontal lobe influences on delusions: A clinical perspective. *Schizophrenia Bulletin*, **16**, 403–411.

Bentall, R.P. (1991) Explaining and explaining away insanity. In: *Pursuit of Mind* (Eds R. Tallis, H. Robinson), pp. 149–170, Carcanet, Manchester.

Bentall, R.P., Slade, P. (1985) Reality testing and auditory hallucinations: A signal detection analysis. *British Journal of Clinical Psychology*, **24**, 159–169.

Bentall, R.P., Baker, G.A., Havers, S. (1991) Reality monitoring and psychotic hallucinations. *British Journal of Clinical Psychology*, **30**, 213–222.

Benton, A.L., Hamsher, K.D.S., Varney, N., Spreen, O. (1983) *Contributions to Neuropsychological Assessment: A Clinical Manual*, Oxford University Press, Oxford.

Berson, R.J. (1983) Capgras' syndrome. *American Journal of Psychiatry* (Special Article), **140**, 969–979.

Bick, P.A. (1986) The syndrome of intermetamorphosis. *Bibliotheca Psychiatrica*, **164**, 131–135.

Bodamer, J. (1947) Die Prosop-Agnosie. *Archiv für Psychiatrie und Nervenkrankheiten*, **179**, 6–54.

Bornstein, B. (1963) Prosopagnosia. In: *Problems of Dynamic Neurology* (Ed. L. Halpern), pp. 283–318, Hadassah Medical School, Jerusalem.

Bruce, V. (1988) *Recognising Faces*, Erlbaum, Hove, UK.

Bruce, V., Young, A.W. (1986) Understanding face recognition. *British Journal of Psychology*, **77**, 305–327.

Bruce, V., Burton, A.M., Craw, I. (1992) Modelling face recognition. *Philosophical Transactions of the Royal Society, London*, **B335**, 121–128.

Bruyer, R. (1991) Covert face recognition in prosopagnosia: A review. *Brain and Cognition*, **15**, 223–235.

Bruyer, R., Laterre, C., Seron, X., Feyereisen, P., Strypstein, E., Pierrard, E., Rectem, D. (1983) A case of prosopagnosia with some preserved covert remembrance of familiar faces. *Brain and Cognition*, **2**, 257–284.

Burton, A.M., Bruce, V., Johnston, R.A. (1990) Understanding face recognition with an interactive activation model. *British Journal of Psychology*, **81**, 361–380.

Burton, A.M., Young, A.W., Bruce, V., Johnston, R., Ellis, A.W. (1991) Understanding covert recognition. *Cognition*, **39**, 129–166.

Campbell, R. (1989) Lipreading. In: *Handbook of Research on Face Processing* (Eds A. Young, H. Ellis), pp. 187–205, North-Holland, Amsterdam.

Campbell, R., Landis, T., Regard, M. (1986) Face recognition and lipreading: A neurological dissociation. *Brain*, **109**, 509–521.

Candido, C.L., Romney, D.M. (1990) Attributional style in paranoid vs. depressed patients. *British Journal of Medical Psychology*, **63**, 355–363.

Capgras, J., Reboul-Lachaux, J. (1923) Illusion de sosies et complexe d'Oedipe. *Annales Mèdico-Psychologiques*, **82**, 48–68.

Caramazza, A. (1992) Is cognitive neuropsychology possible? *Journal of Cognitive Neuroscience*, **4**, 80–95.

Christodoulou, G.N. (1975) *The Syndrome of Doubles*, Associate Professorship Thesis, University of Athens, Athens.

Coltheart, M. (1984) Editorial. *Cognitive Neuropsychology*, **1**, 1–8.

Costello, C.G. (1992) Research on symptoms versus research on syndromes: Arguments in favour of allocating more research time to the study of symptoms. *British Journal of Psychiatry*, **160**, 304–308.

Courbon, P., Fail. G. (1927) Illusion of Frégoli syndrome and schizophrenia. *Societé Clinique de Medécine Mentale*, January.

Courbon, P., Tusques, J. (1932) Illusion d'intermetamorphose et de charme. *Annales Medico-psychologiques* (Paris), **90**, 401–405.

Crichton, P., Lewis, S. (1990) Delusional misidentification, AIDS and the right hemisphere. *British Journal of Psychiatry*, **157**, 608–610.

Critchley, E.M.R. (1989) The neurology of familiarity. *Behavioural Neurology*, **2**, 195–200.

Cutting, J. (1990) *The Right Cerebral Hemisphere and Psychiatric Disorders*, Oxford University Press, Oxford.

David, A.S. (1993) Cognitive neuropsychiatry? *Psychological Medicine*, **23**, 1–5.

de Haan, E.H.F., Young, A., Newcombe, F. (1987) Face recognition without awareness. *Cognitive Neuropsychology*, **4**, 385–415.

de Pauw, K.W., Szulecka, T.K., Poltock, T.L. (1987) Frégoli syndrome after cerebral infarction. *Journal of Nervous and Mental Diseases*, **175**, 433–438.

Dougherty, F.E., Bartlett, F.S., Izard, C.E. (1974) Response of schizophrenics to expressions of fundamental emotions. *Journal of Clinical Psychology*, **30**, 243–246.

Ekman, P., Friesen, W.V. (1976) *Pictures of Facial Affect*, Consulting Psychologists Press, Palo Alto.

Ekman, P., Friesen, W.V., Ellsworth, P. (1972) *Emotion in the Human Face: Guidelines for Research and Integration of Findings*. Pergamon, New York.

Ellis, A.W., Young, A.W. (1988) *Human Cognitive Neuropsychology*, Erlbaum, London.

Ellis, H.D. (1983) The role of the right hemisphere in face perception. In: *Functions of the Right Hemisphere* (Ed. A.W. Young), Academic Press, London.

Ellis, H.D. (1986) Processes underlying face recognition. In: *The Neuropsychology of Face Perception and Facial Expression* (Ed. R. Bruyer), Erlbaum, Hillsdale, NJ.

Ellis, H.D. (1991) *The cognitive neuropsychiatric origins of the Capgras delusion*. Paper presented at the International Symposium on the Neuropsychology of Schizophrenia, Institute of Psychiatry, London.

Ellis, H.D., de Pauw, K.W. (1994) The cognitive neuropsychiatric origins of the Capgras delusion. In: *The Neuropsychology of Schizophrenia* (Eds A. David, J. Cutting), ch. 18, pp. 317–335, Erlbaum, Hove, UK.

Ellis, H.D., Shepherd, J.W. (1992) Face memory: Theory and practice. In: *Aspects of Memory* (Eds M. Gruneberg et al), Routledge, London.

Ellis, H.D., Young, A.W. (1990) Accounting for delusional misidentifications. *British Journal of Psychiatry*, **157**, 239–248.

Ellis, H.D., de Pauw, K.W., Christodoulou, G.N., Milne, A.B., Joseph, A.B. (1993) Responses to facial and non-facial stimuli presented tachistoscopically in either or' both visual fields by patients with the Capgras delusion and paranoid schizophrenia. *Journal of Neurology, Neurosurgery and Psychiatry*, **56**, 215–219.

Enoch, M.D., Trethowan, W.H. (1991) *Uncommon Psychiatric Syndromes* (3rd edn), John Wright, Bristol.

Fleminger, S. (1992) Seeing is believing: The role of "preconscious" perceptual processing in delusional misidentification. *British Journal of Psychiatry*, **160**, 293–303.

Flor-Henry, P. (1976) Lateralised temporal–limbic dysfunction and psychopathology. *Annals of the New York Academy of Science*, **280**, 777–795.

Förstl, H., Almeida, O.P., Owen, A.M., Burns, A., Howard, R. (1991a) Psychiatric, neurological and medical aspects of misidentification syndromes: A review of 260 cases. *Psychological Medicine*, **21**, 905–910.

Förstl, H., Burns, A., Jacoby, R., Levy, R. (1991b) Neuroanatomical correlates of clinical misidentification and misperception in senile dementia of the Alzheimer type. *Journal of Clinical Psychiatry*, **52**, 268–271.

Hay, D.C., Young, A.W. (1982) The human face. In: *Normality and Pathology in Cognitive Functions* (Ed. A. Ellis), Academic Press, New York.

Hécaen, H. (1981) The neuropsychology of face recognition. In: *Perceiving and Remembering Faces* (Eds G. Davies, H. Ellis, J. Shepherd), Academic Press, London.

Joseph, A.B. (1986) Focal central nervous system abnormalities in patients with misidentification syndrome. *Bibliotheca Psychiatrica*, **164**, 68–79.

Kahlbaum, K.L. (1866) Die Sinnes delirien. C. Die Illusion. *Allgemeine Zeitschrift für Psychiatrie*, **23**, 56–78.

Kaney, S., Bentall, R.P. (1989) Persecutory delusions and attributional style. *British Journal of Medical Psychology*, **62**, 191–198.

Kraepelin, E. (1913) *Dementia Praecox and Paraphrenia* (translated by R.M. Barclay, 1919), Livingstone, Edinburgh.

Kurucz, J., Feldmar, G. (1979) Prosopo-affective agnosia as a symptom of cerebral organic disease. *Journal of the American Geriatrics Society*, **27**, 225–230.

Kurucz, J., Feldmar, G., Werner, W. (1979) Prosopo-affective agnosia associated with chronic organic brain syndrome. *Journal of the American Geriatrics Society*, **27**, 91–95.

Lewis, S.W. (1987) Brain imaging in a case of Capgras' syndrome. *British Journal of Psychiatry*, **150**, 117–121.

Luaute, J.P., Bidault, E., Thionville, M. (1978) Syndrome de Capgras et organicité cérébrale: A propos d'une malade étudiée par un test de reconnaissance des visages et par la scanographie. *Annales Mèdico-Psychologiques*, **5**, 803–815.

MacCallum, W. (1973) Capgras symptoms with an organic basis. *British Journal of Psychiatry*, **123**, 639–642.

Magaro, P.A., Chamrad, D.L. (1983) Information processing and lateralization in schizophrenia. *Biological Psychiatry*, **18**, 29–44.

Maher, B.A. (1974) Delusional thinking and perceptual disorder. *Journal of Individual Psychology*, **30**, 98–113.

Maher, B.A. (1988) Anomalous experience and delusional thinking: The logic of explanations. In: *Delusional Belief* (Eds T. Oltmanns, B. Maher), pp. 15–33, Wiley, New York.

Malliaras, D.E., Kossovitsa, Y.T., Christodoulou, G.N. (1978) Organic contributors to the inter-metamorphosis syndrome. *American Journal of Psychiatry*, **135**, 985–987.

Mandler, G. (1980) Recognising: The judgment of previous occurrence. *Psychological Review*, **87**, 252–271.

McDonald, J., McGurk, H. (1976) Visual influence on speech perception processes. *Perception and Psychophysics*, **24**, 253–257.

McGhie, A., Chapman, J. (1961) Disorders of attention and perception in early schizophrenia. *British Journal of Medical Psychology*, **34**, 103–116.

Morrison, R.L., Tarter, R.E. (1984) Neuropsychological findings relating to Capgras syndrome. *Biological Psychiatry*, **19**, 1119–1128.

Morrison, R.L., Bellack, A.S., Mueser, K.T. (1988) Deficits in facial-affect recognition and schizophrenia. *Schizophrenia Bulletin*, **14**, 67–83.

Myslobodsky, M.S., Goldberg, T., Johnson, F., Hicks, L., Weinberger, D. (1992) Lipreading in patients with schizophrenia. *Journal of Nervous and Mental Disease*, **180**, 168–171.

Nathan, P. (1967) *Cues, Decisions and Diagnoses*, Academic Press, New York.

Novic, J., Luchins, D.J., Perline, R. (1984) Facial affect recognition in schizophrenia: Is there a differential deficit? *British Journal of Psychiatry*, **144**, 533–537.

Parry, F.M., Young, A.W., Saul, J.S.M., Moss, A. (1991) Dissociable face processing impairments after brain injury. *Journal of Clinical and Experimental Neuropsychology*, **13**, 545–558.

Pick, A. (1903) On reduplicative paramnesia. *Brain*, **26**, 344–383.

Pilowsky, I., Bassett, D. (1980) Schizophrenia and the response to facial emotions. *Comprehensive Psychiatry*, **21**, 236–244.

Rhodes, G. (1985) Literalised processes in face recognition. *British Journal of Psychology*, **76**, 249–271.

Sergent, J., Poncet, M. (1990) From covert to overt recognition of faces in a prosopagnosic patient. *Brain*, **113**, 989–1004.

Shallice, T. (1988) *From Neuropsychology to Mental Structure*, Cambridge University Press, Cambridge.

Shannon, A. (1970) Unpublished PhD thesis, University of California. Cited by Novic et al.

Shraberg, D., Weitzel, W.D. (1979) Prosopagnosia and the Capgras syndrome. *Journal of Clinical Psychiatry*, **40**, 313–316.

Slade, P., Bentall, R.P. (1988) *Sensory Deception: A Scientific Analysis of Hallucinations*, Croom-Helm, London.

Sno, H.N., Linszen, D.H. (1990) The déjà vu experience: Remembrance of things past? *American Journal of Psychiatry*, **147**, 1587–1595.

Tranel, D., Damasio, A.R. (1985) Knowledge without awareness: An autonomic index of facial recognition by prosopagnosics. *Science*, **228**, 1453–1454.

Tranel, D., Damasio, A.R., Damasio, H. (1988) Intact recognition of facial expression, gender, and age in patients with impaired recognition of face identity. *Neurology*, **38**, 690–696.

Tzavaras, A., Hécaen, H., Le Bras, H. (1970) Le problème de la spécificité du déficit de la reconnaissance du visage humain lors des lésions hémisphériques unilatérales. *Neuropsychologia*, **8**, 403–416.

Tzavaras, A., Luaute, J.P., Bidault, E. (1986) Face recognition dysfunction and delusional misidentification syndromes (DMS) In: *Aspects of Face Processing* (Eds H.D. Ellis, M.A. Jeeves, F. Newcombe, A. Young), pp. 310–316, Martinus Nijhoff, Dordrecht.

Van Lancker, D. (1991) Personal relevance and the human right hemisphere. *Brain and Cognition*, **17**, 64–92.

Warrington, E.K. (1984) *Recognition Memory Test*, NFER-Nelson, Windsor.

Wilcox, J., Waziri, R. (1983) The Capgras symptom and nondominant cerebral dysfunction. *Journal of Clinical Psychiatry*, **44**, 70–72.

Wright, S., Young, A.W., Hellawell, D.J. (1993) Frégoli delusion and erotomania (letter). *Journal of Neurology, Neurosurgery and Psychiatry*, **56**, 322–323.

Young, A.W. (1992) Face recognition impairments. *Philosophical Transactions of the Royal Society, London*, **B335**, 47–54.

Young, A.W., Bruce, V. (1991) Perceptual categories and the computation of "grandmother". *European Journal of Cognitive Psychology*, **3**, 5–49.

Young, A.W., de Haan, E.H.F. (1992) Face recognition and awareness after brain injury. In: *The Neuropsychology of Consciousness* (Eds A.D. Milner, M.D. Rugg), pp. 69–90, Academic Press, London.

Young, A.W., Ellis, H.D. (1989) Childhood prosopagnosia. *Brain and Cognition*, **9**, 16–47.

Young, A.W., Hay, D.C., Ellis A.W. (1985) The faces that launched a thousand slips: Everyday difficulties and errors in recognising people. *British Journal of Psychology*, **76**, 495–523.

Young, A.W., Ellis, H.D., Szulecka, T.K., de Pauw, K.W. (1990) Face processing impairments and delusional misidentification. *Behavioural Neurology*, **3**, 153–168.

Young, A.W., Reid I., Wright, S., Hellawell, D.J. (1993) Face processing impairments and the Capgras delusion. *British Journal of Psychiatry*, **162**, 695–698.

Zuroff, D.C., Colussy, S.A. (1986) Emotion recognition in schizophrenic and depressed patients. *Journal of Clinical Psychology*, **42**, 411–417.

Part E

TREATMENT AND COGNITIVE IMPAIRMENTS

20

Medication and Cognitive Functioning in Schizophrenia

DAVID J. KING and JONATHAN F. GREEN

> Although a patient under the influence of chlorpromazine at first glance presents the aspect of a heavily drugged person, one is surprised at the absence of clouding of consciousness. The higher psychic functions are preserved to a remarkable degree, and the patients are capable of sustained attention, reflection, and concentration . . . the drug seems to have little effect on those psychological functions which have their representation in the cortex, but appears to affect selectively those subcortical structures that are concerned with maintaining psychomotor drive and wakefulness.
>
> (Lehmann & Hanrahan, 1954)

INTRODUCTION

The most remarkable aspect of the neuropsychological effects of neuroleptics is that these drugs usually improve cognitive functioning in schizophrenic patients but impair information processing in normal healthy volunteers (King, 1990). This may be because the resultant improvement in psychopathology in these patients compensates for any drug-induced cognitive impairment, or that improved motivation accompanies the improvement in clinical state, or that the drugs have a primary effect on some attentional mechanism which is defective in schizophrenia. In the latter case we do not yet know whether such a beneficial effect is an indirect result of a general effect on arousal or attention (Tecce & Cole, 1972), or even of "psychic indifference" (Healy, 1989), suppression of "released" limbic dopamine hyperactivity (King, 1990), or a more direct, selective effect on a primary and specific attentional disorder, such as defective filtering of information (Hemsley, 1975; Joseph et al, 1979) or attentional shifting (Berger et al, 1989; Clark et al, 1989).

To avoid the confounding effects of illness, studies in normal healthy volunteers are necessary and these have been reviewed elsewhere (King, 1990, 1992). The earlier studies in schizophrenic patients have also been reviewed previously (King,

Schizophrenia: A Neuropsychological Perspective. Edited by C. Pantelis, H.E. Nelson and T.R.E. Barnes
© 1996 John Wiley & Sons Ltd

1990) and by several other authors as well (Heaton & Crowley, 1981; Medalia et al, 1988; Spohn & Strauss, 1989; Cassens et al, 1990). These have generally examined neuroleptic effects as adverse drug reactions with confounding effects on the results of neuropsychological test batteries. After a brief summary of these reviews some more recent studies will be examined, together with some studies of the effect of anticholinergic drugs – the other main medication commonly used in the treatment of schizophrenic patients.

This chapter will be limited to conventional tests of cognition. A specific memory deficit has been demonstrated in schizophrenia occurring in patients with acute and chronic illness (McKenna et al, 1990). This disorder, thought to have a pattern similar to classical amnesic syndrome (Tamlyn et al, 1992), is not reviewed here (see Chen and McKenna, chapter 7). For neuroleptic effects on EEG parameters the reader is referred elsewhere (Fink, 1969; Saletu et al, 1986, 1987; Merrin et al, 1988; Bartel et al, 1988; Kemali et al, 1991; Nakagawa et al, 1991; Roth et al, 1991). A brief summary of some of this pharmaco-EEG work, however, is given at the end of the conclusion section.

PREVIOUS REVIEWS

Persistent problems in interpreting the literature are: difficulties in controlling for the dose and duration of treatment; variables due to intelligence, practice effects, motivation, and type and severity of schizophrenic illness. The latter may be particularly important in view of the recent findings that three distinct schizophrenic syndromes can be identified with different patterns of altered cerebral metabolism (Liddle et al, 1992; see also Liddle, chapter 15).

Heaton & Crowley (1981) reviewed 12 studies in schizophrenic patients from the point of view of neuroleptics causing misleading neuropsychological test results. They thought that three attributes of neuroleptic drugs – sedation, anticholinergic action (particularly blurring of vision) and extrapyramidal symptoms – might be expected to lead to impaired test results. However, they found that few significant changes occurred once patients were stabilised on neuroleptics and, on balance, these drugs enhanced performance on tests of attention.

Medalia et al (1988) classified their review of neuroleptic effects according to different neuropsychological tests. They found consistent reports of impaired memory and fine motor co-ordination, which were probably related to muscarinic and dopamine receptor antagonism, respectively. Some studies reported impaired planning, as measured by various maze tests. Tests of language, intelligence and attention, including the Halstead–Reitan test battery, however, gave equivocal results. Two studies which found improvement in a backward visual masking task (Braff & Saccuzzo, 1982) and both EEG and psychometric tests (Saletu et al, 1986), however, were not included in this review.

Spohn & Strauss (1989) estimated that the relevant literature in this field exceeded 400 published reports. They extensively reviewed 109 of these and noted the great variability in experimental design and the importance of this in the interpretation of test results. They concluded that neuroleptic treatment was associated with normalisation of disordered thinking and of attention/information-processing dysfunction but that no direct cause and effect relationship could be inferred. Indeed, they cited evidence that very high doses may have deleterious effects on measures that otherwise improve at moderate dose levels. Furthermore, they found that some neuropsychological and psychophysiological measures are unaffected by treatment and may therefore be trait markers, viz. the reaction time crossover effect, orientating-response non-responding and impaired smooth-pursuit eye movements.

Cassens et al (1990) also reviewed this literature and, like Medalia et al (1988), classified the studies according to individual test results and provided several very useful tables. They contrasted the effects of acute with chronic neuroleptic drug treatment in chronic schizophrenic patients. They concluded that chronic dosing was associated with improved performance on sustained attention and visuomotor function, and that there were no residual impairments unrelated to motor effects.

King (1990) found that of 30 early studies of cognitive or psychomotor function in schizophrenic patients undergoing neuroleptic treatment, ten reported no change or variable effects, six reported impairments, and 14 found improvements in at least some tests. Following the work of Kornetsky et al (1959) and Latz and Kornetsky (1965) (reviewed by Kornetsky, 1972), the continuous performance test (CPT) of Rosvold et al (1956) was frequently used as a test of attention which distinguished schizophrenic patients from normal controls and which was "normalised" by neuroleptic treatment. They proposed that chlorpromazine acted preferentially on that portion of the ascending reticular activating system responsible for tonic (sustained) cortical arousal as opposed to phasic (brief) cortical arousal. Thus cortical function would be relatively spared and phasic arousal could be increased, via descending corticoreticular pathways, for the performance of brief cognitive tasks (digit symbol substitution test) but not for tasks which required more sustained (tonic) attention such as the CPT (Mirsky & Kornetsky, 1964). Subsequently, however, as noted by Medalia et al (1988), the CPT gave inconsistent results.

Thus, apart from Medalia et al (1988), there appears to have been a consensus that chronic neuroleptic drug effects in schizophrenic patients are associated with modest improvements in at least some neuropsychological tests. However, because of the confounding problems of the illness variables already alluded to, it is important to try to address two questions:

1. Is it possible to identify changes which are independent of clinical state?
2. Is it possible to identify which particular cognitive function(s) are affected by neuroleptics?

STUDIES OF NEUROLEPTICS AND COGNITIVE FUNCTION IN SCHIZOPHRENIA

With the above two questions in mind, a further review of some more recent studies was undertaken. Twenty-five studies, which were published between 1981 and 1991, are summarised in Table 20.1, and the findings of more recent studies involving clozapine are listed in Table 20.2.

Overall inspection of Table 20.1 shows that very variable effects of neuroleptic treatment on different types of cognitive function have been reported. Improvements are reported in the majority (13), impairments in four, no change in five and mixed effects in three studies.

PRACTICE EFFECTS

In two of the studies reporting improvements the effects of practice could not be excluded (Fields et al, 1988; Calvert et al, 1990). Two of the studies reporting no change attributed improvements on WAIS scores to practice (Killian et al, 1984; Gold & Hurt, 1990). Two studies which controlled for practice by repeated practice sessions before testing nevertheless found further improvements attributable to neuroleptics (Earle-Boyer et al, 1991; Nestor et al, 1991).

STATISTICAL ISSUES

The studies reviewed here differ greatly in their structures and in the nature of the analysis attempted with the data obtained. This affects whether a change in a cognitive measure is considered to have occurred or not. The use of very large test batteries is common and makes the occurrence of false positive results more likely. Some of the studies use statistical techniques to account for this, but it appears that some do not; a considerable issue in view of the powerful effect of Bonferroni correction or similar procedures on statistical significance. Similarly, many studies put emphasis on trends (results approaching but not reaching statistical significance). These variations are not surprising bearing in mind the practical problems involved in this type of study and because trends and borderline results may be consistent with the findings of previous work. Nevertheless, the extent of the variation in statistical methods and interpretation in this field is of major importance when comparing studies that may appear superficially similar.

EFFECTS OF DOSE

Attempts to investigate the effects of neuroleptic dose were only reported in five of these studies. In two of them increasing impairments were found with increasing dose (Spohn et al, 1985a; Cutmore & Beninger, 1990); impairments were associated with sedation in another (Erickson et al, 1984); improvement was dose-dependent in one study (Strauss et al, 1985); and in another study no relationship with dose was found (Bartkó et al, 1989). Since most studies have been carried out in chronically ill patients, this problem is confounded by the effects of tolerance during chronic dosing, which were noted in the earliest studies (Kornetsky et al, 1959). Furthermore, in such patients high doses probably intercorrelate with the severity of illness. Therefore, no firm conclusions can be drawn about this point.

TYPE OF TEST

The variation in reported neuroleptic effects appears to apply equally to all tests. Thus, CPT performance was reported to be improved by neuroleptics in four of these studies (Walker, 1981, 1983; Serper et al, 1990; Earle-Boyer et al, 1991; Nestor et al, 1991) but impaired in two (Erickson et al, 1984; Harvey et al, 1990). Even within one group of workers variable findings were reported (Harvey et al, 1990; Serper et al, 1990; Earle-Boyer et al, 1991). The SAT was improved in two studies (Marder et al, 1984; Spohn et al, 1985b) and impaired in one (Spohn et al, 1985a). Visual backward masking was improved in one (Braff & Saccuzzo, 1982) and impaired in another (Harvey et al, 1990). As argued previously, it seems likely that non-specific aspects of the test such as its duration and experimental design are as important as the specific details of the task used, in detecting neuroleptic drug effects (King, 1990, 1992).

RELATIONSHIP TO CLINICAL STATE

In those studies in which the degree of psychopathology was measured, nine (Braff & Saccuzzo, 1982; Killian et al, 1984; Spohn et al, 1985a; Fields et al, 1988; Cutmore & Beninger, 1990; Harvey et al, 1990; Serper et al, 1990; Earle-Boyer et al, 1991; Nestor et al, 1991) found that the changes in cognitive function (in three of which this was an impairment: Spohn et al, 1985a; Cutmore & Beninger, 1990; Harvey et al, 1990) were independent of clinical state, while three (Wahba et al, 1981; Spohn et al, 1985b; Classen & Laux, 1989) found improvements in cognitive function correlated with improvements in clinical state. Spohn et al have reported conflicting findings. Initially they found improvements in a number of tests which paralleled clinical recovery (Spohn et al, 1977), but later modified this view in the light of their multiple regression analyses which controlled for measures of motivation ("general deficit functioning"), tardive dyskinesia, and drug dose (Spohn et al, 1985a). A further study reported concomitant improvements in SAT and BPRS scores (Spohn et al, 1985b). In their review they say that both thought disorder and some measures of attention (or information processing) are improved while some are unchanged, and that no simple cause and effect relationship can be deduced (Spohn & Strauss, 1989).

A relationship may occur between clinical state and cognitive function but be separated in time. Hagger et al (1993) stated that BPRS negative symptoms and total score predicted changes in cognitive test score, but found that the times at which these improvements occurred were separated by weeks to months. These authors also pointed out that the correlation between clinical state and cognitive function was often not present for those cognitive tests that showed the greatest amount of change.

The types of measures of clinical state used in these studies have been quite limited; most employ only the BPRS. It is possible that different scales, particularly those which emphasise social functioning, may give rise to results more closely linked to cognitive function. For example, one group reported that while the BPRS was a poor predictor of cognitive improvement with clozapine, the

Table 20.1. Effects of neuroleptics on cognitive function in schizophrenic patients (1981–1991)

Study	Design	Neuroleptics	Tests of clinical state	Tests of cognition	Neuroleptic effect[b]	Comment/conclusion
1. Wahba et al. (1981)	44 acute inpatients on 3 dose levels, tested before and after treatment (10 days). 23 normal controls	HPL (10–100 mg/day)	BPRS	Proverbs Vocabulary Digit span	↑ ↑ ↑	Improvement with improvement in clinical state. No change in controls
2. Braff & Saccuzzo (1982)	20 medicated, 16 drug-free patients and 20 depressed "controls", tested on one occasion	Various (400–5000 mg CPZ equivalents per day)	CGI	Visual backward masking task	↑	Improved information processing with medication in spite of greater psychopathology
3. Walker (1981, 1983)	15 acute schizophrenic, 15 schizoaffective and 15 affective disorder in-patients, (11 drug-free), tested on one occasion	Various (no details provided)	–	CPT	↑	Non-significant trend in secondary data analysis
4. Erickson et al (1984)	11 adolescent inpatients randomly assigned to 2 drugs, tested before and 35 days after treatment	Thioridazine (0.23 mg/kg) thiothixene (2.2 mg/kg)	BPRS CGI	CPT	→	Impairment associated with sedation
5. Killian et al (1984)	34 inpatients after 3-week washout and after 4 weeks on medication. 13 inpatients continued on medication. 26 normal controls	Various (no details provided)	BPRS CGI	Block design[a] DSST[a] Object assembly[a] Picture completion[a] Rod and figure Embedded figures Stroop Size estimation Schematizing SOMT CFFT	– – – – – – – – – – –	Practice effects only. Improvement independent of degree of clinical change

No.	Authors	Sample	Drug/dose	Rating scale	Test	Effect	Comments
6.	Marder et al (1984)	13 acute patients before and after 14 days treatment. 18 chronic stabilised outpatients on 2 occasions 3 months apart	HPL (10 mg/day) FPZ (5–37.5 mg i.m. every 14 days)	BPRS BPRS	SAT SAT	↑ —	Poor information processing predicted poor clinical response to neuroleptics
7.	Spohn et al (1985a)	72 medicated and 12 drug-free chronic inpatients	Various (mostly HPL, thiothixine or FPZ)	BPRS, General deficit functioning scale	SAT Skin conductance Eye movements Simple RT	→ → → →	Correlational and stepwise multiple regression analyses indicated that high doses impaired performance
8.	Spohn et al (1985b)	64 chronic patients after drug withdrawal and 36 on continued medication, tested on 4 occasions every 2 weeks	(No details provided)	BPRS, General deficit functioning scale	SAT TDIw TDIr	↑ — —	Neuroleptics decreased effect of distraction and improved BPRS
9.	Strauss et al (1985)	25 chronic outpatients	Various (serum levels: 2–190 ng/ml CPZ equivalents)	Mini PSE	Simple RT Digit Span ± distraction	↑ ↑	High serum levels associated with less distractibility
10.	Berman et al (1986)	24 medicated and 18 drug-free (4 weeks) chronic inpatients and 26 normal controls, tested during rCBF study	HPL (0.4 mg/kg per day) in 17 patients – rest on various neuroleptics	—	WCST NM CPT	— — (not reported)	No changes in WCST or rCBF with neuroleptics, rCBF in DLPFC reduced in patients compared to controls during WCST but not NM or CPT
11.	Saletu et al (1986)	20 acute male patients tested before and after acute and chronic treatment, as part of quantitative EEG study	HPL (5–20 mg/day) Fluperlapine (100–520 mg/day)	—	ART Pauli Test Numerical Memory RT Archimedean Spiral CFFT	↑ ↑ ↑ — —	Acute treatment caused some impairments in attention but chronic treatments were associated with improvements

continued over

Table 20.1. Continued

Study	Design	Neuroleptics	Tests of clinical state	Tests of cognition	Neuroleptic effect[b]	Comment/conclusion
12. Classen & Laux (1988)	50 acute inpatients tested once	HPL (10–30 mg/day) FLU (5–20 mg) Clozapine (150–500 mg/day)	–	Motor skill Auditory and visual RT Stroop IQ	– – – –	NS trend for better performance on 2 Stroop subtests, with clozapine
13. Fields et al (1988)	10 male inpatients tested before and after 3 weeks treatment	Clonidine (0.4–1.4 mg/day)	BHPRS	Wechsler MQ Delayed memory PPVT DSST Trials A Trials B	↑ ↑ – – – ↑	No change in psychosis ratings. Practice effects not excluded
14. Barkó et al (1989)	98 chronic inpatients, open study, tested after 28 days	HPL and various others. Mean dose 615 mg CPZ equivalents/day	CGI	MMS	–	No relationship between neuroleptic dose and cognitive performance
15. Classen & Laux (1989)	29 acute inpatients, double-blind, parallel groups. Tested at beginning and end of 4 weeks treatment	HPL (12–22.5 mg/day) or RMX (270–480 mg/day)	BPRS	Finger tapping Auditory RT Visual RT Stroop	↓ (HLP and RMX) ↓ (RMX) ↑ (HPL) ↓ (RMX) ↑ (HPL)	RMX group had more benzodiazepines; HPL group had more anticholinergics. Performance correlated with improvement in BPRS scores
16. Calvert et al (1990)	7 schizophrenic, 5 "other psychotic", 4 "non-psychotic" inpatients, and 16 controls, tested drug-free and after 4–6 weeks open treatment	Various (drugs and doses not specified)	–	Object naming tests	↑	Effects of practice, illness and drugs cannot be distinguished (controls performed perfectly on both occasions)

Study	Sample	Medication	Clinical scale	Tests		Results/comments
17. Cleghorn et al (1990)	37 medicated chronic outpatients; 27 drug-free acute in-patients; 27 normal controls; tested on one occasion	Various (details provided)	SAPS SANS	WAIS Immediate recall Rey figure Trials A and B WCST Peg board Finger tapping Spatial block span Porteus mazes CPT	— ↑ → — → — → — →← ↑	Clinical symptoms, including thought disorder, less in treated than drug-free patients. Therefore, impairment on some tests due to neuroleptics rather than thought disorder. However, patient groups not comparable (medicated patients had longer illness, more episodes and larger VBRs)
18. Cutmore & Beninger (1990)	(i) 20 male outpatients, and 14 normal male controls	Depot HPL (0.092 mg/kg per day) or depot FLU (0.047 mg/kg per day)	BPRS	Pursuit rotor OPAT PAL Finger tapping RT	→ → → — —	PAL correlated with BPRS (thought disorder) score. Other impairments independent of psychopathology
	(ii) 26 chronic inpatients, and 11 normal controls	Various (mean 12 mg CPZ equivalent/kg per day) Mean serum prolactin: 30.7 µg/l (patients) 11.9 µg/l (controls)	BPRS	Pursuit rotor OPAT PAL Finger tapping RT	→ → — → →	Multiple regression found impairments in all tests (except PAL) predicted by either CPZ or prolactin level. Therefore, incentive, but not associative learning, impaired by neuroleptics

continued over

Table 20.1. Continued

Study	Design	Neuroleptics	Tests of clinical state	Tests of cognition	Neuroleptic effect[b]	Comment/conclusion
19. Gold & Hurt (1990)	19 acute inpatients tested before and 26 days after treatment	HPL (dose not given)	BPRS	WAIS TDIw	— ↑	Tests only correlated at baseline. Improvement in WAIS (6 points) consistent with practice effect. Neuroleptics affect thought disorder but not cognition. Thought disorder causes apparent cognitive impairment and not vice versa
20. Harvey et al (1990)	14 medicated and 14 drug-free inpatients and outpatients, 15 normal controls, tested on one occasion	HPL (20 mg/day) + benztropine (2 mg/day) for 2 weeks	BPRS	CPT Visual backward masking task	↓ ↓	Differences between medicated and drug-free patients only significant on one measure. Tests said, therefore, to be trait markers. However, BPRS scores were almost identical in 2 patient groups
21. Serper et al (1990)	4 medicated and 4 drug-free male, chronic inpatients, and 4 normal controls, tested 16 times over 3 weeks	HPL (20 mg/day) + benztropine (2 mg/day) for 2 weeks	BPRS	CPT ± Word Shadowing task	↑	Automation of dual task of divided attention normalised in medicated but not drug-free patients. Since BPRS scores were unchanged and similar in both groups throughout, neuroleptic effect was independent of clinical state

Study	Sample / Design	Treatment	Rating scales	Cognitive tests	Outcome	Comments
22. Strauss & Klieser (1990)	18 chronic inpatients with acute exacerbations tested before and after 4 weeks treatment in double-blind comparative trial	HPL (16 mg/day) or RMX (375 mg/day)	BPRS	IQ Memory Concentration	↑ (RMX) → (HPL) ↑ (RMX) → (HPL) ↑ (RMX) → (HPL)	No significant differences when baseline differences controlled by ANCOVA
23. Earle-Boyer et al (1991)	17 medicated and 17 drug-free chronic inpatients, and 19 normal controls tested on one occasion after 10 practice sessions	HPL (20 mg/day) + benztropine (2 mg/day) for 2 weeks	SATLCD SANS	CPT (visual) CPT (auditory) Motor proficiency	↑ ↑ —	Both patient groups worse than normals in all tasks. Medicated better than drug-free patients on non-lexical tasks. No differences in clinical ratings between patient groups. Neuroleptics improve attentional capacity independent of clinical state
24. Goldberg et al (1991)	21 chronic inpatients tested on 2 occasions ± D-amphetamine (0.25 mg/kg) in double-blind, placebo-controlled crossover design	HPL (0.4 mg/kg per day)	POMS CGI (videotaped interview)	WCST CPT Stroop Verbal Fluency Selective Reminding Comprehension Spontaneous rotation Finger tapping Trail making Design drawing Eye blinking	— — — — — — — — — — —	NS trend for improvement in WCST with amphetamine. (? Enhanced DLPFC activity with D1 stimulation; ? reversal of HPL-induced dysphoria and dyskinesia)

continued over

Table 20.1. Continued

Study	Design	Neuroleptics	Tests of clinical state	Tests of cognition	Neuroleptic effect[b]	Comment/conclusion
25. Nestor et al. (1991)	13 chronic male patients on medication and 12 chronic male patients drug-free (22 days), tested on one occasion after 200 practice trials on standard CPT	CPZ (798 mg CPZ equivalents/day)	BPRS	CPT – standard – blurred	– ↑	Drug-free patients had greater decline in sensitivity of detection over time, independent of non-specific factors (motivation, fatigue) or clinical state (BPRS identical in 2 groups). Neuroleptics improve attention independently of clinical state

Key: [a]WAIS tests.   [b]↑   improvement in cognitive function
                            ↓   impairment in cognitive function
                            –   no change in cognitive function

QLS was closely related to such improvements, particularly in memory function (Buchanan et al, 1994). On balance, however, most studies agree that changes in cognitive function are independent of changes in clinical state: clinical improvement can occur in spite of impairments in cognition (Spohn et al, 1985a; Cutmore & Beninger, 1990) and cognitive improvement may occur with no change in clinical state (Braff & Saccuzzo, 1982; Serper et al, 1990; Earle-Boyer et al, 1991; Nestor et al, 1991).

CLOZAPINE

Clozapine has shown greater efficacy in improving symptoms of schizophrenia than the conventional neuroleptics and may have a different mechanism of action. It has been suggested that clozapine might, therefore, have more efficacy in improving cognitive dysfunction in psychosis. However, Classen & Laux (1988) found only a trend towards improvement in two Stroop subtests with clozapine. Similarly, Goldberg et al (1993) found that, in 15 patients treated with clozapine for 15 months, although there was a 38% fall in the ratings of psychopathology, there was no change in intelligence, Wechsler Memory Quotient, the Wisconsin Card Sorting Test, Digit Symbol Substitution or a trail making test. Furthermore, since there was no change in social adjustment over this time (occupation or living arrangements) it appeared that cognitive function rather than psychopathology was the principal determinant of successful rehabilitation. However, interpretation of this study is difficult because of major variation in the times of testing (3–24 months) and because of changes in other psychoactive medications.

In contrast to the above findings Hagger et al (1993) showed a significant improvement in some cognitive functions when they examined the effects of clozapine on 36 patients with treatment refractory schizophrenia. These findings were roughly paralleled by a second study in which selective improvements in performance with clozapine were also found (Buchanan et al, 1994). Comparison of these two papers yields some interesting contrasts. Buchanan et al (1994) found less improvement in memory than in other tests which would be in keeping with the strong anticholinergic properties of clozapine. However, Hagger et al (1993) found clear improvements in memory tests and suggested that this reflected a partial cholinergic agonist effect of clozapine *in vivo*. They also demonstrated a tentative link between BPRS negative symptoms and cognitive function whereas Buchanan et al (1994) emphasised a link with the QLS.

Zahn et al (1994) examined reaction time paradigms closely in patients with chronic schizophrenia treated with clozapine. The authors concluded that the processing of certain types of stimuli may be affected by clozapine, perhaps because of reduction in hallucinations. The principal finding was that clozapine does not affect attention.

In conclusion, the results of the studies in this area are contradictory (summarised in Table 20.2). It may, however, be of significance that the Hagger and Buchanan studies were methodologically superior to the others and concurred in showing improvement in cognitive function with clozapine.

Table 20.2. Effects of clozapine on cognitive function in schizophrenic patients (key as for Table 20.1)

Study	Design	Neuroleptics	Clinical tests	Tests of cognition	Drug effect	Comments and conclusions
1. Goldberg et al (1993)	15 patients: 13 schizophrenic, 1 schizoaffective and 1 psychosis NOS. Assessed while on conventional neuroleptic then again after average 15 months on clozapine	Clozapine 250–750 mg; various conventional neuroleptics (drugs and doses provided). Much use of other psychotropic medication: lithium, fluoxetine, valproate, thyroxine, primidone	BPRS CGI	WAIS-R	—	Marked improvement in BPRS and CGI. Cognitive deficits independent of psychotic symptoms, and not affected by medication. Considerable changes in non-neuroleptic psychotropic medication between phases. Raters not blind
				WMS Form II	—	
				WMS visual reproduction	→	
				Digit symbol	—	
				Trails B	—	
				Category test	—	
				WCST	—	
				Facial recognition	—	
				Line orientation	—	
				WRAT	—	
2. Hagger et al (1993)	36 treatment-resistant schizophrenics; 26 controls. Assessed at baseline, and after 6 weeks and 6 months of clozapine treatment	Clozapine: at 6 weeks mean dose 363 mg ± 221 mg; at 6 months mean dose 403 mg ± 208 mg	BPRS	Digit symbol (WAIS-R)	—	↑ a	First column 6 weeks, second column 6 months. All measures impaired in schizophrenics at baseline. Improvement in psychopathology predated cognitive improvement by weeks to months.
				Consonant trigram	a	—	
				VLL – immediate recall	—	a	
				VLL – delayed recall	—	↑	
				COWA	↑	↑	
				Category instance generation	—	a	
				WCST – number of categories	—	—	
				WCST – % perseverative errors	—	—	
				WISC-R maze	—	a	

				Test		Comments
3. Buchanan et al (1994)	41 schizophrenic patients fulfilling neuroleptic partial response criteria. Assessed at baseline, after a 10-week double-blind parallel groups study and then after a 1-year open study	Clozapine 200–600 mg (mean 410.5 mg) or HPL 10–30 mg (mean 24.5 mg) for 10 weeks; then clozapine mean dose 437.9 mg for 1 year	BPRS SANS	COWA	— ↑	First column 10 weeks; second column 1 year. Cognitive changes not related to positive or negative symptoms but were related to Quality of Life Score. Less beneficial effect on memory tests possibly due to anticholinergic properties
				WCST	— —	
				Stroop colour–word	— ↓	
				Trails B	↓[b] →	
				Category fluency	— ↑	
				Mooney faces closure	— —	
				Benton judgement of lines	↓[b] ↑	
				WAIS-R block design	— —	
				WMS – figural memory	— —	
				WMS logical memory	— —	
				WMS – visual pairs	— —	
				WMS – verbal pairs	— —	
				WMS – visual reproduction	— —	
4. Zahn et al (1994)	25 schizophrenic patients; crossover design; variable time on each drug; variable dropout rate (clozapine $n = 25$, FPZ $n = 22$, placebo $n = 17$)	Clozapine mean dose $444 \pm$ SD 189 mg, FPZ $23.0 \pm$ SD 14.8 mg and placebo. Two patients on TDZ instead of FPZ	BPRS BHPRS	RT	—	Clozapine impaired RT with visual stimuli compared to auditory. Clozapine improved ability to process simultaneous stimuli, related to a reduction in hallucinations. Treatments were given in a fixed order

Key: [a]Denotes measures which were significant before, but not after, Bonferroni correction.
[b]Denotes worsening of performance with HPL but no change with clozapine.

NEUROLEPTICS, ATTENTION AND THOUGHT DISORDER

It can be argued that there are two distinct types of cognitive dysfunction, or central processing, in schizophrenia (Spohn et al, 1985b; Gold & Hurt, 1990), one related to formal thought disorder and the other to attention (or "information processing", which has been the preferred term used by many authors since the 1970s; see Oades, 1982a). However, two conflicting views of the relationship between these two, and their response to neuroleptics, have emerged. Originally, Spohn et al (1977) proposed that neuroleptics reduced schizophrenic symptoms by enhancing information processing. Killian et al (1984) took a similar view and regarded the cognitive deficits in schizophrenia as secondary to impaired motivation, attention and vigilance. However, since a measure of information processing (SAT) improved with neuroleptics but thought disorder did not (Spohn et al, 1985b), these authors argued that a deficit in information processing was not the primary pathophysiological abnormality, and that neuroleptics only had an indirect effect on thought disorder by improving information processing. Gold & Hurt (1990), however, reported opposite results. They found that thought disorder but not WAIS scores improved with neuroleptics. They therefore argued that the principal effect of neuroleptics was on the clinical state, including thought disorder, and that any effects on information processing were secondary. Both groups now seem to agree that thought disorder causes apparent cognitive impairment, due to disruption of information processing, rather than vice versa. They disagree as to which of these is principally improved by neuroleptic drugs.

Clearly, attention as measured by the CPT, SAT, CFFT, Stroop or the visual backward masking task is not the same as cognition as measured by such tests as the WAIS, proverbs, memory, PAL or PPVT, and neither is the same as clinical thought disorder as assessed by the TDIw, TDIr or conceptual disorganisation on the BPRS. They must, nevertheless, be closely interrelated and it seems very difficult to design studies which can distinguish which of these is the principal target for neuroleptic drugs. The differences between the Spohn et al (1985b) and Gold & Hurt (1990) studies may therefore be due to the fact that, while a similar measure of thought disorder was used (TDIw), the measures of attention were different (SAT and WAIS). Furthermore, of course, not all schizophrenic patients have formal thought disorder.

A variety of different attentional processes have been described such as: sustained attention, rapid automatic information processing, covert involuntary attention, voluntary selective attention, and voluntary switching of attention. These different attentional mechanisms may be localised in different areas of the brain (Posner et al, 1987, 1988; Posner & Petersen, 1990). Dopamine seems to be principally involved in conscious attention (Joseph et al, 1979) or in the switching of attention (Oades, 1982b; Berger et al, 1989; Clark et al, 1989). Thus, neuroleptics would be expected to have different effects depending upon the nature of attention being studied. However, different tests designed to measure the same type of attention can give very different results depending on other aspects of the test situation. Thus, using a covert attention task of the effects of valid and invalid cueing, Clark et al (1989) found droperidol enhanced the shifting of attention in normal volunteers, whereas Berger et al (1989) came to the opposite conclusion using card-sorting and word-fluency tests to study the effect of haloperidol in spasmodic torticollis.

One can also assume that the aetiology of the cognitive impairment (whether due to thought disorder or attentional dysfunction) will influence the response to neuroleptics. If this is irreversible, such as brain damage or a developmental aberration, little change with neuroleptics would be expected. The cognitive deficits measured by the Withers and Hinton scale, which correlate with negative symptoms and neurological soft signs (Johnstone et al, 1978; Crow, 1980; King et al, 1991), would belong to this category.

CONCLUSIONS

A wide variety of results have been reported in the 25 studies of the cognitive effects of neuroleptics in schizophrenic patients reviewed over the past decade. This is because of the wide number of variables involved and the lack of consistency in the tests and study designs used by different groups of workers. On balance, tests of sustained attention, such as the CPT and SAT, appear to be improved, independently of the clinical response to treatment. There is no agreement as to the nature of the link between attentional mechanisms and thought disorder, or on which of these neuroleptics have their primary effect. It seems likely from studies in animals and normal volunteers that neuroleptics act principally to enhance conscious attention, influencing the ability to decide to concentrate or to switch attention. An optimum dose and duration of treatment may be required to adapt to impairments due to other aspects of drug effects such as decreased alertness.

NEUROLEPTICS AND LATERALITY

The recent studies of the effects of neuroleptics on laterality in schizophrenia are no more conclusive than the above. The two questions posed are whether the reported changes could be secondary to neuroleptic effects and whether neuroleptics act to normalise an abnormality in functional lateralisation in schizophrenia. There appears to be a risk here of adapting the theory to fit the findings.

Tomer et al (1982) started with the hypothesis that schizophrenia was associated with left hemisphere hyperarousal (associated with increased lateral eye movements towards the right) but that, since neuroleptics could have asymmetric effects on the brain, the previous findings could have been an artefact of medication. They examined lateral eye movement bias in response to verbal and spatial emotional questions in 35 right-handed schizophrenics, seven of whom were drug-free. They found that the patients on piperazine phenothiazines had right lateral eye movements in contrast to the normal left eye movements in drug-free patients and patients on non-piperazine drugs. Piperazine drugs could, therefore, have been responsible for the previous reports on preferential orientation of eye movements towards the right. However, it is not clear whether this was thought to be brought about by improvement of left or suppression of right hemisphere function. Further problems with this study were that 15 different neuroleptics were being taken, together with a variety of antidepressants, benzodiazepines and anticholinergic drugs, and the majority of the patients were "non-responders" (i.e. lateral eye movements occurred in response to less than 25% of the questions).

Two further studies from the same group have supported the general hypothesis that neuroleptics normalise asymmetrical temporohippocampal function. Using the Mesulam Cancellation Test in which the accuracy of the cancellation of verbal and non-verbal targets on the left and right halves of sheets of paper can be compared, Tomer & Flor-Henry (1989) found that the effect of neuroleptics in 29 patients was to change inattention to the right to inattention to the left, that is, from an apparent impairment of left hemisphere function to impaired right hemisphere function. It was, therefore, argued that left hemisphere hyperarousal impaired performance in drug-free patients and neuroleptics impaired right hemisphere function in medicated patients. Tomer (1990) then studied 12 acutely psychotic patients before and 30 days after neuroleptic medication using tactile discrimination tasks designed to distinguish inter- and intra-hemispheric transfers of information. In comparison to 12 normal controls the patients made more errors whether or not on medication. Neuroleptics improved the performance of intra-hemispheric tasks with the right, but not with the left hand, and had no effect on inter-hemispheric tasks. Thus, the previously reported hemisphere asymmetries are not likely to be a drug effect but neuroleptic drugs did seem to improve left hemisphere function.

Finally, Frazier et al (1989) carried out a large study using four lateralisation scales from the Luria–Nebraska Neuropsychological Battery, on 52 schizophrenic (21 of whom were drug-free) and 39 manic-depressive patients. Effects of gender and medication, diagnosis and laterality were distinguished by analyses of variance. They found that the deficits in both diagnostic groups were bilateral, consistent with other evidence in the literature which is more supportive of bilateral rather than unilateral brain dysfunction in psychiatric disorders (Seidman, 1983). Neuroleptic treatment was associated with putative left hemisphere cognitive and perceptual impairments in both male and female patients with schizophrenia. No measures of clinical severity were provided and this finding could, therefore, be explained by the more seriously ill patients being on medication.

Taken together there seems little consistency in the findings of these studies. The later study (Tomer, 1990) had the best design and seems to have been more rigorous than the others. It appears, therefore, that if there is any inter-hemisphere asymmetry in schizophrenia it is neither affected by medication nor an artefact of it. Left hemisphere function as measured by tactile tests (Tomer, 1990) improved, while unilateral cognitive and perceptual skills may be impaired (Frazier et al, 1989), by neuroleptic drugs. Recent studies of neuroleptic effects on metabolic rate using positron emission tomography (PET) have not clarified the situation but, if anything, seem to add to the confusion. For instance, Buchsbaum et al (1991) found clozapine increased metabolism in the right putamen, whereas thiothixine decreased metabolism in the right caudate, in schizophrenics during a visual vigilance task.

ANTICHOLINERGIC DRUGS AND COGNITIVE FUNCTION

Clearly, patients with schizophrenia are frequently taking many other drugs, apart from neuroleptics, which might alter their cognitive function. These include antidepressants, lithium, benzodiazepines and anticholinergics. It is beyond the scope of any one chapter to deal with all of these, but since the commonest and the most likely to alter cognition are the anticholinergics, these are reviewed briefly below. In their review, Medalia et al (1988) found, as one might expect, that these drugs were the probable reason for reports of memory deficits in patients with schizophrenia. Furthermore, the majority of neuroleptics in clinical use have an in-built anticholinergic effect in addition to dopamine receptor antagonism (Snyder et al, 1974). This is particularly true, of course, for clozapine and thioridazine.

Tune et al (1982) first demonstrated that serum anticholinergic levels (measured by a radioreceptor assay (RRA) method and expressed in atropine equivalents) were significantly correlated with memory performance on a 10-item word list learning test ($r = 0.51$, $p < 0.01$), in 24 chronic schizophrenic outpatients. They suggested that anticholinergic drugs might have a narrow therapeutic window since the mean level was 12 pmol/ml and a previous study had shown that a level of 10 pmol/ml was required to reduce extrapyramidal symptoms.

A second group has reported two similar studies with conflicting findings. Katz et al (1985) found no correlation between serum anticholinergic levels and memory (Buschke selective reminding test using six trials for learning 12 words) in a mixed group of 22 chronic psychiatric outpatients. In this study there were only eight schizophrenic patients taking medication with anticholinergic activity and their mean serum level was only 3.6 pmol atropine equivalents/ml. They also demonstrated a wide individual variation in the association between memory deficits and serum anticholinergic activity. In longitudinal observations in two patients, one (a 20-year-old male with an acute psychosis) had profound short-term memory deficits associated with 60 pmol atropine equivalents/ml, whereas in the other (a 40-year-old female with chronic schizophrenia) memory function was intact in spite of anticholinergic levels of 44 and 53 pmol/ml. It seems, therefore, that anticholinergic levels can vary widely and that tolerance to the anticholinergic drug effects on memory are likely to occur in chronic patients. In the second study a detailed, 1-hour neuropsychological test battery was carried out in 17 chronic schizophrenic inpatients and the results compared with serum anticholinergic and neuroleptic levels using the same RRA technique (Perlick et al, 1986). On this occasion the mean serum anticholinergic levels were 10.6 pmol atropine equivalents/ml (very similar to those reported by Tune et al, 1982) and inversely correlated with learning of a 20-word list ($r = -0.54$, $p = 0.01$) (again remarkably similar to Tune et al, 1982). Since, however, no other cognitive tests, particularly a measure of recognition memory (the Mattis–Kovner Memory Inventory), correlated with the serum anticholinergic levels, these authors concluded that anticholinergic activity did not impair primary memory functioning but had a secondary effect on cognition by exacerbating attentional and motivational deficits. If this is so then the question arises as to what other cognitive deficits, apart from memory function, might be impaired by anticholinergic effects?

The inconsistencies in the findings of these three studies raise a number of questions. Why were the mean levels in the two studies from the New York group so different? The doses of the drugs were not given (neither for the neuroleptics nor the anticholinergics) and so we do not know if the different findings are due to variations in pharmacokinetics or, perhaps, in the assay. The RRA is a difficult technique and the coefficient of variation reported by Katz et al (1985) was 14%. If this method could be more widely used it would be interesting to see what other cognitive deficits in schizophrenia could be attributed to anticholinergic effects.

This is important work with both theoretical and practical implications. From the theoretical point of view it identifies a confounding variable which might account for some of the inconsistencies reported in the studies of neuroleptics and cognition reviewed above. The clinical relevance of these findings is that subtle, sub-clinical memory deficits, which could go unrecognised by either the doctor or the patient, might occur with therapeutic doses of anticholinergic medication and, more particularly, with unnecessary "as required" doses as prescribed in Katz et al's (1985) first case. It is also important to bear in mind that the bulk of the serum anticholinergic activity may be due to the neuroleptics themselves rather than to additional anticholinergic drugs (Perlick et al, 1986).

CONCLUSIONS AND PROSPECTS

What then can be said about neuroleptic medication and cognitive functioning in schizophrenia? At the present time only the most general conclusions are possible. It also depends upon what is meant by "cognition".

1. It is widely agreed that neuroleptic medication does not account for the cognitive deficits found in patients with schizophrenia.
2. Tests of cognition which depend on attention (particularly voluntary sustained attention or switching of attention) or information processing have generally been found to improve with neuroleptic treatment independently of overall clinical response, although there are several reports which contradict this assertion.
3. Cognition as measured by the WAIS and unpaced tests (such as the DSST, WCST and Stroop tests; see Table 20.1) are less susceptible to change.
4. It is unclear whether the primary effect of neuroleptics is on attentional mechanisms (such as filtering or shifting) or on some other process which is associated with thought disorder. It has been argued before that attention may be improved indirectly as a result of suppression of "released" hyperactivity of the limbic system (King, 1990). The results of Gold & Hurt (1990) are consistent with this view.

5. Previous reports of hemisphere asymmetries in schizophrenia are not an artefact of medication. Tactile tests of left hemisphere function improved with neuroleptic treatment, but unilateral cognitive and perceptual skills may be impaired.

6. Anticholinergic effects are an important confounding variable and probably account for short-term memory deficits (although several memory tests were, in fact, improved with neuroleptic treatment; see Table 20.1), and possibly other cognitive deficits as well. Indeed, we have found, in a healthy volunteer study, that benzhexol (5 mg) caused more cognitive and psychomotor impairments than haloperidol (1 mg) (King & Henry, 1992).

FUTURE DIRECTIONS

It seems that further clarification is unlikely to come from studies of cognition in patients on a variety of treatment regimens, using different test batteries. More robust information about neuroleptic effects should be possible with the development of more precise tests of attention. It is most important to move away from patient studies and towards healthy volunteer studies. Only in such controlled laboratory conditions can improved rigour of experimental design be achieved, allowing the exclusion of variability of results caused by illness, tolerance and the effects of other drugs.

Perhaps, however, more direct measures of brain function would improve our understanding of the level at which neuroleptics have their principal effects. Recently, PET studies of the effects of neuroleptics on regional glucose metabolism have been reported but with ambiguous results. Increases in metabolism in the cerebral cortex and basal ganglia after neuroleptics (DeLisi et al, 1985); increased metabolism in the corpus striatum but no change in cortical activity after chronic treatment (Szechtman et al, 1988); and no change with either thiothixine (Volkow et al, 1986) or CPZ (Wik et al, 1989), have all been reported. None of these studies appears to have adequately controlled for the cognitive state during the PET. So the "chicken and egg" problems remain or, in fact, are compounded by another variable, that is, whether the drugs primarily affect cerebral metabolism, clinical symptoms or cognition. If, as it appears from the study by Wik et al (1989), that cerebral metabolism varies inversely with clinical symptomatology but is relatively unaffected by medication, then it seems that neuroleptics do not act primarily on cerebral metabolic rate.

PHARMACO-EEG STUDIES

What about neuroleptic effects on EEG measures of cognition? The pharmaco-EEG literature would require a separate review and the reader has already been referred to a few of the more recent papers in this area.

The sophistication in this field has improved with computerised techniques which use signal averaging to record event related potentials (ERPs) (auditory or visual evoked potentials) in the time domain and fast Fourier transformations to record power spectra analyses and brain electrical activity mapping (BEAM) in the frequency domain. By using different paradigms the amplitude and latency of the early (N100) and late (P300) components of ERPs can be measured. The paradigms can be active or passive and the "odd-ball" paradigm (detection of a rare tone during a series of tones of similar pitch) can be used to elicit the P300 wave which is usually associated with active cognition. Thus, the great advantage of these techniques is that they can detect brain events rapidly and during the first 50–600 ms of the response to external stimuli. The disadvantages are (i) the familiar one of being unable to distinguish effects due to drugs from those due to illness or other extraneous factors, and (ii) the inability to localise the source of the electrical activity which tends to be "smeared" over a wide area in scalp EEG recordings.

The data on neuroleptic effects in schizophrenic patients appears, so far, to be inconclusive. Using both power spectral analysis and ERP measures respectively, Merrin et al (1988) and Kemali et al (1991) reported improved left hemisphere function following neuroleptics in schizophrenic patients. On the other hand, Nakagawa et al (1991) found no differences between medicated and drug-free schizophrenic patients in EEG $\alpha2$ topography during auditory and visual "odd-ball" paradigms. Bartel et al (1988) found single doses of CPZ (100 mg) increased both the latency and amplitude of all visual evoked potentials (P100, N200, P200 and N300) in healthy volunteers, but Roth et al (1991) found medicated schizo-phrenics had smaller N120 and P200 amplitudes, shorter P200 latencies and longer P320 latencies, than controls or drug-free patients.

This work is patchy and at an early stage. Nevertheless, it seems to have great potential provided future studies are conducted with proper attention to the details of medication status (type, dose and duration of drug treatment), patient characteristics and concomitant measures of psychopathology. If exact brain activity correlates of cognition can be identified then we should be a step nearer exploring and understanding the point at which neuroleptic drugs act on informa-tion processing.

ACKNOWLEDGEMENT

We wish to thank Mrs Helen Hunter for her patience and expertise in typing the manuscript and tables.

REFERENCES

Bartel, P., Blom, M., van der Meyden, C., Sommers, de K. (1988) Effects of single doses of diazepam, chlorpromazine, imipramine and trihexyphenidyl on visual-evoked potentials. *Neuropsychobiology*, **20**, 212–217.

Bartkó, G., Frecska, E., Zador, G., Herczeg, I. (1989) Neurological features, cognitive impair-ment and neuroleptic response in schizophrenic patients. *Schizophrenia Research*, **2**, 311–313.

Berger, H.J.C., van Hoof, J.J.M., van Spaendonck, K.P.M., Horstink, M.W.I., van den Bercken, J.H.L., Jaspers, R., Cools, A.R. (1989) Haloperidol and cognitive shifting. *Neuropsychologia*, **27**, 629–639.

Berman, K.F., Zec, R.F., Weinberger, D.R. (1986) Physiologic dysfunction of dorsolateral prefrontal cortex in schizophrenia. II. Role of neuroleptic treatment, attention, and mental effort. *Archives of General Psychiatry*, **43**, 126–135.

Braff, D.L., Saccuzzo, D.P. (1982) Effect of antipsychotic medication on speed of information processing in schizophrenic patients. *American Journal of Psychiatry*, **139**, 1127–1130.

Buchanan, R.W., Holstein, C., Breier, A. (1994). The comparative efficacy and long-term effect of clozapine treatment on neuropsychological test performance. *Biological Psychiatry*, **36**, 717–725.

Buchsbaum, M.S., Tafalla, R.J., Reynolds, C., Trenary, M., Burgwald, L., Potkin, S., Bunney, W.E. (1991) Drug effects on brain lateralization in the basal ganglia of schizophrenics. In: *The Mesolimbic Dopamine System: From Motivation to Action* (Eds P. Willner, J. Scheel-Krüger), pp. 529–538, Wiley, Chichester.

Calvert, J.E., Babiker, I.E., Harris, J.P., Phillipson, O.T., Ford, M.F., Antebi, D.L. (1990) Object-name selection in psychiatric patients before and after neuroleptic therapy. *Journal of Psychopharmacology*, **4**, 75–82.

Cassens, G., Inglis, A.K., Appelbaum, P.S., Gutheil, T.G. (1990) Neuroleptics: Effects on neuropsychological function in chronic schizophrenic patients. *Schizophrenia Bulletin*, **16**, 477–499.

Clark, C.R., Geffen, G.M., Geffen, L.B. (1989) Catecholamines and the covert orientation of attention in humans. *Neuropsychologia*, **27**, 131–139.

Classen, W., Laux, G. (1988) Sensorimotor and cognitive performance of schizophrenic inpatients treated with haloperidol, flupenthixol, or clozapine. *Pharmacopsychiatry*, **21**, 295–297.

Classen, W., Laux, G. (1989) Comparison of sensorimotor and cognitive performance of acute schizophrenic inpatients treated with remoxipride of haloperidol. *Neuropsychobiology*, **21**, 131–140.

Cleghorn, J.M., Kaplan, R.D., Szechtman, B., Szechtman, H., Brown, G.M. (1990) Neuroleptic drug effects on cognitive function in schizophrenia. *Schizophrenia Research*, **3**, 211–219.

Crow, T.J. (1980) Molecular pathology of schizophrenia: More than one disease process? *British Medical Journal*, **280**, 66–68.

Cutmore, T.R.H., Beninger, R.J. (1990) Do neuroleptics impair learning in schizophrenic patients? *Schizophrenia Research*, **3**, 173–186.

DeLisi, L.E., Holcomb, H.H., Cohen, R.M., Pickar, D., Carpenter, W., Morihisa, J.M., King, A.C., Kessler, R., Buchsbaum, M.S. (1985) Positron Emission Tomography in schizophrenic patients with and without neuroleptic medication. *Journal of Cerebral Blood Flow & Metabolism*, **5**, 201–206.

Earle-Boyer, E.A., Serper, M.R., Davidson, M., Harvey, P.D. (1991) Continuous performance tests in schizophrenic patients: Stimulus and medication effects on performance. *Psychiatry Research*, **37**, 47–56.

Erickson, W.D., Yellin, A.M., Hopwood, J.H., Realmuto, G.M., Greenberg, L.M. (1984) The effects of neuroleptics on attention in adolescent schizophrenics. *Biological Psychiatry*, **19**, 745–753.

Fields, R.B., van Kammen, D.P., Peters, J.L., Rosen, J., van Kammen, W.B., Nugent, A., Stipetic, M., Linnoila, M. (1988) Clonidine improves memory function in schizophrenia independently from change in psychosis. *Schizophrenia Research*, **1**, 417–423.

Fink, M. (1969) EEG and human psychopharmacology. *Annual Review of Pharmacology*, **9**, 241–258.

Frazier, M.F., Silverstein, M.L., Fogg, L. (1989) Lateralized cerebral dysfunction in schizophrenia and depression: Gender and medication effects. *Archives of Clinical Neuropsychology*, **4**, 33–44.

Gold, J.M., Hurt, S.W. (1990) The effects of haloperidol on thought disorder and IQ in schizophrenia. *Journal of Personality Assessment*, **54**, 390–400.

Goldberg, T.E., Bigelow, L.B., Weinberger, D.R., Daniel, D.G., Kleinman, J.E. (1991) Cognitive and behavioral effects of the coadministration of dextroamphetamine and haloperidol in schizophrenia. *American Journal of Psychiatry*, **148**, 78–84.

Goldberg, T.E., Greenberg, R.D., Griffin, S.J., Gold, J.M., Kleinman, J.E., Pickar, D., Schulz, S.C., Weinberger, D.R. (1993) The effect of clozapine on cognition and psychiatric symptoms in patients with schizophrenia. *British Journal of Psychiatry*, **162**, 43–48.

Hagger, C., Buckley, P., Kenny, J.T., Friedman, L., Ubogy, D., Meltzer, H.Y. (1993). Improvement in cognitive functions and psychiatric symptoms in treatment-refractory schizophrenic patients receiving clozapine. *Biological Psychiatry*, **34**, 702–712.

Harvey, P.D., Keefe, R.S.E., Moskowitz, J., Putnam, K.M., Motts, R.C., Davis, K.L. (1990) Attentional markers of vulnerability to schizophrenia: Performance of medicated and unmedicated patients and normals. *Psychiatry Research*, **33**, 179–188.

Healy, D. (1989) Neuroleptics and psychic indifference: A review. *Journal of the Royal Society of Medicine*, **82**, 615–619.

Heaton, R.K., Crowley, T.J. (1981) Effects of psychiatric disorders and their somatic treatments on neuropsychological test results. In: *Handbook of Clinical Neuropsychology* (Eds S.B. Filskov, T.J. Boll), Ch. 15, pp. 481–525, Wiley, Chichester.

Hemsley, D.R. (1975) A two-stage model of attention in schizophrenia research. *British Journal of Social and Clinical Psychology*, **14**, 81–89.

Johnstone, E.C., Crow, T.J., Frith, C.D., Stevens, M., Kreel, L., Husband, J. (1978) The dementia of dementia praecox. *Acta Psychiatrica Scandinavica*, **57**, 305–324.

Joseph, M.H., Frith, C.D., Waddington, J.L. (1979) Dopaminergic mechanisms and cognitive deficit in schizophrenia. *Psychopharmacology*, **63**, 273–280.

Katz, I.R., Greenberg, W.H., Barr, G.A., Garbarino, C., Buckley, P., Smith, D. (1985) Screening for cognitive toxicity of anticholinergic drugs. *Journal of Clinical Psychiatry*, **46**, 323–326.

Kemali, D., Galderisi, S., Maj, M., Mucci, A., Di Gregorio, M. (1991) Lateralization patterns of event-related potential and performance indices in schizophrenia: Relationship to clinical state and neuroleptic treatment. *International Journal of Psychophysiology*, **10**, 225–230.

Killian, G.A., Holzman, P.S., Davis, J.M., Gibbons, R. (1984) Effects of psychotropic medication on selected cognitive and perceptual measures. *Journal of Abnormal Psychology*, **93**, 58–70.

King, D.J. (1990) The effect of neuroleptics on cognitive and psychomotor function. *British Journal of Psychiatry*, **157**, 799–811.

King, D.J. (1992) Measures of neuroleptic effects on cognition and psychomotor performance in healthy volunteers. In: *Human Psychopharmacology: Measures and Methods* (Vol. IV) (Eds I. Hindmarch, P.D. Stonier), Wiley, Chichester.

King, D.J., Henry, G. (1992) The effect of neuroleptics on cognitive and psychomotor function. A preliminary study in healthy volunteers. *British Journal of Psychiatry*, **160**, 647–653.

King, D.J., Wilson, A., Cooper, S.J., Waddington, J.L. (1991) The clinical correlates of neurological soft signs in chronic schizophrenia. *British Journal of Psychiatry*, **158**, 770–775.

Kornetsky, C. (1972) The use of a simple test of attention as a measure of drug effects in schizophrenic patients. *Psychopharmacologia*, **24**, 99–106.

Kornetsky, C., Pettit, M., Wynne, R., Evarts, E.V.A. (1959) A comparison of the psychological effects of acute and chronic administration of chlorpromazine and secobarbital (quinalbarbitone) in schizophrenic patients. *Journal of Medical Science*, **105**, 190–198.

Latz, A., Kornetsky, C. (1965) The effects of chlorpromazine and secobarbital under two conditions of reinforcement on the performance of chronic schizophrenic subjects. *Psychopharmacologia*, **7**, 77–88.

Lehmann, H.E., Hanrahan, G.E. (1954) Chlorpromazine. New inhibiting agent for psychomotor excitement and manic states. *AMA Archives of Neurology and Psychiatry*, **71**, 227–237.

Liddle, P.F., Friston, K.J., Frith, C.D., Hirsch, S.R., Jones, T., Frackowiak, R.S.J. (1992) Patterns of cerebral blood flow in schizophrenia. *British Journal of Psychiatry*, **160**, 179–186.

Marder, S.R., Asarnow, R.F., van Putten, T. (1984) Information processing and neuroleptic response in acute and stabilized schizophrenic patients. *Psychiatry Research*, **13**, 41–49.

McKenna, P.J., Tamlyn, D., Lund, C.E., Mortimer, A.M., Hammond, S., Baddeley, A.D. (1990) Amnesic syndrome in schizophrenia. *Psychological Medicine*, **20**, 967–972.

Medalia, A., Gold, J., Merriam, A. (1988) The effect of neuroleptics on neuropsychological test results of schizophrenics. *Archives of Clinical Neuropsychology*, **3**, 249–271.

Merrin, E.L., Floyd, T.C., Fein, G. (1988) Task-related EEG alpha asymmetry in schizophrenic patients prior to and after neuroleptic treatment. *Schizophrenia Research*, **1**, 283–293.

Mirsky, A.F., Kornetsky, C. (1964) On the dissimilar effects of drugs on the digit symbol substitution and continuous performance tests. A review and preliminary integration of behavioral and physiological evidence. *Psychopharmacologia*, **5**, 161–177.

Nakagawa, M., Takeda, K., Kakimoto, Y. (1991) Characteristic distribution of alpha-2 wave in electroencephalograms of schizophrenic patients during discriminative tasks: Support for the hypofrontality hypothesis of schizophrenia. *Acta Psychiatrica Scandinavica*, **83**, 105–114.

Nestor, P.G., Faux, S.F., McCarley, R.W., Sands, S.F., Horvath, T.B., Peterson, A. (1991) Neuroleptics improve sustained attention in schizophrenia. A study using signal detection theory. *Neuropsychopharmacology*, **4**, 145–149.

Oades, R.D. (1982a) *Attention and Schizophrenia. Neurobiological bases*, pp. 30–36, Pitman, London.

Oades, R.D. (1982b) *Attention and Schizophrenia: Neurobiological bases*, pp. 159–172, Pitman, London.

Perlick, D., Stastny, P., Katz, I., Mayer, M., Mattis, S. (1986) Memory deficits and anticholinergic levels in chronic schizophrenia. *American Journal of Psychiatry*, **143**, 230–232.

Posner, M.I., Petersen, S.E. (1990) The attention system of the human brain. *Annual Reviews of Neuroscience*, **13**, 25–42.

Posner, M.I., Walker, J.A., Friedrich, F.A., Rafal, R.D. (1987) How do the parietal lobes direct covert attention? *Neuropsychologia*, **25**, 135–145.

Posner, M.I., Petersen, S.E., Fox, P.T., Raichle, M.E. (1988) Localization of cognitive operations in the human brain. *Science*, **240**, 1627–1631.

Rosvold, H.E., Mirsky, A.F., Sarason, I., Bransome, E.D., Beck, L.H. (1956) A continuous performance test of brain damage. *Journal of Consulting Psychology*, **20**, 343–350.

Roth, W.T., Goodale, J., Pfefferbaum, A. (1991) Auditory event-related potentials and electrodermal activity in medicated and unmedicated schizophrenics. *Biological Psychiatry*, **29**, 585–599.

Saletu, B., Küfferle, B., Grünberger, J., Anderer, P. (1986) Quantitative EEG, SPEM, and psychometric studies in schizophrenics before and during differential neuroleptic therapy. *Pharmacopsychiatry*, **19**, 434–437.

Seidman, L.J. (1983) Schizophrenia and brain dysfunction: An integration of recent neurodiagnostic findings. *Psychological Bulletin*, **94**, 195–238.

Saletu, B., Grünberger, J., Linzmayer, L., Anderer, P. (1987) Comparative placebo-controlled pharmacodynamic studies with zotepine and clozapine utilizing pharmaco-EEG and psychometry. *Pharmacopsychiatry*, **20**, 12–27.

Serper, M.R., Bergman, R.L., Harvey, P.D. (1990) Medication may be required for the development of automatic information processing in schizophrenia. *Psychiatry Research*, **32**, 281–288.

Snyder, S., Greenberg, D., Yamamura, H.I. (1974) Antischizophrenic drugs and brain cholinergic receptors. *Archives of General Psychiatry*, **31**, 58–61.

Spohn, H.E., Strauss, M.E. (1989) Relation of neuroleptic and anticholinergic medication to cognitive functions in schizophrenia. *Journal of Abnormal Psychology*, **98**, 367–380.

Spohn, H.E., Lacoursiere, R.B., Thompson, K., Coyne, L. (1977) Phenothiazine effects on psychological and psychophysiological dysfunction in chronic schizophrenics. *Archives of General Psychiatry*, **34**, 633–644.

Spohn, H.E., Coyne, L., Lacoursiere, R., Mazur, D., Hayes, K. (1985a) Relation of neuroleptic dose and tardive dyskinesia to attention, information-processing and psychophysiology in medicated schizophrenics. *Archives of General Psychiatry*, **42**, 849–859.

Spohn, H.E., Coyne, L., Mittleman, F., Larson, J., Johnston, M., Spray, J., Hayes, K. (1985b) Effect of neuroleptic treatments on attention, information processing, and thought disorder. *Psychopharmacology Bulletin*, **21**, 582–587.

Strauss, W.H., Klieser, E. (1990) Cognitive disturbances in neuroleptic therapy. *Acta Psychiatrica Scandinavica*, **82** (Suppl. 358), 56–57.

Strauss, M.E., Lew, M.F., Coyle, J.T., Tune, L.E. (1985) Psychopharmacologic and clinical correlates of attention in chronic schizophrenia. *American Journal of Psychiatry*, **142**, 497–499.

Szechtman, H., Nahmias, C., Garnett, S., Firnau, G., Brown, G.M., Kaplan, R.D., Cleghorn, J.M. (1988) Effect of neuroleptics on altered cerebral glucose metabolism in schizophrenia. *Archives of General Psychiatry*, **45**, 523–532.

Tamlyn, D., McKenna, P.J., Mortimer, A.M., Lund, C.E., Hammond, S., Baddeley, A.D.

(1992). Memory impairment in schizophrenia: Its extent, affiliations and neuropsychological character. *Psychological Medicine*, **22**, 101–115.

Tecce, J.J., Cole, J.O. (1972) Psychophysiologic responses of schizophrenics to drugs. *Psychopharmacologia*, **24**, 159–200.

Tomer, R. (1990) Neuroleptic effects on interhemispheric and intrahemispheric performance of tactile discrimination tasks by schizophrenic patients. *Psychiatry Research*, **32**, 289–296.

Tomer, R., Flor-Henry, P. (1989) Neuroleptics reverse attention asymmetries in schizophrenic patients. *Biological Psychiatry*, **25**, 852–860.

Tomer, R., Mintz, M., Myslobodsky, M.S. (1982) Left hemisphere hyperactivity in schizophrenia: Abnormality inherent to psychosis or neuroleptic side-effects? *Psychopharmacology*, **77**, 168–170.

Tune, L.E., Strauss, M.E., Lew, M.F., Breitlinger, E., Coyle, J.T. (1982) Serum levels of anticholinergic drugs and impaired recent memory in chronic schizophrenic patients. *American Journal of Psychiatry*, **139**, 1460–1462.

Volkow, N.D., Brodie, J.D., Wolf, A.P., Angrist, B., Russell, J., Cancro, R. (1986) Brain metabolism in patients with schizophrenia before and after acute neuroleptic administration. *Journal of Neurology, Neurosurgery & Psychiatry*, **49**, 1199–1202.

Wahba, M., Donlon, P.T., Meadow, A. (1981) Cognitive changes in acute schizophrenia with brief neuroleptic treatment. *American Journal of Psychiatry*, **138**, 1307–1310.

Walker, E. (1981) Attentional and neuromotor functions of schizophrenics, schizoaffectives, and patients with other affective disorders. *Archives of General Psychiatry*, **38**, 1355–1358.

Walker, E. (1983) Cognitive changes in schizoaffective patients. *Archives of General Psychiatry*, **40**, 1255.

Wik, G., Wiesel, F-A., Sjögren, I., Blomqvist, G., Greitz, T., Stone-Elander, S. (1989) Effects of sulpiride and chlorpromazine on regional cerebral glucose metabolism in schizophrenic patients as determined by positron emission tomography. *Psychopharmacology*, **97**, 309–318.

Zahn, TP, Pickar, D. and Haier, R.J. (1994) Effects of clozapine, fluphenazine, and placebo on reaction time measures of attention and sensory dominance in schizophrenia. *Schizophrenic Research*, **13**, 133–144.

ABBREVIATIONS

NEUROPSYCHOLOGICAL AND PSYCHOMOTOR TESTS

ART: Alphabetical Reaction Test
CFFT: Critical Flicker Fusion Test
COWA: Controlled Oral Word Association Test
CPT: Continuous Performance Test
CRT: Continuous Reaction Time
DSST: Digit Symbol Substitution Test
MMS: Mini Mental State
NM: Number Matching
OPAT: Operant Avoidance Task
PAL: Paired Associated Learning Test
PPVT: Peabody Picture Vocabulary Test
RT: Reaction Time
SAT: Span of Apprehension Test
SOMT: Spatial Orientation Memory Test
TDIr: Thought Disorder Index (Rorschach)
TDIw: Thought Disorder Index (WAIS)
VLL: Verbal List Learning
WAIS: Wechsler Adult Intelligence Scale
WCST: Wisconsin Card Sorting Test
WISC: Wechsler Intelligence Scale for Children
WMS: Wechsler Memory Scale
WRAT: Wide Range Achievement Test

CLINICAL RATINGS

BHPRS: Bunney–Hamburg Psychosis Rating Scale
BPRS: Brief Psychiatric Rating Scale
CGI: Clinical Global Impression
GDFS: General Deficit Functioning Scale
POMS: Profile of Mood States
QLS: Qualify of Life Score
SANS: Schedule for Assessment of Negative Symptoms (Andreasen)
SAPS: Schedule for Assessment of Positive Symptoms (Andreasen)
SATLCD: Schedule for Assessment of Thought, Language and Communication Disorders (Andreasen)

DRUGS

CPZ: Chlorpromazine
FLU: Flupenthixol
FPZ: Fluphenazine
HPL: Haloperidol
RMX: Remoxipride
TDZ: Thioridazine

MISCELLANEOUS

BEAM: Brain electrical activity mapping
rCBF: Regional cerebral blood flow
DLPFC: Dorsolateral prefrontal cortex
ERP: Event-related potentials
NS: Non-significant
PET: Positron emission tomography
RRA: Radioreceptor assay
VBR: Ventricular–brain ratio

21

Treatment Strategies for the Remediation of Neurocognitive Dysfunction in Schizophrenia

RODNEY MORICE and ANN DELAHUNTY

INTRODUCTION

Many neuropsychological/neurocognitive impairments in schizophrenia have been described in this volume. Others have been discussed in a review by Levin et al (1989) and yet more in a vast array of papers in the psychological and psychiatric literature. Two in particular have been of interest to the authors: cognitive inflexibility and low-level planning impairments.

These were brought into focus by earlier research into prefrontal cortical functioning in schizophrenia. Following studies which examined language (syntactic) impairments in schizophrenia (Morice & Ingram, 1982, 1983; Morice & McNicol, 1985, 1986), Morice speculated that the described and replicated changes could be due to prefrontal executive dysfunction, rather than to focal Broca's or Wernicke's dysfunctions (Morice, 1986). In order to examine prefrontal cortical functioning in schizophrenia, two neuropsychological tests were selected, the Wisconsin Card Sorting Test (WCST) (Berg, 1948; Heaton, 1981) and the Tower of London (Shallice, 1982).

The WCST has long been used as a measure of prefrontal damage following head injury (e.g. Milner, 1963; Drewe, 1974; Nelson, 1976), and of putative prefrontal dysfunction in schizophrenia (Fey, 1951; Malmo, 1974). More recently, it has been used to suggest specific left dorsolateral prefrontal dysfunction in schizophrenia (Weinberger et al, 1986; Goldberg et al, 1987).

The Tower of London was developed as a specific test of planning and, initially, poor performance on this task was demonstrated in a group of patients with left frontal lesions. In a subsequent study, Shallice (1988) found no difference in performance between a left anterior lesion group and normal controls when IQ

Schizophrenia: A Neuropsychological Perspective. Edited by C. Pantelis, H.E. Nelson and T.R.E. Barnes
© 1996 John Wiley & Sons Ltd

was controlled for, although this, of course, begs the question of the effect of prefrontal damage on measured IQ.

Further, each test seemed to measure functions relevant to the activities of daily living. Shifts between ideas and behaviours are inherent in almost everything we do. The ability to plan ahead (measured by the Tower of London) is also essential in many daily activities, such as dressing, preparing a meal, shopping and keeping an appointment, activities in which many people with schizophrenia are relatively disabled. Impairments in one or all of these abilities, especially if of severe dimensions, could have a devastating effect on daily functioning and on interpersonal relationships.

The results examining WCST performance in schizophrenia have been published (Morice, 1990). Sixty patients with schizophrenia, diagnosed according to DSM-III criteria, with none in a stage of acute decompensation and 37 (62%) tested while "in remission" and living in the community, were included in the study, and contrasted with 34 non-psychiatric controls and 20 manic subjects. The patients with schizophrenia, as a group, demonstrated marked cognitive inflexibility and reduced planning abilities. Of the group, 88.3% were impaired on one or both tests, while only 11.7% were not impaired on either test.

The results not only supported hypotheses of prefrontal dysfunction in schizophrenia (Morice, 1986; Weinberger, et al 1986; Robbins, 1990; see also Gourovitch & Goldberg, chapter 5; Pantelis and Brewer, chapter 16) but, perhaps more importantly, indicated a high prevalence of specific neurocognitive impairments which could contribute to disabilities affecting many activities of daily living, impairments which if uncorrected, could form an impediment to successful biopsychosocial rehabilitation.

SCHIZOPHRENIA REHABILITATION

Conventional rehabilitation in schizophrenia in more recent years has been directed mostly at problems associated with the activities of daily living, or living skills. Inpatient and community-based programs devoted to personal hygiene and self-care, to cooking, to household cleaning and to money management have flourished. In some centres, these have been joined by specific programs in psychoeducation, symptom control, medication management, social and communication skills, and prevocational and vocational training (e.g. Hogarty et al, 1986).

In a scrutiny of the rehabilitation literature, rarely have neurocognitive impairments been linked to higher-level disabilities, and even fewer studies have used strategies in an attempt to ameliorate them, nor have they been successful (e.g. Goldberg et al, 1987). Ciompi (1983) referred to problems with the handling of "complex information", which he postulated could have been "the common denominator of the multiple *cognitive disorders*" (p. 54), but his treatment/rehabilitation approach referred only to "the simplification of any information input" (p. 57) rather than to any specific programs aimed at ameliorating the basic cognitive problems. He did, however, develop an extremely comprehensive psychosocial program. Similarly, at least until recently, the rehabilitation work of Liberman and colleagues in California focused on behavioural approaches and social skills training (Liberman, 1982; Wong et al, 1986). Bellack, known for his work in social skills training in schizophrenia, recently adopted a more neuropsychological perspective to social problem solving, but suggested further research rather than formulating actual rehabilitation programs (Bellack et al, 1989).

Almost alone in recognising the importance of neurocognitive impairments in actual mainstream rehabilitation programs, Brenner (1987) not only proposed an hierarchical model for the development of symptoms and problem behaviours in schizophrenia, but also designed and implemented an hierarchical and modular approach to therapy. His model proposed that covert attentional, perceptual and neurocognitive impairments produced overt behavioural disabilities. His initial therapy program comprised five modules, given in the following order: cognitive differentiation, social perception, verbal communication, social skills and interpersonal problem-solving. Positive effects of the program (Brenner et al, 1988) and of the cognitive differentiation model alone (Olbrich & Mussgay, 1990) have been reported.

THE NEWCASTLE PROGRAMS

Neurocognitive rehabilitation was introduced to Newcastle, Australia in 1988. Three different programs have now been used. Each will be described in brief and some results presented for the three groups of seven patients who completed them.

THE MODIFIED BRENNER PROGRAM

The first program to be used was a modified version of the five-module program of Brenner (1987). After pre-training neuropsychological assessment, the identified patient completed four modules, based on Brenner's first four modules. In parallel, the patient's family received a family intervention program (Falloon et al, 1984), which was divided into modules. Use was made of videotapes developed by Liberman and his group in California (Liberman, 1982). Patient and family came together for the final problem-solving module. Post-training assessments were conducted at the completion of that module. The patient modules each comprised four 1-hour sessions per week for 2 weeks.

THE COMPUTER-ASSISTED PROGRAM

The literature on patients with brain injury demonstrates the utility of neurocognitive rehabilitation to supplement and enhance the more conventional physical rehabilitation programs (Weinberg et al, 1977; Bracy, 1983; Sbordone, 1985). In particular, computers have been used for this purpose. Apart from postulating that programs used with patients with frontal executive dysfunction following closed head injury might be useful for patients with frontal executive problems due to schizophrenia, we believed that the use of computers could eventually provide a more cost-effective approach to neurocognitive rehabilitation.

Selected items from seven modules of the Bracy Cognitive Rehabilitation Program (Bracy, 1987) were used (Foundations I and II, Visuospatial I and II, Memory I and II, and Problem Solving), as reported by Delahunty et al (1991). As with the Modified Brenner cognitive differentiation module, the computer modules addressed attentional, perceptual and reasoning deficits. However, memory training was more evident in the Bracy packages. Training with the computer modules occurred 4 days each week, over an 8- to 12-week period, depending on the patient's progress.

While the Computer-Assisted Program addressed only neurocognitive impairments, for future planning it was always seen as the first module in a fully integrated and comprehensive rehabilitation program that would subsequently address issues related to psychoeducation, activities of daily living and psychosocial functioning.

Post-training results from the two programs (Modified Brenner and Computer-Assisted) indicated that there were enhancements in some subtest scores of the WAIS-R (see Tables 21.2 and 21.3), which were in excess of expected practice effects (Wechsler, 1981). Though some improvements in mean scores for the WCST and the Tower of London were noted, they were far from dramatic, and many of the patients were left, after training, with substantial cognitive inflexibility and planning impairments. Because of these persistent deficits, a program was developed specifically to address the impairments of frontal executive function, especially cognitive set shifting and planning abilities.

THE FRONTAL/EXECUTIVE PROGRAM

This program comprised two modules, a Cognitive Shift Module and a Planning Module. Their development and application had been predicated upon theoretical notions of frontal/prefrontal neural network processing and the particular cognitive dysfunctions that accompany circuit specific abnormalities. The Cognitive Shift Module concentrated on set maintenance and set shifting. The Planning Module addressed the processes of data organisation, strategy usage, reasoning, sequencing, working memory and dual tasking.

Both the Cognitive Shift and Planning Modules have been designed to engage as many as possible of the posterior/basal systems of Stuss & Benson (1986) and to provide repetitive practice of executive control processes. Where practicable, the selective processes targeted were each exercised daily, using a range of oculomotor, fine motor, perceptual (visual, spatial, verbal, auditory), attentional and conceptual tasks. Both arousal and alertness are implicated in the processes of sustaining attention, initiating action and deploying inhibitory control. The multiple areas of executive functioning were addressed daily, each in a number of modalities.

The Cognitive Shift Module comprised eight 1-hour training sessions over a 2-week period, and the Planning Module consisted of 24 1-hour sessions over a 6-week period. The decision to use one or both modules was usually based upon

WCST and Tower of London results, however, the seven patients reported here undertook both Modules. It is important to note that neither Module attempted to teach patients directly to perform the relevant test.

RESULTS

Data are presented for 21 patients with chronic schizophrenia, divided into three groups. Each group consisted of seven patients who completed one of the three programs. All were diagnosed according to DSM-III-R criteria (APA, 1987) and each had a duration of illness of at least 2 years. All were living in the community at the time of training. All were on medication, were medication compliant, and no patient was acutely psychotic during the testing and training periods. No patient had a history of epilepsy, serious head injury, primary mental retardation or drug or alcohol dependence. Age, education and duration of illness data are presented in Table 21.1. One-way ANOVAs detected no significant differences between the groups.

Symptoms were measured using the Expanded Brief Psychiatric Rating Scale (BPRS) (Lukoff et al, 1986) and daily functioning was assessed using the Life Skills Profile (LSP) (Rosen et al, 1987). As with the WCST, Tower of London, and WAIS-R, ratings were made before and after training. Mean scores and standard deviations for the groups (programs) pre- and post-training are presented in Table 21.2.

Pre- and post-training scores were analysed statistically using separate 3×2 (Program × Time) ANOVAs. Results are listed in Table 21.3. Newman–Keuls *post hoc* tests were performed on all significant ($p < 0.05$) main effects and on all interactions with $p < 0.1$. Statistical trends were accepted for interactions because of the small numbers in each program.

Pre-training, the three groups did not differ significantly on the WCST, the Tower of London, nor on any measure of the WAIS-R. Post-training, improvements were recorded for many of the measures.

WISCONSIN CARD SORTING TEST

The significant Time and Program × Time interaction effects for the number of trials to complete the WCST indicated that the Frontal/Executive Program group

Table 21.1. Some demographic characteristics of the three training groups

Variable	Modified Brenner ($n = 7$)	Computer-assisted ($n = 7$)	Frontal/executive ($n = 7$)
	Mean (SD)	*Mean (SD)*	*Mean (SD)*
Age (years)	27.7 (4.1)	31.4 (8.9)	30.7 (6.0)
Education (years)	10 (1.0)	11 (1.9)	9.9 (6.4)
Duration of illness (years)	5.1 (2.1)	7.7 (6.2)	7.1 (4.3)

Table 21.2. Mean scores (standard deviations) pre- and post-training for WAIS-R subtests, Wisconsin Card Sorting Test (WCST), Tower of London*, Expanded Brief Psychiatric Rating Scale (BPRS) and Life Skills Profile (LSP) for subjects in each training program

	Modified Brenner (n = 7)				Computer-assisted (n = 7)				Frontal/executive (n = 7)			
	Pre		Post		Pre		Post		Pre		Post	
	X	(SD)	X	(SD)	X	(SD)	X	(SD)	X	(SD)	X	(SD)
FSIQ	83.6	(7.6)	88.7	(10.2)	86.1	(4.9)	99.0	(8.6)	91.3	(5.5)	111.6	(11.0)
Information	8.7	(2.4)	8.6	(2.1)	8.7	(2.7)	10.3	(3.5)	10.1	(2.4)	10.4	(3.0)
Digit Span	7.6	(1.9)	8.3	(1.9)	8.7	(2.8)	10.9	(2.6)	10.3	(3.2)	13.0	(3.0)
Vocabulary	8.3	(2.0)	8.7	(1.9)	8.9	(2.8)	10.1	(2.4)	9.4	(2.1)	11.7	(3.4)
Arithmetic	8.6	(2.1)	8.1	(1.2)	9.4	(2.1)	10.6	(1.5)	7.7	(1.9)	10.9	(2.7)
Comprehension	7.9	(2.2)	8.1	(2.7)	7.7	(2.1)	9.4	(3.2)	8.1	(1.9)	12.6	(1.9)
Similarities	7.3	(1.4)	8.7	(3.0)	8.3	(1.9)	10.0	(2.1)	8.7	(1.5)	13.6	(2.3)
Picture Completion	8.4	(2.9)	9.9	(2.6)	7.6	(1.7)	10.7	(1.0)	9.1	(2.6)	11.9	(1.6)
Picture Arrangement	6.9	(1.2)	9.3	(2.0)	6.6	(0.5)	9.0	(2.8)	7.3	(2.8)	11.7	(3.4)
Block Design	8.0	(2.0)	8.1	(2.5)	8.4	(1.1)	10.6	(1.6)	10.9	(2.2)	11.9	(1.6)
Object Assembly	6.4	(2.4)	8.0	(2.4)	6.6	(3.6)	8.1	(3.4)	9.0	(2.4)	11.7	(1.5)
Digit Symbol	5.6	(1.4)	7.0	(1.0)	6.7	(1.4)	8.6	(1.5)	7.3	(1.8)	7.7	(1.7)
WCST												
No. Trials	107.6	(23.7)	102.6	(27.0)	111.6	(22.4)	109.0	(22.4)	126.9	(3.0)	78.9	(8.3)
Perseverative Errors	21.4	(16.7)	16.6	(10.6)	28.4	(24.9)	17.3	(14.3)	27.4	(17.8)	5.7	(2.4)
Tower of London	66.7	(16.0)	73.9	(16.4)	55.9	(18.7)	70.0	(19.0)	60.1	(14.8)	94.0	(4.9)
BPRS	54.0	(15.3)	32.3	(6.7)	37.8	(9.0)	32.0	(9.0)	34.6	(6.9)	31.4	(8.0)
LSP	108.9	(24.2)	125.1	(25.7)	130.8	(14.6)	138.8	(9.5)	122.7	(16.1)	141.7	(9.4)

*Tower of London results expressed as percentage of solutions achieved in minimum moves.

Table 21.3. Analyses of variance (ANOVAs) for WCST, Tower of London, WAIS-R subtests, BPRS and LSP for Program, Time (pre- and post-training scores), and Program × Time interaction

Test	Main effects — Program		Time		Interaction Program × time	
	F	p	F	p	F	p
WCST						
No. Trials		$p = 0.60$	$F_{(1, 36)} = 9.1$	$p = 0.005$	$F_{(2, 36)} = 5.8$	$p = 0.00$
Perseverative Errors		$p = 0.55$	$F_{(1, 36)} = 6.5$	$p = 0.02$		$p = 0.38$
Tower	$F_{(2, 36)} = 2.8$	$p = 0.07$	$F_{(1, 36)} = 14.4$	$p = 0.001$	$F_{(2, 36)} = 2.7$	$p = 0.07$
WAIS-R						
FSIQ	$F_{(2, 36)} = 12.0$	$p < 0.001$	$F_{(1, 36)} = 24.9$	$p < 0.001$	$F_{(2, 36)} = 2.9$	$p = 0.07$
Subtests						
Information		$p = 0.29$		$p = 0.50$		$p = 0.69$
Digit Span	$F_{(2, 36)} = 7.1$	$p = 0.003$	$F_{(1, 36)} = 5.3$	$p = 0.03$		$p = 0.58$
Vocabulary		$p = 0.10$		$p = 0.09$		$p = 0.61$
Arithmetic		$p = 0.10$	$F_{(1, 36)} = 4.5$	$p = 0.04$	$F_{(2, 36)} = 2.9$	$p = 0.07$
Comprehension	$F_{(2, 36)} = 3.7$	$p = 0.03$	$F_{(1, 36)} = 8.5$	$p = 0.006$	$F_{(2, 36)} = 2.7$	$p = 0.08$
Similarities	$F_{(2, 36)} = 8.0$	$p = 0.001$	$F_{(1, 36)} = 16.9$	$p < 0.001$	$F_{(2, 36)} = 2.9$	$p = 0.07$
Picture Completion		$p = 0.18$	$F_{(1, 36)} = 13.0$	$p < 0.001$		$p = 0.56$
Picture arrangement		$p = 0.13$	$F_{(1, 36)} = 18.8$	$p < 0.001$		$p = 0.43$
Block Design	$F_{(2, 36)} = 10.7$	$p < 0.001$	$F_{(1, 36)} = 3.5$	$p = 0.07$		$p = 0.38$
Object Assembly	$F_{(2, 36)} = 6.0$	$p = 0.000$	$F_{(1, 36)} = 5.5$	$p = 0.03$		$p = 0.81$
Digit Symbol	$F_{(2, 36)} = 3.5$	$p = 0.04$	$F_{(1, 36)} = 7.3$	$p = 0.01$		$p = 0.44$
BPRS	$F_{(2, 32)} = 4.3$	$p = 0.02$	$F_{(1, 32)} = 11.6$	$p = 0.002$	$F_{(2, 32)} = 3.7$	$p = 0.04$
LSP	$F_{(2, 34)} = 3.8$	$p = 0.03$	$F_{(1, 34)} = 6.7$	$p = 0.01$		$p = 0.73$

performed the task in significantly fewer trials after training. *Post hoc* testing demonstrated that this program was superior to the Modified Brenner and the Computer-Assisted Programs at the $p < 0.05$ level of significance.

The analysis of perseverative error scores revealed a significant main effect for Time. All Programs produced a reduction in this measure. However, while not achieving statistical significance, an examination of the means and standard deviations in Table 21.2 revealed that only the patients receiving the Frontal/Executive Program produced perseverative error scores post-training that were substantially below the suggested cut-off scores of 16 or 24 (Heaton, 1981; Morice, 1990). Scores above these cut-offs are considered to be indicative of impairment.

TOWER OF LONDON

The significant main effect for Time indicated that the percentage of tasks completed in the minimum number of moves increased with training. *Post hoc* analyses revealed that the Frontal/Executive Program was superior to the other two, at $p < 0.05$.

WECHSLER ADULT INTELLIGENCE SCALE – REVISED (WAIS-R)

There were significant main effects for Program and Time, and a trend for Program × Time, for full-scale IQ (FSIQ). The Frontal/Executive Program was superior to the other Programs ($p < 0.01$) and the Computer-Assisted Program was superior to the Modified Brenner Program ($p < 0.05$). The mean FSIQ score for the Frontal/Executive group was 20.3 points higher after training, a difference much greater than the suggested practice effect of seven points improvement (Wechsler, 1981). The Computer-Assisted Program produced a mean improvement of 12.9 points.

Training improvements were obtained on eight of the 11 WAIS-R subtests. The Arithmetic, Comprehension and Similarities tests showed interaction effects approaching significance. The Frontal/Executive Program was superior to the other Programs for each of these subtests: Arithmetic ($p < 0.05$), Comprehension ($p < 0.05$) and Similarities ($p < 0.01$).

Main effects for Program and for Time were obtained for Digit Span, Object Assembly and Digit Symbol. The Frontal/Executive group performed better on each of these tasks than the Modified Brenner Group. The Time effect showed that the performance of the three groups was improved post-training. The interaction was not significant. There were significant main effects for Time only for Picture Completion and Picture Arrangement. After training the groups performed better on both tests, the Programs being equally effective.

BRIEF PSYCHIATRIC RATING SCALE (BPRS)

Results for the BPRS were affected by a major floor effect (range of BPRS = 24–168). Only the patients who completed the Modified Brenner Program demonstrated moderate levels of symptomatology before training. Post-training, there was a significant reduction in BPRS score for this group compared with the other groups (post hoc testing $p < 0.01$).

LIFE SKILLS PROFILE (LSP)

Results for the LSP were affected by ceiling effects (range of LSP: 39–156, high scores indicating good daily functioning). There were significant main effects for Program and Time, but no interaction effects. All Programs produced some improvements in daily functioning.

DISCUSSION

The Frontal/Executive Program was designed with the specific intention of ameliorating impairments affecting cognitive flexibility and planning abilities, as measured by the WCST and the Tower of London. In this it has proved successful, at least for the seven schizophrenic patients who had completed the full Program at the time of writing, and it achieved what the two prior versions of neurocognitive training, the Modified Brenner and the Computer-Assisted Programs, had failed to achieve to any significant degree.

The Frontal/Executive program also demonstrated an enhanced efficiency over the other two programs with respect to three subtests of the WAIS-R. While there were significant main effects for Program or Time for all but two of the subtests (Information and Vocabulary), the only Program × Time interactions that approached statistical significance ($p < 0.1$) were for Arithmetic, Comprehension and Similarities, three tests that likely make considerable demands on working memory, an important component of the Planning Module.

Importantly, the modules of the Frontal/Executive Program did not attempt specifically to train patients to perform any of the neuropsychological tests. Rather, the development and application of these modules was predicated upon a number of theoretical notions.

The first assumption was that most neuropsychological tests measure more than one neurocognitive function or process. From a rehabilitation perspective these separate functions may be of extreme importance. Morice and colleagues (unpublished data) found that cognitive flexibility and planning impairments in schizophrenia were distinguishable deficits, suggesting that their remediation could require separate strategies. The design of the modules was driven by hypotheses pertaining to the dysfunctional component cognitive processes rather than by the more global theoretical constructs (such as planning ability) that one attempts to measure.

Effective set flexibility presumably requires the abilities to form, to maintain and to shift attentional and cognitive sets. Accordingly the Cognitive Shift Module addressed those three processes. Planning abilities also appear to involve multiple processing subroutines. The use of principal components analysis in an attempt to fractionate the Tower of London test performance into subprocesses using WAIS-R subtest scores identified three important factors: working memory, cognitive flexibility and reasoning (Morice and colleagues, unpublished data). In addition, it may be that abilities related to inhibitory control, monitoring, the development and use of strategies, sequencing and dual tasking are also important. Disruption to these executive control processes has been reported in patients with schizophrenia (for review: Levin et al 1989) and following prefrontal/frontal lobe damage (for review: Stuss & Benson, 1986).

A second important assumption underlying the development of the Frontal/ Executive Program was that prefrontal functions were not viewed in isolation, but as integral components of a range of neural networks/circuits that permit distributed serial and parallel processing. In particular, impairments of cognitive flexibility have been hypothesised to result from lesions of the "lateral orbitofrontal" circuit and impairments of working memory from lesions of the "dorsolateral prefrontal" circuit (Alexander et al, 1990).

Stuss & Benson (1986) proposed that the executive functions of the prefrontal region find expression via posterior/basal systems, responsible for the following: attention, arousal, visual–spatial processing, autonomic/emotional control, memory, sensation/perception, language, motor function and cognition. Neurophysiological evidence of neural circuits incorporating prefrontal regions, that provide the anatomical connectivities for these posterior/basal systems, has been steadily accumulating (Moruzzi & Magoun, 1949; Nauta 1972; Pandya et al 1981; Alexander et al 1990; Mesulam, 1990). Also, Robbins (1990) recently implicated dysfunctional corticostriatal loops in schizophrenia (see also Pantelis and Brewer, chapter 16).

Possibly, the success of the Frontal/Executive Program was related to its design. Given frontal/prefrontal dysfunction in schizophrenia, it follows that training methods should target executive skills and prefrontal functions. Both patients with frontal/prefrontal lobe damage and patients with schizophrenia are noted for their disorganisation, their rigidity and for disorders of attention and arousal. The Frontal/Executive Program attempted to address each of these processes.

It is always difficult, with any multifaceted program to isolate the factors that produced the achieved effects. It is unlikely that attentional improvement per se could account for the range of test performance enhancements observed. We suggest that the Program's theoretical underpinnings and method of delivery are particularly important.

The Program provided exercise of multiple executive control processes daily, initially with relatively simple material. The critical processes repeatedly addressed were set maintenance, set flexibility, data organisation, strategy usage, sequencing, dual tasking and working memory. Each was viewed as essential for effective planning and complex problem solving, tasks of which were presented in the later sections of the Program. This was in contrast to the Modified Brenner and Computer-Assisted Programs where the aim was not specifically to target executive processes and the therapist addressed areas of cognitive process sequentially rather than simultaneously, according to an hierarchical philosophy.

Further, the therapist delivering the Frontal/Executive Program adopted a facilitatory but interventionist role. The therapist demonstrated orderly information processing practices, sought to restrain impulsivity and ensure attention to all relevant detail, demonstrated how to impose context on problems and how to develop and utilise strategies. Given sufficient information processing resource capacity the patients appeared to internalise the externalised approaches of the therapist. The therapist did not seek to solve/perform the tasks for the patient, but tried to ensure organised information processing practices for at least that one hour of each day. Sacks (1986) described the use of music as a prosthetic organ of succession to facilitate the kinetic melody of neurological patients with motor disorder. It appears that one hour a day training/participation in organised thinking activities 4 days a week helped to organise the disordered thought processes of patients with schizophrenia, inducing a cognitive set that remained beyond the training sessions.

The durability and generalisability of such learning are at this stage unclear. It may be that these core executive control processes are learned/relearned and, thus, the gains may be long lasting. Four patients with schizophrenia who received only the Cognitive Shift Module (and not reported here) were retested 6 months after the completion of training. All had retained their markedly improved levels of performance on the WCST.

It is probable that cognitive flexibility and planning are integral to many of the activities of daily living and that enhanced abilities should contribute to improvements in daily functioning. The LSP was recorded before and after training in an attempt to demonstrate this. While all Programs resulted in increased (improved) measures after training, relative ceiling effects were present, as most of the patients were living in the community at the time of training and were reasonably highly functioning before training commenced. Also, the LSP can provide only a fairly crude measure of daily functioning and the effects of increased cognitive flexibility and improved planning skills may need a more finely tuned instrument to detect functional changes. Ideally, scales to detect perseveration and impaired planning in the activities of daily functioning need to be developed, on which functional changes could be measured.

At the gross clinical level, it is undeniable that many patients with schizophrenia demonstrate a relative inability to shift cognitive set and to plan ahead even the simplest of activities, observations in keeping with the high prevalence of impaired performance on the WCST and the Tower of London. Rehabilitation of these impairments should receive high priority in schizophrenia rehabilitation, as it seems likely that higher-level training (e.g. in housekeeping, cooking, leisure activities, etc.) may be constrained by these lower-level impairments. Neurocognitive rehabilitation could comprise a "front-end" to comprehensive, integrated rehabilitation programs.

While the three programs reported here produced some improvements in neuropsychological performance, the Frontal/Executive Program, albeit with small patient numbers, demonstrated an enhanced efficiency over the Modified Brenner and Computer-Assisted Programs, at least with respect to two extremely important neurocognitive impairments with a high prevalence in schizophrenia. Replication (copies of the Frontal/Executive Program are available on request to the second author) of these results, using a variety of experimental designs, should be attempted independently. If successful, we would urge the inclusion of specific neurocognitive training in schizophrenia rehabilitation programs.

REFERENCES

Alexander, G.E., Crutcher, M.D., DeLong, M.R. (1990) Basal ganglia–thalamocortical circuits: Parallel substrates for motor, oculomotor, "prefrontal" and "limbic" functions. *Progress in Brain Research*, **85**, 119–146.

American Psychiatric Association (1987) Diagnostic and Statistical Manual of Mental Disorders (3rd edn.), American Psychiatric Association, Washington, D.C.

Bellack, A.S., Morrison, R.L., Mueser, L.T. (1989) Social problem solving in schizophrenia. *Schizophrenia Bulletin*, **15**, 101–116.

Berg, E.A. (1948) A simple objective technique for measuring flexibility in thinking. *Journal of General Psychology*, **39**, 15–22.

Bracy, O.L. (1983) Computer based cognitive rehabilitation. *Cognitive Rehabilitation*, **1**, 7–8.

Bracy. O. (1987) *Cognitive Rehabilitation Program*, Psychological Software Services, Indianapolis.

Brenner, H.D. (1987) On the importance of cognitive disorders in treatment and rehabilitation. In: *Psychosocial Treatment of Schizophrenia* (Eds J.S. Strauss, W. Boker, H.D. Brenner), Hans Huber Publications, Bern.

Brenner, H.D., Kraemer, S., Hermanutz, M., Hodel, B. (1988) Cognitive treatment in schizophrenia. In: *Schizophrenia: Models and Interventions* (Eds E. Straube, K. Hahlweg), Springer, Heidelberg.

Ciompi, L. (1983) How to improve the treatment of schizophrenics: A multicausal illness concept and its therapeutic consequences. In: *Psychosocial Intervention in Schizophrenia* (Eds H. Stierlin, L.C. Wynne, M. Wirsching), Springer-Verlag, Berlin.

Delahunty, A., Morice, R., Frost, B., Lambert, F. (1991) Neurocognitive rehabilitation in schizophrenia eight years post head injury: A case study. *Cognitive Rehabilitation*, **9**, 24–28.

Drewe, E.A. (1974) The effect of type and area of brain lesion of Wisconsin Card Sorting Test performance. *Cortex*, **10**, 159–170.

Falloon, I.R.H., Boyd, J.L., McGill, C.W. (1984) *Family Care of Schizophrenia*, Guilford Press, New York.

Fey, E.T. (1951) The performance of young schizophrenics and young normals on the Wisconsin Card Sorting Test. *Journal of Consulting Psychology*, **15**, 311–319.

Goldberg, T.E., Weinberger, D.R., Berman, K.F., Pliskin, N.H., Podd, M.H. (1987) Further evidence for dementia of the prefrontal type in schizophrenia? *Archives of General Psychiatry*, **44**, 1008–1014.

Heaton, R.K. (1981) *A Manual for the Wisconsin Card Sorting Test*, Psychological Assessment Resources, Odessa, FL.

Hogarty, G.E., Anderson, C.M., Reiss, D.J., Kornblith, S.J., Greenwald, D.P., Javna, C.D., Madonia, M.J. (1986) Family psychoeducation, social skills training, and maintenance chemotherapy in the aftercare treatment of schizophrenia. *Archives of General Psychiatry*, **43**, 633–642.

Levin, S., Yurgelun-Todd, D., Craft, S. (1989) Contributions of clinical neuropsychology to the study of schizophrenia. *Journal of Abnormal Psychology*, **98**, 341–356.

Liberman, R.P. (1982) Assessment of social skills. *Schizophrenia Bulletin*, **8**, 62–84.

Lukoff, D., Nuechterlein, K.H., Ventura, J. (1986) Manual for expanded Brief Psychiatric Rating Scale (BPRS). *Schizophrenia Bulletin*, **12**, 594–602.

Malmo, H.P. (1974) On frontal lobe functions: Psychiatric patient controls. *Cortex*, **10**, 231–237.

Mesulam, M.-M. (1990) Large scale neurocognitive networks and distributed processing for attention, language and memory. *Annals of Neurology*, **28**, 597–613.

Milner, B. (1963) Effects of different brain lesions on card sorting. *Archives of Neurology*, **9**, 90–100.

Morice, R. (1986) Beyond language: Speculations on the prefrontal cortex and schizophrenia. *Australian and New Zealand Journal of Psychiatry*, **20**, 7–10.

Morice, R. (1990) Cognitive inflexibility and prefrontal dysfunction in schizophrenia and mania. *British Journal of Psychiatry*, **157**, 50–54.

Morice, R., Ingram, J.C.L. (1982) Language analysis in schizophrenia: Diagnostic implications. *Australian and New Zealand Journal of Psychiatry*, **16**, 11–21.

Morice, R., Ingram, J.C.L. (1983) Language complexity and age of onset of schizophrenia. *Psychiatry Research*, **9**, 233–242.

Morice, R., McNicol, D. (1985) The comprehension and production of complex syntax in schizophrenia. *Cortex*, **21**, 567–580.

Morice, R., McNicol, D. (1986) Language changes in schizophrenia: A limited replication. *Schizophrenia Bulletin*, **12**, 239–251.

Moruzzi, G., Magoun, H.W. (1949) Brain stem reticular formation and activation of the EEG. *Electroencphalography and Clinical Neurophysiology*, **1**, 455–473.

Nauta, W.J.H. (1972) Neural associations of the frontal cortex. *Acta Neurobiologiae Experimentalis*, **32**, 125–140.

Nelson, H.E. (1976) A modified card sorting test sensitive to frontal lobe defects. *Cortex*, **12**, 313–324.

Olbrich, R., Mussgay, L. (1990) Reduction of schizophrenia deficits by cognitive training: An evaluative study. *European Archives of Psychiatry and Neurological Sciences*, **239**, 366–369.

Pandya, D.N., Van Hoesen, G.W., Mesulam, M.-M. (1981) Efferent connections of the cingulate gyrus in the rhesus monkey. *Experimental Brain Research*, **42**, 319–330.

Robbins, T.W. (1990) The case for frontostriatal dysfunction in schizophrenia. *Schizophrenia Bulletin*, **16**, 391–402.

Rosen, A., Parker, G., Hadzi-Pavlovic, D., Hartley, R. (1987) *Developing Evaluation Strategies for Area Mental Health Services in N.S.W.*, State Health Publication, Sydney.

Sacks, O. (1986) *The Man who Mistook His Wife for a Hat*, Pan Books, London.

Sbordone, R. J. (1985) Rehabilitative neuropsychological approach for severe traumatic brain-injured patients. *Professional Psychology: Research and Practise*, **15**, 165–175.

Shallice, T. (1982) Specific impairments of planning. *Philosophical Transactions of the Royal Society of London B*, **298**, 199–209.

Shallice, T. (1988) *From Neuropsychology to Mental Structure*, Cambridge University Press, Cambridge.

Stuss, D.T., Benson, D.F. (1986) *The Frontal Lobes*, Raven Press, New York.

Wechsler, D.A. (1981) *Revised Wechsler Adult Intelligence Scale*, Psychological Corporation, New York.

Weinberg, J., Diller, L., Gordon, W.A., Gerstmann, L.J., Lieberman, A., Lakin, P., Hodges, G., Ezrachi, O. (1977) Visual scanning training effect on reading: Related tasks in acquired right brain damage. *Archives of Physical Medicine and Rehabilitation*, **58**, 479–486.

Weinberger, D.R., Berman, K.F., Zec, R.F. (1986) Physiological dysfunction of dorsolateral prefrontal cortex in schizophrenia. I. Regional cerebral blood flow evidence. *Archives of General Psychiatry*, **43**, 114–124.

Wong, S.E., Massel, D.K., Mosk, M.D., Liberman, R.P. (1986) Behavioural approaches to the treatment of schizophrenia. In: *Handbook of Studies on Schizophrenia: Part 2, Management and Research* (Eds G.D. Burrows, T.R. Norman, G. Rubenstein), Elsevier, Amsterdam.

Index

Index compiled by Caroline Sheard